Comprehensive Textbook on
FOUNDATION OF NURSING-II

Comprehensive Textbook on
FOUNDATION OF NURSING-II

As per the Revised Syllabus for BSc Nursing

Second Edition

Rebecca Nissanka (Jadhav)
RN RM BSc (Nursing) MSc (Child Health Nursing) MA (Sociology) PhD
Principal
Sumantai Wasnik Institute of Nursing
Nagpur, Maharashtra, India

Foreword
Rupa Ashok Verma

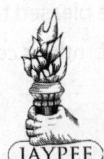

JAYPEE BROTHERS MEDICAL PUBLISHERS
The Health Sciences Publisher
New Delhi | London

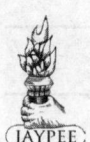

Jaypee Brothers Medical Publishers (P) Ltd.

Headquarters
Jaypee Brothers Medical Publishers (P) Ltd.
EMCA House
23/23-B, Ansari Road, Daryaganj
New Delhi - 110 002, India
Landline: +91-11-23272143, +91-11-23272703
+91-11-23282021, +91-11-23245672
Email: jaypee@jaypeebrothers.com

Corporate Office
Jaypee Brothers Medical Publishers (P) Ltd
4838/24, Ansari Road, Daryaganj
New Delhi 110 002, India
Phone: +91-11-43574357
Fax: +91-11-43574314
Email: jaypee@jaypeebrothers.com

Website: www.jaypeebrothers.com
Website: www.jaypeedigital.com

Overseas Office
J.P. Medical Ltd.
83 Victoria Street, London
SW1H 0HW (UK)
Phone: +44 20 3170 8910
Fax: +44 (0)20 3008 6180
Email: info@jpmedpub.com

© 2023, Jaypee Brothers Medical Publishers (P) Ltd.

The views and opinions expressed in this book are solely those of the original contributor(s)/author(s) and do not necessarily represent those of editor(s) and publisher of the book.

All rights reserved. No part of this publication may be reproduced, stored or transmitted in any form or by any means, electronic, mechanical, photocopying, recording or otherwise, without the prior permission in writing of the publishers.

All brand names and product names used in this book are trade names, service marks, trademarks or registered trademarks of their respective owners. The publisher is not associated with any product or vendor mentioned in this book.

Medical knowledge and practice change constantly. This book is designed to provide accurate, authoritative information about the subject matter in question. However, readers are advised to check the most current information available on procedures included and check information from the manufacturer of each product to be administered, to verify the recommended dose, formula, method and duration of administration, adverse effects and contraindications. It is the responsibility of the practitioner to take all appropriate safety precautions. Neither the publisher nor the author(s)/editor(s) assume any liability for any injury and/or damage to persons or property arising from or related to use of material in this book.

This book is sold on the understanding that the publisher is not engaged in providing professional medical services. If such advice or services are required, the services of a competent medical professional should be sought.

Every effort has been made where necessary to contact holders of copyright to obtain permission to reproduce copyright material. If any have been inadvertently overlooked, the publisher will be pleased to make the necessary arrangements at the first opportunity.

Inquiries for bulk sales may be solicited at: jaypee@jaypeebrothers.com

Comprehensive Textbook on Foundation of Nursing-II

First Edition: 2016

Second Edition: 2023, Reprint : **2024**

ISBN: 978-93-5696-073-2

Printed at Rajkamal Electric Press, Kundli, Haryana.

Dedicated to
My Teachers
Dr Jayseelan Manikan Devdason (Dean)
and
Dr Tamilmani Devdason (Principal)
Annai JKK Sampoorani Ammal College of Nursing
Namakkal, Tamil Nadu, India

FOREWORD

Health care is an exciting and challenging field with plenty of opportunities and advancements.

Training is an integral part of nursing profession.

This book is written exactly according to the revised INC syllabus.

It covers all the topics in the syllabus. The language used is easy for the first year students to understand properly. It includes all the units of Semester II syllabus including first aid management.

I hope the nursing students studying in basic BSc Nursing will be benefited by using this textbook. It gives me immense pleasure and I feel honored to introduce this book.

Rupa Ashok Verma
Principal
MKSSS's Sitabai Nargundkar College of Nursing for Women
Nagpur, Maharashtra, India

PREFACE TO THE SECOND EDITION

It gives me immense pleasure and satisfaction to introduce the Second Edition of *Comprehensive Textbook on Foundation of Nursing-II*.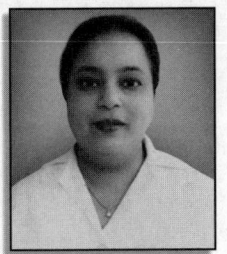

I believe that excellent nursing requires an equal mix of knowledge, thought and action. It is knowledge and its application not just the tasks nurses do that delineate the various level of nursing. Even so, skilful performance of tasks is essential to full attainment of nursing role.

The nursing institutes a major force in the healthcare delivery system. To maintain nobility of the profession in the new millennium, it needs new efforts to reform healthcare. Both high-quality and cost-effective care given is radically transforming the culture of care giving. Although nurses need to reassure the essence of nursing and what has traditionally served nursing well, they also need to change healthcare culture.

The goals of nursing education are to prepare today's student nurses to meet tomorrow's challenges. Nursing as a science, is characterized by growing body of knowledge that links technical and interpersonal interventions to decide client outcome, as an art, nursing demands of its practitioner's sufficient competency to creatively design individual strategies to assist client (patient).

In this changing world of healthcare delivery system, nurses will need a broad knowledge from which to provide the expert care needed in nursing profession. The students first master theories and skills, and then develop and refine ability to apply analytical thinking to clinical situation. I believe that changes in the healthcare present exciting challenges to nurses and it is felt that there is a need for good nursing text of Indian origin to assist nurses to meet this challenge in the Indian context, since their obvious need for nursing text to fit the Indian situation. The book has been written while taking into considerations the revised syllabus of First BSc Nursing (Second Semester).

The Second Edition of *Comprehensive Textbook on Foundation of Nursing-II* has been designed to provide today's students with solid foundations of nursing principles to prepare them to meet the challenges of tomorrow. The comprehensive coverage of the book provides concepts and components of nursing skills and techniques of nursing practice and firm foundation of nursing and also, it presents the theoretical and practical information necessary to make sound judgment while emphasizing cognitive, affective and psychomotor skills needed to carry out fundamentals of nursing activity.

I am aware that for manifold reasons, errors might have crept in and I shall feel obliged, if such errors are brought to my notice. Your suggestions for improvement would be gratefully accepted. I sincerely welcome constructive criticisms from both teachers and students that would help me to enrich myself.

Rebecca Nissanka (Jadhav)

PREFACE TO THE FIRST EDITION

It gives me immense pleasure and satisfaction to introduce *Comprehensive Textbook on Foundation of Nursing*.

I believe that excellent nursing requires an equal mix of knowledge, thought and action. It is knowledge and its application not just the tasks nurses do that delineate the various level of nursing. Even so, skillful performance of tasks is essential to full attainment of nursing role.

The nursing institutes a major force in the healthcare delivery system. To maintain nobility of the profession in the new millennium, it needs new efforts to reform healthcare. Both high-quality and cost-effective care given is radically transforming the culture of care giving. Although nurses need to reassure the essence of nursing and what has traditionally served nursing well, they also need to change healthcare culture.

The goals of nursing education are to prepare today's student nurses to meet tomorrow's challenges. Nursing as a science, is characterized by growing body of knowledge that links technical and interpersonal interventions to decide client outcome, as an art, nursing demands of its practitioner's sufficient competency to creatively design individual strategies to assist client (patient).

In this changing world of healthcare delivery system, nurses will need a broad knowledge from which to provide the expert care needed in nursing profession. The students first master theories and skills, and then develop and refine ability to apply analytical thinking to clinical situation. I believe that changes in the healthcare present exciting challenges to nurses and it is felt that there is a need for good nursing text of Indian origin to assist nurses to meet this challenge in the Indian context, since their obvious need for nursing text to fit the Indian situation. The book has been written while taking into considerations the revised syllabus of first year BSc (Nursing).

Comprehensive Textbook on Foundation of Nursing has been designed to provide today's students with solid foundations of nursing principles to prepare them to meet the challenges of tomorrow. The comprehensive coverage of the book provides concepts and components of nursing skills and techniques of nursing practice and firm foundation of nursing. And also, it presents the theoretical and practical information necessary to make sound judgment while emphasizing cognitive, affective and psychomotor skills needed to carry out fundamentals of nursing activity.

I am aware that for manifold reasons, errors might have crept in and I shall feed obliged, if such errors are brought to my notice. Your suggestions for improvement would be gratefully accepted. I sincerely welcome constructive criticisms from both teachers and students that would help me to enrich myself.

Rebecca Nissanka (Jadhav)

ACKNOWLEDGMENTS

Nursing is a profession devoted to human and social welfare. All the members of this profession must understand that it is his/her duty to add something to the body of nursing knowledge. It was my heartfelt wish from the beginning of my career to write a book according to the prescribed syllabus. It is because of the cooperation, motivation and help at all times by my teachers and dear ones that I was able to complete *Comprehensive Textbook on Foundation of Nursing-II*.

I am greatly and sincerely indebted to God, the almighty for showering his blessings to complete this book.

I owe my heartfelt gratitude and sincere thanks to Jayseelan Manikan Devdason, Dean, Annai JKK Sampoorani Ammal College of Nursing, Komarapalayam, Tamil Nadu, India, for his strong support and encouragement during my career.

I give my sincere thanks to Tamilmani Devdason, Principal, Annai JKK Sampoorani Ammal College of Nursing, Komarapalayam, for her strong support and encouragement during my career.

I express my debts of gratitude to Shri Jitendar P Vij (Group Chairman), Mr Ankit Vij (Managing Director), Mr MS Mani (Group President), Dr Madhu Choudhary (Director–Educational Publishing), Ms Pooja Bhandari (Production Head), Ms Sunita Katla (Executive Assistant to Group Chairman and Publishing Manager), Ms Samina Khan (Executive Assistant to Director–Educational Publishing), Ms Alisha Talwar (Development Editor), Mr Rajesh Sharma (Production Coordinator), Ms Seema Dogra (Cover Visualizer), Mr Vakil Khan (Proofreader), Mr Jagvir Singh Tomar (Typesetter), Mr Shravan Kumar (Graphic Designer) and all other staff members of M/s Jaypee Brothers Medical Publishers (P) Ltd, New Delhi, India, for having readily consented to publish the book.

I extend my heartfelt blessing to my dearest loving son Arpit for typing, computing and helping in preparing the written materials. I submit my humble salutations to my parents Mr Sudhir Nissanka and Mrs Sadhana Nissanka, for their help, cooperation, support, steadfast prayers and encouragement. I extend my heartfelt thanks to my loving sister and her husband, Mrs Neeta Rao and Mr Akhil Rao, and their children Aradhana and Angel, for their constant prayers and support.

I am grateful to all those helping hands and not mentioning of their names are purely unintentional.

CONTENTS

1. **Health Assessment** 1
   - Interview *1*
   - Interview Technique *1*
   - Observation *2*
   - Observation Techniques *3*
   - Health Assessment *4*
   - Health History *4*
   - Physical Examination *5*
   - General Assessment *8*
   - Documenting Physical Assessment Findings *10*
   - Auscultation *10*
   - General Assessment of Each Body System *10*
   - Cranial Nerve Function *24*

2. **The Nursing Process** 27
   - Definition and Meaning of Critical Thinking *27*
   - Critical Thinking: Thinking and Learning *27*
   - Nursing Process *29*
   - Assessment *29*
   - Nursing Diagnosis *30*
   - Planning *30*
   - Implementations *31*
   - Rationale *31*
   - Formulating the Nursing Care Plan *31*
   - Evaluation *31*
   - Nanda Nursing Diagnosis *32*

3. **Nutritional Needs** 37
   - Introduction to Nutrition *37*
   - Importance *37*
   - Factors Affecting Nutritional Needs *38*
   - Assessment of Nutritional Status *39*
   - Review on Therapeutic Diets *40*
   - Review: Special Diets—Solid, Liquid, Soft *40*
   - Fluid or Liquid Diet *40*
   - Dysphagia *43*
   - Anorexia *44*
   - Nausea and Vomiting *44*
   - Vomiting *44*
   - Meeting Nutritional Needs *46*
   - Feeding a Helpless Patient *47*
   - Enteral Feeding *47*
   - Gastrostomy *50*
   - Jejunostomy *51*
   - Gastrostomy/Jejunostomy Tube Feeding *51*
   - Total Parenteral Nutrition *52*

4. **Hygiene** 55
   - Definition *55*
   - Care of the Skin *55*
   - Back Care *58*
   - Decubitus Ulcer/Pressure Sore/Bedsore *60*
   - Braden Scale *64*
   - The Norton Pressure Sore *66*
   - Performing Nail and Foot Care *67*
   - Oral Hygiene for a Conscious Patient *68*
   - Oral Care for an Unconscious Patient *69*
   - Performing a Bed Shampoo/Hair Wash *71*
   - Pediculosis *72*
   - The Eyes, Ears and Nose *74*
   - Perineal Care/Meatal Care *77*
   - Handling Glasses *78*
   - Care for Contact Lenses and Eyes *79*
   - Care for Removable Dentures *80*
   - Care and Maintenance of Hearing Aid *80*

5. **Elimination Needs** 81
   - Urinary Elimination *81*
   - Facilitating Urine Elimination *85*
   - Providing Urinal *85*
   - Providing Bedpan *85*
   - Condom Drainage *86*
   - Providing Genital Care/Hygienic Perineal Care *87*
   - Catheterization of the Urinary Bladder *88*
   - Care of Urinary Drainage *93*
   - Removing an Indwelling Urinary Catheter *94*
   - Urinary Diversions *95*
   - Bladder Irrigation *96*
   - Bowel Elimination *96*
   - Alterations in Bowel Elimination *100*
   - Collecting a Stool Specimen for Routine Examination *101*
   - Passing a Flatus Tube *101*
   - Enema *102*
   - Suppository *104*
   - Sitz Bath *105*
   - Bowel Wash *106*
   - Digital Evacuation of Feces *107*
   - Colostomy *107*
   - Care of Ostomies *109*
   - Colostomy Irrigation *110*

6. **Diagnostic Testing** 113
   - Diagnostic Test *113*
   - Complete Blood Counts (HEMOGRAM) (Cell Counter) *114*
   - Various Blood Components Measured Under Complete Blood Count *115*
   - Serum Electrolytes *117*

- Liver Function Tests 121
- LFTs to Assessment of Metabolic 122
- Lipids/Lipoprotein Profile 124
- Lipoproteins 125
- Blood Glucose Technologies 126
- Testing Procedures 128
- Stool Examination 130
- Physical Examination 131
- Urine Test for Albumin 135
- Test for Sugar in Urine 136
- Urine Test for Acetone 136
- Urine pH 136
- Specific Gravity 137
- Urine Culture 137
- Collection of Urine Specimen 138
- Nurse's Responsibility in Collecting Urine Specimen 139
- Sputum Culture 139
- Radiological Procedures 140
- Diagnostic Radiology 140
- Endoscopic Procedures 141

7. **Oxygenation Needs** 142
   - Review of Cardiovascular and Respiratory Physiology 142
   - Respiratory System (Physiology) 142
   - Factors Affecting Respiratory Functioning 143
   - Alterations in Respiratory Functioning 144
   - Alterations of Oxygenation 145
   - Nursing Interventions to Promote Oxygenation 145
   - Nebulization Therapy 146
   - Steam Inhalation 148
   - Maintenance of Patent Airway 150
   - Oxygen Administration 150
   - Methods of Oxygen Administration 151
   - Suctioning 153
   - Tracheostomy Suctioning 155
   - Chest Physiotherapy 156
   - Care of Clients with Chest Tubes 162
   - Pulse Oximetry 163
   - Restorative and Continuing Care 165
   - Breathing Exercises 167
   - Respiratory Exercises 167
   - Incentive Spirometry 169

8. **Fluid, Electrolyte, and Acid-Base Balances** 171
   - Review of Physiological Regulation of fluid, Electrolyte and Acid-Base Balances 171
   - Homeostasis: Mechanisms of Controlling Fluid and Electrolyte Movement 171
   - Acid and Base Disturbance 173
   - Factors Affecting Fluid, Electrolyte and Acid-Base Balances 175
   - Disturbances in Fluid Volume 178
   - Fluid Volume Excess 180
   - Electrolytes Regulation and Electrolyte Imbalances 182
   - Metabolic: Acidosis and Alkalosis 188
   - Respiratory: Acidosis and Alkalosis 191
   - Intravenous Infusion/Intravenous Therapy 193
   - Performing a Venipuncture 196
   - Complications of IV Fluid Therapy 197
   - Measuring Intake and Output (Fluid Intake) 198
   - Administering Blood and Blood Components 199
   - Restricting Fluid Intake 204
   - Enhancing Fluid Intake 205

9. **Administration of Medications** 206
   - Medication 206
   - Administration of Medication 206
   - Drugs Nomenclature 206
   - Effects of Drugs on the Body 207
   - Forms of Medications 209
   - Drug Preparations 209
   - Purposes of Medications 210
   - Pharmacodynamics and Pharmacokinetics 210
   - Drug Action 211
   - Factors Influencing Medication Action 212
   - Medication Orders and Prescriptions 213
   - Systems of Measurement 214
   - Medication Dose Calculation 216
   - General Principles for Administration of Medications 217
   - 10 Rights of Medication Administration 218
   - Errors in Medication Administration 219
   - Storage and Maintenance of Drugs 220
   - Terminologies 222
   - Abbreviations 223
   - Developmental Considerations in Medication Administration 224
   - Routes of Drug Administration 225
   - Oral Medication 226
   - Sublingual and Buccal Medication Administration 227
   - Administration of Parenteral Medications 228
   - Routes of Parenteral Therapies 228
   - Intramuscular Injection 230
   - Intravenous Injection 232
   - Intravenous Infusions 234
   - Venipuncture Site 234
   - Subcutaneous Injection 236
   - Intradermal Injection 238
   - Equipments 239
   - Infusion set 242
   - Types of Vials and Ampoules 243
   - Preparing Injectable Medicines from Vials and Ampoules 246
   - Care of Equipment: Decontamination and Disposal of Syringes, Needles, Infusion Sets 248
   - Prevention of Needlestick Injuries 248
   - Topical Administration 250
   - Application to Skin and Mucous Membrane 251
   - Direct Application of Liquids 252

- Insertion of Drug into Body Cavity *252*
- Instillations—Ear, Eye, Nasal, Bladder and Rectal *254*
- Irrigations—Eye, Ear, Nasal, Rectal and Bladder *256*
- Spraying: Nose and Throat *260*
- Inhalations *261*
- Dry Inhalations *261*
- Moist Inhalations *261*
- Epidural Route *264*
- Intrathecal Administration *264*
- Intraosseous Route *265*
- Intraperitoneal Route *266*
- Intrapleural Route *267*
- Intra-arterial Route *267*

10. Sensory Needs 269
- Components of Sensory Experience *269*
- Arousal Mechanism *270*
- Factors Affecting the Sensory Function *270*
- Assessment of Sensory Alterations *271*
- Management *274*
- Unconsciousness *278*

11. Care of Terminally Ill, Death and Dying 281
- Concepts of Loss *281*
- Grief, Bereavement and Mourning *281*
- Types of Grief Responses *282*
- Types of Complicated Grief *283*
- Manifestations of Grief *283*
- Factors influencing Loss and Grief Responses *284*
- Theories of Grief and Loss—Kubler Ross *285*
- The R Process model (Rando's) *286*
- Death *287*
- Signs of Impending Death *287*
- Dying patient's Bill of Rights *288*
- Care of Dying Patient *288*
- Physiological Changes Occurring after Death *290*
- Dying Declaration *291*
- Death Certificate *291*
- Care of Dead Body *291*
- Autopsy *293*
- Embalming *296*
- Counseling and Supporting Grieving Relatives *299*
- Placing Body in the Mortuary *300*
- Releasing Body from the Mortuary *300*
- Ethical and Legal Issues in Death and Dying *301*
- Euthanasia *301*
- Organ Donation *302*

12. Psychosocial Needs: Self-concept 304
- Dimensions of Self-concept *305*
- Components of Self-concept *305*
- Factors that Affect Self-concept *307*
- Nursing Management *309*

13. Psychosocial Needs: Sexuality 311
- Meaning *311*
- Definition *311*
- Sexual Health *311*
- Sexual Orientation *314*
- Prevention of Unwanted Pregnancy *316*
- Avoiding Sexual Harassment and Abuse *317*
- Nursing Management *319*

14. Psychosocial Needs: Stress and Adaptation—Introductory Concepts 320
- Stress *320*
- Stressor *321*
- Sources/Causes of Stress *322*
- Effects of Stress *324*
- Indicators of Stress *325*
- Adaptation *325*
- Stress Adaptation *325*
- General Adaptation Syndrome *326*
- Local Adaptation Syndrome *327*
- Manifestations of Stress *328*
- Nursing Theory and Role of Stress *328*
- Factors Influencing Stress and Coping *328*
- Coping *329*
- Coping Strategies *330*
- Stress Management *330*
- Assist with Coping and Adaptation for Stress Management *332*
- Creating a Therapeutic Environment for Stress Management *332*
- Recreational and Diversional Therapies for Stress Management *333*

15. Psychosocial Needs: Concepts of Cultural Diversity and Spirituality 335
- Cultural Diversity *335*
- Providing Culturally Responsive Care *336*
- Spirituality *337*
- Concepts: Faith, Hope, Religion, Spirituality, Spiritual Wellbeing *337*
- Dealing with Spiritual Distress (Spiritual Care Interventions) *340*
- Nursing Management *340*
- The Five R's of Spiritual Care *341*

16. Nursing Theories: Introduction 342
- Models *343*
- Theories *343*
- Historical Perspective *343*
- Theory *344*
- Nursing Theories *345*

Index 359

SYLLABUS

NURSING FOUNDATION—II

Placement: II SEMESTER
Theory: 6 Credits (120 hours)
Practicum: Skill Lab: 3 Credits (120 hours), Clinical: 4 Credits (320 hours)
Description: This course is designed to help novice nursing students develop knowledge and competencies required to provide evidence-based, comprehensive basic nursing care for adult patients, using nursing process approach.
Competencies: On completion of the course, the students will be able to:

1. Develop understanding about fundamentals of health assessment and perform health assessment in supervised clinical settings
2. Demonstrate fundamental skills of assessment, planning, implementation and evaluation of nursing care using Nursing process approach in supervised clinical settings
3. Assess the nutritional needs of patients and provide relevant care under supervision
4. Identify and meet the hygienic needs of patients
5. Identify and meet the elimination needs of patient
6. Interpret findings of specimen testing applying the knowledge of normal values
7. Promote oxygenation based on identified oxygenation needs of patients under supervision
8. Review the concept of fluid, electrolyte balance integrating the knowledge of applied physiology
9. Apply the knowledge of the principles, routes, effects of administration of medications in administering medication
10. Calculate conversions of drugs and dosages within and between systems of measurements
11. Demonstrate knowledge and understanding in caring for patients with altered functioning of sense organs and unconsciousness
12. Explain loss, death and grief
13. Describe sexual development and sexuality
14. Identify stressors and stress adaptation modes
15. Integrate the knowledge of culture and cultural differences in meeting the spiritual needs
16. Explain the introductory concepts relevant to models of health and illness in patient care

*Mandatory Module used in Teaching/Learning:
Health Assessment Module: 40 hours

COURSE OUTLINE
T – Theory, SL – Skill Lab

Unit	Time (Hrs)	Learning objectives	Content	Teaching learning activities	Assessment methods

I	20 (T)
	20 (SL)
		Describe the purpose and process of health assessment and perform assessment under supervised clinical practice	**Health Assessment**
			• Interview techniques
			• Observation techniques
			• Purposes of health assessment
			• Process of health assessment
			  – Health history
			  – Physical examination:
			    ♦ Methods: inspection, palpation, percussion, auscultation, olfaction
			    ♦ Preparation for examination: patient and unit
			    ♦ General assessment
			    ♦ Assessment of each body system
			    ♦ Documenting health assessment findings
				• Modular Learning
				• ***Health Assessment Module**
				• Lecture cum Discussion
				• Demonstration
					• Essay
					• Short answer
					• Objective type
					• OSCE

Unit	Time (Hrs)	Learning objectives	Content	Teaching learning activities	Assessment methods

II	13 (T) 8 (SL)	Describe assessment, planning, implementation and evaluation of nursing care using Nursing process approach	**The Nursing Process**
			• Critical thinking competencies, attitudes for critical thinking, levels of critical thinking in nursing
			• Nursing process overview
			   – **Assessment**
			      • Collection of data: Types, sources, methods
			      • Organizing data
			      • Validating data
			      • Documenting data
			   – **Nursing Diagnosis**
			      • Identification of client problems, risks and strengths
			      • Nursing diagnosis statement—parts, types, formulating, guidelines for formulating nursing diagnosis
			      • NANDA approved diagnoses
			      • Difference between medical and nursing diagnosis
			   – **Planning**
			      • Types of planning
			      • Establishing priorities
			      • Establishing goals and expected outcomes—purposes, types, guidelines, components of goals and outcome statements
			      • Types of nursing interventions, selecting interventions: Protocols and standing orders
			      • Introduction to nursing intervention classification and nursing outcome classification
			      • Guidelines for writing care plan
			   – **Implementation**
			      • Process of implementing the plan of care
			      • Types of care—direct and indirect
			   – **Evaluation:** Evaluation process, documentation and reporting
				• Lecture
				• Discussion
				• Demonstration
				• Supervised clinical practice
					• Essay
					• Short answer
					• Objective type
					• Evaluation of care plan

III	5 (T) 5 (SL)	Identify and meet the nutritional needs of patients	**Nutritional needs**
			• Importance
			• Factors affecting nutritional needs
			• Assessment of nutritional status
			• Review: special diets—solid, liquid, soft
			• Review on therapeutic diets
			• Care of patient with dysphagia, anorexia, nausea, vomiting
			• Meeting nutritional needs: Principles, equipment, procedure, indications
			   – Oral
			   – Enteral: Nasogastric/orogastric
			   – Introduction to other enteral feeds—types, indications, gastrostomy, jejunostomy
			   – Parenteral—TPN (Total parenteral nutrition)
				• Lecture
				• Discussion
				• Demonstration
				• Exercise
				• Supervised clinical practice
					• Essay
					• Short answer
					• Objective type
					• Evaluation of nutritional assessment and diet planning

IV	5 (T) 15 (SL)	Identify and meet the hygienic needs of patients	**Hygiene**
			• Factors influencing hygienic practice
			• Hygienic care: Indications and purposes, effects of neglected care
			   – Care of the skin—(Bath, feet and nail, hair care)
			   – Care of pressure points
			   – Assessment of pressure ulcers using braden scale and norton scale
			   – Pressure ulcers—causes, stages and manifestations, care and prevention
			   – Perineal care/meatal care
			   – Oral care, care of eyes, ears and nose including assistive devices (eye glasses, contact lens, dentures, hearing aid)
				• Lecture
				• Discussion
				• Demonstration
					• Essay
					• Short answer
					• Objective type
					• OSCE

Unit	Time (Hrs)	Learning objectives	Content	Teaching learning activities	Assessment methods

V	10 (T) 10 (SL)	Identify and meet the elimination needs of patient	**Elimination needs**
			• Urinary Elimination
			– Review of physiology of urine elimination, composition and characteristics of urine
			– Factors influencing urination
			– Alteration in urinary elimination
			– Facilitating urine elimination: assessment, types, equipment, procedures and special considerations
			– Providing urinal/bed pan
			– Care of patients with
			  ♦ Condom drainage
			  ♦ Intermittent catheterization
			  ♦ Indwelling urinary catheter and urinary drainage
			  ♦ Urinary diversions
			  ♦ Bladder irrigation
			• Bowel elimination
			– Review of physiology of bowel elimination, composition and characteristics of feces
			– Factors affecting bowel elimination
			– Alteration in bowel elimination
			– Facilitating bowel elimination: assessment, equipment, procedures
			  ♦ Enemas
			  ♦ Suppository
			  ♦ Bowel wash
			  ♦ Digital evacuation of impacted feces
			  ♦ Care of patients with ostomies (bowel diversion procedures)
				• Lecture
				• Discussion
				• Demonstration
					• Essay
					• Short answer
					• Objective type
					• OSCE

VI	3 (T) 4 (SL)	• Explain various types of specimens and identify normal values of tests • Develop skill in specimen collection, handling and transport	**Diagnostic testing** Phases of diagnostic testing (pre-test, intra-test and post-test) in common investigations and clinical implications • Complete blood count • Serum electrolytes • LFT • Lipid/Lipoprotein profile • Serum glucose – AC, PC, HbA1c • Monitoring capillary blood glucose (Glucometer random blood sugar—GRBS) • Stool routine examination • Urine Testing—albumin, acetone, pH, specific gravity • Urine culture, routine, timed urine specimen • Sputum culture • Overview of radiologic and endoscopic procedures	• Lecture • Discussion • Demonstration	• Essay • Short answer • Objective type
VII	11 (T) 10 (SL)	Assess patients for oxygenation needs, promote oxygenation and provide care during oxygen therapy	**Oxygenation needs** • Review of cardiovascular and respiratory physiology • Factors affecting respiratory functioning • Alterations in respiratory functioning • Conditions affecting – Airway – Movement of air – Diffusion – Oxygen transport	• Lecture • Discussion • Demonstration and Re-demonstration	• Essay • Short answer • Objective type

Unit	Time (Hrs)	Learning objectives	Content	Teaching learning activities	Assessment methods

			• Alterations in oxygenation
			• Nursing interventions to promote oxygenation: Assessment, types, equipment used and procedure
			  – Maintenance of patent airway
			  – Oxygen administration
			  – Suctioning—oral, tracheal
			  – Chest physiotherapy—percussion, vibration and postural drainage
			  – Care of chest drainage—principles and purposes
			  – Pulse oximetry—factors affecting measurement of oxygen saturation using pulse oximeter, interpretation
			• Restorative and continuing care
			  – Hydration
			  – Humidification
			  – Coughing techniques
			  – Breathing exercises
			  – Incentive spirometry		

VIII	5 (T)
	10 (SL)
		Describe the concept of fluid, electrolyte balance	**Fluid, Electrolyte, and Acid-Base Balances**
			• Review of physiological regulation of fluid, electrolyte and acid-base balances
			• Factors affecting fluid, electrolyte and acid-base balances
			• Disturbances in fluid volume:
			  – Deficit:
			    ♦ Hypovolemia
			    ♦ Dehydration
			  – Excess:
			    ♦ Fluid overload
			    ♦ Edema
			• Electrolyte imbalances (hypo and hyper)
			  – Acid-base imbalances
			    ♦ Metabolic—acidosis and alkalosis
			    ♦ Respiratory—acidosis and alkalosis
			  – Intravenous therapy
			    ♦ Peripheral venipuncture sites
			    ♦ Types of IV fluids
			    ♦ Calculation for making IV fluid plan
			    ♦ Complications of IV fluid therapy
			    ♦ Measuring fluid intake and output
			    ♦ Administering blood and blood components
			    ♦ Restricting fluid intake
			    ♦ Enhancing fluid intake
				• Lecture
				• Discussion
				• Demonstration
					• Essay
					• Short answer
					• Objective type
					• Problem solving—calculations

IX	20 (T) 22 (SL)	• Explain the principles, routes, effects of administration of medications • Calculate conversions of drugs and dosages within and between systems of measurements • Administer oral and topical medication and document accurately under supervision	**Administration of Medications** • Introduction: Definition of medication, administration of medication, drug nomenclature, effects of drugs, forms of medications, purposes, pharmacodynamics and pharmacokinetics • Factors influencing medication action • Medication orders and prescriptions • Systems of measurement • Medication dose calculation • Principles, 10 rights of medication administration • Errors in medication administration • Routes of administration • Storage and maintenance of drugs and nurses responsibility • Terminologies and abbreviations used in prescriptions and medications orders • Developmental considerations	• Lecture • Discussion • Demonstration and Re-demonstration	• Essay • Short answer • Objective type • OSCE

Unit	Time (Hrs)	Learning objectives	Content	Teaching learning activities	Assessment methods

			• Oral, sublingual and buccal routes: equipment, procedure
			• Introduction to parenteral administration of drugs—intramuscular, intravenous, subcutaneous, intradermal: Location of site, advantages and disadvantages of the specific sites, indication and contraindications for the different routes and sites.
			• Equipment—syringes and needles, cannulas, infusion sets—parts, types, sizes
			• Types of vials and ampoules, preparing injectable medicines from vials and ampoules
			  – Care of equipment: Decontamination and disposal of syringes, needles, infusion sets
			  – Prevention of needlestick Injuries
			• Topical administration: Types, purposes, site, equipment, procedure
			  – Application to skin and mucous membrane
			  – Direct application of liquids, gargle and swabbing the throat
			  – Insertion of drug into body cavity: Suppository/medicated packing in rectum/vagina
			  – Instillations: Ear, eye, nasal, bladder, and rectal
			  – Irrigations: Eye, ear, bladder, vaginal and rectal
			  – Spraying: Nose and throat
			• Inhalation: Nasal, oral, endotracheal/tracheal (steam, oxygen and medications)—purposes, types, equipment, procedure, recording and reporting of medications administered
			• Other parenteral routes: Meaning of epidural, intrathecal, intraosseous, intraperitoneal, intra-pleural, intra-arterial		

X	5 (T) 6 (SL)	Provide care to patients with altered functioning of sense organs and unconsciousness in supervised clinical practice	**Sensory Needs** • Introduction • Components of sensory experience – reception, Perception and reaction • Arousal mechanism • Factors affecting sensory function • Assessment of sensory alterations—sensory deficit, deprivation, overload and sensory poverty • Management: Promoting meaningful communication (patients with aphasia, artificial airway and visual and hearing impairment) **Care of Unconscious Patients** • Unconsciousness: Definition, causes and risk factors, pathophysiology, stages of unconsciousness, clinical manifestations • Assessment and nursing management of patient with unconsciousness, complications	• Lecture • Discussion • Demonstration	• Essay • Short answer • Objective type
XI	4 (T) 6 (SL)	Explain loss, death and grief	**Care of Terminally ill, Death and Dying** • Loss—types • Grief, bereavement and mourning • Types of grief responses • Manifestations of grief • Factors influencing loss and grief responses • Theories of grief and loss—Kubler Ross • 5 Stages of dying • The R Process model (Rando's) • Death—Definition, meaning, types (Brain and circulatory deaths)	• Lecture • Discussion • Case discussions • Death care/last office	• Essay • Short answer • Objective type

Unit	Time (Hrs)	Learning objectives	Content	Teaching learning activities	Assessment methods
			• Signs of impending death • Dying patient's bill of rights • Care of dying patient • Physiological changes occurring after death • Death declaration, certification • Autopsy • Embalming • Last office/death care • Counseling and supporting grieving relatives • Placing body in the mortuary • Releasing body from mortuary • Overview—medicolegal cases, advance directives, DNI/DNR, organ donation, euthanasia		
			PSYCHOSOCIAL NEEDS (A–D)		
XII	3 (T)	Develop basic understanding of self-concept	**A. Self-concept** • Introduction • Components (Personal identity, body image, role Performance, self-esteem) • Factors affecting self-concept • Nursing management	• Lecture • Discussion • Demonstration • Case discussion/ Role play	• Essay • Short answer • Objective type
XIII	2 (T)	Describe sexual development and sexuality	**B. Sexuality** • Sexual development throughout life • Sexual health • Sexual orientation • Factors affecting sexuality • Prevention of STIs, unwanted pregnancy, avoiding sexual harassment and abuse • Dealing with inappropriate sexual behavior	• Lecture • Discussion	• Essay • Short answer • Objective type

XIV	2 (T)
	4 (SL)
		Describe stress and adaptation	**C. Stress and Adaptation—Introductory Concepts**
			• Introduction
			• Sources, effects, indicators and types of stress
			• Types of stressors
			• Stress adaptation—general adaptation syndrome (GAS), local adaptation syndrome (LAS)
			• Manifestation of stress—physical and psychological
			• Coping strategies/Mechanisms
			• Stress management
			  – Assist with coping and adaptation
			  – Creating therapeutic environment
			• Recreational and diversion therapies
				• Lecture
				• Discussion
					• Essay
					• Short answer
					• Objective type

XV	6 (T)	• Explain culture and cultural norms
		• Integrate cultural differences and spiritual needs in providing care to patients under supervision
			D. Concepts of Cultural Diversity and Spirituality
			• Cultural diversity:
			  – Cultural concepts—culture, subculture, multicultural, diversity, race, acculturation, assimilation
			  – Transcultural nursing
			  – Cultural competence
			  – Providing culturally responsive care
			• Spirituality:
			  – Concepts—faith, hope, religion, spirituality, spiritual wellbeing
			  – Factors affecting spirituality
			  – Spiritual problems in acute, chronic, terminal illnesses and near-death experience
			  – Dealing with spiritual distress/problems
				• Lecture
				• Discussion
					• Essay
					• Short answer
					• Objective type

XVI	6 (T)	Explain the significance of nursing theories	**Nursing Theories: Introduction** • Meaning and definition, purposes, types of theories with examples, overview of selected nursing theories–Nightingale, Orem, Roy • Use of theories in nursing practice	• Lecture • Discussion	• Essay • Short answer • Objective type

CHAPTER 1

Health Assessment

■ INTERVIEW

Interview is a systematic process of obtaining data or information from the person with one-on-one communication.

Definition

The interview is usually an organized, systematic communication with the purpose of obtaining subjective data.

The interview is structured communication with the purpose of obtaining subjective information.

■ INTERVIEW TECHNIQUE

Interview technique is the method of used to assess the general condition of the client and collect information about past and present illness of condition.

Definition

Interview technique is the method used to assess the present and past health status of a patient either in Out Patient Department (OPD) or ward.

Purposes

- ❖ To collect specific information required for diagnosis and planning
- ❖ To establish a client-nurse relationship
- ❖ To allow the client to participate in goal settings.
- ❖ To assist the nurse to gain insight into the client's ability to function.

Phases of Nursing Interviews

Professional interpersonal and interviewing skill are necessary to obtain a valid nursing health history. The nursing interview is a communication process that focuses on the patient's development, psychological, physiological, sociocultural and spiritual responses that can be treated with nursing and collaborative interventions. The nursing interview has three basic phases **(Fig. 1.1)**:

1. **Introductory phase:** The introductory phase is the time to introduce yourself to patient, put him/her at ease, and explain the purpose of interview and the time frame needed to complete it. Questions should be non-probing

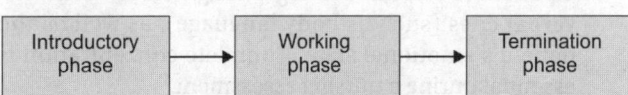

Fig. 1.1: Phases of interview.

and patient centered. Provide comfort, privacy and confidentiality.

2. **The working phase:** The working phase is often where data collection occurs. It is usually very structured. It is also the longest phase. Make sure to allot enough time to working phase. Use critical thinking skills to listen for and observe cues, and to interpret and validate information received from the patient. Collaborate with the patient to identify problems and goals. Although nurses needs to take notes and may be focused on taking minimal notes and documenting data after the interview rather than during it.

3. **The termination phase:** The end of the interview is the termination phase, nurse need to summarize and restate findings. This provides opportunity to clarify the data and share feelings with patient. Based on the information nurse and patient can discuss follow-up plans.

Strategies of Interview Technique

Collecting patient data is a core step in the nursing process. Systemically collect patient health information so the patient can receive the care they need. It is the gateway to building an effective nurse patient relationship that will make patient feel at ease, supported and empowered. The most effective health assessment interview techniques include **(Fig. 1.2)**.

- ❖ **Active listening (Fig. 1.3):**
  - Nurses must do more than simply listen when conducting a health history assessment, they must actively listen.

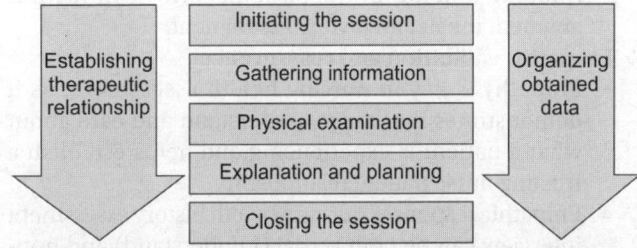

Fig. 1.2: Components of health assessment interview techniques.

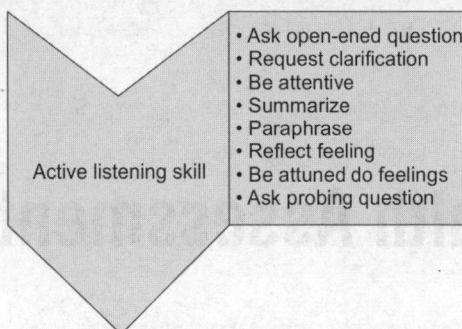

Fig. 1.3: Components of active listening skill.

- Actively listening involves fully comprehending what a patient is communicating through verbal and non-verbal cues (such as body language), as well as the patient's emotional state. Complete concentration is essential during a nursing assessment.
- Listen carefully using verbal and non-verbal prompts to encourage the patient to expand on his or her symptoms and the circumstances sur rounding them.

❖ **Adaptive questioning:**
- Also referred as a guided questioning, adaptive questioning helps to encourage patient to fully communicate without interrupting the flow of his or her narrative.
- Start with general questions, making patient more specific as we move through interview.
- Health assessment in nursing require questioning that elicits a graded response versus a yes or no reply.
- Series of questions, asked one at a time often help patients open up, as does offering multiple choices for answers.
- Request additional information, when necessary, by asking the patient to clarify their statements.
- Repeating his/her statements (a technique called echoing) is also helpful, as is using verbal and non-verbal continuers, such as nodding head or saying things, like "Go On".

❖ **Non-verbal communication:**
- Nursing assessment also require that nurse be in tune with patient's non-verbal communication, such as posture, eye contact, facial expression, and the like.
- Reading and understanding nonverbal cues help nurses understand patients more fully and using non-verbal communication of their own such as mirroring a patient's position or using therapeutic physical contact (placing a hand on the patients' arm) can further augment the health history assessment.

❖ **Empathy, validation and reassurance:**
- Empathy is key in nursing health assessment, as it demonstrates that nurse, understand and care about what a patient is experiencing and helps establish a trusting nurse patient relationship.
- Empathic responses during a health history assessment interview can be both verbal (I understand) and non-verbal (such as offering a tissue if the patient is crying).
- Beyond being empathic be sure to validate patient's feelings to help reassure them that their emotions are natural and understood and will be fully addressed.

❖ **Partnering and summarization:**
- Another essential element of a nursing health assessment is expressing to the patient that nurse committed to forgoing a continuing partnership dedicated to his or her wellness.
- When conducting an interview, summarizing what the patient has said is also helpful, as it demonstrates that nurse in listening and can fill in holes in the patient's story.

❖ **Transition and empowerments:**
- Health problems can elicit feelings of anxiety in patients; one way to put their fears at ease is to use transitions during their health history assessment to let them know what they should expect next, such as change in subject matter or a physical examination.
- Patients also feel vulnerable when they are experiencing health problems, making it essential to empower then with the idea that their participation in the process and working closely with their medical team can make a positive difference in their outcomes.

OBSERVATION

Observation is the method of data collection through the use of senses, ie sight, smell, hearing and touch. Observation is the skill that required practice
Nurses adopt this method in an attempt to understand patients' values, rituals, symbols, beliefs, and emotions.

Characteristics

- ❖ Observation is systemic and scientific
- ❖ It is specific, selective and purposeful.
- ❖ It is quantitative.
- ❖ Recorded immediately.
- ❖ Done by an expert.
- ❖ Results can be checked and verified.

Types

❖ **Structured and unstructured observation:**
- When observation is done by characterizing style of recording the observed information, standardized conditions of observation, definition of the units to be observed, selection of pertinent data of observation then it is structured observation.
- When observation is done without any thought before observation then it is called as unstructured observation.

❖ **Participant and non-participant observation:**
- *Participant observation:*
  - When the observer is the member of the group in which he/she is observing then it is participant observation.
  - In participant observation nurse can record natural behavior of group, nurse can verify the truth of statements given by patient in the content of questionnaire. It is difficult to collect information

through this method because nurse may loose objectivity of data due to emotional feelings.
- *Non-participant observation:* When nurse is observing patient without giving any information to them.

❖ **Controlled or uncontrolled observation:**
- When the observation takes places in natural condition, i.e., uncontrolled observation. It is done to get spontaneous picture of patient.
- When observation takes place according to definite pre-arranged plans, with experimental procedures then it is controlled observation. It is generally done in laboratory under controlled conditions.

Advantages
❖ Directness
❖ Natural environment
❖ Longitudinal analysis
❖ Non-verbal behavior
❖ Data gathered can be very reliable.
❖ Relatively inexpensive compared with other techniques.

Disadvantages
❖ Lack of control.
❖ Difficulties in quantification.
❖ Timing may be inconvenient.
❖ Some tasks cannot always be performed the same way.
❖ Possible observer bias.
❖ No opportunity to learn from past.

OBSERVATION TECHNIQUES

Observation is a technique that involves systematically recording behavior and characteristics of living beings, selecting, watching, listening, reading, touching and objects, or phenomena.

Levels of Observation

All services should have explicit policies on observation types and frequencies and communication of observations. Since observation, assessment and interventions are interlinked, nurses sighting people and talking with them is implicit in describing levels of observation. One possible model with four defined levels of observation is outlined below:

1. **Constant arm's length**—periods of one-to-one nursing observation, with the person within an arm's length of an experienced nurse at all times
2. **Constant visual** periods of one-to-one nursing observation, with the person within the vision of an experienced nurse at all times
3. **Intermittent an** experienced nurse (or mentored, less experienced nurse) engages with a person at regular intervals. The identified risk factors and purpose of observation will determine the frequency (for example, several times per hour) and pattern of observations (for example, equal or random lengths of time between observations)
4. **Negotiated** nurses negotiate the frequency of engagement with people who do not have identified risk factors requiring intermittent or constant observation.

Principles

There are several core principles that underlie the practice of nursing observation. The principles hold that:
❖ Nursing observation is multifaceted
❖ Observation and assessment are interrelated
❖ Observation is grounded in therapeutic engagement with the person
❖ Nurses appreciate how inpatient environments influence behavior
❖ Observations are communicated between colleagues
❖ There is a clear process of documentation that is timely and descriptive

Observation Techniques during a Health Assessment

During the health assessment, nurses need to have an analytical ability to observe and interpret the nonverbal activities of the client. Nonverbal activities are important because they provide a clue to understanding the feelings. Nurses should observe the following things during health assessment:

Physical Appearance
❖ Person's physical appearance can provide lots of information about the client. According to Hans Selye, a person's physical condition can be also known through his appearance.
❖ For example, a person who looks sick may have some internal disease. Inattention to dressing and grooming suggests a person has some problem, for that he/she does not have the energy to maintain his grooming.
❖ Choice of clothing also represents the role of the person, such as (student, worker and professionals).

Posture
❖ In the beginning, nurses need to observe the posture and position of the client.
❖ An open posture exposing the large muscle group of the client suggest his/her feeling of relaxation. It shows he/she is comfortable with the interviewer.
❖ A closed position, such as crossed legs and closed arms suggests the client is defensive and anxious he/she does not want to share any information with the interviewer.
❖ Changing position during interview indicates the comfort level with new topics.
❖ For example, a client was in an open posture at starting of the interview, when the interviewer asked about the relationship with his wife, he sat in a closed posture. It shows client is comfortable with the 'relation topic.

Gesture
❖ Gesture shows the interest of the interviewer towards the client. Nodding head, open posture, accepting client, showing attention, or agreement is favorable gestures.

- ❖ Whereas fidgeting of hand and picking nails shows anxiety. So nurses must observe the gestures of the client to recognize the feelings of the client.

Facial Expression
- ❖ When we meet any person, the first thing we see is a higher facial expression.
- ❖ The facial expression also tells many things about that person, character, and personality. Some physical conditions, such as pain, sadness are also reflected through facial expressions.

Eye Contact
- ❖ During the interview, eye contact is very important to show how much confident you are.
- ❖ Lack of eye contact indicates the person is shy, withdrawn, depressed, bored, and confused.
- ❖ Casual eye contact should be there, eye contact should not be penetrating.

Voice
- ❖ The interviewer must aware of the tone of the voice of the client.
- ❖ Not only do spoken words give meaning, but also voice characteristics, such as intensity, rate of speech, pitch, and any pauses give meaning to the conversation.
- ❖ Anxious people speak louder and faster than normal.
- ❖ A soft voice may indicate the person's shyness and fear. Even pauses also give meaning to the discussion.

Touch
- ❖ The meaning of touch is different according to different cultures, past experiences, age, gender, and current setting.
- ❖ In Western culture, it is regarded as an expression of love. But some cultures avoid touch or it is misinterpreted.
- ❖ Do not use touch if you do not know how another person will take it.

HEALTH ASSESSMENT
- ❖ Health assessment is a regular and continuous process. This is an important tool to determine the health status of an individual.
- ❖ It consists of systematic and orderly collection of information pertaining to and about the health status of patient.
- ❖ Assessment includes subjective data through interviewing the patient and obtaining objective data by physically examining the patient.
- ❖ Subjective data are those symptoms, values and information that only the patient can state and validate.
- ❖ Objective data can be directly observed or measured such as vital signs or appearance.

Purposes
- ❖ To establish a database for the patient's normal abilities, risk factors and any current alteration in function.
- ❖ To plan strategies to encourage continuation of healthy patterns, prevent potential health problems and alleviate or manage existing health problems.
- ❖ To provide a holistic view of the patient.
- ❖ To formulate a conclusion or a problem statement, such as a nursing diagnosis.
- ❖ To provide an essential foundation for the care of the patient.
- ❖ To develop (obtain baseline data) and expand the data base from which subsequent phases of the nursing process can evolve.
- ❖ To identify and manage a variety of patient problems (actual and potential).
- ❖ To evaluate the effectiveness of nursing care
- ❖ To enhance the nurse-patient relationship.
- ❖ To make clinical judgments.

Process of Health Assessment
- ❖ A thorough inspection or detailed inspection on entire body or some part of the body to determine the general physical conditions or the conditions of some part of the body or its function is called physical examination.
- ❖ A complete health assessment includes a comprehensive history and a complete physical assessment.

HEALTH HISTORY

Biographical Data
Includes name, address, phone number, contact person, age, birth date, place of birth, gender, race/ethnicity nationality, religion, marital status, number of dependents, educational level occupation, social security number, health insurance, source of history/reliability, referral, advance directive.

Current Health Status
Includes symptom analysis for chief complaint and current medication. At primary level of health care when the patient does not have an acute problem, current health status should include, usual state of health, any major health problems, usual patterns of health care and any health concerns.

Past Health History
Includes childhood, illnesses, surgeries, hospitalizations, serious injuries, medical problems, medications, allergies, immunizations, and recent travel or military service.

Family History
Includes patient spouse, children siblings, parents, aunts, uncles, and grandparents' health status, or if deceased, age and cause of death.

Review of Systems
Includes questions specific to each body system and analysis of any positive symptoms.

Psychosocial Profile
Includes health practices and beliefs, typical day, nutritional patterns, activity/exercise patterns, recreation. Pets/hobbies, sleep/rest patterns, personal habits, occupational health patterns, socioeconomic status environmental health

patterns, roles/relationships, sexuality patterns, social supports and stress/coping patterns.

PHYSICAL EXAMINATION

Approach

Two methods are used for completing a total physical assessment, a systems approach and a head to toe approach.

- ❖ A systems approach allows for a thorough assessment of each system, doing all assessments related to one system before moving on to the next, better for a focused assessment.
- ❖ A head-to-toe assessment includes the same examinations as a systems assessment, but you assess each region of the body before moving on to the next.
- ❖ No matter which approach you use, be systematic and consistent. All four assessment techniques—inspection, percussion, palpation, and auscultation are used to perform a complete assessment.
- ❖ **Remember:**
  - Inspect for abnormalities and normal variations of visible body parts.
  - Palpate to identify surface characteristics areas of pain, or tenderness, organs and abnormalities, including masses and fremitus.
  - Percuss to determine the density of underlying tissues and to detect abnormalities in the underlying organs.
  - Auscultate for sounds made by body organs, including heart, lungs, intestines, and vascular structures.

Assessment data are usually charted by systems (e.g., respiratory or neurological) and by regions to a limited extent (e.g., head/neck). Your documentation can focus only on positive findings or on both positive and negative findings. No matter which format you use, always be brief and to the point and avoid generalizations.

Performing a Head-to-Toe Physical Assessment

Here are some helpful hints to keep in mind as you conduct the assessment.

- ❖ Wash your hands, before you begin.
- ❖ Listen to your patient.
- ❖ Provide a warm environment.
- ❖ If your patient has a problem, start at your point.
- ❖ Work from head-to-toe.
- ❖ Compare side-to-side.
- ❖ Let your patient know your findings.
- ❖ Use your time not only to assess but also to teach your patient.
- ❖ Leave sensitive or painful areas until the end of the examination.

Techniques of Physical Examinations

Observation

- ❖ The basic techniques of physical examination are inspection, palpation, percussion, and auscultation, together referred to as observation.
- ❖ These skills enable you to collect data systematically using the senses of sight, touch, hearing and smell. Physical appearance, behavior, communication patterns, and activity abilities can all be observed, as can a person's environment and events that affect him/her.
- ❖ Observing facial expression for signs of discomfort, detecting odors that indicate infection, listening to chest sounds to determine airway patency, and touching the skin to determine body temperature are all examples of observation.

Inspection

- ❖ Inspection is systematic and deliberate visual observation to determine health status.
- ❖ Begin the physical examination with a general survey or inspection of the client, including an assessment of age posture, stature, body weight, grooming and mobility patterns.
- ❖ Next carryout a more though observation in a head-to-toe fashion.
- ❖ Note the shape and size of the head, hair distribution, general skin condition, and facial expressions. Inspect the face for symmetry of eyes and balance of facial expression.
- ❖ While inspecting the neck note visible pulsations, bulges, or venous distention. Inspect the chest and abdomen, noting symmetry, masses, pulsations, skin condition and visible signs of discomfort, such as holding the abdomen.
- ❖ Inspect the lower extremities, noting especially ankle swelling and skin integrity.
- ❖ Following the general survey, more detailed observations are made as the physical examination progresses to specific body parts or systems. Inspection always precedes palpation, percussion, or auscultation of a particular area.
- ❖ Effective inspection is facilitated by good lighting and exposure.
- ❖ Occasionally, instrument such as the ophthalmoscope and auroscope may be used as well.

Palpation

- ❖ With palpation you rely on the sense of touch to make judgments about the size, shape, texture and mobility of structures and masses, the quality of pulses, the condition of bones and joints, the extent of tenderness in injured areas or structures, skin temperature and moisture, fluid accumulations and edema, and chest wall vibrations.
- ❖ Different parts of the hand are used to palpate different types of structures.
  - Breasts, lymph nodes and pulses should by palpated with the fingertips, where nerve endings are most concentrated.
  - The thumb and index fingertips are used to evaluate tissue firmness.
  - Temperature can be quickly assessed with the back of the hand, where temperature sensory nerves are most concentrated and the skin is thin.
  - Vibrations can be felt most strongly with the palm of the hand especially along the metacarpal joints.

- ❖ Palpation should be carried out in such a way as to avoid discomfort.
- ❖ Your hands should be warm and the client relaxed to avoid muscle tensing.
- ❖ Palpate painful areas last.
- ❖ The amount of pressure you apply is governed by the type of structure you are examining and the degree to which palpation may cause discomfort.
- ❖ Any expression of distress or pain should prompt you to palpate lightly.
- ❖ Palpation may be light, deep, or bimanual.
  - *Light palpation* (**Fig. 1.4**):
    - The safest and least uncomfortable palpation involves exerting gentle pressure with the fingertips of your dominant hand, moving them in a circular motion.
    - Place your hand parallel to the part of the body surface you are examining and extend your fingers to depress the skin surface approximately 0.5–0.75 inches (1–2 cm).
    - Exert and release fingertip pressure several times over an area. Exerting continuous pressure would tend to dull the tactile discrimination senses.
  - *Deep palpation* (**Fig. 1.5**):
    - It is done after light palpation, and is used to detect abdominal masses.
    - The technique is similar to light palpation except that the fingers are held at a greater angle to the body surface and the skin is depressed about 1.5–2 inches (4–5 cm).
    - A variation of this technique involves placing the fingertips of one hand over the fingertips of the palpating hand.
    - The top hand should press and guide the bottom hand to detect underlying masses.
  - *Bimanual palpation:* It involves using both hands to trap a structure between them. This technique can be used to evaluate the spleen, kidneys, breasts, uterus, and ovaries.

Percussion (Fig. 1.6)

- ❖ Percussion involves trapping the body lightly but sharply to determine the position, size, and density of underlying structures, as well as to detect fluid or air in a cavity.
- ❖ Tapping the body creates a sound wave that travels 2–3 inches (5–7 cm) toward underlying areas.
- ❖ Sound reverberations assume different characteristics depending on the features of the underlying structures.
- ❖ Percussing the right upper abdominal quadrant, for example, will usually elicit dull sounds.
- ❖ Indicating the presence of the liver, tapping over the lungs should reveal resonant sounds associated with air-filled spaces. Percussion should usually be performed after an area has been palpated.
- ❖ Three percussion methods can be used, i.e., mediate or indirect, immediate, and fist percussion. The method chosen depends on the area to be percussed.
  1. "Mediate or indirect percussion" should be used to percuss the abdomen and thorax, and can be performed by using the finger of one hand as a plexor (striking finger) and the middle finger of the other hand as a pleximeter (the finger being struck).
  2. "Immediate percussion", used mainly to evaluate the sinuses or an infant's thorax, involves striking the surface directly with the fingers of the hand only.

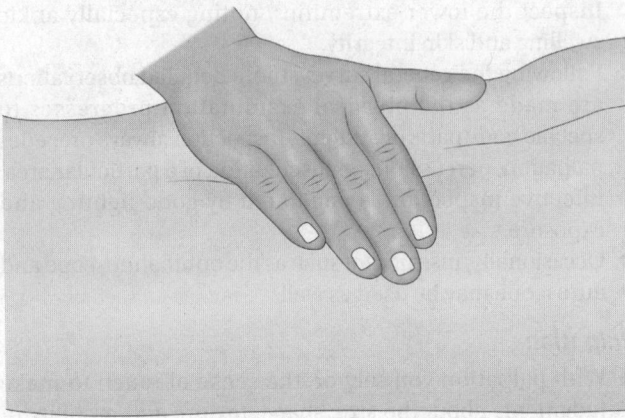

Fig. 1.4: Light palpation.

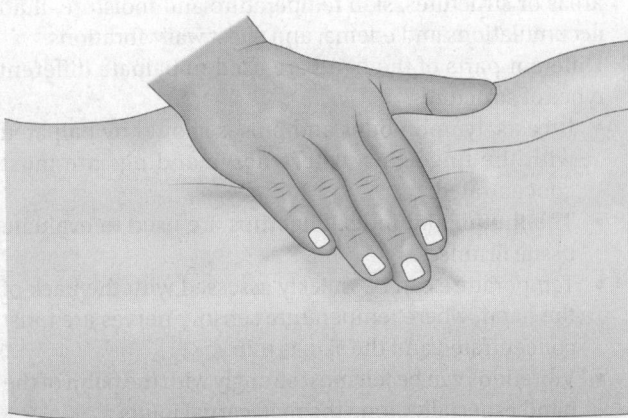

Fig. 1.5: Deep palpation.

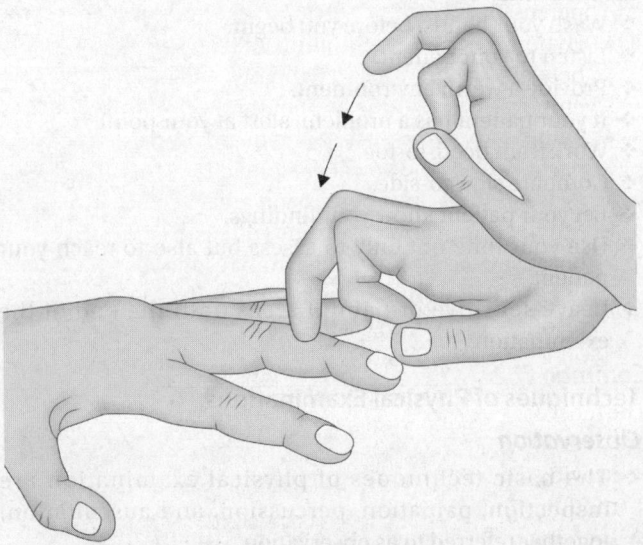

Fig. 1.6: Percussion.

3. "First percussion", used to evaluate the back and kidneys for tenderness, involves placing one hand flat against the body surface and striking the back of the hand with a clenched fist of the other hand.
- ❖ Procedure mediate or indirect percussion is the basic technique or percussion and is performed as the following.
  - Place the pad of the middle finger of your nondominant hand firmly against the surface being percussed.
  - The other fingers as well as the heel of this hand, should be raised to avoid contact with the body surface.
  - Hold the finger firmly against the body surface throughout percussion, even when it is not being tapped by the other hand.
  - Use the middle finger of your dominant hand as the plexor.
  - Hold the forearm horizontal to the surface being percussed.
  - Keep the forearm stationary and use wrist motion to make striking movements.
  - Quickly strike the distal phalanx of the finger that is positioned on the body surface with the tips of the finger of the other hand.
  - Use only the wrist to generate motion, and quickly remove the striking hand after percussing to avoid muffling the percussion sound.
  - You may percuss a single area two or three times before moving to the next area.
  - Light tapping is more effective than heavy tapping.
  - Identify the percussion sound.
  - Skillful percussion reveals one of percussion sounds, depending on the density of underlying structure, i.e., flatness, dullness, resonance, hyperresonance, and tympany.
  - A flat sound is elicited by percussing over solid masses such as bone or muscle.
  - A dull sound which has a lower pitch than a flat sound, is elicited when high density structures, such as the liver, are percussed.
  - Resonance is a hollow sound, heard, for example, by percussing the lung.
  - Hyperresonance is an abnormal sound with a pitch between resonance and tympany, and may indicate an emphysematous lung or pneumothorax.
  - Tympany is a drum-like sound heard over air-filled body parts, such as the bowel or stomach.
  - Proceed to the next percussion area.
  - Move from more resonant to less resonant areas, because detecting a change from resonance to dullness is easier than detecting a change from dullness to resonance.

Common Error in Percussion

The most common errors in performing immediate percussion are as follows:
- ❖ Moving the forearm of the dominant hand. Remember, all motion should be generated from the wrist.
- ❖ Pressing the striking finger into the positioned finger.
- ❖ Remove the striking finger immediately after tapping.
- ❖ Causing injury to oneself or the client by in advertently striking the client or your own hand with along finger nail.
- ❖ The fingernail of the flexor finger should be kept short.
- ❖ Failing to hear the percussion note.
- ❖ Eliminate environmental noise including noise caused by bracelets or loose fitting watches.
- ❖ If the note is still difficult to hear, check your technique.

Auscultation

- ❖ Auscultation is the skill of listening to body sounds created in the lungs, heart, blood vessels, and abdominal viscera.
- ❖ Auscultation is usually the last technique used during the examination.
- ❖ The sequence usually progresses from inspection to palpation, percussion, and auscultation, except during the abdominal examination, when auscultation is the second step (following inspection).
- ❖ "Immediate auscultation" involves placing one's ear directly on the skin, such as over the mental noise frequently interferes with hearing.
- ❖ The usual method is "mediate auscultation", or using a stethoscope to detect sounds.
- ❖ The best results are gained using a good quality stethoscope.
- ❖ You should eliminate extraneous noise such as televisions, voices, and equipment sounds before performing auscultation.
- ❖ Do not create noise by moving the stethoscope over the body hair or clothing or by touching the stethoscope tubing.
- ❖ Auscultated sounds are described in terms of pitch, intensity, duration and quality.

Preparation for Examination: Patient and Unit

Unit
- ❖ Maintain good ventilation and privacy.
- ❖ Provide adequate light.
- ❖ Arrange a separate examination room.
- ❖ Provide a special examination table with mattress and pillow or an ordinary cot and sheets for draping.
- ❖ Articles should be arranged conveniently at the bedside.

Articles Required for Examination
- ❖ Sphygmomanometer
- ❖ Stethoscope
- ❖ Flash light
- ❖ Tongue depressor
- ❖ Tape measure and skin pencil
- ❖ Percussion hammer
- ❖ Safety pin
- ❖ Tuning fork
- ❖ Cotton applicators
- ❖ Specimen bottles
- ❖ Test tubes
- ❖ Culture bottles and slides if needed
- ❖ Kidney tray
- ❖ Ophthalmoscope
- ❖ Ear speculum
- ❖ Cotton wool
- ❖ Nasal speculum
- ❖ Head mirror.

Patient

- **Mental preparation:** The patient may be quite new to the hospital situation and he may be anxious and worried about his future life as well as his family. It is the duty of the nurse to allay his anxieties and fears by proper explanation of the advantages and purpose of the examination and treatment and try to win his confidence.
- **Physical preparation:** Keep the patient clean. Help the patient to empty the bladder. Loosen the garments, expose only the needed area and provide privacy. Keep the patient in a comfortable position and convenient to the doctor for examination. Avoid all unnecessary exposure.
- **Assistance with the examination:** Never leave the patient alone during the physical examination especially female, win the confidence and cooperation of the patients so that it will be easy for the doctor to do the examination.
- Prepare the patient and get the equipment ready.
- Secure privacy.
- Keep the patient ready for examination.
- Nurse should stand on the opposite side of the doctor to assist him.
- Adjust the position according to the need. Expose parts of the patients as needed for the examination.
- Avoid unnecessary exposure by proper draping.
- Handle the equipment to the doctors as needed.
- Turn the patient's head to the opposite side of the doctor especially during the chest examination.
- After finishing the examination, keep the patient in comfortable position and replace the articles to the proper place after cleaning them. Send specimens to the laboratory immediately if any taken.

GENERAL ASSESSMENT

Get anthropometric data and vital signs, and evaluate patient's clothing, hygiene, state of well-being nutritional status, emotional status, speech patterns, level of consciousness, affect, posture, gait, coordination, balance, and gross deformities.

Skin/Hair/Nails

- Inspect and palpate patient's visible skin for color, lesions, texture, and warmth. Continue observation throughout the examination.
- Note hair color, texture, and distribution over body.
- Observe hands and nails for clubbing or other abnormalities.

Head/Face

- Note head size, shape, and position.
- Note scalp tenderness, lesions, or masses.
- Observe the facial symmetry and note facial expressions (cranial nerve CN VII).
- Test sensation on face (CN V).
- Palpate temporomandibular joint for popping or tenderness.
- Test range of motion (ROM) of neck and assess muscle strength.

Eyes

- Test visual acuity (CN II) with Snellen test or pocket vision screener.
- Perform test of extraocular movements (CNs III, IV, VI).
- Perform cover test and corneal light reflex test.
- Test visual fields by confrontation.
- Inspect cornea, iris, and lens with oblique lighting.
- Observe sclera and conjunctivae.
- Perform papillary reaction to light and accommodation.
- Perform fundoscopic examination to rest for red reflex and to observes disks and retinal vessels.

Ears

- Inspect external ear and canal.
- Inspect position and angle of attachment.
- Palpate tragus, mastoid, and helix for tenderness.

Nose

- Test for patency of each nostril.
- Test sense of smell (CN I).
- Palpate for sinus tenderness.
- Observe nasal mucosa, septum, and turbinates with speculum.

Mouth/Pharynx

- Inspect and palpate lips and oral mucosa.
- Inspect teeth, gingiva and palate.
- Inspect pharynx and tonsils.
- Test gag and swallow reflexes and have patient say "ah"(CNs IX, X).
- Test taste on anterior and posterior tongue (CNs VII, XII).

Neck

- Inspect and palpate thyroid gland.
- Inspect for masses, abnormal pulsations, or tracheal deviation.
- Palpate carotid pulse and listen for bruits.
- Inspect jugular veins.
- Measure jugular venous pressure.
- Palpate lymph nodes in head, neck, and clavicular are as.
- Test ROM of neck.
- Test muscle strength of neck and shoulder muscles (CNXI).

Upper Extremities

- Test of ROM muscle strength.
- Inspect joints for swelling, redness, and deformities.
- Test and grip.
- Test superficial and deep sensations.
- Palpate radial, ulnar, and brachial pulses.
- Test for deep tendon reflexes of biceps, triceps, and brachioradialis.
- Test coordination, rapid alternating movements, and finger thumb opposition.
- Inspect and palpate nails, checking capillary refill and angle of attachment.
- Test for pronator drift.
- Test for a accuracy of movements with point-to-point-movements.

Posterior Thorax/Back
- Palpate thyroid from behind (if not done previously).
- Inspect spine and palpate muscles along spine.
- Percuss and auscultate lung fields.
- Fist/blunt percuss costovertebral angle tenderness.
- Palpate and percuss chest excursion.
- Note normal curvatures of spine.
- Palpate tactile fremitus.
- Check ROM of spine.

Anterior Thorax
- Inspect, palpate, percuss and auscultate lungs.
- Inspect and palpate precordium for pulsations, point of maximal impulse and thrills.
- Auscultate heart.
- Inspect and palpate breasts.
- Palpate axillary and epitrochlear lymph nodes.

Abdomen
- Inspect for shape, scars, movements, and abnormalities.
- Auscultate for bowel sounds and vascular sounds.
- Percuss abdomen and organs for size.
- Obtain a liver measurement.
- Palpate lightly for tenderness.
- Palpate deeply for masses and enlarged liver, spleen, kidneys, and aorta.
- Palpate femoral arteries and inguinal lymph nodes.
- If ascites suspected, percuss for shifting dullness.

Lower Extremities
- Inspect for skin color, hair distribution, temperature, edema, and varicose veins.
- Test for ROM, muscle strength, and superficial and deep sensations.
- Palpate pulses.
- Test deep tendon reflexes and plantar reflex.
- Observe gait, toe walk, heel walk, heel-to-toe-walk, and deep knee bend.
- Perform Romberg's test and proprioception test.
- Test coordination with toe tapping and heel down skin.
- If indicated test knees, for fluid with bulge sign or patellar tap.
- If indicated, test for torn meniscus with Apley's or McMurray's test.
- Observe ROM of lower extremities.
- Test muscle strength of lower extremities.

Female Genitalia/Rectum
- Inspect and palpate external genitalia and inguinal lymph nodes.
- Perform internal examination: Inspect vagina and cervix, collect Pap smear and cultures.
- Palpate uterus and adnexa.
- Inspect perianal area and palpate anal canal and rectum.
- Test stool for occult blood.

Cardiovascular System

Physical Assessment
History collection

General Appearance
- Level of distress
- Level of consciousness
- Level of answering thinking (cerebral perfusion)
- Behavioral changes
- Anxiety level.

Blood Pressure
- Hypertension/hypotension
- Auscultation of BP.
- The diaphragm is placed over the brachial artery.
- The cuff is deflated 2–3 mm of Hg/second.
- On listening of tapping sounds which indicate systolic BP.
- These sounds are called Korotkoff sounds.
- Suddenly the sound increase and disappears and muffled sound is heard and is recorded called: Tripartite pressure, e.g., /20/80/60.
- Sometimes a temporary disappearance of sound occurs when auscultating the blood pressure. This is called auscultator gap.

Postural or Orthostatic Hypotension

Examination of Pulse
- Pulse rate
- Pulse rhythm
- Pulse deficit
- Pulse quality
- Pulse configuration
- Sinus dysrhythmia (Pulse increased on inspiration and decreased on expiration)
- Vessel quality.

Hands
- Peripheral cyanosis
- **Pallor:**
  - Capillary refill
  - Hand temperature and moistness
  - Edema
  - Reduced skin turgor
  - Clubbing of the fingers and toes.

Head and Neck
Jugular vein dissipation
Lips and earlobes: Peripheral cyanosis.

Heart Sounds–S1 and S2
- S1 and S2—Systole decreased.
- S2 and S1—Systole increased.
- First heart sound S1—Closure of the mitral and tricuspid valve.
- Second heart sound S2—Closure of aortic and pulmonic valve.
- Gallops—First and second heart sounds usually trip cells.

- ❖ Snaps and clicks—stenosis of mitral valve resulting from rheumatic heart disease gives rise to an unusual sound very rarely is diastole that is high pitched, best heard, left sterna border—opening snap.
- ❖ Stenosis of the aortic valve gives rise to a short high pitched sound immediately after the first hear sound is called—Ejection click.
- ❖ Murmurs—due to turbulent flow of blood time, location, intensity, pitch, radiation of sound.

DOCUMENTING PHYSICAL ASSESSMENT FINDINGS

Document physical assessment findings by system, using the following sequence:

- ❖ General survey, including anthropometric measurements and vital signs
- ❖ Integumentary
- ❖ Head, face and neck
- ❖ Eyes
- ❖ Ears, nose, and throat
- ❖ Respiratory
- ❖ Cardiovascular
- ❖ Breasts
- ❖ Abdomen
- ❖ Male/female genitourinary
- ❖ Musculoskeletal
- ❖ Neurologic
- ❖ Focused assessments are only partial ones, dealing only with systems that relate to the patient's problem, so less data are collected
- ❖ Focused assessments are used when the patient's condition or time restraints preclude a comprehensive assessment

A focused physical assessment should include:

- ❖ A general survey with vital signs and weight
- ❖ Assessment of level of consciousness
- ❖ Assessment of skin, color, temperature, and texture
- ❖ Testing of gross motor balance and coordination
- ❖ Testing of extraocular movements
- ❖ Testing of papillary reaction
- ❖ Testing of gross vision of hearing
- ❖ Inspection of oral mucosa as patient says "ah"
- ❖ Auscultation of anterior and posterior breath sounds
- ❖ Palpation of apical impulse, point of maximal impulse
- ❖ Auscultation of heart sounds
- ❖ Inspect abdomen
- ❖ Auscultation of abdomen
- ❖ Percussion of abdomen
- ❖ Palpation of abdomen
- ❖ Testing sensation to touch on extremities
- ❖ Palpation of muscle strength of upper and lower extremities.

AUSCULTATION

Heart

- ❖ **Aortic area:** Second intercostals space to the right side of sternum.
- ❖ **Pulmonary area:** Second intercostals space to the left side of sternum.
- ❖ **Erb's point:** Third intercostals space to left of sternum.
- ❖ **Right ventricular (tricuspid area):** Fourth and fifth intercostals space to the left of the sternum.
- ❖ **Left ventricular (apical area):** Fifth intercostals space on the left of the sternum.
- ❖ **Epigastric area:** Below the xiphoid process.
  - *Inspection:* Apical pulse or of point of marsupial impulse (PMI)
  - *Palpation:* Left ventricular leave.
  - *Percussion:* Cardiomegaly.
  - *Friction rub:* Harsh grating sound both systole and diastole is called friction rub.

Other Assessment Parameters

- ❖ **Lungs:**
  - Tachypnea
  - Cheyne stokes respirations.
  - Cough
  - Crack lets
  - Wheezes
  - Rales and rhonchi
  - Breath sounds
  - Tactile vocal fremitus.
- ❖ **Abdomen:**
  - Hepatojugular reflex
  - Bladder distension.
- ❖ **Feet and legs:**
  - Thrombophlebitis
  - Pedal edema—right ventricular failure.
  - Temperature
  - Cyanosis
  - Sensation.

Investigations

- ❖ **Cardiac:** Enzymes
- ❖ Creatinine kinase are and its enzymes (CK-MB)
- ❖ **Myocardial infarction:** Lactose dehydrogenase (LDH)

Blood Chemistry

- ❖ Lipid profile:
- ❖ Triglycerides
- ❖ Lipoproteins
  - Total cholesterol <200 mg dL
  - High density of lipoproteins (HDL)
  - Low density of lipoproteins (LDL)

Serum Electrolytes

- ❖ Serum Sodium—hypo/hypernatremia
- ❖ Serum Calcium—hypercalcemia
- ❖ Serum Potassium—hypo/hyperkalemia.
- ❖ Blood urea nitrogen BUN
- ❖ Blood glucose

GENERAL ASSESSMENT OF EACH BODY SYSTEM

Equipments

- ❖ Cotton applicator stick
- ❖ Flashlight

- Oto-ophthalmoscope
- Reflex hammer
- Safety pin
- Sphygmomanometer
- Stethoscope
- Thermometer
- Tongue blade
- Tuning fork
- Additional items may include disposable gloves and lubricant for rectal examination and a speculum for examination of female pelvis.

Vital Signs

Importance: Many major therapeutic decisions are based on the vital signs; therefore, accuracy is essential.

Temperature
- Routinely, where accuracy is not crucial an oral temperature will suffice.
- A rectal temperature is the most accurate.
- Unless contraindicated (as in a patient with a severe cardiac arrhythmia), a rectal temperature is often preferred.

Findings
Temperature may vary with the time of day.
- **Oral:**
  - 98.6°F (37°C) is considered normal.
  - May vary from 96.4–99.1°F (35.8–37.3°C)
- **Rectal:**
  - Higher than oral by 0.7–0.9°F (0.4–0.5°C)

Pulse
- Palpate the radial pulse and count for at least 30 seconds.
- If the pulse is irregular count for a full minute and note the number of irregular beats per minute.
- Note whether the beat of the pulse against your finger is strong or weak, bounding or thready.

Findings
- Normal adult pulse is 60–80 beats/minute; regular in rhythm.
- Elasticity of the arterial walls, blood volume and mechanical action of the heart muscle are some of the factor that effect strength of the pulse wave which normally is full and strong.

Respiration
- Count the number of respirations taken in 15 seconds and multiply that by 4.
- Note rhythm and depth of breathing.

Findings
Respiration: Normally 16–20 respirations per minute.

Blood Pressure
- Measure the blood pressure in both arms.
- Document the patient's position.
- Palpate the systolic pressure before using the stethoscope in order to detect on auscultatory gap.
- Apply the cuff firmly; if it is too loose, it will give a falsely high reading.
- Use an appropriate sized cuff, a pediatric cuff for children; a large cuff or a leg cuff for obese people.
- The cuff should be approximately 1 inch (2.5 cm) above the antecubital fossa.

Findings
- Normal blood pressure is <120/80 mm Hg.
- A difference of 5–10 mm Hg between arms is common.
- Systolic pressure is lower extremities is usually 10 mm Hg higher than reading in upper extremities.
- Going from a recumbent to a standing position can cause the systolic pressure to fall 10–15 mm Hg and the diastolic pressure to rise slightly (by 5 mm Hg).

Height and Weight
- Determine the patient's height and weight. Use a measuring
- Stick or tape rather than asking the patient's height.

General Appearance
Begin observation on first contact with the patient (in the waiting room or while the patient is in bed); continue throughout the interview systematically.

Auscultatory Gap
- The first sound of blood in artery is usually followed by continuous sound until nothing is audible with the stethoscope.
- Occasionally, the sound is not continuous and there is a gap after the first sound, after which the sound of blood in the vessel is heard again.
- If one uses only the auscultatory method and pumps the cuff up until the sound is no longer heard, it is possible, when there is a gap in the sound or when the sound is not continuous, to get a falsely low systolic reading.

General Appearance
Inspection: Observe for race, sex, general physical development, nutritional state, mental alertness, affect, evidence of pain restlessness, body position, clothes, apparent age, hygiene, grooming.

Finding
Careful observations of the general state of the individual provides many clues about a person's body image, how he behaves, and also some idea of how well or ill he is.

Skin
- Examination of the skin's correlated with the information obtained in the history and other parts of the physical examination.
- Examine the skin as you proceed through each body system.

Inspection
Observe for skin color, pigmentation, lesions (distribution, type, configuration, size), jaundice, cyanosis, scars, superficial vascularity, hydration edema, color of mucous membrane, hair distribution, nails.

Palpation
Examine skin for temperature, texture, elasticity, turgor.

Findings
- "Normal" varies considerably depending on racial or ethnic background, exposure to sun, complexion, pigmentation tendencies (such as freckles).
- The skin is normally warm, slightly moist, and smooth, and returns quickly to its original shape when picked up between two fingers and released.
- There is a characteristic hair distribution over the body associated with gender and normal physiologic function.
- Nails are present and smooth and care for in same way).

Head
Inspection
Observe for: Symmetry of face, configuration of skull, hair color and distribution and scalp.

Palpation
Examine hair texture, masses, swelling or tenderness of scalp, configuration of skull.

Findings
- Normally the skull and face are symmetric, with distribution of hair varying from person to person.(However, determine by history if there has been any change).
- The scalp should be free of flaking, with no signs of nits(small, white louse eggs), lesions, deformities or tenderness.

Eyes and Vision
Equipment
- Ophthalmoscope.
- Snellen chart for visual acuity

Anatomic Landmarks
- Globes
- Palpebral fissures
- Lid margins
- Conjunctivae
- Sclerae
- Pupils
- Iris.

Inspection
- Globes—for protrusion.
- Palpebral fissures (longitudinal openings between the eyelids) for width and symmetry.

Findings
Appear equal in size when the eye are open.
- **Upper lid:** Covers a small portion of the iris and cornea.
- **Lower lid:** Margin is just below the junction of the cornea and sclera (limbus).
- **Ptosis:** Drooping of eyelids.
- **Lid margins:** For scaling, secretions, erythema, position of lashes. Lid margins are clear, the lacrimal duct opening (puncta)are evident at the nasal ends of the upper and lower lids.
- **Bulbar and palpebral conjunctivae:** For congestion and color.
  - *Bulbar conjunctiva:* Membranous covering of the sclera (contains blood vessels). It consists of transparent red blood vessels, which may become dilated and produce the characteristic "bloodshot" eye.
  - *Palpebral conjunctiva:* Membranous covering of the inside of the upper and lower lids (contains blood vessels). Palpebral conjunctiva are pink and clear.
- **Conjunctivitis:** Inflammation of the conjunctival surfaces.

Sclerae and Iris
For color.

Findings
Sclerae should be white and clear.

Pupils
For size, shape, symmetry, reaction to light and accommodation (ability of the lens to adjust to objects at varying distance).

Findings
Pupils normally constrict with increasing light and accommodation. Pupils are normally round and can range in size from very small ("pinpoint") to large (occupying the entire space of the iris).

Eye Movement
Extraocular movements, nystagmus, convergence. (Nystagmus: rapid, lateral, horizontal, or rotary movement of the eye). (Convergence: ability of the eye to turn in and focus on a very close object).

Findings
Extraocular movement—movement of the eyes in conjugate fashion. (Six muscles control the movement of the eye). Eyes normally move in conjugate fashion, except when converging on an object that is moving closer.

Nystagmus
It may be seen briefly on lateral movement as are sult of eye fatigue, however, vertical nystagmus or prolonged nystagmus should be evaluated.

Convergence
Fails when double vision occurs, usually 4-6 inches (10–15 cm) from the nose.

Gross Visual Fields
By confrontation.

Findings
Peripheral vision—is full (medially and laterally, superiorly and inferiorly) in both eyes.
- **Visual acuity:** Check with a Snellen chart (with and without glasses).
- **Findings:** Normal vision—20/20.
- **Myopia:** Nearsightedness
- **Hyperopia:** Farsightedness.

Palpations
- Determine the strength of the upper lids by attempting to open closed lids against resistance.
- Palpate globes through closed lids for tenderness and tension.

Findings
The examiner should not be able to open the lids when the patient is squeezing them shut. Globes normally are tender when palpated.

Funduscopic Examination
- **Red retinal reflex:** Check the transparency of the anterior and posterior chambers.
- **Cornea:** Check for transparency.
- **Lens:** Check for transparency.
- **Retina:** Check for color, pigmentation, hemorrhages, and exudates.
- **Optic disc:** Check color, distinction of margins, pigmentation, degree of elevation, cupping.
- **Macula:** Check for color, (lies at a distance of 2 optic disk diameters laterally from the optic disc).
- **Blood vessels:** Check for diameter, arteriovenous (AV) ratio, origin and course, venous-arterial crossings (Both arteries and veins are present and move outward from the disk nasally and temporarily).

Findings
- **Red retinal reflex:** It can be spotted by the examiner while standing 1 foot (30 cm) from the eye.
- **Cornea:** It should be transparent with the light directed at the pupil.
- **Lens:** It should be transparent (retina can be seen).
- **Retina:** Color varies according to the amount of pigment present. There should be no hemorrhages or exudates.
- **Optic disc:** It is circular and has a yellowish pink color, although disk appearance may vary, the margins are normally distinct and regular, with varying amounts of pigment.
- Macula because it is free of blood vessels, it is lighter in color than the rest of the retina.

Use of the Ophthalmoscope
- Hold the instrument in your right and use your right eye to examine, the patients right eye.
  - Reverse the procedure to the patients left eye.
  - This approach allows you to get close to the patient without bumping noses.
- Hold the instrument so your last two fingers are straight, rather than curved around the handle. You can place these fingers against the patient's cheek to steady the instrument and to avoid hitting the patient with it.
- Begin the funduscopic examination standing about 1 foot (30 cm) away from, and on the same level as, the patient, the room should be darkened.
- Turn the dial on the head of the ophthalmoscope to 0 diopters.
- Turn on the ophthalmoscope light and place the eyepiece up to your eye. If you wear glasses or contact lenses, it is best to wear them during the examination so you do not have to accommodate for your vision by turning dial on the ophthalmoscope.
- Aim the light at the pupil of the eye. You should see the red reflex immediately.
- Slowly move in toward the patient, continuing to look through the eyepiece and keeping the light directed at the pupil beyond which is fundus.
- With the index finger of the hand holding the ophthalmoscope turn the dial counterclockwise (to the minus diopters) to focus if the patient is nearsighted, or clockwise (toward the plus diopters) to focus if the patient is farsighted.
  - This allows you to focus on the various chambers of the eye.
  - A way to find the eye and pupil is to put your hand on top of the patient's head and your thumb at your outer corner of the eye. If you lose the fundus, you can return to your thumb and get your bearings by moving medially from the thumb nail.
- Once your hand is resting on the patient's cheek, continue to turn the dial until you can focus on the retina, and the blood vessels and the optic disk appear sharp.
- Once you are focused on the optic disk it is possible to follow the blood vessels out from the disk inferiorly and superiorly, medially and laterally.

Findings
- Absence of the red reflex suggests capacity of the lens (contract) detached retina, or retinoblastoma (rarely).
- Abnormal findings include hemorrhages, exudates and papilledema.

Ears and Hearing
Equipments
- Tuning fork
- Otoscope.

To Examine with Otoscope
- Hold the helix of the ear and gently pull the pinna upward and back toward the occiput to straighten the external canal.
- Gently insert the lighted otoscope using an earpiece that is a comfortable size for the patient.
- Once the otoscope is in place put your eye up to the eyepiece and examine the external canal.

Inspection
- **Pinna:** Examine for size, shape, color, symmetry, placement on the head, lesions, and masses.
- **External canal:** Examine with the otoscope for discharge, impacted cerumen, inflammation, masses, or foreign bodies.
- **Tympanic membrane:** Examine for color, luster, shape position transparency, integrity, and scarring.
- **Landmarks:** Note cone of light, umbo, handle and short, process of the malleus, pars flaccida, and pars tensa.

Gently move the otoscope to observe the entire drum. (Cerumen may obscure visualization of the drum)

Palpation
Pinna examine for tenderness, consistency of cartilage, swelling.

Findings
- External canal is normally clear with perhaps minimal cerumen.
- **Tympanic membrane and landmarks:** Junction of incus and stapes, chorda tympani nerve, posterior malleolar folds, pars flaccida, anterior malleolar folds, short
- process of malleus, manubrium (handle), umbo, pars, tensa, right ear drum, cone of light.

Mechanical Test
- Test each ear for gross hearing acuity using a whispered word or a watch. Cover the ear not being tested.
- **Weber test:** Test for lateralization of vibration. Top the tuning fork against a hard surface to make it vibrate. Then, place the tuning fork in the center of the scalp near forehead.
- **Rinne test:** Compares air and bone conduction.
  - Place vibrating tuning fork on the mastoid process
  - behind the ear and have the patient tell you when the vibration stops.
  - Then quickly hold the buzzing end of the tuning fork near the ear canal and ask patient can hear it.

Findings
- A personal with normal hearing can hear a whispered word from approximately 15 feet (4.5 m) and a watch from 1 foot (30 cm). The patient should hear the sound equally well in both ears, that is there is no lateralization.
- Sound should be heard equally in both ears.
- Sound should be heard after vibration can no longer be left, that is, air conduction, is greater than bone conduction. Lateralization and conduction findings are altered by damage to the cranial nerve VIII and damage to the ossicles in the middle ear.

Nose and Sinuses
Equipment
- Otoscope
- Nasal speculum.

Inspection
- Observe for general deformity.
- With nasal speculum (otoscope, if speculum is unavailable), examine for:
  - Nasal septum (position and perforation)
  - Discharge (anteriorly and posteriorly)
  - Nasal obstruction and airway patency
  - Turbinate for color and swelling.

Findings
- **Nasal septum:** It is normally straight and not perforated.
- **Discharge:** None should be present.
- Airways are patent.
- **Mucous membranes:** These are normally pink

- **Turbinates:** Three bony projections on each lateral wall of the nasal cavity covered with well-vascularized mucous-secreting membranes. They warm the air going into the lungs and may become swollen and pale with colds and allergies.

Palpation
- Sinuses (frontal and maxillary)—for tenderness.
- Frontal direct manual pressure upward toward the wall of the sinus. Avoid pressure on eyes. Maxillary—with thumbs, direct pressure upward over lower edge of maxillary bones. (Tenderness of sinuses may indicate sinusitis.

Mouth
Equipments
- Flashlight
- Tongue blade
- Gloves
- Gauze sponges.

Inspection
- Observe lips for color, moisture, pigment, masses, ulcerations, fissures.
- **Use tongue blade and penlight to examine:**
  - *Teeth:* Number, arrangement, general condition.
  - *Gums:* For color, texture, discharge, swelling or retraction.
  - *Buccal mucosa:* For discoloration, vesicles, ulcers, masses.
  - *Pharynx:* For inflammation, exudates, and masses.
  - *Tongue (protruded):* For size, color, thickness lesions, moisture, symmetry, deviations from midline, fasciculations.
  - *Salivary glands:* For patency. Parotid glands.
  - *Uvula:* For symmetry when patient says "ah"
  - *Tonsils:* For size, ulceration, exudates, inflammations.
  - *Voice:* For hoarseness.
  - *Breath:* For odor.

Findings
- **Teeth:** An adult normally has 32 teeth.
- **Gums:** Commonly recede in adult. Bleeding is fairly common and may result from trauma, gingival disease, of systemic problems (less common).
- **Tongue:** It is normally midline and covered with papillae which vary in size from the tip of the tongue to the back. (The circumvallated papillae are large and posterior).
- **Parotid glands:** Open in the buccal pouch at the level of the upper teeth halfway back. Sublingual and submaxillary glands-open underneath the tongue. Lingual tonsils-can often be seen on the posterior portion of the tongue.

Palpations
- Examine the oral cavity with a gloved hand for masses and ulceration. Palpate beneath the tongue and laterally explore the floor of the mouth.
- Grasp the tongue with a gauze sponge to retract it, inspect the sides and undersurface of the tongue and the floor of the mouth.

Finding
Entire oral cavity should be pink and without ulcers deep red color, lesions, palpable masses, or swelling. An indurated mass raises the suspicion of malignancy.

Neck

Equipment
Stethoscope.

Inspections
- Inspect all areas of the neck anteriorly and posteriorly for muscular symmetry, masses, unusual swelling or pulsations, and range of motion.
- **Thyroid:** Ask the patient to swallow and observe for movement of an enlarged thyroid gland at the suprasternal notch.
- **Muscular strength:**
  - *Cervical muscles:* Have the patient turn his chin forcefully against your hand.
  - *Trapezius muscles:* Exert pressure on the patient's shoulders while he shrugs his shoulders.

Findings
- **Range of motion:** Normally, the chin can touch the anterior chest, the head can be extended at least 45° from the vertical position and can be rotated 90° from middle to side.
- **Thyroid:** It is not usually visible, except in extremely thin person.
- **Strength:** The neck and shoulder muscle strength should be symmetric.

Palpations
- Palpate the 10 areas for cervical lymph nodes.
- **Trachea:** Palpate at the sternal notch. Place one finger along the side of the trachea and note the space between it and the sternomastoid. Compare to the other side.
- **Thyroid:**
  - Stand behind the patient and have him flex the neck slightly to relax the muscles.
  - Place the fingertips of both hands on either side of the trachea just below the circoid cartilage. Have the patient, swallow and feel for any glandular tissue rising under your fingertips.
  - Palpate the area over the trachea for the isthmus and laterally for the right and left lobes.
  - Note any enlargement, masses, consistency.
- **Carotid arteries:**
  - Palpate the carotids one side at a time.
  - The carotids lie anterolaterally in the neck—avoid palpating the carotid sinuses at the level of the thyroid cartilage, just below the angle of the jaw, because this may cause slowing of heart rates.
  - Note the symmetry of pulsations, strength and amplitude.

Findings
- **Cervical nodes:** In the adult, the cervical lymph nodes are not normally palpable unless the patient is very thin, in which case the nodes are felt as small, freely movable masses. Tender nodes suggest inflammation, hard, fixed, nodes, suggest malignancy.
- **Trachea:** It should be midline, spaces measure by fingers should be symmetrical. Tracheal deviation may be caused by neck mass or problems within the chest.
- If the thyroid is palpable, it is normally smooth, without nodules, masses, or irregularities.
- A thrill (humming-like vibration) usually indicates arterial narrowing.

Auscultation
Use the diaphragm of the stethoscope to listen for bruits (murmur-like sound) over the carotid arteries.

Findings
A bruit may indicate arterial narrowing with turbulent blood flow. A cardiac murmur may also be referred to the carotid arteries.

Lymph Nodes
- It is important at some point in the examination to palpate all areas where lymphadenopathy might appear.
- Typically, this is done as each region of the body is examined, for example, the cervical nodes are studied when the neck is examined and inguinal nodes are inspected when the abdomen is examined.

Findings
Lymph nodes are normally nonpalpable or felt as small, non-tender, freely moveable masses.

Inspection
Note size, shape, mobility, consistency, tenderness, and inflammation.

Palpations
- Cervical, supraclavicular, and infraclavicular nodes.
- **Axillary nodes (usually done during breast exam):**
  - Examine the patient while patient is sitting.
  - Place the patients' arm at his side and examine the apex of the patient's axilla. (Use the fingers of your right hand to examine the left axilla and vice versa).
  - Rotate the examining hands so the fingers can palpate the anterior and posterior axillary fossae pressing against the chest wall. Press against the humerus bone in the axilla to examine the lateral fossae for nodes.

  Conclude the axillary examination by moving the fingers from the apex of the axilla downward in the midline along the chest wall.
- **Inguinal nodes:** These are located in the groin and are usually examined when the abdomen is examined.
- **Epitrochlear nodes:** These are palpated just above the medical epicondyle, between the biceps and triceps muscles.

Findings
- **Supraclavicular and infraclavicular nodes:** Not normally palpable. Enlargement may indicate a thoracic problem.
- **Axillary nodes:** Normally nonpalpable. Enlargement may occur with a breast or arm problem.

- **Inguinal nodes:** A few may be felt. Enlargement and acute tenderness may indicate a genital or lower extremity problem.
- **Epitrochlear nodes:** These are normally palpable enlargement may indicate and arm or systemic problem.

Breasts (Male and Female)

Female Breast

Inspection (with the patient sitting, arms relaxed at sides.

- Inspect the areolae and nipples for position pigmentation, inversion, discharge, crusting and masses. Extra or supernumerary, nipples may occur normally, most commonly in the anterior axillary region or just below the normal breasts.
- Examine the breast tissue for size, shape, color, symmetry, surface, contour, skin characteristics, and level of breasts; Note any retraction or dimpling of the skin.
- Ask the patient to elevate her hands over her head; repeat the observations.
- Have the patient press her hands to her hips; repeat the observation.

Findings

- The nipples should be at the same level and protrude slightly. An inverted nipple (one that turns inward) if present since puberty, may be normal.
- **Breast size:** In the female, it is not uncommon to find a difference In the size of two breasts. Normal asymmetry has usually been present since puberty and is not a recent phenomenon.
- If there is a mass attached to the pectoral muscles, contracting the muscle will cause retraction of the breast tissue.

Palpation

This is best done with the patient in a recumbent position.

- The patient with pendulous breasts should be given a pillow to place under the ipsilateral scapula of the breast being palpated so the tissue is disturbed more evenly over the chest wall.
- The arm on the side of the breast being palpated should be raised above the patient's head.
- Palpate one breast at a time. Beginning with the "asymptomatic" breast if, the patient complains of symptoms.
- To palpate, use the palmar aspects of the fingers in a rotating motion, compressing the breast tissue against the chest wall. Do not forget to include the "tail" of the breast tissue, which extends into the axillary region in the upper outer quadrant of the breast.
- Note skin texture, moisture temperature, or masses.
- Gently squeeze the nipple and note any expressible discharge.
- Repeat the examination on the opposite breast and compare findings.

Findings

- This allows the examiner to palpate the "normal" breast first and then compare the "symptomatic" breast to it.
- Breast texture varies according to the amount of subcutaneous tissue present.
  - In young females, tissue is fairly soft and homogeneous; is postmenopausal women, tissue may feel nodular or stringy.
  - Consistency also varies with menstrual cycle, being more nodular and edematous just prior to menstruation.
- **Masses:** If a mass is palpated, its location size, shape, consistency, mobility, and associated tenderness are reported.
- **Discharge:** In the normal nonpregnant or nonlactating female, there is usually no nipple discharge.

Male Breast

Examination of the male breast can be brief but may be important.

- Observe the nipple and areola for ulceration, nodules, swelling or discharge.
- Palpate the areola for nodules and tenderness.
- Palpate axillary lymph nodes.

Findings

- There should be no discharge.
- Enlargement of glandular tissue is gynecomastia, related to hormone imbalance.

Thorax and Lungs

- Methodical inspection of the thorax requires reference to established "landmark" to locate specific structures and to report significant findings.
- The same structural landmarks are used in examining both the lung and the heart.
- It is important to visualize the underlying structures and organs when examining the thorax.

Posterior Thorax and Lungs

Begin the examination with the patient seated; examine posterior chest and lungs.

Inspection

- Inspect the spine for mobility and any structural deformity.
- Observe the symmetry of the posterior chest and posture and mobility of the thorax on respiration. Note any bulges or retractions of the costal interspaces on respiration or any impairment of respiratory movement.
- Note the anteroposterior diameter in relation to the lateral diameter of the chest.

Findings

- The thorax is normally symmetric; it moves easily and without impairment on respiration. There are no bulges or retractions of the intercostals spaces.
- The anteroposterior (AP) diameter of the thorax in relation to the lateral diameter is approximately 1:2.

Palpations

- Palpate the posterior chest with the patient sitting; identify areas of tenderness, masses, inflammation.
- Palpate the ribs and costal margins for symmetry and vertebral position.

- To assess respiratory expansion, place thumbs or the level of the 10th vertebra. With hands held parallel to the 10th ribs as they grasp the lateral rib cage, ask the patient to inhale deeply. Observe the movement of the thumbs while feeling the range and observe the symmetry of the hands.
- To elicit vocal and tactile fremitus (palpable vibrations transmitted through the bronchopulmonary system on speaking.
  - Ask the patient to say "99"; palpate and compare symmetric areas of the lungs with the ball of one hand. Begin at the upper lobes and move downward.
  - Note any areas of increased or decreased fremitus.
  - If fremitus is faint, ask the patient to speak louder and in a deeper voice.

Findings
- On palpation there should be no tenderness, chest movement should be symmetric and without lag or impairment. Tenderness may indicate musculoskeletal strain, fracture, or other problems.
- Posteriorly, fremitus is generally equal throughout the lung fields. It may be increased near the large bronchi due to consolidation of tissue resulting from pneumonia. It may be decreased or absent anteriorly and posteriorly when vocal loudness is decreased, when posture is not erect or when excessive tissue or underlying structures are present, or incases of pneumothorax and other pathology.

Percussion
As with palpation, the posterior chest is optimally percussed with the patient sitting.
- Percuss symmetric areas, comparing sides.
- Begin across the top of each shoulder and proceed down between the scapulae and then under the scapulae, both medially and laterally in the axillary lines.
- Note and localize any abnormal percussion sound.
- For diaphragmatic excursion, percuss by placing the pleximeter (stationary) finger parallel to the approximate level of the diaphragm below the right scapula.
  - Ask the patient to inhale deeply and hold his breath; percuss downward to the point of dullness. Mark this point.
  - Let the patient breathe normally and then ask patient to exhale deeply; percuss upward from the mark to the point of resonance.
  - Mark this point and measure between the two marks normally 2-21/2 inches (5-6 cm).
  - Repeat the procedure on the opposite side of the chest.

Findings
- Percussion normally reveals resonance over symmetric area of the lung. Percussion sound may be altered by poor posture or the presence of excessive tissue.
- Dullness may indicate mass or consolidation due to pneumonia.
- The lower border of the lungs approximately at the level of the 10th thoracic spinous process on normal respiration. Unilateral abnormality of decreased excursion may indicate pleural effusion, atelectasis, or paralysis of one side of the diaphragm.

Auscultation
- Aids in assessing airflow through the lungs the presence of fluid or mucus, and the condition of the surrounding pleural space.
- Have the patient sit erect. (if the patient is unable to sit without assistance for examination of the posterior chest and lungs, position him first on one side and then on the other as you examine the lung fields).
- With a stethoscope, listen to the lungs as the patient breathes more deeply than normally with his mouth open (Let the patient pause, as needed, to avoid hyperventilation).
- Place the stethoscope in the same areas on the chest wall as those percussed and listen to a complete inspiration and expiration in each area.
- Compare symmetric areas methodically from the apex to the lung bases.
- It should be possible to distinguish three types of normal breath sounds.

Findings
On auscultation, breath sounds vary according to proximity of the large bronchi (**Table 1.1**):
- They are louder and coarser near the large bronchi and over the anterior.
- They are softer and much finer (vesicular) at the periphery over the alveolae.
- Breath sound also vary in duration with inspiration and expiration.
- Sounds may normally decrease in obese individuals.
- Pathology will alter the normal bronchial, bronchovesicular, and vesicular breath sounds.
- Adventitious sounds may indicate crackles, wheezes, and rhonchi.

Anterior Thorax and Lungs
The patient should be recumbent with his arms at his sides and slightly abducted.

TABLE 1.1: Lung sounds and its characteristics.

Breath sounds	Duration of inspiration and expiration	Pitch of expiration	Intensity of expiration	Normal location
Vesicular	Insp. >Exp.	Low	Soft	Most of lungs
Bronchovesicular	Insp. = Exp.	Medium	Medium	Near the main stem bronchi below the clavicles and between the scapulae, especially on the right
Bronchial or tubular	Exp. >Insp.	High	Usually loud	Over the trachea

Inspections

- Inspect the chest for any structural deformity.
- Note the width of the costal angle.
- Observe the rate and rhythm of breathing, any bulging or retraction of intercostal spaces on respiration, and use of accessory muscles of respiration (sternocleidomastoid and trapezius on inspiration and abdominal muscles on expiration).
- Note any asymmetry of chest wall movement of respiration.

Findings

- The angle of the tip of the sternum is determined by the right and left rib margins at the xiphoid process. Normally the angle is less than 90°.
- There are no bulges or retractions of the intercostals spaces.
- The thorax is normally symmetric and moves easily without impairment on respiration.

Palpations

- To assess expansion, place your hands along the costal margins and note symmetry and degree of expansion as the patient inhales deeply.
- Palpate for fremitus with the ball of the hand anteriorly and laterally (Underlying structures (heart, liver) may damp, or decrease fremitus).
- Compare symmetric areas.
- If necessary, displace the female breast gently.

Percussions

- With patient's arm resting comfortably at his sides, percuss the anterior and lateral chest. Begin just below the clavicles and percuss downward from the interspace to the next, comparing the sound from the interspace on one side with that of the contralateral interspace.
- Displace the female breast so breast tissue does not damp the vibration. Continue, downward, noting the intercostals space where hepatic dullness is percussed on the right and cardiac dullness on the left.
- Note the effect of underlying structures.

Findings

- A tympanic sound is produced over the gastric air bubble on the left somewhat lower than the point of liver dullness on the right.
- Percussion over heart will produce a dull sound. The upper border of the liver will be percussed on the right side, producing a dull note.

Auscultation

Listen to the chest anteriorly and laterally for the distribution of resonance and any abnormal or adventitious sounds.

Heart

General Approach

- The examiner must visualize the position of the heart under the sternum and the ribs and know certain landmarks for identification of specific structures and significant findings.
- It is also important to identify those "areas" on the chest wall that will yield the most information initially about the function of heart and its valves.
- In locating the intercostal spaces, begin by identifying the angle of Louis, which is felt as a slight, ridge approximately 1 inch (2.5 cm) below the sternal notch. Where the manubrium and the body of the sternum are joined.
- The 2nd ribs extend to the right and left of this angle.
- Once the 2nd rib is located palpate downward and obliquely away from the sternum to identify the remaining ribs and intercostals spaces.

Inspections

- Inspect the precordium of any bulging, heaving, or thrusting.
- Look for the apical impulse in the 5th or 6th intercostal space at or just medial to the midclavicular line.
- Note any other pulsations. Tangential lighting is most helpful in detecting pulsations.

Findings

- Normally, there are no bulges or heaves; these indicated pathology.
- An apical impulse, may or may not be observable.
- There should be no other pulsations.

Palpations

- Use the ball of the hand to detect vibrations, or "thrills", which may be caused by murmurs (Use the fingertips or palmar surface to detect pulsations).
- Proceed methodically through the examination so no area is omitted. Palpate for thrills and pulsations, in each area (aortic, pulmonic, tricuspid mitral).
- Begin in the aortic area (2nd right intercostal space close to the sternum) and proceed to the pulmonic area (2nd left intercostals space) and then downward to the apex of the heart. (The mitral area is concerned the apex of the heart.
- In the tricuspid area, use the palm of the hand to detect any heaving or thrusting of the precordium (tricuspid area-5th intercostal space next to the sternum.
- In the mitral area (5th intercostals space at or just medial to the midclavicular line) palpate for the apical beat; identify the point of maximal impulse (PMI) and note its size and force.

Findings

There should be no thrills or other pulsation. (Thrills are vibrations caused by turbulence of blood moving through valves that are transmitted through the skin, which feels, similar to a purring cat).

- Ordinarily, to heaving of the ventricle is felt except, possibly, in the pregnant.
- The apical pulse should be felt approximately in the 5th intercostals space at or just medial to the midclavicular line. In a young, thin person, it is a sharp, quick impulse no larger than the intercostals space. In an older person, the impulse may be less sharp and quick. An apical impulse displaced laterally may indicate left ventricular hypertrophy.

Percussion

- Outline the heart border or area of cardiac dullness.

- The left border generally does not extend beyond 4, 7, and 10 cm left of the midsternal line in the 4th, 5th, and 6th intercostals spaces respectively.
- The right border usually lies under the sternum.

❖ Percuss outward from the sternum with the stationary finger parallel, to the intercostals space until dullness is no longer heard. Measure the distance from the midsternal line in centimeters.

Auscultation

❖ Place the stethoscope in the pulmonic or aortic area.
❖ Begin by identifying the first (S1) and second (S2) heart sounds.
  - (S1) is caused by the closing of the tricuspid and mitral valves.
  - (S2) result from the closing of the aortic and pulmonary valves.
❖ Once the heart sounds are identified count the rate and note the rhythm as discussed under vital signs. If there is an irregularity, try to determine if there is any pattern to the irregularity in relation to the intervals, heart sounds, or respirations.
❖ Once rate and rhythm are determined, listen in each of the four areas and at Erb's point (3rd left intercostals space, close to the sternum) systematically, first with the diaphragm (detects lower pitched sounds). In each area, listen to S1 and then to S2 for intensity and splitting.

Findings

❖ The two sounds are separated by a short systolic interval, each pair of sounds is separated from the next pair by a longer, diastolic interval. Normally two sounds are heard- "lub", "dub".
  - In the aortic and pulmonic areas, S2 is usually louder than S1. In this way, each of the paired sounds can be distinguished from the other.
  - In the tricuspid area, S1 and S2 are of almost equal intensity and in the mitral area, S1 is often slightly louder than S2.
❖ Normally, the heart sounds are regular with a rate of 60–80 beats/minute (in the adult). In the athlete or jogger the resting pulse may be between 40–60 beats/minute.
❖ An extra "woosh" sound between S1 and S2 indicates systolic murmur. Note the area of its greatest intensity (aortic, pulmonic, mitral, tricuspid). An extra sound of short duration usually indicates on S3 or S4 gallop.
❖ Occasionally, there may be slitting of S2 in the pulmonary area. This is normal. Splitting of S2 (two contiguous sounds are heard instead of one) is best heard at the end of inspiration. When right ventricular stroke volume is sufficiently increased to delay closure of the pulmonic valve slightly behind closure of the aortic valve.

Peripheral Circulation

Jugular veins: Evaluation of jugular venous distention is most useful in patients with suspected compromise of cardiac function.

TABLE 1.2: Comparison of internal jugular pulsation and carotid pulsation.

Internal jugular pulsations	Carotid pulsations
Rarely palpable	Palpable
Pulsation eliminated by light pressure on the vein just above the sterna end of the clavicle	Pulsation not eliminated
Level of pulsation barely descends with inspiration	Pulsation is unchanged position
Pulsation vary with position	Pulsations are changed by position

Inspection

Inspect neck for internal jugular venous pulsations.

Findings

Jugular venous pulsations can be distinguished from carotid pulsations by the following charges **(Table 1.2)**.

Note the highest point at which pulsations are seen and measure the vertical line between the point and the sternal angle. With the head raised 30°, the internal jugular venous pulsations should not be visible more than 1 inch (3 cm) above the sternal angle. Increased level of internal jugular pulsations indicates right heart failure.

Extremities

Inspection

❖ Observe skin over extremities for color, hair distribution, pallor, rubor, and swelling.
❖ Inspect for any superficial vessels.

Findings

Extremities should be symmetrically even in color, warmth, and moisture without swelling. Swelling of feet may occur after prolonged standing or sitting, but will disappear readily when extremity is elevated (dependent edema).

Palpations

❖ Note the temperature of the skin over extremities, comparing one side to the other.
❖ Palpate pulses (radial, femoral, posterior tibial, dorsalis pedis), comparing symmetry from side-to-side.
❖ Palpate the skin over the tibia for edema by squeezing the skin between for 30–60 seconds. Run the pads of your fingers over the area pressed and not indentation. If indentation is noted, repeat the procedures, moving up the extremity, and note the point at which no more swelling is present.

Findings

❖ Absence of peripheral pulses indicates peripheral vascular disease.
❖ Edema is usually from trace to 3+ or 4+ pitting. Trace is a slight indentation that disappears in a short time. Grade 3+ or 4+ is deep pitting that does not disappear readily. At best, these are subjective measurements, which are tried and confirmed through practice and comparison of findings with associates.

Abdomen

General Approach
- Make sure the patient has an empty bladder.
- The patient should be lying comfortably with his arms on his side. Bending the knees slightly will help to relax the abdominal muscles and make palpation easier.
- Expose the abdomen fully. Make sure your hands and the stethoscope diaphragm are warm.
- Be methodical in visualizing the underlying organs as you inspect, auscultate, percuss, and palpate each quadrant or region of the abdomen.

Inspection
- Observe the general contour of the abdomen (flat, protuberant, scaphoid, or concave, local bulges). Also note symmetry, visible peristalsis, aortic pulsations.
- Check the umbilicus for contour or hernia and the skin for rashes, striae and scares.

Findings
The abdomen may or may not have any scars and should be flat or slightly rounded in the nonobese person.

Auscultation
- This is done before percussion and palpation because palpation may alter the character of bowel sounds.
- Note the frequency and character of bowel sounds (pitch, duration).
- Listen over the aorta, renal arteries (upper quadrants) and iliac arteries (lower quadrants) for bruits.

Findings
- Anywhere from 5-35 bowel sounds per minute. May have familiar sound of "growling".
- Bruits indicate arterial narrowing.

Percussion
- Percussion provides a general orientation to the abdomen.
- Proceed methodically from quadrant to quadrant, noting tympany and dullness.
- In the right upper quadrant (RUQ) in the midclavicular line, percuss the borders of the liver.
  - Begin at a point of tympany in the midclavicular line of the right lower quadrant (RLQ) and percuss upward to the point of dullness (the lower liver border); mark the point.
  - Percuss downward from the point of lung resonance above the RLQ to the point of dullness (the upper border of the liver); mark the point
  - Measure in centimeters the distance between the two marks in the midclavicular line (the lifespan).
  - Tympany of the gastric air bubble can be percussed in the left upper quadrant (LUQ) over the anterior lower border of the rib cage.
- Assess for and enlarged by percussion the lowest interspace of the right anterior axillary line (should be tympanic). Ask the patient to take a deep breath and repeat (should still be tympanic).

Findings
- Tympany usually predominates, possibly with scattered areas of dullness due to fluid and feces.
- Percussion of the liver should help guide subsequent palpation. The liver border in the midclavicular line should normally range from 2 ½-4½ inches (6-11 cm).
- Change in percussion note to dullness on inspiration indicates an enlarged spleen.

Palpations
- Perform light palpation in an organized manner to detect any muscular resistance (guarding), tenderness, or superficial organs or masses.
- Perform deep palpation to determine location, size shape, consistency, tenderness, pulsations, and mobility of underlying organs and masses.
- Move slowly and gently from one quadrant to the next to relax and reassure the patient.
- Use two hands if the abdomen is obese or muscular, with one hand on top of the other. The upper hand exerts pressure downward while the lower hand feels the abdomen.

Findings
- Tenderness and involuntary guarding indicate peritoneal inflammation.
- Rebound tenderness (pain on quick withdrawal of the fingers following palpation) suggests peritoneal irritation, as in acute appendicitis.
- Palpate painful areas last.

Liver
Palpates the liver by placing the left hand under the patient's lower right rib cage and the right hand on the abdomen below the level of liver dullness. Press gently inward and upward with your fingertips while the patient takes a deep breathe.

Findings
A normal edge may be palpable as a smooth, sharp, regular surface. An enlarged liver will be palpable and may be tender, hard or irregular.

Spleen
Place your left hand around and under the patient's left lower rib cage and press your right hand below the left costal margin inward toward the spleen while the patient takes a deep breathe.

Findings
A normal spleen is usually not palpable. Be sure to start low enough to as not to miss the border of an enlarged spleen.

Kidney
- Next palpate for the left and right kidneys.
- Place the left hand under the patient's pack.
- Support the patient while you palpate the abdomen with the right palmar surface of the fingers facing the left side of the body.

- ❖ Palpate by bringing the left and right hands, together as much as possible slightly below the level of the umbilicus on the right and left.
- ❖ If the kidney is felt, describe its size and shape and note any tenderness.
- ❖ Costal vertebral angle tenderness is palpated with the patient sitting, usually during the examination of the posterior chest. Locate the costal vertebral angle in the flank region and strike firmly with the ulnar surface of your hand. Note any tenderness over the area.

Findings
- ❖ The kidney is usually felt only in persons with very relaxed abdominal muscles (the very young, the aged, and multiparous women). The right kidney is slightly lower than the left. The kidney is felt as a solid, firm, smooth elastic mass.
- ❖ There should be no costal vertebral angle tenderness.

Palpation
Aorta
- ❖ Palpate for the aorta with the thumb and index finger.
- ❖ Press deeply in the epigastric region (rough in the midline) and feel with the fingers for pulsations, as well as for the contour of the aorta.

Findings
The aorta is soft and pulsatile.

Other Findings
- ❖ Palpation of the RLQ may reveal the part of the bowel called the cecum.
- ❖ The sigmoid colon may be palpated in the LLQ.
- ❖ The inguinal and femoral areas should be palpated bilaterally for lymph nodes.

Findings
- ❖ The cecum will be soft.
- ❖ The sigmoid colon is rope-like and vertical and, if filled with feces, may be quite firm.
- ❖ Often small inguinal nodes are present, they are non-tender, freely movable, and firm.

Male Genitalia and Hernias
The part of the examination, especially for hernias, is best done with the patient standing. (A hernia is the protrusion of a portion of the intestine through an abnormal opening).
- ❖ Drape the patient's chest and abdomen.
- ❖ Expose the groin and genitalia.

Inspections
- ❖ Inspect the public hair distribution and the skin of the penis.
- ❖ Retract the foreskin, if present.
- ❖ Observe the glans penis and the urethral meatus. Note any ulcers, masses, or scars.
- ❖ Note the location of the urethral meatus and any discharge.
- ❖ Observe the skin of the scrotum for ulcers.
- ❖ Inspect the inguinal areas and groin for bulges (with and without the patient bearing down, as thought having a bowel movement.

Findings
- ❖ The foreskin of the penis, if present, should be easily retractable.
- ❖ The skin of the glans penis is smooth without ulceration.
- ❖ The urethral meatus normally is located ventrally on the end of the penis. Normally, there is no discharge from the urethra.
- ❖ The scrotum descends approximately 1½ inches (4 cm) in the adult; the left side is often larger than the right side.

Palpation
Wear Gloves
- ❖ Palpate any lesions, nodules, or masses, noting tenderness, contour, size and induration. Palpate the shaft of the penis for any indurations (firmness in relation to surroundings tissues).
- ❖ Palpate each testis and epididymis separately between the thumb and first two fingers. Noting size, shape consistency and undue tenderness (pressure on the testis normally produces pain).
- ❖ Palpate the spermatic cord, including the vas deferens within the cord, form the testis to the inguinal ring Note any nodules or tenderness.
- ❖ Palpate for inguinal hernias, using the left hand to examine the patient's right side.
  - Insert the right index finger laterally invaginating the scrotal sac to the external inguinal ring.
  - If the external ring is large enough, insert the finger along the inguinal canal toward the internal ring and ask the patient to strain down, noting any mass that touches the finger.
  - Palpate the anterior thigh for a herniating mass in the femoral canal. Ask the patient to strain down. (The femoral canal is not palpable; it is potential opening in the anterior thigh, medial to the femoral artery below the inguinal ligament).

Findings
- ❖ The testes are usually rubbery and of approximately equal size, the epididymis is located posterolaterally on each testis and is most easily palpable on the superior portion of the testis.
- ❖ Normally, there is not palpable herniating mass in the inguinal area.
- ❖ Ordinarily, there is no palpable mass in the femoral area.

Female Genitalia
Equipments
- ❖ Perineal drape
- ❖ Vaginal specula
- ❖ Water-soluble lubricant
- ❖ Sterile gloves
- ❖ Long swab sticks
- ❖ Papanicolaou (Pap) smear equipment
- ❖ Adequate lighting.

Procedure
Preparatory Phase
- ❖ Have the patient void before positioning on examining table, and remove clothing from waist to knees.

- ❖ **Position the patient on examining table:**
  - Have buttock at edge of table.
  - Position feet in stirrups to assume dorsal lithotomy position.
  - Make the patient as comfortable as possible with a small pillow under her head.
  - Drape the patient to permit minimal exposure (but adequate for examine).
- ❖ Encourage the patient to relax, tell her what you are doing and what she may feel.
- ❖ Adjust light for maximum focus.
- ❖ Offer the patient a mirror to watch the examination to teach vulvar self-examination and to teach about contraceptives as appropriate.

Performance Phase
- ❖ Be gentle, and take your time, wash hands, put on clean gloves, lubricate finger with water.
- ❖ Observe external genitalia for apparent abnormalities, gently separate labia and continue visual inspection.
- ❖ To encourage relaxation in the patient, gently place the tip of one or two fingers into introitus.
- ❖ Identify cervix manually and depress the perineum downward with fingers of one hand.
- ❖ Lubricate speculum with warm water with your other hand.
- ❖ Gently insert warm speculum horizontally passing it over your fingers and aiming it toward the cervix.
- ❖ Slowly open the speculum and lock into position. With slow manipulation, the speculum can be turned to permit visualization of the vaginal walls.
- ❖ Inspect the cervix, which should be pink. Normally, the os is a closed, round indentation, unless the woman has had children, in which case a slit is noted.
- ❖ If Pap test is to be done, newer automated systems can increase the accuracy of Pap result.
- ❖ If indicated, swab cervix, with Schiller's iodine solution to detect epithelial change. Or, swab vagina and cervix with acetic acid solution to detect lesions caused by human papillomavirus (HPV).
- ❖ When removing speculum hold it open until cervix is cleared, then withdraw speculum downward, applying pressure to posterior vaginal wall and allowing speculum to close as it is withdrawn.
- ❖ **Bimanual examination of pelvic examination:**
  - Insert two fingers of dominant hand into vagina (one finger for vaginal introitus).
  - Place second hand midline lower abdomen. Gently capture the uterus between your two hands to feel and size and to elicit tenderness.
  - Move hands to either side of midline to palpate the adnexa, feeling for swelling masses, or tenderness of the ovaries and fallopian tubes.

Follow-up Phase
- ❖ Gently wipe the perineal area with soft tissue or gauze, using firm strokes from the pubic area back to beyond the rectum.
- ❖ Instruct and assist the patient to remove feet from stirrups.
- ❖ Elevate the lower third of the examining table to receive legs. Keep the patient covered with a sheet.
- ❖ Assist the patient in sliding toward head end of table; provide a wide-based stool for her to step on as she gets off table.
- ❖ Assist the patient in dressing if necessary. Answer any questions she may have.

Rectum

Equipment
- ❖ **Glove:** Lubricants

Techniques of Examination: Male
General Approach
- ❖ If the patient is ambulatory, have him stand and bend over the edge of the table with his toes pointed inward.
- ❖ It is also possible to examine the anus and rectum with the patient lying on the left side, knees drawn up and buttocks close to the edge of the table.
- ❖ The patient should be draped so only the buttocks are exposes.

Inspection
Spread the buttocks and inspect the anus, perineal region, and sacral region for inflammation, nodules. Scars, lesions, ulcerations or rashes. Ask the patient to bear done; note any bulges.

Palpations
- ❖ Palpate any abnormal area noted on inspection.
- ❖ Lubricate the index finger of the gloved hand. Rest the finger over the anus as the patient bears down and, as the sphincter relaxes, insert your finger slowly into the rectum.
- ❖ Note sphincter tone, any nodules or masses, or tenderness.
- ❖ Insert the finger further and palpate the walls of the rectum laterally and posteriorly while rooting your index finger. Note irregularities, masses, nodules, tenderness.
- ❖ Anteriorly palpate the two lateral lobes of the prostate gland and its median sulcus for irregularities, nodules, swelling, or tenderness.
- ❖ If possible, palpate the superior portion of the lateral lobe, where the seminal vesicles are located. Note induration, swelling or tenderness.
- ❖ Just above the prostate anteriorly, the rectum lies adjacent to the peritoneal cavity. If possible, palpate this region for peritoneal masses and tenderness.
- ❖ Continue to insert the finger as far as possible and have the patient bear down so more of the bowel can be palpated.
- ❖ Gently withdraw your finger. Any fecal material on the glove should be tested for occult blood.

Findings
- ❖ The anal canal is approximately 1 inch (2.5 cm) long; it is bordered by the external and internal anal sphincters.
- ❖ The wall of the rectum in males and females is smooth and moist.
- ❖ The male prostate gland is approximately 1 inch long, smooth, regular, nonmovable, nontender and rubbery.
- ❖ The seminal vesicles are generally not palpable unless swollen.
- ❖ There is normally no occult blood in the stools.

General Approaches
- The examination is usually performed following the pelvic examination with the patient. Still in the lithotomy position.
- If only the rectal examination is done, the patient may be positioned laterally, as for examination of the male. The lateral position permits better visualization of the sacral region.
- The technique is basically the same for the female as for the male.
- Anteriorly, the cervix and perhaps a retroverted uterus, may be felt.

Findings
Anteriorly, the cervix is round and smooth.

Musculoskeletal System
General Approach
- Examine the muscles and joints, keeping in mind the structure and functions of each.
- Observe and palpate joints and muscles for symmetry and examine each joint individually as indicated.
- The examination is performed with the joints both at rest and in motion, moving through a full range of motion, joint and supporting muscles and tissues are noted.

Inspections
- Inspect the upper and lower extremities for size, symmetry, deformity and muscle mass.
- Inspect the joints for range of motion (in degrees), enlargement and redness.
- Note gait and posture; observe the spine for range of motion, lateral curvature or any abnormal curvature.
- Observe the patient for signs of pain during the examination.

Palpations
- Palpate the joints of the upper and lower extremities and the neck and back for tenderness, swelling, warmth, any bony overgrowth or deformity and range of motion.
- Hold the palm of your hand cover the joint as it moves, or note any crepitation (crackling feeling within the joint).
- Palpate the muscles for size, tone, strength, any contractures, and tenderness.
- Palpate the spine for bony deformities and crepitation. Gently tap the spine with the ulnar surface of your fist from the cervical to the lumbar region and note any pain or tenderness.

Neurologic System
Equipments
- Safety pin
- Cotton
- Tuning fork
- Reflex hammer
- Flashlight
- Tongue blade
- Ophthalmoscope
- Vision screener
- Cloves, coffee or other scented items.

General Informations
- The examination describe in this section is a screening neurologic examination. It is performed on individuals without specific neurologic complaints.
- The examination is performed with the patient in either the sitting or supine position.
- Much of the neurologic examination can be performed as different regions of the body are being examined. This facilitates the flow of the entire examination.

Components of the Neurologic Examination
There are five components of the neurologic examination:
1. Mental status (cerebral function)
2. Cranial nerve function
3. Motor function
4. Sensory function
5. Deep tendon reflexes (DTRs).

The screening neurologic examination involves testing all of these components at least superficially. Learning these components in order will help in organizing the examination and in avoiding the omission of any part.

Basic Principles
- Symmetry of function and findings on both sides of the body are important to note. Always compare one side of the body with the other side (for example compare degree of motor strength of the right biceps with that of the left biceps).
- Integrating the neurologic examination into the examination of the various body regions is advisable, although the results of the neurologic findings should be recorded together as an entity.

Mental Status
Components of the mental status examination include the following:
- State of consciousness (alert, somnolent, stuporous, comatose)
- Memory (short-term, long-term, intermediate)
- Affect (mood)
- Ideational content (hallucinations).

In a screening examination, mental status is evaluated by observing the patient's affect during the history and the content of what he/she says:
- While recording the history, ask the patient for identifying information (how to spell his name, where he lives), and ask what the date is. This tests orientation.
- The patient's ability to remember is also evaluated as the history is taken; ask for his past medical history (long-term memory) and dietary habits: "What did you eat for breakfast?" (intermediate memory).
- Cognition and ideational content are evaluated throughout the history by what the patient says and by his articulateness, consistency, and reliability in reporting events.
- Affect or mood is evaluated by observing the patient's verbal and nonverbal behavior in response to questions asked, sudden noises, and interruptions. For example—does the patient laugh or smile when talking about normally sad events; is he easily startled by unexpected noises?

Findings

- Normally the individual is alert, knows who he is and where he lives, and can tell you the date.
- The patient remembers recent and past events consistently, and willingly admits forgetting something. Elderly people often have much better long-term memory than recent memory.
- Mood should be appropriate to the content of the conversation.

CRANIAL NERVE FUNCTION

First (Olfactory) Nerve

The olfactory nerve is not usually tested unless the patient complains of a disturbance in sense of smell.
- The airway must be patent.
- Occlude one nostril; ask the patient to close his eyes and then present various substances to smell (coffee, tobacco) Occlude the other nostril and repeat.

Findings

The patient should be able to identify common smells such as cinnamon coffee. Second (optic) nerve—includes tests of visual acuity and of gross visual fields and examination of the optic disk with a funduscope.

Visual Acuity

- Visual acuity is tested with the use of a Snellen chart (patient uses glasses if required).
- Have the patient cover one eye at a time and read the smallest print possible on the chart from a distance of 20 feet (6 m).

Findings

Normal vision and corrected vision should be 20/20.

Visual Fields

- Have the patient cover his right eye with the right hand. (You cover your left eye with your left hand).
- Stand approximately 2 feed (60 cm) from the patient and have him fix his gaze on your nose.
- Bring two wagging fingers in from the periphery (in a plane equidistant from the patient and you) in all quadrants of the visual field and ask the patient to tell you when he sees your wagging fingers.

Findings

Assuming your visual fields are grossly normal the patient and you should see the wagging fingers approximately simultaneously. (The patient's peripheral vision should approximate the examiner's assuming that it is normal).

Optic Disk

- The optic disk is visualized as part of the funduscopic examination.
- Third (oculomotor), fourth (trochlear), and sixth (abducens) nerves
- These nerves are tested together. They control the movements of the extraocular muscles of the eye-the superior and inferior oblique and the medial and lateral rectus muscles. The oculomotor nerve also controls pupillary constriction.
  - Hold your index finger approximately 1 foot (30 cm) from the patient's nose. Ask the patient to hold his head steady.
  - Ask the patient to follow your finger with his eyes.
  - Move your finger to the right as far as the patient's eye moves. Before bringing your finger back to the center, move it up and then down, so that the patient glances up and peripherally and then down and peripherally.
  - Repeat, the test, moving your finger to the left.

Fifth (Trigeminal) Nerve

The trigeminal nerve controls muscles of mastication and has a sensory component that controls sensations of the face.

Motor

Have the patient clench teeth while palpating the temporal and masseter muscle of the jaws with both hands.

Findings

Muscle strength in the face should be present and should be symmetric.

Sensory

Sensation to light touch.
- Have the patient close eyes.
- Touch first one side of the patient's face and then the other (forehead, cheek, and chin), asking the patient if the sensation is present and feels the same on both sides.
- Sensation to pain (pinprick) is tested similarly.

Findings

Sensation should be present and symmetrical. Always demonstrate to the patient how and with what your are testing sensation- to avoid starting the patient and to encourage cooperation.

Seventh Facial Nerve

- Motor function is tested by observing facial expressions and symmetry of facial movement.
- Ask the patient to frown, close his eyes, and smile.

Findings

The facial muscles should look symmetric, when the patient frown, closes his eyes, and smiles. Notice particularly the symmetry of the nasolabial folds.

Eighth (Acoustic) Nerve

- The acoustic nerve has two branches.
- Cochlear (mediates hearing)
- Vestibular (helps control equilibrium)
- **Romberg test:** Have the patient stand erect with his eyes closed and feet close together.

Findings

Slight swaying may occur but the patient so you can assist if he begins to fall.

Ninth (Glossopharyngeal) and Tenth (Vagus) Nerves

These nerves are tested together because they both have a motor portion innervating the pharynx.
Ninth: Test the presence of the gag reflex.
Tenth: Ask the patient to say "ah" and observe the movement of the uvula and palate for deviation and asymmetry.

Findings

- The gag reflex should be present, and there should be no difficulty in swallowing.
- The palate and the uvula should move symmetrically without deviation.

Eleventh (Spinal Accessory) Nerve

The spinal accessory nerve mediates the sternocleidomastoid and upper portion of the trapezius muscles.
- Ask the patient to turn his head to the side against resistance while you apply pressure to the jaw.
- Palpate the sternocleidomastoid muscle on the opposite side.
- Have the patient shrug his shoulders while you place your hands on his shoulders and apply slight pressure.

Findings
Neck and shoulder muscle strength should be symmetric.

Twelfth (Hypoglossal) Nerve

This nerve innervates muscle of the tongue. It is tested by noting articulation and by having the patient stick out his tongue, noting any deviation or asymmetry.

Findings
The tongue should be symmetric and should not deviate.

Cerebellar Functions

Purpose: To screen for coordination.
- Observe posture and gait.
- Ask the patient to walk forward (and then backward) in a straight line.
- To test for muscle coordination in the lower extremities, have the patient run his right heel down his left shin and vice versa.
- To test coordination in upper extremities, have the patient close his eyes and touch his nose with his index finger. (Starting position: arms outstretched) first left, then right, in rapid succession.

Findings
- The patient should be able to perform all the tests described with smooth, even movement and without losing balance.
- The normal person can do this with rapid, smooth movements without undershooting or overshooting the target.

Motor Function

Tested in conjunction with the skeletal system because any bony deformity will affect motor function. Evaluate muscle mass, tone, strength and any abnormal movements (tics, fasciculation twitching).
- To assess muscle mass, not symmetry between sides of the body and distribution distally and proximally.
- Test muscle tone by noting the resistance the muscle offers to movement on passive motion.
- Have the patient do deep knee bends' walk on his toes and then his heels, hop on one foot and then the other.
- Have the patient squeeze your fingers with both hands; compare sides of the body. Also, apply resistance to the patient's outstretched arms and when the patient flexes the wrist and elbow' compare sides.
- Unusual muscle movements, if present are noted both when muscle is at rest and when it is moving.

Findings
- Muscle mass is usually considered in relation to sex and body build and to use of various muscle groups.
- Generally, there is slight resistant to passive movement of muscles as opposed to flaccidity (no resistance) or rigidity (increased muscle tone).
- Strength will vary from person to person but should be equal bilaterally.
- Normally, tremors, tics, or fasciculation are not presents either at rest or with movement.

Sensory Function

Should test sensitivity to light touch (cotton), pain (pinprick), vibration (tuning fork), and position. Compare both sides of the body.
- Ask the patient to close eyes. Brush skin with a piece of cotton (on the back of hands, forearms, upper arms, dorsal portion of foot laterally and medially, and along the tibia and thigh laterally and medially). Ask the patient to indicate when he/she feels the cotton and to compare the sensation bilaterally.
- Use a safety pin; touch the skin as lightly as possible to elicit a sharp sensation.
- Test vibration sense by placing a vibrating tuning fork on a bony prominence (wrist, medical and lateral malleoli). Ask the patient to tell you when he no longer feels the vibration. Stop the vibration with your hand.
- **Test position sense by having the patient close his eyes:**
  - Move the patient's digit (finger, great toe) up or down and ask the patient to say in what direction his finger or toe is pointing.
  - Place your thumb and index finger on either side of the digit being move so the patient will not sense any pressure from your finger in the direction in which you are moving the digit.

Findings
- Patient should feel light touch bilaterally.
- Pain should be felt bilaterally.
- The patient should normally feel no vibration within a very short time.
- Normally, the patient can tell you without hesitation in what direction his digit is pointing.

Deep Tendon Reflexes

- Place your right thumb on the patient's right biceps tendon (located in the antecubital fossa) with the patient's arm slightly flexed.
- Strike your thumb with the pointed end of the hammer head. Hold the hammer loosely so it pivots in your hand when it is moved with a wrist action.
- Strike your thumb with the least amount of pressure needed to elicit the reflex.

Findings

- Amplitude of the reflex may vary for different tendons but is equal bilaterally.
- The forearm may move, and your thumb should feel the tendon jerk.

Triceps Tendon

- Have the patient hang his or her arm freely while support it with your nondominant hand or rest the slightly flexed arm in the patient's lap.
- With the elbow flexed, strike the tendon directly, using the pointed end of the hammer.
(If the reflexes are diminished symmetrically, have the patient grasp hands and contract arm muscles to relax the lower extremities, or tap feet on the floor to relax the upper extremities).

Findings
The forearm should move slightly.

Brachioradialis Tendon

- Strike the forearm with the hammer about 1 inch (2.5 cm) above the wrist over the radius.
- Be sure the forearm is supported and relaxed.

Findings
The thumb is observed moving downward.

Lower Extremities

Quadriceps Reflex

- Have the patient sit with his leg hanging over the edge of the table or lay down while you support the legs at the knee (slightly bent).
- Strike the tendon just below the patella.

Achilles Reflex

- Support the foot in dorsiflexed position.
- Tap the achilles tendon with the hammer.

Findings
The foot should move downward into your hand.

Plantar Reflex

Stroke the sole of the patient's foot with a flat object such as a tongue blade.

Findings

Toe normally flex. Dorsiflexion of the great toe and fanning of the other toes is known as a positive Babinski response and indicates a central nervous system problem.

CHAPTER 2: The Nursing Process

■ INTRODUCTION

- ❖ In every clinical situation, it is important for a nurse to think critically and make sound judgment so that client ultimately receives the very best nursing care.
- ❖ Critical thinking is a process acquired only through hard work, commitment and an active curiosity towards learning.
- ❖ *"Ideally, critical thinking becomes a habit of mind, a part of each nurse's character".*—**Facione and Facione (1996).**

■ DEFINITION AND MEANING OF CRITICAL THINKING

"Critical thinking is the active, organized, cognitive process used to carefully examine one's thinking and the thinking of others."
—**Chaffee 1994**

"Critical thinking involves use of the mind informing, conclusions, making decisions, drawing inferences and reflecting. It means taking nothing for granted."
—**Gordon 1995**

Meaning

- ❖ A critical thinker identifies and challenges, assumptions, considers what is important in a situation, imagines and explores alternatives, applies reason and logic, and thus makes informed decisions, for a new student nurse, critical thinking begins when the student seriously questions, and in a continuing way tries to answer again and again.
- ❖ Critical thinking presupposes a certain basic level of intellectual humility, (e.g., acknowledging one's own ignorance) and a commitment to think clearly, precisely and accurately and to act on the basis of genuine knowledge.
- ❖ When the nurse directs critical thinking towards understanding and assisting clients in finding solutions, to their health problems, the process becomes purposeful and goal oriented.
- ❖ Every clinical experience becomes a lesson that informs the nurse about the next practice experience.
- ❖ No nursing action or interaction with a client is trivial or ordinary. Although the responsibility of making clinical decisions may seem frightening to a new student it is what makes nursing rewarding and challenging profession

■ CRITICAL THINKING: THINKING AND LEARNING

Critical Thinking Model

- ❖ Models help to explain concepts. Because critical thinking in nursing is complex, a model can help to explain all of the factors involved in making decisions and judgments about clients.
- ❖ Kataoka-Yahiro and Saylor (1994) have developed a model of critical thinking for nursing judgement based in part on previous work by Paul (1993), Glaser (1941), Perry (1979) and Miller and Malcolm (1990).
- ❖ **The model defines the outcome of critical thinking:** Nursing judgment that is relevant to nursing problems in a variety of settings.
- ❖ According to this model, there are five components of critical thinking—knowledge base, experience, competence, attitudes, standards and the critical thinking competency of the nursing process.
- ❖ The elements of the model combine to explain how nurses make clinical judgment that is necessary for safe, effective, nursing care.

Components of Critical Thinking in Nursing

- ❖ Specific knowledge base in nursing
- ❖ Experience in nursing
- ❖ **Critical thinking competencies:**
  - General critical thinking competencies
  - Specific critical thinking competencies in clinical situation
  - Specific critical thinking competency in nursing.
- ❖ **Attitudes for critical thinking:**
  - Confidence
  - Independence
  - Fairness
  - Responsibility
  - Risk taking
  - Discipline
  - Perseverance
  - Creativity
  - Curiosity
  - Integrity
  - Humility

Chapter 2: The Nursing Process

❖ **Standards for critical thinking:**
- *Intellectual standards*
  - Clear
  - Logical
  - Precise
  - Deep
  - Specific
  - Broad
  - Accurate
  - Complete
  - Relevant
  - Significant
  - Plausible
  - Adequate (for purpose)
  - Consistent
  - Fair
- *Professional standards:*
  - Ethical criteria for nursing judgement
  - Criteria for evaluation
  - Professional responsibility

Critical Thinking Attitudes and Applications in Nursing Practice

Confidence
Learn how to introduce yourself to a client. Speak with conviction when you begin a treatment or procedure. Do not lead a client to think that you are uncertain of being able to perform care safely, especially when there are different views on the same subject.

Thinking independently
Read the nursing literature, especially where there are deferent views on the same subject. Talk with colleagues and share ideas about nursing interventions.

Fairness
Listen to both sides in any discussion. If client or family members complain about a colleague, listen to the story and then speak with the colleague as well.

Responsibility and authority
Ask for help if you are uncertain about an aspect of client care. Report any problems immediately. Follows standards of practice in your care.

Risk taking
If your knowledge causes you to question a physician's order, do so. Be willing to recommend alternative approach to nursing care when colleagues are having little success with client.

Discipline
Be thorough in whatever you do.

Use Known Scientific and Practice-based Criteria
for activities, such as assessment and evolution. Take time to be thorough, and manage your time effectively.

Perseverance
Beware of an easy answer. If colleagues give you information about a client, and some fact seems to be missing, go clarify information or talk to the client directly. If problem of the same type continues to occur on a nursing division, bring colleagues together, look for a pattern, and find a solution.

Creativity
Look for different approaches if interventions are not working. A client we need a different positioning technique or a different instructional approach that will suit his or her unique needs.

Curiosity
Always ask why. A clinic sign or symptoms can indicate a variety of problems. Explore and learn more about the client so as to make appropriate clinical judgment.

Integrity
Recognized when your opinion may conflict with those of a client, review your position, and decide how best to proceed to reach usually beneficial outcome. Do not compromise nursing standard or honesty in delivering nursing care.

Humility
Recognized when you need more information to make a decision when you are newly assigned to clinical division and you are unfamiliar with the client, ask to be oriented to the area. Ask RNs regularly assigned to the area for assistance. Read the professional generals regularly to keep updated on new approaches to care.

Levels of Critical Tinking in Nursing
The ability to think critically expands as a nurse gains new knowledge and experience and matures into a competent professional.

Critical Thinking in Nursing
By Kataoka Yahiro and Baylor (1994)
According to this model there are three levels of critical thinking in nursing:
1. Basic
2. Complex
3. Commitment.

Basic Critical Thinking
❖ At the basic level of critical thinking, a learner trusts that experts have the right answers for every problem.
❖ Thinking is concrete and based on a set of rules or principles.
❖ For basic critical thinkers, answers to complex problems are either right or wrong and one right answer usually exists for each problem.
❖ This is an early step in the development of reasoning ability, revealing that the individual has had limited critical thinking experience.
❖ Despite the tendency to be governed by others, a person learns to accept the diverse opinions one values of experts.

- However, in experience, weak competencies, and inflexible attitudes can restrict a person's ability to move to the next level of critical thinking.

Complex Critical Thinking
- A person begins to detach from authorities and analyze and examine alternatives more independently at the complex level of critical thinking.
- The nurse's best answer to a problem at this level is "It depends".
- The person's thinking ability and initiative to look beyond expert opinion begin to change.
- A nurse realizes that alternative and perhaps conflicting, solutions do exist.
- In complex critical thinking each solution has benefits and risks that the nurse weighs before making a final decision.
- There are options.
- Thinking can become more creative and innovative.
- There is a willingness to consider deviations from standard protocols or policies when complex situations develop.
- Nurses learn a variety of different approaches for the same therapy.

Commitment
- The third level of critical thinking is commitment.
- The individual anticipates the need to make choices without assistance from others and then assumes accountability to them.
- At this level the nurse does more than first counter the complex alternatives a problem poses.
- At the commitment level the nurse chooses an action or belief based on the alternative available and stands by it.
- Sometimes an action may be no action, or the nurse may choose to delay an action until a later time, but does it as a result of experience and knowledge, because the nurse assumes accountability for the decision, alternation, is given to the results of the decision and a determination of whether it was appropriate.

■ NURSING PROCESS

The nursing process has been accepted as the essence of nursing.

Definition
"Nursing process is a deliberate, problem-identification, and problem-solving approach to meeting the health care and nursing needs of patient." —**Brunner and Suddarth**

"Process as a whole is cyclic different steps is involved interdependent, interrelated, and recurrent till the patient is satisfied." —**Brunner and Suddarth**

"Nursing process is a data–collecting, decision–making process that incorporates evaluation and subsequent modification as feedback mechanisms that promote the ultimate resolution of the patient's nursing diagnoses."

■ ASSESSMENT

"Assessment involves the systematic collection of data about the patient's health status, analysis of the data to determine his actual and potential health needs, and use of the data to formulate nursing diagnosis." —**Brunner and Suddarth**

"Nursing process is a system of inter-related and interdependent problem-solving steps directed at meeting the needs of people." —**Luckman and Sorenson**

"Nursing assessment is a systematic collection and ordering of information to identify unmet human needs and a person's responses to actual and potential health problems. It involves data gathering, problem reinter relation and establishing a nursing diagnosis."

Steps
- Conduct the health history.
- Perform the health assessment.
- Interview the patient's family or significant others.
- Study the health record. Organize, analyze, synthesize and summarize the collected data which help to formulate the nursing diagnosis.

Health History
The health history is carried out for the purpose of determining the patient's state of wellness or illness and is best accomplished as part of a planned interview. Interview requires wisdom, judgment, tact and experience.

Skills for Interviewing Includes
- Listening and questioning
- Observing and interpreting
- Synthesizing
- Incorporating what is learned into a plan of care.

Suggestions for Interviewing the Patient
- At the beginning of the interview, focus on what is most troublesome to the patient.
- Learn about the patient's background and experience in order to determine his needs.
- As certain what can be done to support the patient and help him to make the best use of his resources.

Health Assessment (Physical Examination)
The health assessment of the patient may be carried out prior to, during or following the health history, depending on the patient's physical and emotional state, his response to his illness and hospitalization, and the immediate priorities of his illness situation.

Purposes
- Identify those parameters of physical, psychological, and emotional functioning that indicates that a nursing need exists.
- It requires the use of the senses of sight, hearing, touch, and smell as well as the appropriate interview skills and techniques.

Other Components of the Data Base
Following the health history and the health assessment, the nurse seeks additional relevant, information from the patient's family or significant others, from other members of the health team, and from the patient's health record or chart.

Recording of the Data Base

After completion of the health history and health assessment the information obtained must be recorded in the patient's permanent record.

Function of Record

- Provides a means of communication between the members of the health care team and facilitates coordinated planning and continuity of care.
- It serves as the legal record for the hospital and for the professional staff responsible for the patient's care.
- It serves as a basis for evaluating the quality and appropriateness of care as well as for renewing the effective use of patient care health practices.

Therapeutic Communication Techniques

- Listening
- Silence
- Establishing guidelines
- Open ended comments
- Reducing distance
- Acknowledgement
- Restating
- Reflecting
- Seeking unification
- Sorting consensual validation
- Focusing
- Summarizing
- Planning

NURSING DIAGNOSIS

"Those actual or potential health problems that are amenable to resolution by nursing actions are identified as nursing diagnosis."

"A nursing diagnosis is a diagnoses judgment about, individual, family, or community response to actual or potential health problems/life processes. Nursing diagnosis produces the basis for selection of nursing interventions to achieve out comes for which the nurse is accountable."

A well-worded nursing diagnosis has 2 parts:
1. Problem
2. Etiology of the problem.

Recording the Nursing Diagnosis

- The patient's nursing diagnoses are recorded on the nursing care plans well as in the patient problem list.
- "A problem is defined as anything that concerns the patient, endangers his health, requires management and concerns any member of the health care team."
- The problems are used by all concerned members for writing the progress notes.

Steps

- Identify the patient's nursing problem.
- Identify the defining characteristic of the nursing problems.
- Identify the etiology of the nursing problem.
- State nursing diagnosis concisely and precisely.

Brunner and Suddarth 1970s

Brought a surge of professional activity aimed at making nursing diagnosis a function for which the nurse is held legally responsible and accountable.

"A large number of nurse practice acts were revised to include nursing diagnosis as a nursing function."

1973

Nursing diagnosis was included in the American Nurses Association (ANA) standards of nursing practice and in the standards developed by many nursing specialty organizations. The National Conferences on the classification of nursing diagnosis held regularly since 1973 have proved an impetus for the identification and classification of nursing diagnoses according to symptomatology.

1982

At the fifth conference, held in 1982, a major step was taken toward coordinating the work of developing nursing diagnoses.

"A new organization, the North American Nursing Diagnosis Association (NANDA) was formulated.

1986

NANDA approved its first taxonomy for classification of nursing diagnosis, this taxonomy sometimes to be further developed.

1990

At the NANDA Biennial Conference, the association officially adopted a definition for nursing diagnosis.

Objectives of Care and Goals that Reflect Outcome (May be Short-term or Long-term Goals)

- **Short-term goals:** Used for actual problem.
- Intermediate goals.
- **Long-term goals:** Used for potential problem.

PLANNING

- "Development of goal and a plan of care designed to assist the patient in resolving the nursing diagnosis."
- Once the nursing diagnosis is identified the planning component of the nursing process is developed.
- In this phase, it is the responsibility of the nurse to communicate to appropriate persons any assessment data indicative of health needs that can be best met by other members of the health care team.

Definition

"During planning phase, of nursing process, the nurse establishes priorities of care, writes desired patient's outcome (goals), selects and converts nursing interventions into nursing orders, and communicates the plan of care."

Steps of Planning

- ❖ Assign priority to the nursing diagnosis.
- ❖ **Specify the goals:**
  - Develop immediate; intermediate and long-term goals.
  - State the goals in realistic and measurable terms.
- ❖ Identify nursing interventions appropriate for goal achievement
- ❖ Establish expected outcome:
  - Make sure that the outcomes are realistic and measurable.
  - Identify critical times for attainment of outcomes.
- ❖ **Develop the written nursing care plan:**
  - Include nursing diagnosis, goals, nursing interventions, expected outcomes at critical times.
  - Write all entries precisely, concisely and systematically.
  - Keep the plan current and flexible to meet the patient's changing problems and needs.
  - Involve the patient, his family or significant others, nursing team members and other health team members in all aspects of planning.

■ IMPLEMENTATIONS

- ❖ "Implementations is actualization of the plan of care through nursing interventions or supervision of others to do the same."
- ❖ "Nursing interventions are those actions that should promote the achievement of the desired patient's outcome."

They are classified into 2 types:

1. **Independent interventions:** These are those that nurse can perform without direction from others.
2. **Dependent interventions:** These are prescribed by the physician and carried out by the nurse. They are aimed at reducing or eliminating the causative factors affecting health. The nurse uses judgment and decision-making talks in relation of appropriate interventions that are based on physiologic principles. All nursing interventions are patient focused and goal-directed. They are based on scientific principles and implemented with compassion, confidence and a willingness to accept and understand the patient's response.

Steps

- ❖ Put the nursing care plan into action.
- ❖ Coordinate the activities of the patient his family or significant others, nursing team members and other health team members.
- ❖ Record the patient's responses to the nursing actions.

Patient's Progress Notes

Are written in a narrative form using the acronym **SOAPIE**:
S—Subjective Data
O—Objective Data
A—Assessment
P—Plan
I—Interventions
E—Evaluations

■ RATIONALE

Are the scientific principles and have a physical or pathophysiological basis.

- ❖ Implementation phase of the nursing process follows the formulation of the nursing care plan.
- ❖ The nurse assumes responsibility for the implementation, but includes the patient and his family and other members of the nursing team and the health care team as appropriate in implementation, and coordinated by the nurse.
- ❖ The nursing care plan serves as the basis for un-implementation.
- ❖ The immediate, intermediate and long-term goals are used as a focus for the implementing of the designed nursing interventions.
- ❖ While implementing nursing care, the nurse continually assesses the patient and his response to the nursing care.
- ❖ Alternations are made in the care plan as the Patient's condition, problems, and responses change and as reassignment of priorities are required.
- ❖ Implementation includes all the nursing interventions that are directed toward resolution of the patient's nursing diagnosis and meeting his health needs.

■ FORMULATING THE NURSING CARE PLAN

The entire planning phase of the nursing process culminates in the formulation, of the patient's nursing care plan by the professional nurse.

The nursing care plan serves to communicate the following information to all members of the nursing team:

- ❖ The nursing diagnosis and their priorities.
- ❖ The goals of the nursing interventions.
- ❖ The nursing interventions which are expressed in the form of nursing orders.
- ❖ The expected outcomes, which identify the expected behavioral responses for the patient.
- ❖ The critical time period within which each outcome must be met.

■ EVALUATION

"It is the determination of the patient's responses to the nursing interventions and the extent to which the goals have been achieved." —Brunner and Suddarth

- ❖ The nurse receives the patient-centered goals or desired patient outcome.
- ❖ The nurse reassesses the patient to gather data including the patient's actual response to the nursing interventions.
- ❖ The nurse compares the actual outcome with the desired outcome and makes critical judgment about whether the patient-centered goal or desired patient outcome was achieved. (Outcome criteria).

Steps

- ❖ Collect objective data.
- ❖ Compare the patient's behavioral outcomes with the expected outcomes.

- Determine the extent to which the goals were achieved.
- Include the patient his family and significant others, nursing team members, and other health care team members in evaluation.
- Identify alterations that are to be made in the nursing diagnosis, goals, and nursing interventions and expected outcomes.
- Continue all steps of nursing process assessment, nursing diagnosis, planning, implementation and evaluation.
- Evaluation is the final component of the nursing process and is directed toward determining the patient's response to the nursing interventions and the extent to which the goals have been achieved.
- The nursing care plan provides the basis for evaluation.
- The nursing diagnoses, goals, nursing interventions, and expected outcomes provide the specific guidelines that dictate the focus of the evaluation.

Evaluation will answer the following question:
- Were the nursing diagnoses accurate?
- Did the patient reach the expected outcome?
- Did the patient attain the expected outcomes within the critical time periods?
- Has the patient's nursing diagnosis been resolved?
- Have the patient's nursing needs been met?
- Should the nursing interventions be retained, alerted or discontinued?
- Have new problems evolved for which nursing interventions have not been planned or implemented?
- What factors influenced the achievement or lack of achievement of the goals?
- Do priorities need to be reassigned?
- Should changes be made in the goals and expected outcomes?
- Objective data that answer their questions must be collected from all available sources.
- This data should be available in the patient's record and should be substantiated by direct observation of the patient.

NANDA NURSING DIAGNOSIS (TABLE 1.1)

1. Health Promotion

Class 1. Health Awareness
- Decreased diversional activity engagement (Nursing care plan)
- Readiness for enhanced health literacy sedentary lifestyle (Nursing care plan)

Class 2. Health Management
- Frail elderly syndrome (Nursing care plan)
- Risk for frail elderly syndrome
- Deficient community health
- Risk-prone health behavior
- Ineffective health maintenance (Nursing care plan)
- Ineffective health management
- Readiness for enhanced health management
- Ineffective family health management
- Ineffective protection

TABLE 1.1: NANDA classification.

Domain	Health promotion	Nutrition	Elimination/ exchange	Activity	Perception/ cognition	Self-perception	Role relationship	Sexuality	Coping/ stress tolerance	Life principles	Safety/ protection	Comfort	Growth/ development
Class 1	Health awareness	Ingestion	Urinary function	Sleep/rest	Attention	Self-concept	Caregiving roles	Sexual identity	Post trauma responses	Values	Infection	Physical comfort	Growth
Class 2	Health Management	Digestion	Gastro-intestinal function	Activity/exercise	Orientation	Self esteem	Family relationships	Sexual function	Coping responses	Beliefs	Physical injury	Environmental comfort	Development
Class 3		Absorption	Integumentary function	Energy balance	Sensation/ perception	Body image	Role performance	Reproduction	Neuro behavioural stress	Value/belief/action congruence	Violence	Social comfort	
Class 4		Metabolism	Respiratory function	Cardiovascular/ pulmonary responses	perception						Environmental hazards		
Class 5		Hydration		Self-care	Cognition						Defensive processes		
Class 6					Communication						Thermo-regulation		

2. Nutrition

Class 1. Ingestion
Imbalanced nutrition:
- Less than body requirements (Nursing care plan)
- Readiness for enhanced nutrition
- Insufficient breast milk production
- Ineffective breastfeeding (Nursing care plan)
- Interrupted breastfeeding (Nursing care plan)
- Readiness for enhanced breastfeeding
- Ineffective adolescent eating dynamics
- Ineffective child eating dynamics
- Ineffective infant feeding dynamics
- Ineffective infant feeding pattern (Nursing care plan)
- Obesity
- Overweight
- Risk for overweight
- Impaired swallowing (Nursing care plan)

Class 2. Digestion
This class does not currently contain any diagnoses

Class 3. Absorption
This class does not currently contain any diagnoses

Class 4. Metabolism
- Risk for unstable blood glucose level (Nursing care plan)
- Neonatal hyperbilirubinemia
- Risk for neonatal hyperbilirubinemia
- Risk for impaired liver function
- Risk for metabolic imbalance syndrome

Class 5. Hydration
- Risk for electrolyte imbalance
- Risk for imbalanced fluid volume
- Deficient fluid volume (Nursing care plan)
- Risk for deficient fluid volume
- Excess fluid volume (Nursing care plan)

3. Elimination and Exchange

Class 1. Urinary Function
- Impaired urinary elimination
- Functional urinary incontinence
- Overflow urinary incontinence
- Reflex urinary incontinence
- Stress urinary incontinence
- Urge urinary incontinence
- Risk for urge urinary incontinence
- Urinary retention

Class 2. Gastrointestinal Function
- Constipation (Nursing care plan)
- Risk for constipation
- Perceived constipation
- Chronic functional constipation
- Risk for chronic functional constipation
- Diarrhea
- Dysfunctional gastrointestinal motility
- Risk for dysfunctional gastrointestinal motility
- Bowel incontinence

Class 3. Integumentary Function
This class does not currently contain any diagnoses.

Class 4. Respiratory Function
Impaired gas exchange

4. Activity/rest

Class 1. Sleep/Rest
- Insomnia Sleep deprivation
- Readiness for enhanced sleep
- Disturbed sleep pattern

Class 2. Activity/Exercise
- Risk for disuse syndrome
- Impaired bed mobility
- Impaired physical mobility
- Impaired wheelchair mobility
- Impaired sitting
- Impaired standing
- Impaired transfer ability
- Impaired walking

Class 3. Energy Balance
Imbalanced energy field fatigue wandering

Class 4. Cardiovascular/Pulmonary Responses
- Activity intolerance
- Risk for activity intolerance
- Ineffective breathing pattern
- Decreased cardiac output
- Risk for decreased cardiac output
- Impaired spontaneous ventilation
- Risk for unstable blood pressure
- Risk for decreased cardiac tissue perfusion
- Risk for ineffective cerebral tissue perfusion
- Ineffective peripheral tissue perfusion
- Risk for ineffective peripheral tissue perfusion
- Dysfunctional ventilatory weaning response

Class 5. Self-care
- Impaired home maintenance
- Bathing self-care deficit
- Dressing self-care deficit
- Feeding self-care deficit
- Toileting self-care deficit
- Readiness for enhanced self-care
- Self-neglect

5. Perception/cognition

Class 1. Attention
Unilateral neglect

Class 2. Orientation
This class does not currently contain any diagnoses.

Class 3. Sensation/Perception
This class does not currently contain any diagnoses.

Class 4. Cognition
- Acute confusion
- Risk for acute confusion
- Chronic confusion
- Labile emotional control
- Ineffective impulse control
- Deficient knowledge
- Readiness for enhanced knowledge
- Impaired memory

Class 5. Communication
- Readiness for enhanced communication
- Impaired verbal communication

6. Self-perception

Class 1. Self-concept
- Hopelessness
- Readiness for enhanced hope
- Risk for compromised human dignity
- Disturbed personal identity
- Risk for disturbed personal identity
- Readiness for enhanced self-concept

Class 2. Self-esteem
- Chronic low self-esteem
- Risk for chronic low self-esteem
- Situational low self-esteem
- Risk for situational low self-esteem

Class 3. Body Image
Disturbed body image

7. Role Relationship

Class 1. Caregiving Roles
- Caregiver role strain
- Risk for caregiver role strain
- Impaired parenting
- Risk for impaired parenting
- Readiness for enhanced parenting

Class 2. Family Relationships
- Risk for impaired attachment
- Dysfunctional family processes
- Interrupted family processes
- Readiness for enhanced family processes

Class 3. Role Performance
- Ineffective relationship
- Risk for ineffective relationship
- Readiness for enhanced relationship
- Parental role conflict
- Ineffective role performance Impaired social interaction

8. Sexuality

Class 1. Sexual Identity
This class does not currently contain any diagnoses.

Class 2. Sexual Function
Sexual dysfunction: Ineffective sexuality pattern

Class 3. Reproduction
- Ineffective childbearing process
- Risk for ineffective childbearing process
- Readiness for enhanced childbearing process
- Risk for disturbed maternal-fetal dyad

9. Coping/Stress Tolerance

Class 1. Post-trauma Responses
- Risk for complicated immigration transition
- Post-trauma syndrome
- Risk for post-trauma syndrome
- Rape-trauma syndrome
- Relocation stress syndrome
- Risk for relocation stress syndrome

Class 2. Coping Responses
- Ineffective activity planning
- **Risk for ineffective activity planning:** Anxiety (Nursing care plan)
- **Defensive coping:** Ineffective coping
- **Readiness for enhanced coping:** Ineffective community coping
- Readiness for enhanced community coping
- Compromised family coping
- Disabled family coping
- Readiness for enhanced family coping
- Death anxiety
- **Ineffective denial:** Fear
- Grieving complicated grieving
- Risk for complicated grieving
- Impaired mood regulation
- Powerlessness
- Risk for powerlessness
- Readiness for enhanced power
- Impaired resilience
- Risk for impaired resilience
- Readiness for enhanced resilience
- Chronic sorrow
- Stress overload

Class 3. Neurobehavioral Stress
- Acute substance withdrawal syndrome
- Risk for acute substance withdrawal syndrome
- Autonomic dysreflexia
- Risk for autonomic dysreflexia
- Decreased intracranial adaptive capacity
- Neonatal abstinence syndrome
- Disorganized infant behavior
- Risk for disorganized infant behavior
- Readiness for enhanced organized infant behavior

10. Life Principles

Class 1. Values
This class does not currently contain any diagnoses.

Class 2. Beliefs
Readiness for enhanced spiritual well-being

Class 3. Value/Belief/Action Congruence
- Readiness for enhanced decision-making
- Decisional conflict
- Impaired emancipated decision-making
- Risk for impaired emancipated decision-making
- Readiness for enhanced emancipated decision-making
- **Moral distress:** Impaired religiosity
- Risk for impaired religiosity
- Readiness for enhanced religiosity
- Spiritual distress
- Risk for spiritual distress

11. Safety/protection
Class 1. Infection
Risk for infection: Risk for surgical site infection

Class 2. Physical Injury
- Ineffective airway clearance
- Risk for aspiration
- Risk for bleeding (Nursing care plan)
- Impaired dentition
- Risk for dry eye
- Risk for dry mouth
- Risk for falls
- Risk for corneal injury
- Risk for injury
- Risk for urinary tract injury
- Risk for perioperative positioning injury
- Risk for thermal injury
- Impaired oral mucous membrane integrity
- Risk for impaired oral mucous membrane integrity
- Risk for peripheral neurovascular dysfunction
- Risk for physical trauma
- Risk for vascular trauma
- Risk for pressure ulcer
- Risk for shock
- Impaired skin integrity (Nursing care plan)
- Risk for impaired skin integrity
- Risk for sudden infant death
- Risk for suffocation
- Delayed surgical recovery
- Risk for delayed surgical recovery
- Impaired tissue integrity
- Risk for impaired tissue integrity
- Risk for venous thromboembolism

Class 3. Violence
- Risk for female genital mutilation
- Risk for other-directed violence
- Risk for self-directed violence
- Self-mutilation
- Risk for self-mutilation
- Risk for suicide

Class 4. Environmental Hazards
- Contamination
- Risk for contamination
- Risk for occupational injury
- Risk for poisoning

Class 5. Defensive Processes
- Risk for adverse reaction to iodinated contrast media
- Risk for allergy reaction
- Latex allergy reaction
- Risk for latex allergy reaction

Class 6. Thermoregulation
- Hyperthermia
- Hypothermia
- Risk for hypothermia
- Risk for perioperative hypothermia
- Ineffective thermoregulation
- Risk for ineffective thermoregulation

12. Comfort
Class 1. Physical Comfort
- Impaired comfort
- Readiness for enhanced comfort
- Nausea
- Acute pain
- Chronic pain
- Chronic pain syndrome
- Labor pain

Class 2. Environmental Comfort
- Impaired comfort
- Readiness for enhanced comfort

Class 3. Social Comfort
- Impaired comfort
- Readiness for enhanced comfort
- Risk for loneliness
- Social isolation

13. Growth/development
Class 1. Growth
This class does not currently contain any diagnoses

Class 2. Development
Risk for delayed development

Comparison Between Nursing and Medical Diagnosis
See **Table 2.2**.

Chapter 2: The Nursing Process

TABLE 2.2: Shows the comparison between the nursing diagnosis and medical diagnosis.

Parameters of comparison	Nursing diagnosis	Medical diagnosis
Focus	This type of diagnosis focuses more on care for a patient	This type of diagnosis focuses more on the etiologic of a patient
Meaning	There is a process of identification in this type of diagnosis of all the possibilities of risks and problems in a patient	There is a process of identification in this type of diagnosis of a clear medical entity that caused the illness to a patient
Identification	This identifies the signs and symptoms of an illness of a patient	This identifies the pathology that caused the illness to a patient
Main feature	This helps to focus on the reactions in physical and psychological reactions of a patient	This helps to focus on the actual illness of a patient
Example	Diagnosis of heartbeats	Diagnosis of infarction

Nursing Process

Patient Name: **Date:** /   /   **Ward**

Date	Assessment	Nursing diagnosis	Objective	Plan of care	Implementation	Rationale	Evaluation

CHAPTER 3

Nutritional Needs

■ INTRODUCTION TO NUTRITION

- Nutrition is the science of food, the nutrients and other substance, their intake, their action, interaction and their relationship to various diseases.
- The process by which organism ingest, digest, absorb, transport, utilize and excrete out the waste end products are covered under nutrition.
- Food is essential for life.
- To sustain life, the nutrients in food must perform three functions within the body—build tissue, regulate metabolic processes and provide a source of energy.
- A proper diet is essential for good health.
- A well-nourished person is more likely to be well developed, mentally and physically alert and better able to resist infectious diseases than one who is not well nourished.
- Proper diet creates a healthier person and extends the years of normal bodily functions.
- Diet therapy is the application of nutritional science to promote human health and treat disease.
- A "nutritionally adequate diet will contain all the essential nutritive substances in the amounts and proportions required to maintain life and health.
- These essential nutrients are carbohydrates, proteins, fats, minerals, vitamins and water.
- Carbohydrates, proteins and fats are the basic fuels for cellular activity.
- Minerals are inorganic substances that help to regulate body processes.
- Some work with the enzymes, some act as catalysts and some work within the buffer systems.
- Vitamins are organic nutrients that function to regulate physiological processes, such as growth and metabolism.
- Water is an important nutrient with many functions. It acts as a coolant, a lubricant, a suspending medium and as a reactant in chemical processes.
- Since the food we eat cannot be used for fuel in its consumed form, it must be broken down (digested) to the molecular level.
- In molecular form, the chemicals can be transported and absorbed through the cell membranes for utilization by the body cells. This process of digestion consists of both mechanical and chemical breakdown.
- Mechanical digestion includes chewing, swallowing, peristalsis and defecation.
- Chemical digestion is the enzymatic breakdown of the food stuffs into chemically simple molecules that can be absorbed and utilized by the cells.

■ IMPORTANCE

- A healthy diet is essential for good health and nutrition.
- A healthy lifestyle can be attained by maintaining a balanced diet and keeping into consideration to meet all the essential nutrients required by the body.
- A proper meal plan helps to attain ideal body weight and reduce the risk of chronic diseases like diabetes, cardiovascular diseases and different types of cancer.
- Balanced diet is a diet that offers all the essential nutrients to help the body function properly.
- Calories are indicators of the energy content in the food. The calories are consumed when a person walks, thinks, or breathes.
- On average, a person may require about 2000 calories a day to maintain the body weight.
- Generally, a person's calorie need may depend on his gender, age, and physical activity.
- Moreover, men need more calories than women.
- People who are more into exercising require more calories in comparison to people who do not.
- Eating a healthy diet is all about feeling great, having more energy, improving health, and boosting the mood.
- Good nutrition, physical activity, and healthy body weight are essential parts of a person's overall health and well-being.
- Unless a person maintains a proper diet for a healthy body, he may be prone to diseases, infection, or even exhaustion
- The importance of nutritious food for children especially needs to be highlighted since otherwise they may end up being prone to several growth and developmental problems.
- Some of the most common health problems that arise from lack of a balanced diet are heart diseases, cancer, stroke, and diabetes.
- Being physically active manages many health problems and improves mental health by reducing stress, depression, and pain.

- Regular exercise helps to prevent metabolic syndrome, stroke, high blood pressure, arthritis, and anxiety.
- In some illnesses, such as diabetes mellitus or hypertension, diet therapy may be the major treatment for disease control.
- Nutritional status represents meeting of human body needs for nutritive and protective substances and the reflection of these in physical, physiological and biochemical characteristics, functional capability and health status Nutritional assessment can be defined as the interpretation from dietary laboratory, anthropometric and clinical studies.
- It is used to determine the nutritional status of individual or population groups as influenced by the intake and utilization of nutrients.
- It is essential for identification of potential population group at risk of deficiency or for formulation of recommendations for nutrient intake.
- Optimal nutritional status is the state of the body with respect to each nutrient and overall body weight and condition; is a powerful factor in promoting health and preventing and treating diseases.
- Nutritional status affects immune response and response to medical therapies.

The importance of nutritional assessment includes:
- Identification of people at risk of malnutrition for early intervention or referral before they become malnourished.
- Identify malnourished patients for treatment.
- The malnourished people who are not treated early have longer hospital stays, slower recovery from infection and complications, and higher morbidity and mortality
- For tracking child growth and detecting practices that can increase the risk of malnutrition and infection.
- For providing information regarding nutrition education and counseling.

FACTORS AFFECTING NUTRITIONAL NEEDS

Age/Development
- People in rapid period growth (e.g., infancy and adolescence) have increased needs for nutrients.
- Elders (Old age), on other hand, need fewer calories and dietary changes.
- During the growth period, the BMR is high, therefore during infancy the energy need per kg of body weight is highest than during adulthood.
- The period at which the basal metabolism reaches its highest level is between the ages of 1–2 years.
- A gradual decline occurs between the ages of 2–5 years, with a more rapid decline until adult age.

Gender
- Nutrients requirements are different for men and women because of body composition and reproductive functions.
- Men require greater need of calories and protein because of larger body mass.
- Women require more iron because of menstruation.
- Pregnant and lactating mothers have increased caloric and fluid needs.
- The BMR is higher in adolescent boys and adult males as compared to adolescent girls and adult females though it is not due to direct influence of sex differences, but are due to the differences in body composition.
- Males have a greater amount of muscles and glandular tissues which is metabolically more active whereas, females have greater adipose tissues which is metabolically less active
- Hence energy requirement of males is higher than of females.

Ethnicity and Culture
- Ethnicity often determines food preference.
- Cultural beliefs and customs vary from state to state and even the staple food is not the same.
- A person in South India will have rice and Jowar as his staple food.
- A person in North India will have wheat as his staple food.
- Even the variety of rice is different, as the people in Tamil Nadu eat white rice
- A person in Kerala eats red/brown rice, which is more nutritious.
- Most of communities in India that women and girls eat only after men and boys finish their eating.
- Curd and citrus food is not taken by a person suffering from cold and cough.

Social Factors/Superstition
- Many people believe in superstition and try to avoid certain food.
- Papaya is avoided during pregnancy, as it is believed to cause abortion.
- Pregnant women drink milk with saffron to have a fair baby.
- Consumption of garlic will increase milk secretion.
- Some food, such as papaya, meat, eggs, and legumes are believed to increase heat in the body.

Religious Factor
- Many Hindus are vegetarian.
- Jains do not eat after sunset.
- Muslims are prohibited from eating pork.
- Hindus do not eat beef.
- Traditional factors
- The traditional cooking practice also acts as a barrier to achieving a balanced diet.
- Ex-using polished rice draining away a rice water
- Boiling of vegetables adds to great loss of nutrients.
- Doing a fasting

Economic Factors
- Food selection is based upon a affordability.
- A daily wage earner will spend more on staple food than fruits and vegetables.
- They depend on cereals, low cost green leafy vegetables and root and tubers.
- An effluent person will consume a variety of foods.

Geographical areas
- People in coastal areas of Karnataka, Kerala, Goa and west Bengal consume a lot of sea food.
- Rice is staple food in south India (Andhra Pradesh, Kerala, Tamil Nadu)
- Wheat is staple food of northern and eastern regions. As wheat is the main crop in temperate regions.

Production and Transport
Locally grown foods are consumed more and the availability of the locally grown product is cheaper.

Lifestyle
- Food forms important part of festivals, parties and celebration.
- The way person lives his life influence his food habits.
- The work routine and the timings at work also affects the food habits.

Climate
- It is known that the BMR is lower in tropics then in temperate zones.
- Hence the energy cost of work is slightly higher when the temperature falls.

Body Size
- It will have an important effect on energy needs because a larger body has a greater amount of muscles and glandular tissue to maintain, thus requiring higher energy allowances.
- A tall thin individual has a greater surface area than an individual of the same weight who is short and fat and the former will therefore, have a higher basal metabolic rate.

Secretion of Endocrine Glands
- The thyroid gland in particular exerts a marked influence on the energy requirement.
- If it is overactive (hyperthyroidism), the BMR will increase
- If the activity of the gland decreases (hypothyroidism), the BMR will be reduced.

Status of Health
- During the periods of fever as well as malnutrition, the BMR of an individual is affected.
- Illness involving an elevation of body temperature markedly increases the basal heat production thus increasing the BMR, hence increased energy requirement.

Altered Physiological States
- During pregnancy and lactation, the energy needs are increased because of an elevated BMR.
- In pregnancy, this additional energy is needed to support the growth of fetus and maternal tissues.
- During lactation energy is required for synthesis of milk.

Effect of Food
- A certain amount of work is expended in the digestion of food, its absorption transfer to the tissues and utilization.
- The increased heat production as a result of the ingestion of food is known as the specific dynamic action of the food.
- Protein when eaten alone has been shown to increase the metabolic rate by 30%.
- On the basis of the mixed diets, which are usually consumed, the specific dynamic action of food is approximately 10% of the energy requirement.

Extent of Physical Activity
- Any kind of physical activity increases the energy expenditure above the basal energy need.
- Energy for the performance of all types of physical activities ranks next to basal metabolism in amount of energy expended.
- Sleep causes a reduction of about 10% in the BMR depending on the number of hours spent in sleeping and its manner, i.e., restless/peaceful.
- The energy need is determined by the nature and duration of physical activity.
- Sedentary work, which includes once work, book keeping, typing, teaching, etc., calls for lesser energy than moderate work (more active and strenuous occupations) such as nursing, homemaking, or gardening.

ASSESSMENT OF NUTRITIONAL STATUS

Nutritional status of an individual can be assessed by following techniques:

Clinical Examination
- Nutritional assessment gives direct evidence of under nutrition and signs and symptoms of diseases.
- The nutritional status of a person can be known by examination of weight, height, eyes, nose, ears, skin, hair, mouth, muscles, abdomen and bones.
- A standard score-card can also be used for diagnosis of various signs and symptoms.

Biochemical Examination
- Nutritional status and abnormalities of metabolism can be diagnosed by biochemical examination.
- For this purpose, estimation of serum, vitamin A, serum globulin, serum albumin, serum protein, hemoglobin in blood is carried out.
- Urine is examined for presence of creatinine, thiamine, riboflavin, iodine, etc.
- Even in the absence of clinical manifestations of dietary malnutrition, these investigations can help in assessment of nutritional status.

Anthropometric Measurement
- Under anthropometric measurement, age, height and weight, circumference of head, circumference of chest and arm and skin fold thickness are measured.
- The nutritional status of the person is assessed on the basis of standards.
- Age wise height and weight charts of average Indian males and females, serves as guidelines for this purpose.

Radiological Examination

- ❖ Generally, this method is not used for nutritional assessment.
- ❖ But in order to get additional information about changes in skeletal, body or cellular tissue, radiological examination is undertaken. This method is more useful

Food Intake Assessment

- ❖ Nutritional assessment can be done by measuring the amount of nutrients, their quality, frequency of meals and the diet consumed.
- ❖ The diet and nutrients consumed by the person can be measured by food record or by 24 hour recall method.
- ❖ The figures so obtained, can help in nutritional assessment.
- ❖ Besides this, nutritional assessment can also be done by environmental studies, and by knowing the health and vital statistics.
- ❖ It may be mentioned that more than one method may be useful in proper and accurate assessment.

■ REVIEW ON THERAPEUTIC DIETS

Therapeutic Diets

Dietary management refers to managing a disease condition using dietary means. It focuses on practical aspects of normal diets, application, adaptation or modification of these diets to the disease conditions.

Definition

"Diets which are adapted or modified for therapeutic purpose are called therapeutic diets."

Objectives of Therapeutic Diets

- ❖ To maintain good nutritional/health status.
- ❖ To correct deficiencies.
- ❖ To give rest to the body or any specific organ.
- ❖ To meet the requirement of specific conditions.
- ❖ It should be kept in mind that therapeutic diets are especially prepared for each patient and these require individualized dietary care.

Responsibilities of Nurse in Therapeutic Diet

Responsibilities of Nurse in Therapeutic Diet

- ❖ Low intake or refusal for food is a problem in individuals suffering from a disease.
- ❖ Under this condition, it is the main duty of a nurse to provide nutritious diet to the patient.

The duties of the nurse in diet therapy are as follows:
- ❖ Assessing the nutritional requirements of the patient.
- ❖ Helping the patient in taking his diet.
- ❖ Providing nutrition to helpless patient and arranging for artificial feeding, when needed.
- ❖ Create interest and motivate the patient towards diet.
- ❖ Planning proper diet for the patient and implementing it.
- ❖ Modifying the diet according to his taste, considering the need and the objectives of therapeutic diet.
- ❖ Preparing the patient and his relatives for following diet limitations or prohibitions (such as salt restricted diet).
- ❖ Observing the effects of therapeutic diet and taking necessary steps after its evaluation.

■ REVIEW: SPECIAL DIETS—SOLID, LIQUID, SOFT

- ❖ The diet of a patient beside the other factors depends on his disease.
- ❖ The type and preparation of diet is controlled by the principles and objectives of diet therapy.

The diet served during hospitalization or their common preparation can be classified as follows:
- ❖ Liquid/Fluid diet
- ❖ Absolute liquid or residue free diet
- ❖ Full liquid diet or residual diet
- ❖ Light or soft diet
- ❖ Bland/Nonirritant diet
- ❖ Full or normal diet
- ❖ Special diet

■ FLUID OR LIQUID DIET

- ❖ Fluid or liquid diet is a constituent of diet which can be given in squid form.
- ❖ This type of diet is used for those patients, who are unable to receive or tolerate solid diet.

Types of Fluid Diets

- ❖ **Clear fluid diets (Absolute liquid diet):**
  - Clear fluid diets are used when the patient is unable to tolerate foodstuff or roughage.
  - As in this type of diet, no residue is left; it is called as residual free diet. Clear fluid diet has extremely less or no nutritional or caloric value but has important role in maintaining the fluid balance of the body.
  - Patient cannot be kept on such a diet for long, as it can lead to nutritional deficiencies and symptoms of disease.
  - This includes light tea with less milk, light black coffee, clear soups, soda water or soft drinks.
- ❖ **Full fluid diet:**
  - When liquid diet is to be given for a longer time, the patient is kept on full fluid diet.
  - Full fluid diet is given when the patient is unable to accept solid food or is on tube feeding.
  - The main constituent of full fluid diet is milk which can be mixed with egg or custard.
  - Vitamins, minerals, sugar, glucose or starch can also be given with milk.
  - This way, full fluid diet can fulfill the caloric and nutritional requirements of the patient.

Foodstuff as Liquid Diet

Beverages

- ❖ Water is the main constituent of all beverages.
- ❖ These can be classified as hot and cold.
- ❖ Beverages include milk, butter milk, lassi tea, coffee, coke, fruit juices, sugarcane juice, soft drinks, etc.

- ❖ Alcoholic beverages (beer, rum, wine, whiskey, spirits, etc.) are generally harmful for the body.
- ❖ Hence, hospital diet has no place for them.

Some beverages used as diet are as follows:

❖ **Tea and coffee:**
- Tea and coffee are very popular beverages.
- People use these for relieving fatigue and mental distress. Caffeine found in tea and coffee has stimulating effect.
- Average caffeine content in one cup (150 mL) of brewed coffee is 80–120 mg, instant coffee is 50–65 mg, while tea contains 30–65 mg caffeine.
- Low doses (20–200 mg) of caffeine produce mild energetic effect but higher dose (more than 200 mg) can create negative effects, such as anxiety, nervousness, etc., so caffeine content should not exceed the tolerable limits.
- Tannin is another component found in tea and coffee, which interfere with iron absorption. So tea and coffee should be avoided following iron supplements.

❖ **Tea:**
- Tea can be light, strong or very strong.
- Tea can be prepared from dried leaves or green leaves, sugar and milk increase its nutritive value.
- Beside caffeine, tea contains theobromine and theophylline, they promote circulation.
- Flavonoids and other anti-oxidant polyphenols present in tea, are known to reduce the risk of coronary heart disease and stomach cancer.
- However, caffeine in excess amount is dangerous to health.
- Hence decaffeinated tea is much safer.

❖ **Coffee:**
- Coffee contains tannic acid and caffeine.
- Black coffee (sugar and milk free), cold coffee can also be used as a beverage.
- Coffee stimulates the nervous system.
- Nutritive or caloric value of coffee depends on amount of milk and sugar.
- Excess use of coffee can elevate blood pressure and causes problems of heartbeat.
- It has been found that there is an association between coffee intake and raised levels of total and bad or LDL cholesterol, triglycerides and heart disease.
- So the persons with heart disease and experiencing adverse effects from caffeine should avoid drinking coffee.

❖ **Soft drinks**
- Soft drinks can be kept under two categories—natural soft drinks and artificial or synthetic soft drinks.
- Natural fruit juices in addition to energy, provide some vitamins (beta-carotenes, vitamin C) and minerals (calcium, potassium, etc.).
- Fruit juices rich in potassium are fruitful for hypertensive persons.
- Synthetic drinks do not contain nutrients unless they are fortified.
- These are prepared using preservatives, artificial colours and flavors, such as cola, orange, mango, lime, and most of them are carbonated.
- If taken in excess these drinks can damage teeth and affect digestive system.

❖ **Fruit juices:**
- Fruit juices are extensively used in diet therapy.
- The caloric value depends on the type of fruit. Fruit juices yield carbohydrates for energy, good amount of vitamin C, some amount of vitamin D and minerals.
- Lime, grapes, apple, mangoes, orange and pineapple are commonly used for fruit juices. Sugar can be added for taste.
- Coconut water, sugarcane juice, etc., are also used in hospital diet therapy.
- Their caloric value is comparatively better.

❖ **Barley water:**
- This can be prepared from whole barley or its flour.
- Barley is mixed with about 500 mL of water and slightly heated. When water is reduced to 300 mL, it is filtered and used after mixing with lemon and sugar.
- In the other method, barley flour is mixed with cold water, then in 500 mL of water for 30 minutes.
- It is used after filter and is mixed with lemon juice and salt. (When permitted).

❖ **Synthetic drinks:** Their caloric value is negligible and the taste is affected by additives (e.g., sugar, citric acid, carbon di-oxide, etc.).

❖ **Coconut water:**
- Coconut water is popular, tender, nutritious beverage.
- It works as a rehydration solution and keeps the body cool.
- It has a caloric value of 17.4 per 100 g.
- Tender coconut water contains most of the minerals such as potassium, sodium, calcium, magnesium, phosphorus, iron, copper, etc.
- Coconut water is not recommended in cases of renal failure, acute adrenal insufficiency and patients with low urine output.

Milk Products in Liquid Form

- ❖ This includes milk, curd, butter milk, lactic acid milk, vegetable milk, shakes, etc.
- ❖ **Whey:** 500 mL of milk is heated to 37°C and lemon juice is added to it. 15–20 minutes later, when the milk sours and stabilizes, the supernatant water is boiled and used.
- ❖ **Curd water also comes in this category:**
  - *Lassi:* Curd can be used as liquid diet after dilution. This is a diet which is digestible and of high caloric value, but its nutritive value depends on the amount of water added. Sugar can be mixed in this or even salted curd can be used. Raita is a popular preparation of curd.
  - *Butter milk:* Curd is churned in a churner or a mixer and the butter is removed. Desired amount of water can be added to the remaining fluid. Butter milk can be sweet or salty. Butter milk can be used in place of water. Butter milk is a low fat liquid diet.
  - *Shakes:* Shakes are very common liquid preparation which are made by mixing fruits, chocolate, cocoa, ice cream, etc., in the milk. Yogurt can also be used for making shakes. Protein shake can be used as a therapeutic diet.

Other milk products, such as vegetable milk, toned milk, skimmed milk, fortified milk, milk prepared from whole milk powder, etc., can also be used as a liquid diet.

Egg Preparations as Liquid Diet

Following preparations of egg can be used as liquid diet:

- **Egg flip or nog:** Whole egg (white and yellow) is nicely stirred and then mixed with milk in the ratio of 250 mL per egg and vigorously shaken. Orange juice, sugar, tea or coffee can also be mixed with the mixture. This is a protein rich liquid diet.
- **Albumin water:** The white of egg is strained and without stirring, albumin jell is prepared by mixing lemon juice, water and sugar which is useful in fever. The albumin water can also be mixed with other diets.

Soups

Soup is used as full liquid diet. Some soups are described below:

- **Bone soups:** The base of this soup is stock or meat water (prepared by warming bones and meat for a long time). Bones are broken into small pieces and meat is grinded and then they are warmed in water. Salt is added after foam appears. The mixture is warmed for 2–3 hours. From time to time, the foam is removed. After this, the mixture is strained through a fine strainer (filter) to remove fat and solids. Soup is served hot.
- **Vegetable soup:** There are different methods of making vegetable soups. Vegetables are washed and cut into fine pieces. They are then cooked over steam or by boiling in water till they become soft. The soup can be used after straining and mixing salt, sugar or light spices. Tomato soup is prepared by boiling tomatoes along with the skin. Then the skin is removed and the bulk is nicely squeezed in boiled water. With the help of strainer the soup is separated which can be made tasty by addition of salt, spices, etc.
- **Non-vegetarian soup:** Vegetable pieces are heated with butter in a saucepan. For taste, salt, chillies and boiled meat water is mixed and the vegetable pieces are boiled till they become soft. This can be used after straining. Vegetable cream soup can also be prepared. One or more vegetables can be used in preparing soup.
- **Pulse soup:** 40–50 g of finely grounded pulse is mixed with about 300 mL of water and boiled for 20–30 minutes. This mixture can be used as liquid diet by mixing salt or directly after straining.
- Similarly, meat and liver soup can also be used as liquid diet.

Light or Soft Diet

- Soft diets are comparable with full diet but the food articles served in it can be easily chewed, swallowed and digested.
- Soft diets are more useful for old age, those with less digestive power and convalescing patients.
- This diet is between full diet and full liquid diet.

Some of the soft diets are described below:

Diet Prepared from Egg

- In this, roasted egg, boiled or poached egg can be used as soft diet.

- **Omlette** is also prepared for the same purpose.
- **Boiled egg:** 3–4 eggs are put in the water in a pot. Then water is heated. After 10–12 minutes, eggs are boiled, cooled and served.
- **Poached egg:** A poached egg is an egg that has been cooked by poaching, that is, in simmering liquid. Egg for poaching should be fresh otherwise the white will separate from the yolk during simmering. The egg is cracked into a bowel and then gently slides into a pan of simmering water and cooked until the egg white has mostly solidified, but the yolk remains soft. Other methods are also used for poaching egg.
- **Scrambled egg:** Scrambled eggs are prepared by using milk, salt, pepper and butter. Egg is beaten then milk, salt and pepper is mixed and blended. Butter is heated and egg mixture is poured. As it begins to set, eggs are pulled across the pan and large soft curds are formed. Cooking is continued till mixture is thickened and no visible liquid egg remains. Scrambled eggs are served hot.
- **Porridge:**
  - Cereals are coarse grinded and boiled in sufficient quantity of water.
  - This can be made more balanced and delicious by adding milk and sugar.
  - Porridge is commonly prepared from wheat, bajra, maize, etc.
  - Wheat porridge can be roasted with ghee on a frying pan before boiling.

Other Soft Preparations

- **Double boiled rice:**
  - In double boiled rice, rice is boiled with milk to such an extent that the mixture is turned into a paste.
  - This is served after mixing sugar.
- **Khichadi:**
  - Khichadi is prepared by mixing rice with green gram (2:1) and boiled for sufficient time.
  - This can be sweetened or salted. Vegetable pieces can also be mixed.
- **Idlies:**
  - Idlies are prepared over steam from the fermented mixture of rice and blackgram which is finely grinded
  - This South Indian dish is prevalent in North India as a soft diet.
- **Kheer:** Kheer prepared by mixing milk and sugar with is also a digestible and palatable soft diet.
- **Rice water:**
  - Rice water (Conjee) is prepared by nicely boiling rice in water and straining it or by mixing rice flour in water and boiling it for 15 minutes.
  - Milk and sugar can also be added to this.
  - Khichadi can also be prepared by mixing sago with rice and Kheer by addition of milk to sago.

Vegetables, Salads, Jellies, Custard

- **Salads:**
  - Delicious and digestible salads can be prepared from boiled vegetables or cutting carrot, radish, tomato, cucumber etc. and mixing these with spices.

- Pieces of fruits can also be mixed with this or fruit salad can be prepared separately, vegetables can be taken as a salad in their raw forms.
- **Jelly:**
  - It can be made of fruits or milk.
  - Sugar and gelatin powder is mixed with fruit juices and the mixture is gradually warmed, stirring continuously.
  - The then is stabilized in a refrigerator and served cold.
- **Custard:**
  - Custard is a variety of culinary preparations based on a cooked mixture of milk or cream and yolk
  - Most common custards are used as dessert and include sugar and vanilla.
  - Flour, corn starch or gelatin can be added as in pastry cream.
  - Eggless vegetarian custards can also be prepared.
  - Many types of readymade custards are available in the market which can be served in the diet.

Soft diets also include liquid diets which can serve as supplementary to main diet.

Some preparations of toast, meat and liver, steamed fish, ice cream, kulfi, bread, biscuits light pudding are also included in soft diet.

Bland or Non-irritant Diet

Bland or non-irritant diet is prepared from such articles of food which are easily digestible, are free from stimulation of stomach or intestine, have a low roughage.

Some Facts Related to Bland Diet

- Diets are not fried.
- They are cooked by boiling, warming, roasting or steaming.
- Increased quantity of milk should be used in a bland diet.
- Stimulating beverages, such as tea, coffee, kulfi, soup, curry, alcohol, etc., are not included in bland diet.
- The diet should be completely free from chemical and mechanical stimulants.
- Mechanical stimulants consist of fruits with cellulose, skins of vegetables, seeds, fibers, etc., while chemical stimulants include chilies, black pepper, ginger and other strong spices.
- Bland diet consists of vegetables without skins, bulk of fruits and fibreless articles.
- Beverages containing excessive sugar are not used in bland diet.
- Similarly, excessive use of fat is also prohibited.
- Bland and non-stimulating diets are generally given to patient suffering from disturbances of digestive system.

Full Diet

- This is a regular, normal and balanced diet which can be either vegetarian or non-vegetarian.
- Full diet is served to those patients in whom diet modification is not necessary
- Full diet is prepared depending upon the patient's age group, his nutritional and energy requirement.

Low Cost Preparations

- In our country, so many dishes are prevalent which are nutrient rich and can be obtained on low cost.
- Sometimes substitutes may be helpful in lowering the price without compromising the nutritive value.

Here two such preparations are mentioned:
1. **Chikki:** It is prepared by mixing various types of nuts and other ingredients either with jaggery or sugar. Ground nut chikki is nutricious and popular in our country. Ingredients of groundnut chikki are peanuts, ghee and jaggery or sugar.
2. **Multigrain roti:** Various combinations and formulas are used to prepare this recipe.

One formula is given here:
- Whole wheat—2 kg.
- Chana dal—100 g
- Maize—100 g
- Bajra—50 g
- Barley—50 g
- Ragi—50 g
- Soyabeen—50 g
- Oats—100 g

Except wheat, all grains are roasted. Then all are mixed and grinded to form a smooth powder. After sieving, coarse is discarded. Flour is used to make roti.

Special Diet

- Special diet is one, in which for therapeutic purpose, one or more nutrients are removed or added.
- This is done in those patients, in whom normal physiological functions are disturbed or changed.

DYSPHAGIA

It is defined as difficulty in swallowing as a result of an obstruction or blockage.

Causes

- Cancer (oral or esophageal)
- Gastroesophageal reflux disorder (GERD)
- Neurological condition (stroke)
- Esophagitis
- Radiotherapy (it causes scar tissue)
- Facial paralysis

Assessment

- Assess ability to swallow, check for coughing or choking during eating and drinking. These signs indicate aspiration.
- Assess ability to swallow a small amount of water.
- Nurses should check for food or fluid regurgitation as regurgitation indicate decreased ability to swallow food or fluids and an increased risk for aspirations.
- Determine patient's readiness to eat. Patient needs to be alert, able to follow instructions, hold head erect and able to move tongue in mouth as cognitive deficits can results in aspiration.

The nursing interventions for dysphagia and its rationale are shown in **Table 3.1**.

TABLE 3.1: Nursing interventions and its rationale for dysphagia.

Interventions	Rationale
Provide for adequate rest before meal time	Fatigue leads to swallowing impairment
Eliminate any environmental stimuli, e.g., TV, radio	The patient can more concentrate when external stimuli are removed
Provide oral care before feeding	Optimal oral care promotes appetite and eating
If patient has impaired swallowing, consult a speech pathologist for bedside evaluation as soon as possible	Speech pathologists provides specialized care and initiation of nutritional support
Place suction equipment at the bedside and suction, as needed	With impaired swallowing reflexes secretions accumulate in the posterior pharynx and upper trachea, increasing the risk of aspiration
Position patient upright at a 90° angle with the head flexed forward at a 45° angle	This position allow the trachea to close and esophagus to open which makes swallowing easier and reduces the risk of aspiration
Ensure patient is awake, alert and able to follow sequenced directions before attempting to feed	As the patient becomes less alert the swallowing response decreases which increases the risk of aspiration
Provide small amount of food alternate serving of liquid and solids	To prevent foods from being left in the mouth
If oral intake is not possible or inadequate, initiate alternative feedings (e.g., nasogastric feedings or gastrostomy feedings)	For maintaining the nutrition pattern
Weight patient weekly	This is to help evaluate nutritional status
Encourage the patient for exercise of the and tongue to enhance swallowing	Muscle strengthening in facilitates greater chewing ability

ANOREXIA

It is classified as a loss of appetite or an inability to eat. It can be serious psychological disorder which causes an abnormal fear of being fat leading to very poor eating habits and is termed as anorexia nervosa.

Causes

- Genetics
- Dieting or starvation
- Transitions (e.g., new school or job)
- Psychological

NAUSEA AND VOMITING

- **Nausea:** It is the feeling of uneasiness in stomach that causes the urge to vomit.

TABLE 3.2: Nursing interventions and its rationale for nausea and vomiting.

Interventions	Rationale
Measure patient weight	This will accurately monitor the response to therapy
Monitor the patient's food intake	To determine the amount of food that is consumed
Provide a diverse diet according to his needs	This will stimulate the appetite of the patient
Monitor for bloating	To ensure adequate fluid and electrolyte levels
Provide small frequent meals to the patient	Bloating may inhibit so, it should be treated.
Provide parenteral fluids, as ordered	It with promote digestion and increase appetite
Educate and guide the patient	To improve patient's confidence

- **Vomiting:** It is defined as the forceful expulsion of the gastric content.

Causes

- Indigestion
- Intense pain
- Early pregnancy
- Emotional stress
- Food poisoning
- Certain odors
- Motion sickness

Assessment

- Record the patient's hydration status, BP, intake and output
- Assessing skin turgor
- Assessing the patient with the cause of nausea.
- Perform a thorough assessment and evaluation of nausea that can help determining interventions to lessen or case the problem.

The nursing interventions for nausea and vomiting and its rationale are shown in **Table 3.2**.

VOMITING

- Vomiting is the forceful expulsion of the contents of the upper gastrointestinal tract which results from contraction of muscles in the gut and abdominal wall
- Vomiting is the common gastrointestinal signs and symptoms which can be caused by numerous conditions.
- It is a vague, but pleasant sensation of sickness or queasiness.
- Nausea and vomiting often occur together but may occur independently.
- They are the part of the body's protective mechanisms.
- They are usually a response to chemical, bacterial or viral insults to the body's integrity.

Etiology

- The most common cause of nausea and vomiting which may occur separately or together with gland other problems are given below:

- General anesthesia
- Migraine
- Morning sickness
- Viral gastroenteritis
- Intestinal obstruction
❖ Medications including aspirin, NSAIDS, oral contraceptives and antibiotics
❖ Peptic ulcer
❖ Meningitis
❖ Severe pain
❖ Meniere's disease (Disorder of the inner ear that can lead to dizzy spells (vertigo) and hearing loss).
❖ Toxic ingestion
❖ **Others:**
  - Appendicitis
  - Alcohol use disorder
  - Brain tumor
  - Depression
  - Food poisoning
  - Generalized anxiety disorder
  - Cholecystitis

Risk Factors

❖ Anesthetic agents
❖ Pain
❖ Hypotension
❖ History of motion sickness
❖ High level of anxiety

Pathophysiology

❖ Vomiting is the complex phenomenon which begins with rhythmic contractions of the respiratory and abdominal muscles.
❖ It may be accompanied by retching or dry heaves and should be distinguished from classic regurgitation which may accompany gastroesophageal reflux.
❖ It presents as a manifestation of different diseases and cancer chemotherapy.
❖ Vomiting center is located in the medulla adjacent to the respiratory and salivary control centers.
❖ It can be stimulated directly by input from different sources
❖ Gastrointestinal tract produced by the following:
  - Distention
  - Irritation
  - Infection
❖ Vestibular system of the ear
❖ Chemoreceptor's outside the blood brain barrier which are stimulated by the following:
  - Drugs
  - Toxins
  - Chemotherapeutic agents
  - Systemic disorders
  - Pregnancy
❖ Higher central nervous system centers in response to certain smells, sights or emotional experiences
❖ Increased intracranial pressure produces vomiting which may or may not be accompanied by nausea.
❖ Vomiting is the response which requires coordinated movements of the thorax and abdominal wall, gut, pharynx and muscles of the mouth and is also coordinated by brain stem.
❖ Vomiting which stimulates vagus nerve or parasympathetic nervous system may be accompanied by the following:
  - Dizziness
  - Hypotension
  - Bradycardia

Clinical Manifestations

❖ Water and essential electrolytes are lost.
❖ Vertigo
❖ Excessive sweating
❖ Abdominal pain
❖ Dry mouth
❖ Chest pain
❖ Confusion

Diagnostic Evaluation

❖ Obtain complete medical history and perform physical examination of patient.
❖ **Laboratory testing:** There is no specific laboratory test to determine the etiology of vomiting. Test should be directed by the medical history or physical examination of patient can determine the exact cause of vomiting.
  - *Pregnancy test:* It should be performed in any woman of childbearing age. It reveals the cause of symptoms.
  - *Radiographic testing:* If there is any concern about a small bowel obstruction, supine or upright abdominal radiographic test should be performed.
  - *Esophagogastroduodenoscopy:* It is used to detect and treat problems of upper GI tract.
  - *Computer tomography:* It is used to detect intestinal obstructions and it also allows the evaluation of surrounding abdominal structures.

Management

Medical Management

❖ **Serotonin-receptor antagonists, such as ondansetron, granisetron:** It suppresses vomiting by blocking the effect of serotonin on vagal afferent nerves which stimulates vomiting center.
❖ **Dopamine antagonists, such as promethazine, haloperidol, droperidol, prochlorperazine:** These drugs help to block dopamine receptors in the chemoreceptor trigger zone. Their primary use is to suppress vomiting associated with surgery, cancer chemotherapy or toxins.
❖ **Antihistamine, such as meclizine, hydroxyzine:** These are used to treat nausea or vomiting associated with motion sickness.
❖ **Cannabinoids, such as nabilone:** It is used to relieve vomiting associated with cancer chemotherapy in patients who have not responded to treat with other antiemetics
❖ **Prokinetic agents:** These agents are useful with gastroparesis and motor dysfunction of the upper gastrointestinal tract.

- **Miscellaneous:**
  - *Trimethobenzamide:* It has a weak antihistamine action. It is believed to act on CTZ.
  - *Benzamide:* It inhibits the stimulation of CTZ

Nursing Management

- Maintain patient safety and assess for sedation or confusion.
- For some patients, acupuncture or acupressure can produce dramatic results
- Prevention of dehydration is also important because appears to worsen the cycle of vomiting
- Elevate head of bed.
- Protect airway with suction and positioning, if patient is not alert.
- Provide frequent mouth care.
- Provide quiet or distraction on the basis of patient response.
- Modify environmental stimuli and response.
- Provide ongoing patient support.
- Administer medicines as ordered by physician.

Complications

- Dehydration
- Weight loss
- Esophagitis
- Oropharyngeal aspiration: Pneumonia
- Hypochloremic metabolic alkalosis
- Hypokalemia

Nursing Care Plan

Nursing Assessment

- Assess the duration, frequency and nature of vomiting
- Observe for the signs of dehydration.
- Monitor vital signs.
- Measure fluid balance.
- Measure the weight as indicated.

Nursing Diagnosis

- Fluid volume deficit related to loss of active liquid.
- **Imbalance nutrition:** Less than body requirements related to absorption disorders.

Planning

Nursing Goals

- To resolve fluid and electrolyte deficit.
- To maintain nutrition balance.

Nursing Interventions

- Measure and record patient's vital signs
- Measure the input and output of fluid.
- Encourage oral hygiene before eating
- Provide a varied diet.
- Administer medicines as ordered.
- Maintain a quiet environment and avoid unnecessary procedures or activities to minimize triggers of vomiting.
- Remove visual stimuli and sources of odors to avoid precipitating triggers of nausea or vomiting.

Patient Education and Health Maintenance

- Encourage patient to maintain his/her oral hygiene.
- Instruct patient to avoid food and beverages that stimulate vomiting
- Advice patient to eat light or bland food, such as saltine crackers or plain bread.
- Instruct patient to avoid fried, greasy or sweet food.
- Advice patient to take medicines exactly as ordered by physician.
- Drink plenty of clear fluid to remain hydrated.
- Encourage patient to get plenty of rest.

Evaluation: Expected Outcomes

- Fluid and electrolyte deficit is restored.
- Nutritional

MEETING NUTRITIONAL NEEDS

Meeting the nutritional needs of a patient by serving normal/regular diet.

Purposes

- To maintain adequate nutrition of the individual.
- To promote optimal nutrition.
- To restore the individual to a satisfactory nutritional status, if his nutritional balance has been disturbed.

Articles

- A tray containing prepared diet (solid/fluid)
- Face towel
- Water.

Procedures

For oral

- Wash hands.
- Help the patient or wash hands and face, in preparation for eating.
- Remove any unpleasant visual stimuli, such as commodes, bedpans and urinals from the unit.
- If possible, raise the head of the patient's bed or have the patient sit in a chair.
- Check to be sure that the food corresponds to what the patient has ordered.
- Be sure the food is in a form the patient can eat. Check for presence of any specialize utensils the patient may require like spoons, forks, etc.
- Check for tubes, braces or dressing that may make eating more difficult.
- Place a napkin or protective cover over the patient is needed.
- Arrange food in a tray and place on the over bed table or in a manner convenient for the patient to eat.
- Cut food into large pieces, open cartons and pour fluids. Open straws if present and place them in glasses.
- Allow patient to make choice regarding the order in which food is eaten, the speed at which patient eats, and the amount patient will eat.
- Do not hurry the patient through the meal.

- Use this time as an opportunity to converse with the patient.
- Do not discuss stressful events with the patient.
- When the patient decides she/he is finished with the meal, remove the tray.
- Encourage the patient to remain in sitting position for at least 15 minutes following the meal.
- Help the patient to clean up following the meal. Allow patient to wash hands and face and clean dentures if needed.
- Wash hands.
- Record the time, type and amount of food taken and tolerance to food.

Special Considerations

- Note any food preferences, allergies or restrictions of diet.
- Note the diet the patient on and indicate any special preparation or utensils the patient needs while eating.
- Not any eating difficulties or how well the patient tolerated the meal.
- Check for medications to be administered before, after and along with the meal, e.g., insulin.

FEEDING A HELPLESS PATIENT

Assisting a helpless patient to take food and fluids.

Purposes

To assist a patient to need his nutritional needs.

Articles

- Tray containing prepared diet
- Face towel and tray
- Kidney tray
- Backrest and cardiac table
- Fork and spoon
- Feeding cup with water.

Procedure

- Explain procedure to the patient and assess how he can participate.
- Position the patient comfortably, preferably in Fowler's position.
- Assist the patient to wash his hands and face.
- Place towel over chest and around the neck.
- Make sure that therapeutic restrictions are considered. Check the diet and ensure that it is the one that was ordered.
- Create a pleasant environment.
- Wash your hands.
- Consider the patient's preferences while feeding and encourage his participation to the extent possible.
- Sit or stand at the side of patient.
- Feed the patient in small spoonfuls waiting for him to chew and swallow one mouthful before next.
- Encourage the patient to take all the food served to him, but do not force.
- Give water in between if patient prefer water.
- When the patient has eaten food and he feels satisfied, stop feeding and give him a glass of water if he prefers.
- Provide articles for rinsing mouth and encourage patient to do so.
- Dry lips and face with towel.
- Replace articles and wash hands.
- Record in nurse's record the type of diet, time of feeding, amount taken and tolerance.
- Record fluid taken, in intake–output record.

Special Considerations

- Patient should be undisturbed by treatments, dressing, visitors, doctors, rounds, unpleasant sounds and odor during meal time.
- Room should be ventilated, quite and comfortable and remove all unappetizing objects like bedpan, urinal, etc., from the premises.
- Encourage patient to eat by himself if possible and to the extent possible.
- When blind patients are fed, they should be told what feed they are being given as patients have the right to know what they are eating.

ENTERAL FEEDING

Nasogastric Intubation

Definition

Nasogastric intubation is the process of placing a soft plastic tube called nasogastric (NG) tube through any of the one nostril of the patient, past the pharynx and down the esophagus into a patient's stomach to provide the feed, when the patient is not able to have food by mouth.

Purposes

- To remove fluid and gas from gastrointestinal tract (decompression).
- Prevent or relieve nausea and vomiting after surgery.
- To obtain a specimen of gastric contents for laboratory studies.
- To treat patients with mechanical obstruction and bleeding of the upper gastrointestinal tract.
- Administer medications
- administer feeding directly into gastro-intestinal tract.

General Instructions

- Do not use force when inserting an NG tube. If resistance occurs, rotate and retract the tube slightly and try again. Forcing the tube can cause traumatic injury to the tissue of the nose, throat or esophagus.
- Always check the tube positioning before giving feed. If the tube is out of place, the patient may aspirate the feeding solution into the lungs,
- Keep the patient in an upright or semi upright sitting position when delivering a tube feeding to enhance peristalsis and avoid regurgitation of the feeding,
- Cap or clamp off the NG tube when not in use to prevent backflow of stomach contents or accumulation of air in the stomach.

- If a patient has severe sinus conditions, nasal obstruction or has had facial surgery, it may be necessary to place an orogastric tube to avoid further nasal trauma.
- If the amount of gastric aspirate is large prior to a bolus or intermittent feeding, notify the physician. The feeding size may need to be decreased if the patient is not digesting it.
- Long-term NG tube usage can cause nasal erosion, sinusitis, esophagitis, gastric ulceration, esophageal-tracheal fistula formation, oral infections and respiratory infections.
- Keep the head of the bed elevated 30° at all times to decrease gastric reflux. Place the head of the bed 30–45° during tube feedings and for 30–60 minutes after intermittent tube feedings if the patient can tolerate this position.

Articles Required
- A tray containing:
- Drawsheet
- Towel with mackintosh
- Nasogastric tube 14–16 Fr
- Sterile gloves
- 50 mL syringe
- Water soluble lubricating jelly
- Adhesive tape
- Glass with water
- Kidney tray
- Stethoscope
- Recording and reporting sheet.

Procedure
- Assess patient for the need for enteral tube feeding. NPO or insufficient intake for more than 5 days, functional GI tract, unable to ingest sufficient nutrients.
- **Assess patient for appropriate route of administration. Evaluate nares for patency:**
    a. Close each nostril alternately and ask patient to breathe for easy insertion of NG tube.
    b. Assess gag reflex to identify the ability to swallow and risk of aspiration.
    c. Inspect nares for any irritation or obstruction.
    d. Review patient's medical history for nasal problems and risk of aspiration. Nurse may seek physician's order to change route of nutritional support or to place tube that pass-through stomach into the intestine with increased risk of aspiration to prevent any complications
- Review physician's order for type of tube and enteral feeding schedule to assess patient's needs.
- Perform hand hygiene to prevent cross infection.
- Explain procedure to the patient This will reduce anxiety and help patient to assist in insertion.
- Stand on same side of bed as nare for insertion and assist patient to high Fowler's position unless contraindicated to reduce the risk of aspiration and promotes effective swallowing.
- Place bath towel over chest. Keep facial tissues within reach. Insertion of tube may produce tearing to prevent soiling of gown.
- Determine length of tube to be inserted and mark with tape. Traditional method, measures distance from

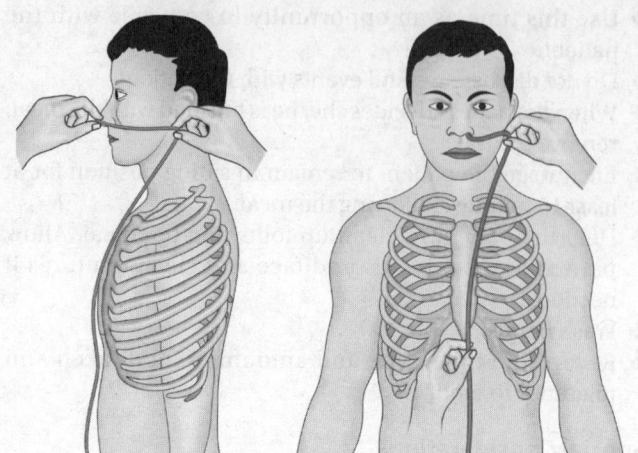

Fig. 3.1: Measurement and insertion of nasogastric tube.

tip of nose to earlobe to xiphoid process of sternum. Length approximates distance from nose to stomach in 98% patients. For duodenal or jejunal placement, an additional 20–30 cm is required **(Fig. 3.1)**.
- Prepare nasogastric or nasointestinal tube for intubation to prevent any trauma to mucous membrane.
- Cut tape 10 cm long to fix the tube and to prevent displacement to tube.
- Put on sterile gloves to reduce transmission of infection.
- Dip tube with surface lubricant into glass of water. Activates lubricant to facilitate passage of tube from nares to GI tract.
- Insert tube through nostril to back of throat (posterior nasopharynx). Aim back and down toward ear. Natural contours facilitate passage of tube into GI tract to reduce gagging by patient.
- Flex patient's head toward chest after tube has passed through nasopharynx to reduces the risk of tube entering into trachea.
- Emphasis on the need to mouth breathe and swallow during the procedure that facilitates the tube.
- Insert tube each time patient swallows until desired length have been passed. Do not force tube. If resistance is met or patient starts to cough, shock, or become cyanotic, stop advancing the tube and pull tube back.
- Check for position of tube in back throat with penlight and tongue blade to check the tube placement because it may be coiled or kinked.
- **Perform measures to verify placement of tube:**
    a. Inject 30 mL of air into the tube and aspirate GI contents with a syringe. Gastric contents are usually cloudy and grassy green or tan to off white in contrast. Intestinal fluid is usually deep golden yellow and is more clear than gastric fluid.
    b. Measure pH of aspirated GI contents. Fasting gastric pH is usually in a range of 1–4 only infrequently is it greater than In contrast, intestinal sites usually have pH of 7 or greater.
- Apply tincture of benzoin or other skin adhesive on tip of patient's nose and tube. Allow to dry. Helps take adhere better

- ❖ **Remove gloves and secure tube with tape, avoiding pressure on nares:**
  a. Split one end of tape lengthwise 5 cm (2 inches). Place the intact end of tape over bridge of patient's nose. Wrap each of the 5 cm strips around tube as it exits nose securing tape to nares prevents tissue necrosis.
  b. Fasten end of nasogastric tube to patient's gown by looping rubber band around tube in slip knot. Pin rubber band to gown. Reduce traction on the nares, if tube moves.
- ❖ For intestinal placement, position the patient on right side when possible until radiological confirmation of correct placement has been verified. Otherwise, assist patient to a comfortable position.
- ❖ Apply gloves and administer oral hygiene. Cleanse tubing at nostril to promotes comfort and integrity of oral mucous membrane.
- ❖ Remove gloves, dispose of equipment and wash hands.
- ❖ Inspect nares and oropharynx for any difficulty in breathing or gagging,

Contraindications
- ❖ Esophageal varices
- ❖ Esophageal surgery
- ❖ GI bleeding
- ❖ Facial fractures
- ❖ Epistaxis
- ❖ Nose and throat surgery
- ❖ Sinusitis
- ❖ Severe coagulopathies

Complications of NG Tubing
- ❖ **Pulmonary aspiration due to:**
  - Feeding tube displacement.
  - Patient in supine position.
  - Deficient gag reflex.
  - Gastroesophageal reflex disease.
  - Delayed gastric emptying
- ❖ **Diarrhea due to:**
  - Hyperosmolar formula or medications.
  - Antibiotic therapy
  - Bacterial contamination
  - Malnutrition/hypoalbuminemia.
  - Malabsorption.
- ❖ **Tube occlusion due to:**
  - Insufficient tube irrigation.
  - Reaction of incompatible medication or formula.
  - Pulverized medications given per tube.
  - Sedimentation formula.
- ❖ **Constipation due to:**
  - Medications.
  - Lack of free water.
  - Inactivity.
  - Lack of fiber.
- ❖ **Abdominal cramping/nausea/vomiting due to:**
  - Lactose intolerance.
  - Delayed gastric emptying.
  - Intestinal obstruction.
  - Rapid increase in rate/volume.
- ❖ **Tube displacement due to:**
  - Not taped securely.
  - Coughing, vomiting.
- ❖ **Delayed gastric emptying due to:**
  - Serious illnesses.
  - Diabetic gastroparesis.
  - Inactivity.
  - Prematurity.
- ❖ **Increased respiratory quotient:** Overfeeding of carbohydrates.
- ❖ **Hyperosmolar dehydration:** Hypertonic formula with sufficient free 10.
- ❖ **Serum electrolyte imbalance due to:**
  - Renal insufficiency
  - Diabetes mellitus.
  - Excess GI losses.
  - Congestive heart failure, edema.
  - Cirrhosis.
  - Dehydration.
- ❖ **Fluid overload due to:**
  - Refeeding syndrome in malnutrition.
  - Excess free water or diluted (hypotonic) formula.

Orogastric Feeding
In this method of enteral feeding, the site of insertion of the tube is by mouth not from the nose. This is mainly practiced in newborns.

Intake and Output is the Record
Intake and output is the recording of all fluid intake and output during a 24-hour period, it is an important indicator critically-ill patients.

Purpose
To maintain an accurate record of fluid intake and output.

Necessary Equipment
- ❖ Intake and output work sheet
- ❖ Measurement glass
- ❖ Pint measure for measuring urine, drainage, etc.
- ❖ Patient's chart

Instructions
- ❖ Intake and output will be recorded in milliliters and totaled at 8:00 AM. Totals are transferred to the appropriate columns in the patient's chart.
- ❖ The work sheet for intake and output will be kept at the bedside affixed on the bedside chart back.
- ❖ The nurse incharge of the patient will be responsible for maintaining the record. However, the patient and his attendant if capable can be taught to do so.

Measuring Intake
- ❖ Fluid intake refers to all fluid entering the patient's body. It also includes foods that are liquid at room temperature, such as ice chips, ice cream and certain beverages.
- ❖ Measure any fluids offered to the patient and make a note of how much the patient drinks and the time of the day at which it is drunk.

- If the patient is drinking from a jug, obtain the total intake by subtracting the fluid remaining in the jug at the end of the day plus any fluid added.
- You can also pre-measure the drinking glasses or bowls most commonly used by the patient. So, when the patient tells you that he had "one glass of water", you will know the amount.
- Measure ice chips by multiplying the volume by 0.5; when melted, the volume of ice is approximately half its previous volume.
- For yogurt, ice cream, gelatin, packed or canned drinks, measure the amount printed on the labels.
- Measure the amount of feeds through nasogastric tube by noting the volume of the bag at the beginning of the feeding and then subtracting the amount left at the end of the feeding. Remember to include any feeding that is added during the day.
- Intravenous intake (drips) can also be measured using the above method.
- If water is used to flush the nasogastric tube, record the amount used for irrigation in the intake and output chart.

Measuring Output
- Fluid output refers to all fluids that leave the patient's body. This includes urine, loose stools, vomitus, aspirated fluid, excessive perspiration and drainage from surgical drains, nasogastric tubes and chest tubes.
- Use a container marked with milliliters (mL) to collect fluid output. Be sure to label the container "for measuring output only" to prevent confusion with intake container.
- Always wear gloves when handling body fluids.
- Any amount not measured due to any reasons, such as patient passed urine while in the toilet should be documented, otherwise the chart becomes inaccurate and misleading.
- In cases, such as vomits or diarrhea, record the number of time, it was passed. For such cases, check with your doctor in advance if it is necessary to measure the exact amount.
- It is also important to make a note of the fact if the patient is sweating.
- If the patient has drainage, record the amount of the drainage. It is important to document the source of the drainage, especially if he has more than one drainage site.
- If patient is on intermittent or continuous irrigation, calculate the true output by measuring the total output and subtracting the total irrigation infused.

GASTROSTOMY
- A gastrostomy is a surgical opening into the stomach, made through an incision in the left, upper abdomen.
- The anterior gastric wall is sutured to the abdomen, preventing leakage of gastric contents into the abdominal cavity.
- The gastrostomy procedure is done when disease or injury of the esophagus makes gastric intubation by way of the esophagus impossible.
- At the time of surgery, the gastrostomy tube, with usually size 20 to 26 catheters, is inserted into the stomach through the incision.
- The distal end is clamped to prevent leakage and the tube is secured at the incision with one or two sutures.
- As healing of the wound takes place, a stoma (artificial opening) is formed and the catheter can then be removed and reinserted.
- Some patients are fitted with a plastic prosthesis instead of the catheter.
- The prosthesis remains in place and a catheter inserted through its lumen for feeding.
- A screw cap seals off the prosthesis opening when the catheter is already in use

Nursing Care of the Patient with a Gastrostomy
- Special attention must be paid to the skin area around the tube since there may be some leakage of gastric secretions and unless the skin is kept clean and dry, it will soon become very irritated.
- When the nursing professional does the gastrostomy feeding, he/she must also know how to carry out the prescribed skin care and dressing procedure.
- For the patient's morale, his feeding procedure should resemble as much as possible a normal meal procedure and not be an activity incidental to the dressing and skin care routine.
- For example, dressing and skin care materials should not be assembled on the same tray with his feeding set.
- When the time intervals for doing all required procedures coincide, plan to do the dressing and skin care procedures first so that the patient is clean, comfortable and relaxed as possible for his meal.
- The teeth and mouth of a patient with a gastrostomy must be kept in optimum condition by frequent oral hygiene measures.
- The teeth and mouth of a patient with a gastrostomy must be kept in optimum condition by frequent oral hygiene measures.
- If permissible, chewing gum may be given to stimulate the flow of saliva and keep the mouth moist.
- If the patient is unable to swallow the saliva, a covered, disposable sputum container should be provided and changed frequently.
- Measurement of expectorated saliva should be recorded on the intake and output worksheet
- The physician may allow the patient to chew food and spit it out. This will stimulate salivation and exercise the gums.
- This measure should only be entrusted to reliable, compliant patients.

Gastrostomy Dressing
- After the original surgical incision has healed, the dressing procedure for the stoma is routinely done by the nursing personnel in accordance with the physician's orders.
- Generally, a minimal number of dry, sterile, gauze compresses are placed around the tube.
- The clamped end of the gastrostomy tube may be coiled on top of the dressing.
- A semi-permeable surgical dressing may also be used to protect the skin from breakdown.

Gastrostomy Tube Feeding

- The gastrostomy tube is a short feeding tube that goes directly into the stomach through a surgical incision called a stoma
- The procedure must never be rushed and the atmosphere should be pleasant and relaxing for the patient
- The prescribed feeding may be a commercially prepared formula or a special preparation from the hospital food service

Indications
- Prematurity
- Post surgical malformations of the mouth, esophagus.
- Inability to swallow
- Digestive disorders.

JEJUNOSTOMY

- It is the surgical procedure of creating an opening (known as stoma) in the wall of jejunum through the skin at the anterior abdomen.
- It is the process of providing feed to the patient from enteral route via a F-shaped tube inserted in the jejunum.

Indications
- Jejunostomy is done when the nutrition cannot be provided through oral route.
- It is done when the artificial route of nutrition has to be used for more than 6 weeks.
- Jejunostomy is preferred when the patient had undergone major GI surgery with prolonged recovery time.

Purpose
The principal purpose of jejunostomy feeding is to maintain the adequate nutrition level of the patient.

Note: Nursing care and feeding technique in jejunostomy is same as gastrostomy.

GASTROSTOMY/JEJUNOSTOMY TUBE FEEDING

Introduction
When the patient is unable to ingest or swallow the food but is still able to digest and absorb nutrients from ingested food, in this case an opening (gastrostomy or Jejunostomy) is made to introduce the food in the GI tract

Definition
It is a procedure in which food is administered in the form of fluid through a tube, which is placed directly into the stomach (gastrostomy) or jejunum (jejunostomy).

Purposes
- To maintain the nutritional status of a patient whose upper gastrointestinal tract is bypassed
- To administer medications
- To nourish the gastrointestinal mucosa
- To maintain intestinal structure and function when compared to parenteral nutrition
- To prevent aspiration/regurgitation

Indications
Patient with:
- Swallowing difficulty
- Obstruction in the upper GI tract (e.g., cancer)
- Any GI surgery (Billroth 1 and 2)
- Extensive burns in upper GI

Types
Feeding method:
- Syringe feeding (intermittent)
- Continuous drip method

Nursing Process

Assessment
- Check the physician's order.
- Assess the indication for gastrostomy and jejunostomy feeding.
- Observe for abdominal distension.
- In case of delayed gastric emptying, increase the risk of regurgitation and pulmonary aspiration.
- Auscultate the bowel sound before feeding, which indicates active peristalsis.

Nursing Diagnosis
- Imbalanced nutrition less than body requirement—deficient fluid volume
- Deficient knowledge
- Risk for aspiration

Expected Outcome
- Patient attains adequate nutritional status
- Demonstrates adequate hydration status
- Exhibits adequate cooperation
- Demonstrates normal respiratory rate

Articles
- Disposable feeding (gavage) bag and tubing
- 60 mL syringe
- Feeding formula
- IV pole
- Stethoscope
- 4 × 4-inch gauze pads
- Container with 60 mL of water
- Gloves

Steps of Procedure
- Explain the procedure and obtain consent from the patient or relatives
- Perform hand hygiene and don apron, mask, and gloves
- Remove the dental appliances and inspect the oral cavity for any dentures/loose teeth
- Measure and mark the distance on the lavage tube between the bridge of the nose and the earlobe and the xiphoid process

- Ensure that unconscious patient is intubated prior to procedure
- Place the patient on a firm surface lying in left lateral position with head down (Trendelenburg position)
- Monitor oxygen saturation
- Apply restraints if indicated and prescribed
- Start the IV line
- Assemble the lavage tubing and fill the irrigating can with fluid
- Place a mackintosh under the patient's head and a plastic sheet over the floor
- Arrange the emergency resuscitation equipment at the bedside
- Lubricate the tube with jelly
- Insert the gastric tube in the mouth or nose if inserted through the mouth, a bite block with a hole for the tube to pass through is preferable
- Check the position of the tube by auscultation/aspirating the content of stomach
- Aspirate the stomach contents and collect in the specimen container
- Test the stomach content with the litmus paper if an urgent report is needed
- Unclamp the tubing between the irrigating can and the patient and allow 200–300 mL of warm fluid to run.
- Re-clamp the tubing (Step 1)
- Unclamp the tube between the patient and the drainage bag by use of gravity. If there is no drain, use the syringe to pull the fluid through the tube. Changing position sometimes helps to drain the fluid (Step 2)
- Avoid continuous suction to remove the fluid
- Repeat steps 1 and 2 until the fluid returns clear if any antidote or charcoal is prescribed, instill before removing the lavage tube
- Provide oral hygiene if required
- Perform hand hygiene
- Monitor the patient's cardio-respiratory status, gag reflex, patency of airway, breathing pattern, and level of consciousness
- Send the collected specimen to the lab with appropriate labeling
- Evaluate the type of return flow from the stomach, the amount and the characteristics of the stomach contents
- Monitor for any complications like Aspiration. Chemical pneumonia, damage to mucous membrane
- Document the procedure (date, time, amount, intake and output, types and color of the stomach contents) and the response of the patient to the procedure.

Evaluation

Patient
- Feels comfort the procedure
- Attains normal nutritional and hydration status
- Remains free of aspiration
- Is free from complications

Precautions
- In case of aspiration, apply suction and obtain chest X-ray film to confirm tube placement.
- In case of diarrhea, nausea, and vomiting, withhold the feeding and inform the physician.
- In case of absence of bowel sounds, inform physician before initiating the feed.

TOTAL PARENTERAL NUTRITION

Introduction
- Total parenteral nutrition, also known as parenteral nutrition (PN) is a form of nutritional support given completely via the bloodstream through intravenous route.
- TPN administers proteins, carbohydrates, fats, vitamins, and minerals.
- It aims to prevent and restore nutritional deficits, allowing bowel rest while supplying adequate caloric intake and essential nutrients.
- The caloric requirements of each patient are individualized according to the degree of stress, organ failure, and percentage of ideal body weight.
- It may be used as short- or long-term therapy and can be used in acute and critical care settings.

Definition
- Total parenteral nutrition (TPN) is a way of supplying all the nutritional needs of the body by bypassing the digestive system and dripping nutrient solution directly into a vein
- Total parenteral nutrition (TPN), the administration of a nutritionally adequate hypertonic solution consisting of glucose, protein hydrolysates, minerals, and vitamins through an indwelling catheter into the superior vena cava or other main vein. Fat is also provided in three in one solution or "piggy-backed". The high rate of blood flow results in rapid dilution of the solution, and full nutritional requirements can be met indefinitely.

Purposes
- To provide nutrients required for normal metabolism, tissue maintenance, repair and energy demands To bypass gastrointestinal (GI) tract for patients who are unable to take food orally
- TPN is used when individuals cannot or should not get their nutrition through eating.
- TPN is used when the intestines are obstructed, when the small intestine is not absorbing nutrients properly, or a gastrointestinal fistula (abnormal connection) is present.
- It is also used when the bowels need to rest and not have any food passing through them.
- Bowel rest may be necessary in Crohn's disease, pancreatitis, ulcerative colitis, and with prolonged bouts of diarrhea in young children.
- It is also used for individuals with severe burns, multiple fractures, and in malnourished individuals to prepare them for major surgery, chemotherapy, or radiation treatment.
- Individuals with AIDS or widespread infection (sepsis) may also benefit from TPN.

Clinical Indications

The indications for parenteral nutrition (PN) include a 10% deficit in body weight (compared with pre-illness weight), an inability to take oral food or fluids within 7 days after surgery, and hypercatabolic situations, such as major infection with fever P indicated in the following situations, such as major infection with fever.

PN is indicated in the following situations:
- The patient's intake is insufficient to maintain an anabolic state (e.g., severe burns, malnutrition, short bowel syndrome acquired immunodeficiency syndrome, sepsis, cancer).
- The patient's ability to ingest food orally or by tube is impaired (e.g., paralytic ileus, Crohn's disease with obstruction, post-radiation enteritis, severe hyperemesis gravidarum in pregnancy).
- The patient is not interested in or is unwilling to ingest adequate nutrients (e.g., anorexia nervosa, postoperative elderly patients).
- The underlying medical condition precludes being fed orally or by tube (e.g., acute pancreatitis, high enterocutaneous fistula).
- Preoperative and postoperative nutritional needs are prolonged (e.g., extensive bowel surgery).
- Critically-ill patients.

Contraindications of TPN
- Functional and accessible GI tract
- Patient is taking oral diet
- Prognosis does not warrants aggressive nutrition support
- Risk exceeds benefit
- Patient expected to meet needs within 14 days.

Routes
TPN can be administered through central or peripheral IV lines.
- **Central parenteral nutrition:** Delivered via a central venous access with catheter tip located in superior vena cava. This is used if length of therapy is long-term (>7 days)
- **Peripheral parenteral nutrition:** Delivered via a peripheral venous access with catheter tip located outside of the inferior or superior vena cava. This is chosen when expected length of therapy is short-term (<7 days).

Components of TPN
- **Carbohydrates:** Glucose solution, i.e., 5% glucose solution for peripheral nutrition or 50–70% (hypertonic) for central parenteral solution, 60–70% of caloric needs.
- **Amino acid:** Provides 3–15% of TPN calories.
- **Lipids (fat emulsion):** Lipid provide up to 30%, if caloric (energy) needs.
- Vitamins
- Minerals
- Water
- Electrolytes
- **Insulin:** To control blood glucose level (as higher concentration of glucose solution is TPN).
- **Heparin:** To reduce build up of fibrous clots at the catheter tip.

Do's of Total Parenteral Nutrition
- Monitor the laboratory investigation results before administering TPN
- Monitor the cannulation site for displacement of catheter
- Monitor strict intake and output record
- Document the whole procedure
- Severe metabolic and electrolyte abnormalities are prevented by increasing the infusion rate of TPN gradually, starting at a rate of no more than 50% of the energy requirements

Precautions
- Individuals need to tell their doctor if they have any allergies, what medications they are taking, if they are diabetic, have had liver, kidney, heart, lung, or hormonal disorders, and if they are pregnant.
- All these factors can affect the type and amount of TPN required.

Don'ts of Total Parenteral Nutrition
- Do not administer cold solution
- Do not administer any other fluid or medicine through same cannula as TPN is not compatible with any other type of IV solution or medication and must be administered by itself
- Do not obtain blood samples or central venous pressure readings from the same port as TPN infusions
- Do not abruptly discontinue TPN because this may lead to hypoglycemia

Articles
- Patients' prescription chart
- Prescribed bag of parenteral nutrition.
- PN solutions should be removed from refrigeration 1 hour prior to Infusion in order to reach approximate room temperature
- Intravenous infusion stand
- Patients' prescription chart
- PN intravenous administration set
- **Filters:** 0.22 micron for TPN (without fat emulsion) and 3.2 micron for fat emulsion TPN
- Sterile dressing pack
- Sterile gloves
- Mask
- Spirit
- Volumetric pump
- Sodium chloride 0.9% for injection
- Sterile 10 mL syringe.

Steps of Procedure

Preprocedural Steps
- Ensure that the intravenous access has been approved for use and is documented in the medical notes before administering PN.
- To ensure that TPN is not mixed with any other solution while delivering
- A single lumen catheter should be used for the administration of PN. If a multilumen catheter is used, PN should be administered via a lumen kept exclusively for this

purpose and strict aseptic technique implemented when handling this men.
- The greater risk of infection if a line is manipulated more
- Explain and discuss the procedure with the patient/caregiver.
- To ensure that the patient understands the procedure and gives their valid consent
- Before administering any PN consult the patient's prescription chart, check patients identity and ascertain the following:
  - Type of parenteral nutrition (Amino acids or lipids)
  - Drugs to be added if any like heparin or insulin
  - Dose/rate
  - Date and time of administration
  - Route and method of administration
  - Validity of prescription
  - Signature of prescriber
  - Wash hands with soap and water or alcohol based hand rub.
- To prevent contamination of medication and equipment
- Inspect the insertion site to detect any signs of inflammation, infiltration, etc.
- If present, take appropriate action
- Collect the needed equipments for the procedure.

Intraprocedural Steps
- Wash hands with soap and water or with alcohol-based hand rub. To minimize the risk of cross-infection
- Put on mask and sterile gloves. To prevent infection
- Using strict aseptic technique, prepare TPN, mix it and attach tubing (with filter) and flush air from the tubing.
- Hang the bag on infusion stand
- Connect the tubing with volumetric pump so that rate of infusion is controlled
- Check patency of the device with syringe, check that no resistance is met, no pain or discomfort is felt by the patient, no swelling is evident, no leakage occurs around the device and there is a good backflow of blood on aspiration.
- Connect the infusion to the central/peripheral line as ordered. To commence treatment
- Adjust the flow rate as prescribed. To ensure that the correct speed of administration is established
- Remove gloves
- Monitor flow rate and device site frequently. To ensure the flow rate is correct and the patient is comfortable, and to check for signs of infiltration
- Monitor for signs and symptoms of complications related to TPN. To act timely, if complications develop
- Complete daily assessments and monitoring for patient on TPN. To assess and compare changes with earlier readings.

Stopping and Disconnecting the Infusion
- Stop the infusion when all the fluid has been delivered. To ensure that all the prescribed mixture has been delivered.
- Put on sterile gloves. To maintain sterility
- Disconnect the infusion set and clean the injection site of the cap with 2% chlorhexidine swab or spirit swab. To minimize the risk of contamination
- Flush the device with 10 mL of 0.9% sodium chloride. To flush any remaining TPN solution catheter.
- Cover the ports in sterile dressing as per hospital policy. To prevent infection
- Remove gloves. To ensure disposal
- Assist the patient into a comfortable position.

Post-procedural Steps
- Discard waste, placing it in the correct containers. For example, sharps into a designated container. To ensure safe disposal and avoid injury to staff.
- Wash hands
- Documentation on patient's charts

Complications
Technical Complications
- Pneumothorax
- Venous thrombus
- Clot and air embolism.

Metabolic Complications
- Hyperglycemia and hypoglycemia
- Electrolyte imbalance
- Fatty acid deficiency
- Liver toxicity
- Excessive weight gain.

Miscellaneous
- Catheter related blood stream infections and sepsis
- Psychological complications (anxiety, depression, oral craving).

Special Considerations
- Check the patient's baseline vital signs; electrolyte, glucose, and triglyceride levels; weight; and fluid intake and output, and investigate any rapid change in such values.
- To identify signs of infection early, be aware of the patient's recent temperature range.
- Use strict aseptic technique when caring for central venous catheters and peripheral lines.
- Do not use old TPN solution, as evidenced by formation of a thick, dense layer of fat droplets on its surface.
- If the solution appears abnormal in any way, request a replacement or consult physician.
- Never try to catch up with a delayed infusion.

Aftercare
During the time, the catheter is in place, patients and caregivers must be alert to any signs of infection, such as redness, swelling, fever, drainage, or pain.

Risks
- TPN requires close monitoring. Two types of complications can develop. Infection, air in the lung cavity (pneumothorax) and blood clot formation (thrombosis) all can develop as a result of inserting the catheter into a vein.
- Metabolic and fluid imbalances can occur, if the contents of the nutritional fluid are not properly balanced and monitored. The most common metabolic imbalance is hypoglycemia, or low blood sugar, caused by abruptly discontinuing a solution high in sugar.

Hygiene

■ DEFINITION

"Hygiene refers to conditions and practices that help to maintain health and prevent the spread of diseases."
—WHO

Factors Influencing Hygienic Practice

The following factors have to be considered by a nurse while providing nursing care to the patients:

- **General condition of the patient:** On the basis of the general condition of the patient, the nurse assesses the need for providing hygiene care to the patient.
- **Self-care ability:** The type of assistance required in maintaining personal hygiene depends upon the self-care ability of the patient.
- **Age of the patient:** The hygiene care varies according to the age. Infants and children are more dependent on others for their hygiene needs. The adult, adolescent and elderly persons will be able to take care of their hygiene needs to quiet an extent.
- **Educational status:** The educated person will be more aware of the need for maintenance of personal hygiene than the illiterate person.
- **Socioeconomic conditions:** People of low socioeconomic conditions live in poor unhygienic conditions and are less aware of the need for maintaining proper hygienic status.
- **Mentally challenged/physically challenged persons:** They are dependent for meeting their hygiene needs.

■ CARE OF THE SKIN

Bathing a Patient in Bed

Types of Bath

- **Bed bath:** Complete bed bath, partial bed bath, self-help bath. The client can have a complete bed bath or a partial bath.
- **Bathroom bath:** In the bathing room, the clients can take a shower bath or a tub bath. The nurse, while sending the clients for a bath in the bathroom, should keep in mind the safety of the clients.
- **Partial bath (back rub):** The clients who are prone to bedsores, must have their back treated two hourly or more frequently. The back is washed with soap and water, dried and massaged with powder.

Definition

Cleansing the entire body of a dependent patient in bed.

Purposes

- To remove transient microorganisms, body secretions, excretions and dead skin cells.
- To stimulate circulation.
- To produce a feeling of well being.
- To promote relaxation and comfort.
- To improve self-esteem.
- To prevent or eliminate bad odor.
- To clean the body off dirt and bacteria
- To increase elimination through the skin
- To prevent bedsores
- To induce sleep
- To provide comfort to the client
- To relieve fatigue
- To give the client a sense of well being
- To regulate body temperature
- To provide active and passive exercises
- To observe objective symptoms
- To give the nurse an opportunity for health teaching
- To establish an effective nurse-client relationship

Nurse's Responsibility in Giving Bed Bath

- Check the physician's orders to see the specific precautions if any, regarding the positioning and movement of the client.
- Assess the client's need for bathing.
- Assess the client's ability for self care.
- Assess the cardiorespiratory functioning check TPR and BP
- Assess the client's mental state to follow directions.
- Check the client's preference for soap, powder, etc.
- Check the linen and equipment available in the client's unit.
- Check whether the client has taken any meal in the previous 1 hour.

Articles

- Bedpan/urinal
- Basin

- Jugs with hot water and cold water (water of 110° to 115°F (43–45°C) for adults and 100–105°F for children).
- Table or trolley.
- Bath blanket/sheet.
- Clean gloves
- Wash clothes (2)
- Soap
- Towels (2)
- Lotions, powders, deodorants (optional)
- Patient's dress (1 set).

Preparation of the Client and Unit

- Explain the sequence of the procedure to the client and explain how the client can assist you.
- Move the unnecessary items from the work area.
- Place the articles needed conveniently on the bedside table.
- Adjust the height of the bed to the comfortable working of the nurse.
- Bring the client to the edge of the bed and towards the nurse to prevent overreaching.
- Check the room temperature and warm, it if necessary.
- Close the windows, if necessary and put off the fan to prevent draughts.
- Provide privacy by the means of curtains.
- Remove the top bed linen or fanfold them to the foot end of the bed, leaving a sheet or bath blanket over the client. Keep if free at the foot end to allow freedom for the legs.
- Offer bedpan or urinal, if necessary (wash hands).
- Keep the client flat if the condition permits. Remove extra pillows and back rest.
- Remove the personal clothing and cover the client with the bath blanket. If the client has IV, remove the gown from the arm without IV, first, then lower the IV, bottle, slide gown up the IV, tubing and over the IV, container. Rehang the IV, container and check the rate of flow.

Procedure

- Wash hands.
- Mix hot and cold water in the basin and check the temperature on the back of the hand. Fill the basin half full.
- Place the towel under the chin. Wash, rinse and dry the areas in the following sequence—face, neck, farthest arm, near arm, chest, abdomen, back, farthest leg, near leg and pubic region.
- Take a wash cloth, wet it, squeeze the excessive water, make a mitten, apply soap on it and clean the face, ears and neck. Put back the wash cloth in the small bowl provided.
- Take the other wash cloth, rinse it in water. squeeze it, make a mitten and clean the area where soap is applied. Repeat the procedure till the area is cleaned thoroughly. Put back the wash cloth in the basin. Observe the eyes, nose, ears, face etc. for any abnormalities.
- Dry the face with a face towel.
- Place the bath towel lengthwise under the farthest arm. Clean and dry the farthest arm as described above. Pay special attention to axilla. Support the arm at the joints.
Note: Observe the skin and look for any palpable lymph nodes in the axilla.
- Repeat the procedure on the near arm.
- Place the basin on the bath towel at the edge of the bed and let the client place hands in the basin. Rinse and dry thoroughly, paying particular attention to the skin between fingers and nails.
- Place one corner of the bath towel over one shoulder and the opposite corner folded back and placed on the other shoulder. Both corners are fixed under the back of the client. Fold bath blanket down to the level of the umbilicus.
- With the left hand raise the towel and the right hand mitted, cleanse the chest as before. Replace the towel over the chest between wash, rinse and dry periods. Remember to wash under the breasts.
- While the towel remaining on the chest, fold back the bath blanket down to the pubic region, clean and dry the abdomen. Give special attention to the cleanliness of the umbilicus and creased folds of abdomen.
- Remove the towel and put hack the bath blanket and cover the client completely
- Change water. The waste water is discarded into the bucket.
- Turn the client to a prone or side-lying position with the face away from the nurse. Make sure that the client will not fall to the ground.
- Fold back the bath blanket from the shoulder to the thighs and tuck the edges securely around the thighs. Place the towel over the bed, close to the back, lengthwise.
- Wash, rinse and dry the back from the shoulders to the buttocks with brisk circular movements. After drying the back give a thorough back rub with methylated spirit and powder. Pay particular attention to the pressure points.
- Put on the upper garments and cover him with the bath blanket.
- Change water.
- Expose the farthest leg. Place the bath towel lengthwise under the leg. Flex the knee so that the sole of the foot is supporting on the mattress. Place the basin on the towel and keep the foot in the basin. Wash and rinse the thigh and leg with the wash clothes. Clean the foot under the water paying particular attention to the toes and nails.
- Remove the basin and dry the entire leg and repeat the procedure on the near leg.
- Wash the pubic area. It can be done by the T client if he is capable. If he is not able to do it for himself, the nurse does it for him, making sure that the entire area is washed thoroughly and dried.

After Care of the Client and Articles

- Replace the client's personal clothing.
- Straighten the bed linen.
- Remove the bath blanket and put it for washing.
- Change the bed linen if needed.
- Offer a hot drink if permitted.
- Cut short the finger nails and the toe nails. The nail cuttings should be received in the kidney tray.
- Comb the hair and arrange the hair.
- Position the client for comfort and proper alignment.
- Take all articles to the utility room. Disinfect the bath basin and the wash clothes. Send the soiled linen to the laundry.

- Put back all the articles in their proper places after cleaning. Personal articles are replaced into the bedside table.
- Wash hands. Record the procedure in the nurse's record with time and date and the type of bath. Record any abnormalities observed.
- Take the opportunity to teach the client or his relatives about personal hygiene.

Special Considerations
- Obtain assistance if required in case of helpless/unconscious patient.
- If patient is obese or cannot move in bed, nurse may move from one side of the bed to the other side to ensure good body mechanics.
- Assess patient's general condition before giving bath. If unstable, refrain from giving bath.
- Bath should not be given immediately after food because it interferes with the process of digestion.

Scientific Principles of Bed Bath
Anatomy and Physiology
- The skin is a soft flexible, membranous covering and is continuous at the natural orifices with the mucous membranes.
- Skin is made up of two layers the epidermis or surface layer, and dermis or true skin.
- The epidermis is composed of stratified squamous epithelium formed in four layers.
- The epidermis varies in thickness in different parts of the body
- The dermis or corium is an underlying layer of connective tissue and contains many glands, blood vessels, nerves and the roots of hairs.
- Sebaccous glands and sweat glands are found in the skin.
- Sebaceous glands secrete oil or sebum. It is an oily, yellowish, semifluid substance.
- The sebaceous glands are located near the hair follicles and are found on all parts of the body except the palms, soles and the last phalanges of the fingers and toes.
- Sweat glands are numerous, especially on the palms and soles, on the forehead and in the axilla.
- The sweat glands also function as excretory organs.
- The activity of all these glands may be influenced by external heat, dyspnea, muscular exercise, strong emotions and the actions of various drugs.
- The skin is provided with variety of nerves, e.g., sense of heat, cold, pain and pressure.
- Bathing stimulate nerve endings and creates a sense of well-being.
- Skin protects the underlying tissues against the invasion of microorganisms and mechanical injury.
- Skin functions as an organ of secretion, excretion, sense organ, and body temperature regulation
- Absorption through the skin is rapid if the solution is above 100.40°F.
- Absorption takes place to the hair follicles.

Microbiology
- The intact skin is impassable barrier to microorganisms
- Many bacteria are found normally on the skin between the superficial horney cells, but they have little invasive power.
- *Staphylococcus albus, Staphylococcus viridans*, gamma type streptococci, diphtheroids, gram-positive bacilli and many varieties of saprophytic fungi are isolated from normal healthy skin.
- These microorganisms enter into the skin when there is a chemical or mechanical injury to the skin.
- Perspiration helps to protect the body from invasion of bacteria.
- Bacteria and yeasts decrease rapidly on dry healthy skin.
- The skin contains the layer of oil, so water cannot wet the skin.
- Soap lowers the surface tension of water and thus penetrates the oil.
- Bacteria and yeasts grow well in moist areas so that, it is necessary to dry the skin thoroughly.
- The nurse must wash her hands before and after the procedure to prevent cross infection.
- Nurse should hold her head at a proper distance from the patient's face to avoid transmission of by droplet infection.

Physics and Chemistry
- Constant pressure of the skin against the mattress may deplete the blood supply at points of uneven pressure so much as to cause injury to the tissue.
- The amount of pressure applied to the surface of the mattress depends upon the weight of the patient and the area of the mattress that he covers.
- An air or sponge rubber mattress produces more even pressure against all parts of the skin.
- Rubber is a good conductor of heat. The rubber sheet prevents evaporation of moisture, and the patient feels hot and comfortable.
- Water is a good conductor of heat, so the heat may be conveyed to the skin by the application of the warm water.
- Friction is reduced by moisture, by a lubricant or by a smooth substance, such as a powder
- Soap lowers the surface tension of water and helps it to unite quickly with the fat and debris on the skin
- Soap has a high capillarity, so that it spreads readily over a surface
- Before starting the sponge the patient should be moved to the working side of the bed to avoid strain and fatigue.
- When carrying the basin, support it by placing the palms flat around the side, use hand and arm muscle to lessen strain.
- Sweat is a watery or fatty clear fluid with a low specific gravity and a faintly acid in reaction.
- The acidity of the sweat is a protection against bacterial infection, chief organic constituent of sweat urea.
- Sweat with high sugar content is an excellent culture medium for microorganisms.
- The skin is a large reservoir of glycogen.
- Sebum contains remnants of epithelial cells, some inorganic salts, fats, soaps and cholesterol.
- Soap acts by lowering surface tension of water which aids in emulsification of fats.
- Powder is used on the skin to keep it dry.

Pharmacology
- The drugs used in the daily skin care are alcohol, powder and a lubricant.
- Alcohol content in solution hardens the skin.
- Skin antiseptics and astringents may be powder or liquid.

Psychology
- Explain what you are going to do.
- Provide privacy throughout the procedure.
- It gives psychological comfort to the patient.
- Talk to the patient while sponging, so that he will be at ease.

BACK CARE

Definition
"Back care means cleaning and massaging back, paying special attention to pressure points."

"Back massage is a scientific form of massaging the back using different massaging strokes to provide cutaneous stimulation and thus promote comfort."

Purpose
- To improve circulation to the back
- To refresh the mood and feeling
- To relieve fatigue, pain and stress
- To induce sleep and relieve insomnia
- To relieve muscle tension
- To stimulate blood circulation
- To assess condition of skin
- To promote physical and mental relaxation
- To prevent pressure sore
- To provide an opportunity to observe the condition of patient's back
- To stimulate and relax muscles
- Specially back massage provides comfort and relaxes the client
- It facilitates the physical stimulation to the skin and the emotional relaxation

Indications
- Bed ridden patients.
- Patients with poor personal hygiene
- Malnourished patient
- Obese patients
- Very thin patients
- Unconscious and serious patients
- Paralyzed patients
- Edematous patients
- Patient with loss of movement

Principles
- Hand washing before the procedure
- Proper explanation and privacy should be maintained
- Back care should be given as a part of morning and evening care and when necessary according the condition and need of the individual patient
- When the skin is greasy, moist and about to break the powder should be used to reduce friction
- When giving back rub, use more pressure on upward strokes towards the head and less pressure on the downward strokes
- The nurse must use good body mechanism while doing procedure
- Keep the patient in proper position
- Consider cultural preferences of patient.

Contraindication
- Patient's with rib fracture
- Burns
- Immediate post operative period
- Spinal injuries
- Surgeries on back

Articles required
- Screen
- **A clean trolley containing:** Basin (medium steel bowl) with warm water: (2)
- **Tray containing:**
  - *Soap with soap dish:* 1
  - *Sponge cloth:* 2, i.e., 1 for wetting the back, 1 for rinsing
  - *Mackintosh:* 1
  - *Big towel:* 1 for covering a Mackintosh
  - Oil/powder (according to the skin condition)

Procedure
- Check the patient's identification and condition
- Explain to the client about the purpose and the procedure
- Wash hands with soap and water
- Assemble all articles required
- Put all required articles to the bed side and set up
- Close all windows and doors and put the screen
- Adjust light, temperature and switch off the fan
- Position the patient in the prone or lateral/side lying or Sim's or prone position with back towards you and observe it
- Expose back, shoulders, upper arms and buttocks and cover the rest of the body
- Place the Mackintosh and towel close to the patient's back or under the back
- Use warm water 105–110°F
- Wash/wet the patient's back thoroughly from cervical spine to the coccyx with the help of sponge towel
- Apply soap on your hands and then rub the back in circular motion over the shoulder, length of the back and buttocks with special attention to bony prominences (both scapulae, right and left iliac crests)
- Clean the soap with sponge clothes

1. Effleurage (Fig. 4.1)
- Apply back rub lotion/oil and apply hands first to sacral area massaging in the circular motion.
- Effleurage is applied in an upwards direction towards lymph nodes.
- Stroke upward from buttocks to shoulders
- Continue using light pressure in one smooth firm stroke from upper back to arms

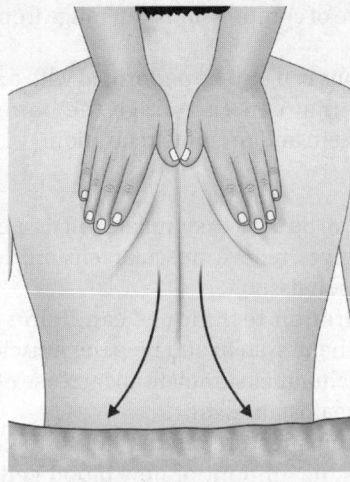

Fig. 4.1: Effleurage.

- Massage over scapula with smooth, firm stroke
- Then move down without circular motion along sides of back, down to iliac crests
- Do not take the hands off from patient's back till the end of the procedure
- Continue for at least 1 minute
- Effleurage must always follow the direction of venous return back to the heart and the direction of lymphatic drainage towards the nearest group of lymphatic nodes.
- Effleurage increases blood circulation towards the heart, using long strokes to help increase temperature of the soft tissues.
- Effleurage is effective to stimulate the lymphatic system.

2. Kneading (Petrissage) (Fig. 4.2)

- Knead gently by grasping tissue between the thumb and fingers.
- Knead upward along one side of spine from buttocks to shoulders and around the nape of the neck
- Knead downward towards the sacrum, repeat along other side of the back
- This activity helps to improve blood circulation to the tissue

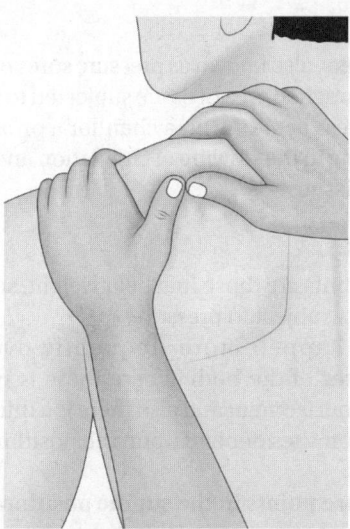

Fig. 4.2: Kneading (Petrissage).

3. Tapotement/Cupping

- Perform tapotement (tapping movements with medial and lateral aspects of hands on side of spine from sacral region upwards)
- It is a massage technique in which local suction is a created on the skin by making the hands cup shaped.
- It increases blood circulation and is effective to release tight muscles, fascia (band of connective tissue) and reduce high tone (tension of muscles).
- By creating suction and vacuum pressure, it can soften tight muscles and tone, loosen adhesions and lift up restrictive connective tissues.
- The specific technique brings hydration and blood flow to the body's tissues.
- It can be used to move deep inflammation to the skin surface for release and drain excess fluid and toxins by opening lymphatic pathways.

Five types of tapotement:
1. Beating (closed fist lightly hitting area), **(Fig. 4.3)**
2. Slapping (use of fingers to gently slap), **(Fig. 4.4)**
3. Hacking (use the edge of hand on pinky finger side) **(Fig. 4.5)**
4. Cupping (make your hand look like a cup and gently tap) **(Fig. 4.6)**
5. Pounding (fist in circular motion) **(Fig. 4.7)**

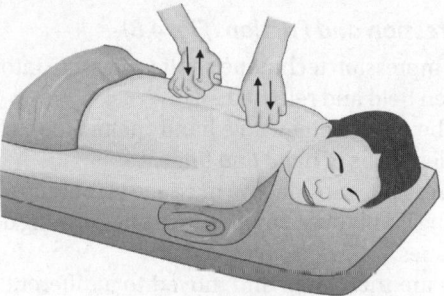

Fig. 4.3: Beating.

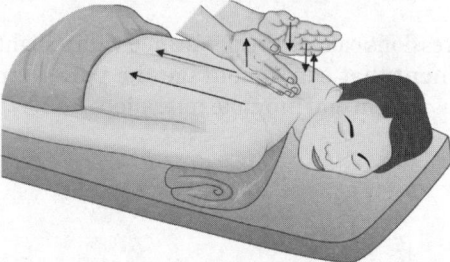

Fig. 4.4: Slapping.

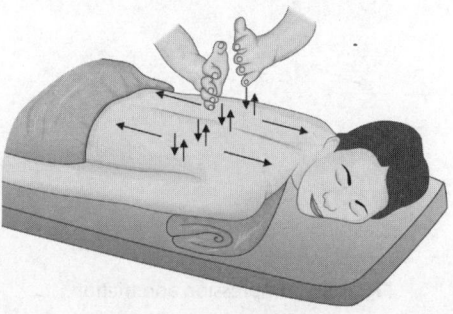

Fig. 4.5: Hacking.

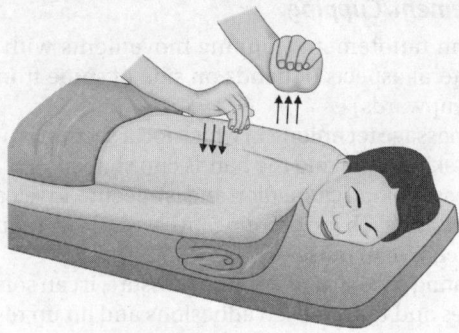

Fig. 4.6: Cupping.

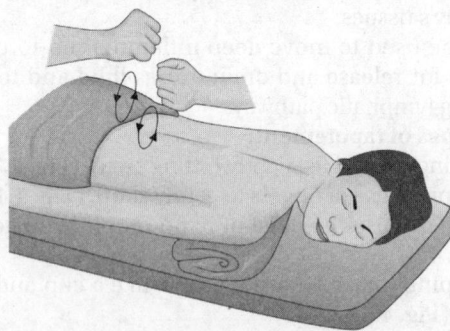

Fig. 4.7: Pounding

4. Compression and Friction (Fig. 4.8)

- The compression technique applies pressure into muscles, it is then held and released.
- It can be done using whole hand (palm side), closed fist, knuckles, heals of hand and fingers
- Compression is an effective massage technique performed by laying hands over a muscle area and pushing down onto the tissues.
- Hands are then lifted and moved to a different area and then repeated.
- The pressure of compressions can range from light to very deep.
- Compressions can also be performed with a slight rocking movement that can encourage the parasympathetic nervous system and promote relaxation.

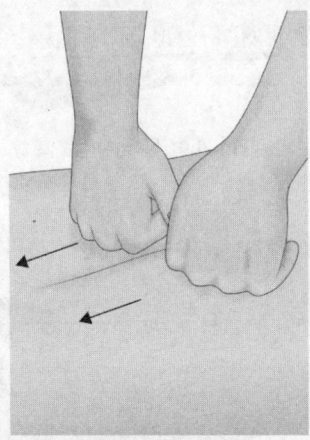

Fig. 4.8: Compression and friction.

- The pressure of compressions can range from light to very deep.
- Compressions can also be performed with a slight rocking movement that can encourage the parasympathetic nervous system and promote relaxation

5. Vibrations

- Vibrations can be used to stimulate soft tissues in the body, stimulate nerves, relieve muscular tension, decrease stress and loosen soft tissue.
- Lighter vibration techniques can help stimulate the parasympathetic system and help the muscles relax.
- Vibration techniques stimulate an increase of temperature by friction against the skin.
- Vibration helps restore circulation to the muscles and it increases the amount of new blood cells to the area stimulating the healing process.
- End the massage with long stroking movements for an additional 1 minute with total time of 3–5 minutes
- Wipe excess lubricant to back as required
- Remove Mackintosh and towel
- Help to put on cloths and tighten the bed, if needed
- Keep the patient in comfortable position and open curtains
- Educate to the patient and family about the importance of cleanliness, dryness, massage and position change
- Replace all equipment in proper place
- Record in the patient's chart including date, time and patient's general and back condition
- Report to the senior staffs if found any abnormalities

Special Considerations

- For patients with history of hypertension and dysrhythmias assess pulse and blood pressure as massage may cause stimulation of autonomic nervous system, which increases heart rate, and BP
- Consider cultural preferences of patient. Some cultures may consider it as an invasion of personal space.
- Do not give massage if any discoloration of skin is present.

DECUBITUS ULCER/PRESSURE SORE/BEDSORE

Definition

Decubitus ulcers, also known as pressure sores or decubiti, are ulcerated or sloughed area of tissue subjected to pressure from lying on mattress or sitting on a chair for a prolonged period of time resulting in the slowing of circulation and finally death (necrosis) of tissues.

Common Sites

- Pressure points are those that bear weight, so that the skin over them is subject to pressure.
- This may happen more frequently over the bony prominences of the body where there is no rich blood supply or nourishment and also there is a thin layer of skin.
- The common sites depend upon the position of the client in bed
- **The pressure points in the supine position (Fig. 4.9):**
  - Back of the head (occiput)
  - Scapula

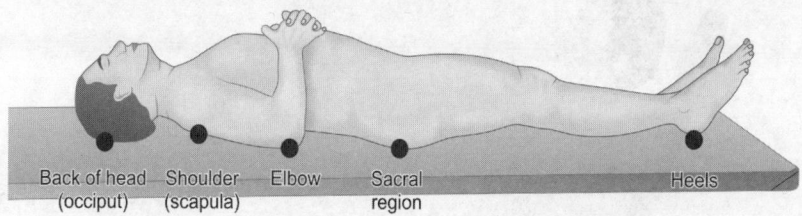

Fig. 4.9: Sites prone to pressure ulcer in supine position.

- Elbow
- Sacral region,
- Heels.

❖ **In a side-lying position (Fig. 4.10):**
- Ears
- Acromion process of the shoulder
- Ribs and elbow
- Greater trochanter of the hip
- Medial and lateral condyles of the knee
- Malleolus of the ankle joint.

❖ **In a prone position (Fig. 4.11):**
- Ears, cheek
- Acromion process
- Elbow
- Breasts (in the females)
- Genitalia (in the males)
- Knees toes.

❖ **In sitting position (Fig. 4.12):**
- Scapula
- Ilium
- Ischial tuberosities

- Back of knee
- Heel

Stages

The stages of pressure ulcers (decubitus ulcers) are (**Fig. 4.13**):

Stage-I

This is the mildest stage the pressure sore only affect the upper most layer of skin.

Symptoms

❖ Pain, burning or itching
❖ The spots are different from the surrounding skin (firmer or softer, warmer or colder)
❖ It could also be seen as red area (erythematous) on the skin which does not get lighter, when pressed this shows lack of blood supply in the area.

Interventions

It consists of help and instruction of the client:
❖ Relieve pressure by changing position using foam pads, pillows or mattresses.

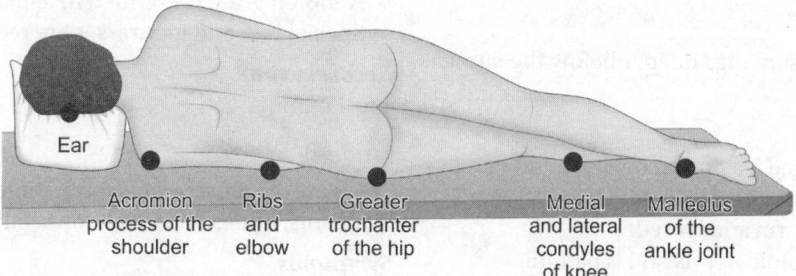

Fig. 4.10: Sites prone to pressure ulcer in side-lying position.

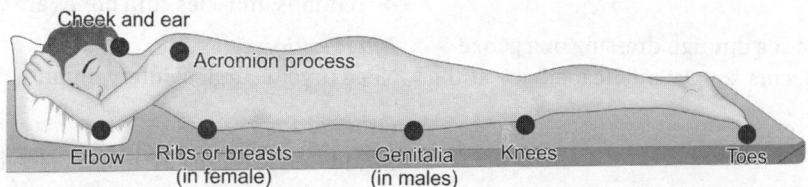

Fig. 4.11: Sites prone to pressure ulcers in prone position.

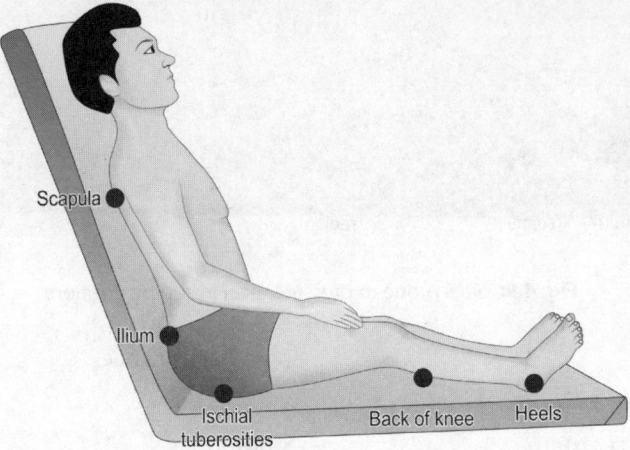

Fig. 4.12: Sites prone to pressure ulcer in sitting position.

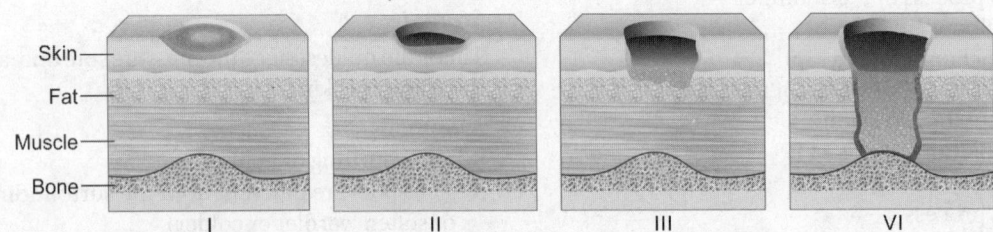

Fig. 4.13: Stages of pressure ulcers.

- Eat high protein diet with sufficient amount of vitamin 'A' and 'C' and minerals such as iron and zinc.
- Drink plenty of water
- Wash sore with mild soap and water and dry it gently

Recovery time
2–3 days

Stage-II
This happens when the sore digs deeper below the surface of the skin.

Symptoms
- Skin integrity penetrated leaving an open wound or a pus filled blister forms
- The area is swollen, warm and/or red.
- A sore may ooze clear fluid or pus and is painful.

Interventions
- Same as stage-I
- Wash with saline or pure water as it an open wound and prone to infection.
- Dry gently and apply a see through dressing or a gauze
- If signs of infection occurs sought medical advice at the earliest.

Recovery time
3 days to 3 weeks

Stage-III
The sore has gone through the second layer of skin into the fat tissue.

Symptoms
- The sore looks like a crater and may have a bad odour
- It has signs of infection, red edges, pus, odor, heat and/or drainage.
- The tissue in/or around the sore in darkened as if died.

Interventions
- Require medical care
- Debridement by a surgeon and dressing may needed
- Antibiotics are prescribed to fight infections
- Special bed and mattresses are required

Recovery time
1 to 4 months

Stage-IV
These are the most serious sores, some may affect the muscles, ligaments, bones and other connective tissues

Symptoms
- Deep large sores
- Skin turned dark
- Prominent sign of infections
- Tendons, muscles, and bones are visible

Intervention
Need urgent surgical intervention

Other stages
In addition to these four main stages, there are two additional stages:
1. **Unstageable:** When bottom of the score cannot be distinguished and debridement is required for distinguishing.
2. **Suspected deep tissue injury (SDTI):** This is when the surface of the score shows signs of 1 or 2 stage but has underling tissue damage equivalent to the 3 and 4 stages.

Solutions used in the treatment of ulcers:
- **Insulin:** Few drops of insulin in the sore promote healing
- **Hydrogen peroxide:** It is used for cleaning purpose alone saline solution.
- Granulating sugar can be filled in the cavity to assist healing.
- Waterproofing ointments, such as zinc oxide can be used to prevent infections.

Causes of Pressure Sores
- Direct or immediate causes
- **Pressure:**
  - Pressure is considered to be primary cause of the pressure sore.
  - In a sick person, the areas of tissue resting against the mattress are vulnerable areas.
  - The pressure in these areas causes depletion of blood supply with the failure of circulation to the weight bearing area resulting in the tissue damage.
  - The pressure over these areas is increased in the following conditions:
  - When there is lumps and creases on the bed
  - Incorrect positioning of the body.
  - Infrequent change of position.
- **Friction:**
  - Friction of the skin with a rough or hard surface can cause tissue damage.
  - Contact with the rough surfaces of the bed, wrinkles on the bed clothes, hard surfaces of the plaster casts and splints, presence of foreign bodies on the bed (e.g., bread crumbs, orange peelings), careless handling of bedpan, pulling sheets under the clients, etc., are frequent causes of friction which cause tissue damage.
  - Friction is also caused due to the rough sponge clothes and prolonged massage without lubricant.
- **Moisture:**
  - The skin contact with moisture for a period of time can lead to maceration of the skin.
  - Clients who are sweating profusely, with incontinence of n urine and stools are liable to pressure sores.
- **Presence of pathogenic organism:** Lack of cleanliness harbors pathogenic organisms and infection settles on the skin.
- **Predisposing causes:**
  - Impaired circulation
  - Lowered vitality
  - Emaciation
  - Obesity
  - Edema

Clients Susceptible to Pressure Sores
- Acutely-ill clients, whose general condition is rapidly deteriorating.
- Elderly bedridden clients, who make very little movements in bed.
- Obese clients.
- Very thin and emaciated clients, having very little subcutaneous tissue to pad the bony prominences
- Sedated clients, who have suffered spinal cord injuries.
- Paralyzed clients, who have suffered spinal cord injuries, e.g., clients with paraplegia, hemiplegia, and quadriplegia.
- These clients are not able to make movements in the bed and very often they have incontinence of urine.
- Neurologic clients with lack of sensation that they cannot feel any irritation of the skin.
- Edematous clients especially those with edema of the sacrum and buttocks.
- Malnourished clients with protein and vitamin deficiencies.
- Agitated clients in restraints.
- Clients on complete bed rest or with limited movements, e.g., clients with fractures, plaster casts, cardiac diseases
- Surgical clients with limited movements.
- Clients with hyperpyrexia who sweat profusely.
- Client's with incontinence of urine and stool
- Clients with excessive bodily discharges or drainage from the wounds
- Diabetic clients.

Prevention of Pressure Sore
- Identification of clients who are particularly prone to the development of decubitis ulcer.
- Daily examination of the decubitus prone clients for redness, discoloration or blister on the pressure points and they should be reported and treated immediately.
- Keep the clients clean and dry.
- Change the position of the client every a hours so that another body surface bears weight.
- Use a bed cradle to take off the weight of the bed linen of the client, so as to enable him to move in bed with ease.
- Keep the client's skin well lubricated to prevent cracking by using powder.
- Protect the damaged skin. Damaged skin can be further irritated and macerated by urine. feces, sweat, etc.
- Provide the client with adequate fluids and with a nourishing diet that is high in protein and vitamins
- Attend to the pressure points as often as necessary to stimulate circulation.
- The clients who are liable to bed sores must have their back treated two hourly or more often.
- The back is washed with soap and warm water, dried and massaged with powder.
- Avoid using excess alcohol for back rub because it dries the skin and cause tissue damage.
- Attending to the back alone is not sufficient but should include the pressure areas at the iliac crests, ankles, heels, elbows and other pressure points.
- Call assistance and lift the client before giving and taking bedpans. If the bedpan is chipped, care should be taken to pad the bedpan to avoid friction.
- Provide a smooth, firm and wrinkle free bed on which the client can take rest.
- Use special mattresses and beds to decrease the pressure on body parts, e.g., air mattresses, water mattresses, etc.
- Cut short the finger nails of the clients to avoid scratching on the skin.

- Use adequate amount of cotton under splints and plaster casts to prevent friction
- Use the comfort devices to take off the pressure from the pressure points, e.g., air cushions, cotton rings, etc.
- Avoid using rubber rings since they compress the area of the skin beneath them, decreasing blood supply around the pressure points.
- Encourage the clients to move in bed as far as it is allowed.
- Change the linen as soon as they become wet. The back and buttocks also must be washed, dried and rubbed with powder. After each urination and defecation the back must be attended.
- Teach the clients and their relatives the hygienic care of the skin.

BRADEN SCALE

- The Braden scale (is a scale that measures the risk of developing pressure ulcers. The scale consists of six subscales that reflect determinants of pressure (sensory perception, activity and mobility) and factors influencing tissue tolerance (moisture, nutrition and friction and shear) **(Tables 4.1 and 4.2)**. Five of the six subscales are rated from 1 (least favourable) to 4 (most favorable); the friction and shear subscale is rated from 1–3. To determine the risk of developing pressure ulcers each subscale has to be rated in reflecting the condition of the patient best.
- The sensory perception subscale has two components, one of measuring level of consciousness and the other involving cutaneous sensation. In those instances in which a person exhibits both decreased level of consciousness and diminishing cutaneous sensation, the condition which results in a lower rating should be used. Although most of the other indicators do not clearly consist of several parts, more than one aspect may be included. In these cases the following rule applies: When in doubt, choose the answer with the lowest score.
- The sum score of the subscales (with a minimum of 6 and a maximum of 23) determines the risk of developing pressure ulcers.
- A low total score indicates a high risk of developing pressure ulcers; a high total score indicates a low risk of developing pressure ulcers.
    - At risk = 15
    - Moderate risk = 13 –14
    - High risk = 10 –12
    - Very high risk = 9 or below

Sensory Perception
Ability to respond meaningfully to pressure related discomfort

1. Completely Limited
Unresponsive (does not moan, flinch or gasp) to painful stimuli, due to diminished level of consciousness or sedation. OR limited ability to feel pain over most of body surface.

2. Very Limited
Responds only to painful stimuli. Cannot communicate discomfort except by moaning or restlessness

3. Slightly Limited
Responds to verbal commands, but cannot always communicate discomfort or need to be turned OR has some sensory impairment which limits ability to feel pain or discomfort in 1 or 2 extremities.

4. No Impairment
Responds to verbal commands. Had no sensory deficit which would limit ability to feel or voice pain or discomfort.

Moisture
Degree to which skin is exposed to moisture

1. Constantly Moist
Skin is kept moist almost constantly by perspiration, urine, etc. Dampness is detected every time patient is moved or turned.

2. Very Moist
Skin is often, but not always moist. Linen must be changed at least once a shift.

3. Occasionally Moist
Skin is occasionally moist, requiring an extra linen change approximately once a day.

4. Rarely Moist
Skin is usually dry. Linen only requires changing at routine intervals.

Activity
Degree of physical activity

1. Bedfast
Confined to bed.

TABLE 4.1: Braden scale.

Sensory perception		Moisture		Activity		Mobility		Nutrition		Friction and shear	
No impairment	4	Rarely moist	4	Walks frequently	4	No limitations	4	Excellent	4		
Slightly limited	3	Occasionally moist	3	Walks occasionally	3	Slightly limited	3	Adequate	3	No apparent problem	3
Very limited	2	Very moist	2	Chair bound	2	Very limited	2	Probably inadequate	2	Potential problem	2
Completely limited	1	Constantly moist	1	Bedbound	1	Completely immobile	1	Very poor	1	Problem	1

TABLE 4.2: Braden scale for predicting pressure sore risk.

					DATE OF ASSESS ➡	1	2	3	4
SEVERE RISK: Total score ≤ 9 **HIGH RISK:** Total score 10-12 **MODERATE RISK:** Total score 13-14 **MILD RISK:** Total score 15-18									
RISK FACTOR	**SCORE/DESCRIPTION**								
SENSORY PERCEPTION Ability to respond meaningfully to pressure-related discomfort	**1. COMPLETELY LIMITED** – Unresponsive (does not moan, flinch, or grasp) to painful stimuli, due to diminished level of consciousness or sedation, OR limited ability to feel pain over most of body surface.	**2. VERY LIMITED** – Responds only to painful stimuli. Cannot communicate discomfort except by moaning or restlessness, OR has a sensory impairment which limits the ability to feel pain or discomfort over ½ of body.	**3. SLIGHTLY LIMITED** – Responds to verbal commands but cannot always communicate discomfort or need to be turned, OR has some sensory impairment which limits ability to feel pain or discomfort in 1 or 2 extremities.	**4. NO IMPAIRMENT** – Responds to verbal commands. Has no sensory deficit which would limit ability to feel or voice pain or discomfort.					
MOISTURE Degree to which skin is exposed to moisture	**1. CONSTANTLY MOIST** – Skin is kept moist almost constantly by perspiration, urine, etc. Dampness is detected every time patient is moved or turned.	**2. OFTEN MOIST** – Skin is often but not always moist. Linen must be changed at least once a shift.	**3. OCCASIONALLY MOIST** – Skin is occasionally moist, requiring an extra linen change approximately once a day.	**4. RARELY MOIST** – Skin is usually dry; linen only requires changing at routine intervals.					
ACTIVITY Degree of physical activity	**1. BEDFAST** – Confined to bed.	**2. CHAIRFAST** – Ability to walk severely limited or nonexistent. Cannot bear own weight and/or must be assisted into chair or wheelchair.	**3. WALKS OCCASIONALLY** – Walks occasionally during day, but for very short distances, with or without assistance. Spends majority of each shift in bed or chair.	**4. WALKS FREQUENTLY** – Walks outside the room at least twice a day and inside room at least once every 2 hours during waking hours.					
MOBILITY Ability to change and control body position	**1. COMPLETELY IMMOBILE** – Does not make even slight changes in body or extremity position without assistance.	**2. VERY LIMITED** – Makes occasional slight changes in body or extremity position but unable to make frequent or significant changes independently.	**3. SLIGHTLY LIMITED** – Makes frequent though slight changes in body or extremity position independently.	**4. NO LIMITATIONS** – Makes major and frequent changes in position without assistance.					
NUTRITION Usual food intake pattern [1]NPO: Nothing by mouth. [2]IV: Intravenously. [3]TPN: Total parenteral nutrition.	**1. VERY POOR** – Never eats a complete meal. Rarely eats more than 1/3 of any food offered. Eats 2 servings or less of protein (meat or dairy products) per day. Takes fluids poorly. Does not take a liquid dietary supplement, OR is NPO[1] and/or maintained on clear liquids or IV[2] for more than 5 days.	**2. PROBABLY INADEQUATE** – Rarely eats a complete meal and generally eats only about ½ of any food offered. Protein intake includes only 3 servings of meat or dairy products per day. Occasionally will take a dietary supplement OR receives less than optimum amount of liquid diet or tube feeding.	**3. ADEQUATE** – Eats over half of most meals. Eats a total of 4 servings of protein (meat, dairy products) each day. Occasionally refuses a meal, but will usually take a supplement if offered, OR is on a tube feeding or TPN[3] regimen, which probably meets most of nutritional needs.	**4. EXCELLENT** – Eats most of every meal. Never refuses a meal. Usually eats a total of 4 or more servings of meat and dairy products. Occasionally eats between meals. Does not require supplementation.					
FRICTION AND SHEAR	**1. PROBLEM** – Requires moderate to maximum assistance in moving. Complete lifting without sliding against sheets is impossible. Frequently slides down in bed or chair, requiring frequent repositioning with maximum assistance. Spasticity, contractures, or agitation leads to almost constant friction.	**2. POTENTIAL PROBLEM** – Moves feebly or requires minimum assistance. During a move, skin probably slides to some extent against sheets, chair, restraints, or other devices. Maintains relatively good position in chair or bed most of the time but occasionally slides down.	**3. NO APPARENT PROBLEM** – Moves in bed and in chair independently and has sufficient muscle strength to lift up completely during move. Maintains good position in bed or chair at all times.						
TOTAL SCORE	Total score of 12 or less represents HIGH RISK								

ASSESS	DATE	EVALUATOR SIGNATURE/TITLE	ASSESS.	DATE	EVALUATOR SIGNATURE/TITLE
1	/ /		3	/ /	
2	/ /		4	/ /	

NAME-Last	First	Middle	Attending Physician	Record No.	Room/Bed

2. Chairfast
Ability to walk severely limited or non-existent. Cannot bear own weight and/or must be assisted into chair or wheelchair.

3. Walks Occasionally
Walks occasionally during day, but for very short distances, with/without assistance. Spends majority of each shift in bed or chair.

4. Walks Frequently
Walks outside the room at least twice a day and inside room at least once every 2 hours during waking hours.

Mobility
Ability to change and control body position

1. Completely Immobile
Does not make even slight changes in body or extremity position without assistance.

2. Very Limited
Makes occasional slight changes in body or extremity position but unable to make frequent or significant changes independently.

3. Slightly Limited
Makes frequent though slight changes in body or extremity position independently.

4. No Limitations
Makes major and frequent changes in position without assistance.

Nutrition
Usual food intake pattern

1. Very Poor
Never eats a complete meal. Rarely eats more than 1/3 of any food offered. Eats 2 servings or less of protein per day. Takes fluids poorly. Does not take a liquid dietary supplement. OR is NBM and/or maintained or clear liquids or IVs for more than 5 days.

2. Probably Inadequate
Rarely eats a complete meal and generally eats only about ½ of any food offered. Eats only 3 servings of protein per day. Occasionally will take a dietary supplement. OR receives less than optimum amount of liquid diet or tube feeding.

3. Adequate
Eats over half of most meals. Eats a total of 4 servings of protein each day. Occasionally will refuse a meal, but will usually take a supplement if offered. OR is on a tube feeding or TPN regimen which probably meets most of nutritional needs.

4. Excellent
Eats most of every meal. Never refuses a meal. Usually eats a total of 4 or more servings of protein per day. Occasionally eats between meals. Does not require supplementation.

Friction and Shear
Friction and Shear

1. Problem
Requires moderate to maximum assistance in moving. Complete lifting without sliding against sheets is impossible. Frequently slides down bed or chair, requiring frequent repositioning with maximum assistance. Spasticity, contractures or agitation lead to almost constant friction.

2. Potential Problem
Moves feebly or requires minimum assistance. During a move, skin probably slides to some extent against sheets or other surfaces. Maintains relatively good position in chair or bed most of the time, but occasionally slides down.

3. No apparent Problem
Moves in bed and in chair independently and has sufficient muscle strength to lift up completely during move. Maintains good position in bed or chair at all times.

■ THE NORTON PRESSURE SORE

- ❖ The Norton Scoring system, shown below, and created in England in 1962, has been the first pressure sore risk evaluation scale to be created, back in 1962, and for this it is now criticized in the wake of the results of modern research. Its ease of use, however, makes it still widely used today.
- ❖ To evaluate the Norton Rating for a certain patient look at the tables below and add up the values beside each parameter which apply to the patient. The total sum is the Norton Rating (NR) for that patient and may vary from 20 (minimum risk) to 5 (maximum risk) **(Table 4.3)**.

TABLE 4.3: The norton rating for pressure sore.

Physical condition	Good	4
	Fair	3
	Poor	2
	Very bad	1
Mental condition	Alert	4
	Apathetic	3
	Confused	2
	Stuporous	1
Activity	Ambulant	4
	Walks with help	3
	Chairbound	2
	Bedfast	1
Mobility	Full	4
	Slightly impaired	3
	Very limited	2
	Immobile	1
Incontinence	None	4
	Occasional	3
	Usually urinary	2
	Urinary and fecal	1

- (Indicatively, a Norton rating below 9 means very high risk, 10-13 means high risk, 14-17 medium risk and above 18 means low risk)
- Greater than 18 low risk
- Between 18 and 14 medium risk
- Between 14 and 10 high risk
- Lesser than 10 very high risk

PERFORMING NAIL AND FOOT CARE

Definition

"Nail care in the nursing interventions classification, defined as promotion of clean, neat, attractive nails and prevention of skin lesions related to improper care of nails."

Purposes

- To keep the feet clean and dry.
- To teach the patient proper way to inspect all surfaces of feet and hands for lesions, dryness or signs of infection.
- To trim nails and keep them short to prevent injury.
- To prevent accumulation of dirt and microorganisms underneath the nails.

Articles

- Wash basin.
- Washcloth.
- Bath or face towel.
- Nail cutter with a nail file.
- Warm water.
- Soap in soap dish.
- Body lotion.
- Clean disposable gloves.
- Paper bag/kidney tray.
- A bowl with cotton swabs.
- Bowl with antiseptic solution.
- Bowl with cotton swabs soaked in antiseptic solution (optional: for diabetic and unconscious patients).

Procedures

- Inspect all surfaces of fingers, toes, feet and nails. Pay particular attention to areas of dryness, inflammation and cracking. Also inspect areas between toes, heels and soles of feet.
- Assess color and temperature of toes, feet and fingers. Assess capillary refill of nails, palpate radial and ulnar pulses of each hand and dorsalis pedis pulse of feet, note character of pulses.
- Observe patient's gait. Have patient walk down the hall or walk in straight line (if able).
- Ask female patients whether they use nail polish and polish remover frequently.
- Assess type of footwear worn by patients.
- Identify patients at risk for foot or nail problems.
  - Older adults.
  - Diabetes mellitus
  - Heart failure and renal disease
  - Cerebrovascular accident or stroke.
- Assess type of home remedies patient uses for existing foot problems.
  - Over the counter liquid preparation to remove corns.
  - Cutting of corns or calluses with razor blade or scissors
  - Application of adhesive tape.
- Assess patient's ability to care for nails or feet, visual alteration, fatigue musculoskeletal weakness, etc.
- Assess patient's knowledge of foot and nail care practices.
- Explain procedure to patient including that the proper soaking requires several minutes. In case of patients who are unconscious, soak nails with wet cotton swabs. In patients with diabetes soak only for a few minutes.
- Wash hands and arrange equipment on the over bed table.
- Pull curtain around bed or close room door.
- Assist ambulatory patient to sit in bedside chair. Help bed-bound patient to supine position with head of bed elevated. Place towel on mattress.
- Fill washbasin, with warm water. Test water temperature and have it about 43-44°C.
- Adjust over bed table to low position and place it over patient's lap (patient may sit in chair or lie in bed).
- Place basin on towel and help patient place feet in basin for soaking toe nails. Place call light within patient's reach.
- Fill basin with warm water and place basin on towel on over bed table for soaking finger nails.
- Instruct patient to place fingers in basin and place arms in comfortable position.
- Allow patient's feet and fingernails to soak for 10-20 minutes and re-warm the water after 10 minutes if necessary.
- Dry hands with towel.
- Clip fingernails straight across and even with top of fingers using nail clipper. Shape nails with file. Wipe each finger tip with cotton dipped in antiseptic solution.
- Move over bed table away from patient.
- Put on disposable gloves and scrub callused areas of feet with washcloth.
- Remove feet from basin and dry thoroughly.
- Clean and trim toenails. Do not file corners of toenails.
- Apply lotion to feet and hands and assist patient back to bed and into comfortable position.
- Remove disposable gloves and place in receptacle. Clean and replace equipment and supplies to proper place. Dispose off soiled linen in hamper. Wash hands.
- Inspect nails and surroundings skin surfaces after soaking and nail trimming. Place nail cutter in a bowl with antiseptic solution for 20 to 30 minutes then washes, dry and replace.
- Record procedure and observations (e.g., breaks in skin, inflammation, ulceration, etc., and patients response).
- Report any breaks in skin or ulcerations to nurse in-charge or physician.

Scientific Principles of Nail Cutting

Anatomy and Physiology

- The nails are the portion of boney layer of the skin. Nails grow from the epithelial cells lying under the lunula at the proximal end of the each nail

- The cells of the nails are translucent parts
- The parts of the nails are the part under the skin is called as nail root, the portion above the nail is called as nail plate; the portion which is cut is called blade and the portion upon which the nail is embedded is called nail bed
- Nails roots have rich supply of blood and nerves. So when there is an injury to the nail bed severe pain and bleeding occurs
- The average growth of nails is approximately 1 mm a week. Excessively hot water, acids and alkalies loosen the nails from their beds.
- Low humidity in winter causes brittleness of the nails.

Microbiology
- Fingernails are transmitters of bacteria
- Dirt accumulated under the fingernails and provides an excellent medium for the growth of all kinds of bacteria
- Biting fingernails introduces dirt into the mouth
- Nails should be cut off close to the skin
- To destroy the microorganisms Dettol lotion 1:20 is used
- Pathogenic organisms may be introduced into the fingertips by dirty manicuring instruments
- The nurse must take care of her nails because nails harbor dirt containing microorganisms, well rounded fingernails prevent punctured wounds which may lead to infection.

Physics and Chemistry
- The nails are made up of keratin, which is insoluble nitrogenous substance
- Nail polish remover contains fat solvents (acetone or ethyl acetate) that removes sebum from the skin and makes the cuticle dry.

Psychology
- Explain the procedure to patient to get cooperation
- Tell him the advantage of nail cutting
- Clean nails on clean hands give a sense of cleanliness
- Nail biting may be caused by emotional maladjustment.

ORAL HYGIENE FOR A CONSCIOUS PATIENT

Definition
"Oral hygiene means assisting the weak or debilitated patient for cleansing mouth by mechanical brushing of the teeth and rinsing of the mouth."

Indications
- Mouth breathers
- Patients on NPO
- Oral surgery patients (sterile special mouth care)
- Patients on oxygen inhalation
- Children under three years
- Patients who are unable to maintain adequate oral hygiene.

Purposes
- To maintain the healthy state of mouth, teeth, gums and lips.
- To clean the mouth off food particles, plaque and bacteria.
- To relieve discomfort resulting from unpleasant odors and tasters.
- To enhance the well-being and comfort and to stimulate appetite.
- To prevent sores, caries and infection to oral tissues.

Nurse's Responsibility in Attending the Mouth of a Client in Illness
- Check the condition of the oral cavity.
- Check the ability of the client for self-care.
- Check the general condition of the client.
- The frequency of mouth care needed.
- Doctor's orders for specific precautions regarding the movement and positioning of the client.
- Articles available in client's unit.

Dentifrices Commonly Used
- Reliable toothpaste or tooth powder with a soft brush.
- Glycerin with lime juice.
- Sodium bicarbonate paste.
- Equal parts of sodium chloride, sodium bicarbonate and calcium carbonate.
- Neem stick.

Solutions Commonly Used
- Potassium permanganate ($KMnO_4$) 1:5000 solution (one crystal to a glass of water to give a pink color and it should be freshly prepared each time).
- Hydrogen peroxide (H_2O_2) 1:8. Sodium chloride (normal saline), 1 teaspoon to a pint of water.
- A number of commercial preparations are available in the market which can be used as mouthwashes.
- **Emollients used:** Cream or butter, Liquid paraffin, Olive oil, White Vaseline, Glycerin borax
- A number of commercial preparations are available in the market, e.g., Nivea cream.

Articles
A clean mouth toilet tray containing:
- Face towel.
- Tumbler/feeding cup containing water.
- Soft bristled toothbrush.
- Toothpaste/tooth powder/available dentifrice.
- Mouthwash solution (according to patient's preference and availability)
  - Sodium chloride
  - Thymol
  - Listerine
  - Chlorhexidine
- Cotton applicators/cotton balls
- Emollient in a container—Glycerin, liquid paraffin, Vaseline, coconut oil.
- K-basin, Emesis basin—2 (one could be a paper bag)
- Small Mackintosh.
- Clean gloves.

Procedure

- Assess the condition of the patient of his mouth and level of consciousness.
- Inspect the integrity of lips, teeth buccal mucosa, gums, palate and tongue.
- Assess the patient's ability to grasp and manipulate toothbrush.
- Explain procedure to patient and encourage him to participate.
- Pull the screen.
- Wash hands and Don gloves.
- Bring patient to edge of the bed nearest to the nurse.
- Position patient in high fowlers/semi Fowler's position as tolerated.
- Place the small Mackintosh with the face towel on the chest.
- Place K-basin close to the patient's chin.
- Apply toothpaste to brush. Holding brush over K-basin pour small amount of water over toothpaste.
- Instruct patient to hold toothbrush bristles at 45° angle to gum line. Brush inner and outer surfaces of upper and lower teeth by brushing from gum to crown of each tooth.
- Clean the biting surface back and forth; farther side first and then nearer side and upper jaw first and then lower jaw.
- Hold the patient hold the brush at the same angle over tongue and brush lightly over surface horizontally taking care not to initiate gag reflex.
- Allow patient to rinse mouth thoroughly by taking mouthful of water and spitting into the K-basin.
- Allow patient to rinse mouth with mouthwash as desired.
- Assist wiping mouth with face towel.
- Apply emollient to lips.
- Assist patient to comfortable position.
- Discard the waste, clean the used articles and replace equipment as appropriate.
- Wash hands.
- Record the procedure including time, solution used and condition of mouth.

ORAL CARE FOR AN UNCONSCIOUS PATIENT

Definition

"Performing mechanical cleansing of the teeth and the mouth, for an unconscious patient"

Purposes

- To maintain integrity of the lips, tongue, and mucous membrane of the mouth.
- To prevent and treat oral infection.
- To clean and moisturize oral mucous membrane.
- To stimulate salivation.
- To prevent dental caries and tooth decay.
- To prevent halitosis.

Articles

- Small Mackintosh and face towel
- Artery forceps
- Dissecting forceps/thumb forceps
- Small bowl with mouthwash solution or normal saline
- Kidney tray
- Emollient
- Tongue depressor
- Disposable gloves
- Cotton applicator
- Mouth gag
- Suction apparatus
- Square gauze piece (2" × 2")
- Small jug with plain water.

Procedure

- Assess patient's oral hygiene.
- Test for presence of gag reflex by placing tongue blade on back half of tongue.
- Check the doctor's order for specific precautions regarding the movement and positioning of patient.
- Explain the procedure to patient and/or relative.
- Pull curtains.
- Raise bed to comfortable working level. Arrange articles by bedside.
- Position the patient on side. Head turned towards you.
- Place towel and Mackintosh under the patients head and spread one towel over chest and an emesis basis under the chin.
- Raise side rails of bed on both sides.
- Wash hands and Don gloves.
- Lower the side rails on the working side
- Do not pour water into the mouth of an unconscious patient.
- Separate the upper and lower teeth with padded tongue depressor by inserting it quickly and gently if required.
- Take gauze piece with the dissecting forceps.
- Wrap the gauze piece around the artery forceps covering its tip. Moisten the gauze piece with normal saline or dip in the cleaning agent (Fig. 4.14).
- Swab each tooth gently but firmly and clean all the sides of the tooth. Clean chewing surface first and then, inner and outer surface from gum to crown.
- Clean lower teeth on both sides followed by upper teeth on both sides (Fig. 4.15).

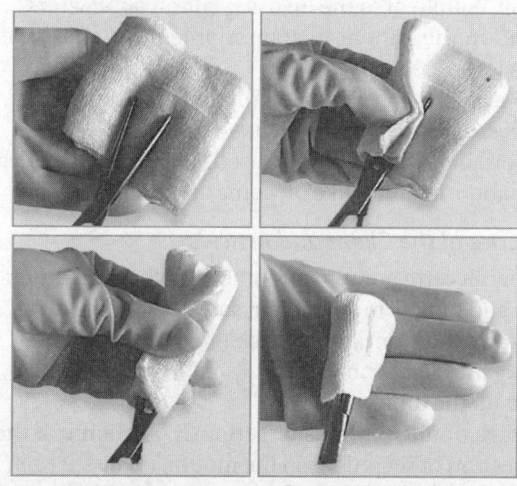

Fig. 4.14: Steps of holding sponge in artery forceps for oral care.

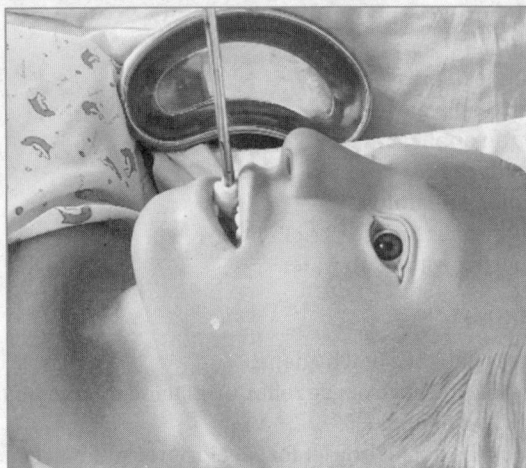

Fig. 4.15: Cleaning the both sides in oral care.

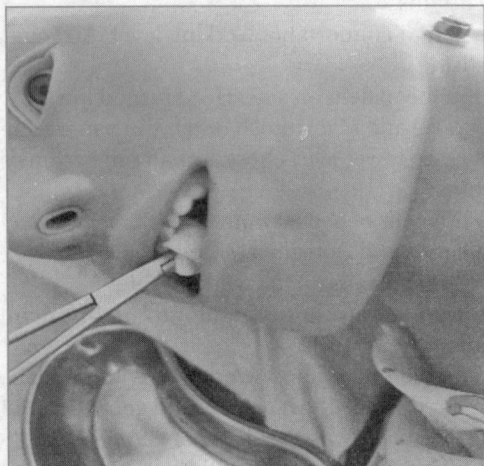

Fig. 4.16: Cleaning the roof of mouth, gums and cheeks in oral care.

- Gently swab roof of the mouth, gums and inner side of cheeks **(Fig. 4.16)**.
- Clean the tongue from back to front using artery forceps covered with gauze.
- Clean the teeth and tongue in similar way using plain water.
- Apply emollient to the lip using cotton applicators.
- Position the patient in comfortable position. Raise side rails lower bed.
- Replace all the articles after discarding the waste, remove gloves, discard it and wash hands.
- Record date, time, solution used, condition of mouth and any abnormalities, like bleeding/inflammation.

After Care of the Client and Articles

- Apply glycerin borax or any other emollient on the cracked lips and tongue to keep them soft.
- Remove the kidney tray, Mackintosh and towel.
- Make the client comfortable.
- Tidy up the unit.
- In case of unconscious or seriously-ill clients, if there is collection of secretions in the mouth, apply suction.
- Take all articles to the utility room. Discard the wastes and clean the articles with soap and water. Boil the forceps and replace them in their proper places. Personal articles are replaced into the bedside table.
- Wash hands.
- Record the time and nature of the treatment and the condition of the mouth on the nurse's record.
- Take the opportunity to teach the client or his in relatives on the principles of oral hygiene.

Scientific Principles of Mouth Wash

Anatomy and Physiology

- **Oral or buccal cavity is formed as follows:** The lips are in front, the cheeks on the sides, and the back communicates with the pharynx.
- The mouth is lined with mucus membrane.
- There are six openings opened in the pharynx. Two openings of the nostrils, one trachea, one esophagus and two are of eustachian tubes.
- The mouth contains the tongue, salivary glands, and teeth.
- **Tongue:**
  - The tongue is made up of skeletal muscles and is covered with mucous membrane.
  - The papillae on the tongue contain taste buds.
  - Sweet taste in the front, bitter at the back and sour and salty taste is at the side of the tongue.
  - The function of the tongue is it helps speaking and in eating.
- **Salivary glands:**
  - There are three sets of salivary glands, in the mouth.
  - Namely parotid, sublingual and submaxillary glands.
  - They secrete saliva when the taste buds are stimulated by the smell, sight, feel and thought of food.
  - Saliva contains ptyalin, which hydrolyzes starch.
- **Teeth:**
  - Temporary or deciduous teeth are 20 in number and permanent teeth are 32 in number.
  - The teeth are covered by a dense fibrous membrane over which is smooth mucous membrane called gums,
  - *Each tooth has three parts*—a root, a neck, and a crown. The outside of the crown is enamel which is the hardest substance in the body and it is affected only by acids.
  - The outside of the root is cement. Under the enamel of the crown and the cement of the root is dentine. Dentine contains tubules which brings nourishment.
  - The pulp of the tooth lies within the dentin. Pulp contains blood vessels and nerve branches from the fifth cranial nerve.
  - For normal development of the teeth mastication of hard fibrous food, firm, raw fruits and vegetables are required.

Microbiology

- Many bacteria are found in normal healthy mouth, among which are the pneumococci, the staphylococci and the streptococci.
- Saliva is mildly bactericidal.
- The mouth represents all requirements for bacterial growth—warmth, moisture, food supply from the residual foods on and between the teeth and a protected environment.
- If oral hygiene is not maintained it will lead to the diseases of the teeth and mouth.

- Mouth washes help to remove food particles after they have brushed from the teeth.
- Oral cleanliness is preventive against dental carries.
- Lactobacillus acidophilus causes dental carries. It acts on carbohydrate material which is left on the surfaces and produces lactic acid that dissolves the tooth structure.
- The molars, the bicuspids and upper incisors are most liable to decay.
- Inflammation of the gums may be caused by poor oral hygiene, bacterial infection or deficiency of vitamin C in the diet. Gingivitis may lead to pyorrhea.
- Sordes is a collection of food, mucus and bacteria in the mouth and on the lips. It may lead to infection in the mouth or adjacent tissues.
- Dentures should be cleaned well, especially in and around the clips

Physics and Chemistry
- Soap is a constituent of most dentifrices, has a low surface tension so that it spreads readily over the teeth and penetrates between them.
- Friction of raw foods against the teeth and gums produces stimulation.
- The force of chewing, pushing the gelatinous bacterial plaque and lactic acid into the pits and crevices. may be partially responsible for the speed of dental decay
- Dentures should be dipped in cold water to avoid friction with the mouth and to make it slide easily into place.
- When a nurse attending mouth care the patient should be near the working side of the bed to prevent strain for the patient and the nurse.
- The nurse should stand erect to avoid strain on back muscles.
- The teeth are formed of calcium and phosphorus. So for healthy growth of the teeth these minerals are necessary.
- Vitamin D helps in the assimilation of the calcium and phosphorus.
- Vitamin A controls the growth of enamel.
- Vitamin C is necessary for formation of dentin.
- Saliva consists of 99.5% water and 0.5% total solids. Its constituents are water, inorganic salts, and mucin, traces of protein and salivary amylase or ptyalin.
- Saliva is slightly acid in reaction and its pH is between 6.35–6.85.
- Sweets increase the acid reaction of the saliva.
- Tartar consists of mineral matter precipitated from saliva mixed with food debris. The pressure of tartar against the gums irritates them and lowers their resistances to bacteria.
- The fluorine.
- Synthetic vitamin K retards the formation of acid in the mouth.
- Dentifrices clean the mouth by mechanical action rather than chemical action on bacteria.

Pharmacology
- Glycerin with lemon juice helps in softening dry lips.
- All liquid dentifrices contain antiseptics such as boric acid, phenol, thymol, etc., and flavored with peppermint, cinnamon cloves, etc.
- Salt solution is a good mouth wash.

Psychology
- A clean mouth makes a person feel fresh, clean and comfortable.
- Daily brushing of teeth is a desirable esthetic habit.
- A set of sound teeth is valuable asset as it contributes to personal appearance.
- Privacy should be provided to the patient while caring for his dentures.

PERFORMING A BED SHAMPOO/HAIR WASH

Definition
"Cleaning of hair with shampoo or soap to remove dirt oil and odor on scalp and hair, for a helpless patient in bed."

Purposes
- To keep hair clean and healthy
- To promote growth of hair
- To prevent loss of hair
- To prevent itching and infection
- To prevent accumulation of dirt, dandruff and oil
- To prevent tangles
- To stimulate circulation
- To enhance personal appearance and self-esteem
- To clean hair after pediculosis treatment
- To observe the scalp
- To provide a sense of well-being.

Contraindications
- Head and neck injuries
- Spinal cord injuries
- Surgeries on back and neck.

Nurses Responsibilities
- Check the physician's orders to see the specific precautions for the client's movement and positioning.
- Assess the general condition of the client and the ability for self care.
- Assess the condition of scalp and hair.
- Assess the client's mental state to follow directions.
- Check the articles available in the client's unit.

Articles
A tray containing
- Bath towels—(2 Nos)
- Washcloth or face towel
- Mackintosh—(2 Nos)
- Nonabsorbent cotton balls
- Bath blanket/sheet
- Oil (optional)
- Shampoo or liquid soap
- Hair comb
- Kidney tray or paper bag
- Basin
- Bucket
- Mug

- Jugs (2 Nos)
- Low stool
- Clean linen
- Newspaper.

Procedure

- Check the physician's order for specific precautions if any for movement and positioning of the patient.
- Assess the general condition of the patient, the scalp, hair and need for shampoo.
- Check the patient's preference for soap/shampoo.
- Explain procedure to the patient.
- Adjust the bed to comfortable height.
- Close windows and put of the fan.
- Pull the curtains
- Fan fold the top linen to the foot end of the bed leaving a sheet or bath blanket over the patient.
- Make a trough with the Mackintosh or just a Kelly's pad if available.
- Unless contraindicated, move the patient's head to the edge of the bed, position patient diagonally with head positioned inside trough.
- Place pillow under the shoulder so that the head is slightly tilted backwards.
- Protect the pillow and bed with a Mackintosh and towel.
- Place the bucket on a low stool close to the side of bed.
- Plug the ears with cotton balls.
- Place a wash cloth or a towel over the eyes.
- Wash hands.
- Loosen and remove tangles.
- Mix cold and hot water and test the temperature with the back of hand.
- Start cleaning at hairline and working towards the back of the head symmetrically using shampoo.
- Rub shampoo and massage the scalp well.
- Rinse thoroughly with water.
- Repeat washing and rinsing until hair is clean, squeeze off water from hair.
- Instruct patient to inform nurse, if any discomfort or pain occurs.
- Dry hair with second towel.
- Remove the trough and place it in the bucket. Discard the cotton plugs used to plug ears into the paper bag.
- Reposition the patient in proper alignment.
- Spread the hair over Mackintosh and towel placed on the pillow and allow it to dry.
- Change linen if wet.
- Offer hot drink.
- Take all articles to the utility room, and clean them. Disinfect the towels, Mackintosh, basin and bucket. Send soiled linen to laundry. Wash hands.
- Return to bedside when the hair is dry. Comb and arrange the hair. Remove Mackintosh and towel from the bed. Make the patient comfortable.
- Record the procedure and report any abnormalities if present.

Special Considerations

- Consider cultural, religious and personal preferences of patients.
- Special precaution should be taken in-positioning patient if central venous lines are present.

PEDICULOSIS

- The term pediculosis is defined as the state of being infected with lice.
- Lice or pediculi (Louse singular) are small wingless blood sucking insects which are parasitic on warm blooded animals.
- They are found on the head (pediculus capitis), the body (pediculus corporis), and the perineal area, eyebrows, eye lashes and beard (pediculus pubis).
- Pediculosis is associated with poor hygiene, crowded living conditions and exposure to other individuals with pediculosis.
- Lice can be transferred from person to person through direct contact or indirect contact. It gets easily transmitted from person to person, perhaps sleeping together, sitting together, etc. They can also be transmitted through clothing, bedding, combs, etc.

Danger of Pediculosis

- The client complaints of severe itching of the scalp and scratches the head continuously giving rise to abscess formation.
- In severe infestations, the hair may appear to be heavily sprinkled with dandruff.
- The itching of the scalp is a source of discomfort to the client causing restlessness and insomnia.
- The lice are blood suckers and cause anemia.
- They spread the disease, e.g., typhus fever, relapsing fever, trench fever.
- Itching of the scalp results in scalp injury and the injured area is subjected to infection which leads to infected glands.

Prevention of Pediculosis

- Prevention is easier than controlling.
- For this, proper personal hygiene concept should be practised by everybody in their life.
- Combing the hair daily, washing it frequently, keeping the skin and clothing clean will solve the problem.
- Any client complaining of itching or if he/she scratches their head, needs thorough examination of the hair and scalp, body and linen to discover lice.
- If lice are found on the client's head or body, follow the prescribed treatment.

Parasiticides used in the Treatment of Pediculosis

- DDT 5% or 10% (Add talcum powder to dilute it).
- Carbolic lotion 1:40 (it is an irritant to the skin).
- Equal parts of kerosene oil and coconut oil.
- Preparations containing gamma benzene hexachloride available in the market.

Application of Parasiticide

- The parasiticides are applied thoroughly on the scalp (to the body if necessary) and is left overnight.
- On the next day, a thorough bath is given and the linen is charged.
- The linen should be thoroughly disinfected to remove the lice from the clothes.
- Since the parasiticides are not effective against the nits (eggs) the procedure is repeated after a week.

Nurse's Responsibility in the Treatment of Pediculus Capitis

- Check the physician's orders to see the specific precautions for the client's movements and positioning,
- Assess the general condition of the client and the ability to follow directions
- Assess the condition of the scalp and the hair.
- Check the articles available in the client's unit.

Preparation of the Client and the Unit

- Explain the sequence of procedure to the client to gain his confidence and cooperation.
- Explain how the client can help you.
- Provide privacy by means of screens.
- Place the articles conveniently on the bedside table.
- Remove the top linen or fanfold it to the foot end of the bed leaving a sheet or bath blanket over the client.
- Keep the client flat if the condition permits
- Remove the extra pillows and back rest leaving one pillow under the head.
- Unless contraindicated, move the client's head and shoulders to the edge of the bed.
- Position the client diagonally to the bed in good alignment.
- Protect the pillow and bed with a Mackintosh and a towel.
- One towel is put on the shoulders to protect the shoulders and the garments.
- Protect the client's eyes with a clean damp wash cloth.
- Put off the fan to prevent the parasiticide spilling over the face during its application.
- Loosen the hair and comb out the tangles.

After Care of the Client and Articles

- Remove the Mackintosh and towels from under the client's head. Towels are put into the antiseptic lotion.
- Tidy up the bed.
- Adjust the position of the client in bed.
- Remove the gown, mask and cap and put them into the antiseptic lotion.
- Take all articles into the utility room. Clean and disinfect the articles. Replace them in their proper place.
- Wash hands.
- Record the procedure with date and time and the observations made.
- The hair is washed in the following morning.
- Apply warm vinegar diluted with equal amount of water to loosen the nits if any.
- Comb the hair with a fine toothed comb

- If living lice are still found on the head repeat the procedure with other parasiticides.
- Repeat the procedure after 1 week because the nits are not affected by the parasiticide.
- Disinfect all the articles that have come in contact with the hair by immersing them in carbolic 1:20 for 1 hour before washing.

Articles

A tray containing:
- Mackintosh (1)
- Bath towels (2)
- Wash cloth (1)
- A cap, a triangular bandage or a towel folded diagonally
- Safety pins
- Kidney tray with disinfectant, e.g., carbolic 1:40
- Paper bag
- Hair comb
- Cotton swabs or gauze piece in a container
- Vaseline
- Gown, mask and cap
- Bucket with antiseptic solution, e.g., carbolic 5%.

Steps of Procedure

- Wash hands. Put on the gown mask and cap.
- Part the hair into small sections and apply the parasiticide on the hair and scalp, rubbing gently. In long hair, the medicine is to be applied along the whole length of the hair.
- Roll up the long hair to the top of the head and cover the head with the cap or triangular bandage or by a towel folded diagonally. Secure it with pins.
- The treatment is done in the evening and left overnight.

Scientific Principles of Hair Care

Anatomy and Physiology

- The hairs are cylindrical, horny structures of the epidermis.
- Hairs develop in the hair follicles and extend downward into the subcutaneous tissue.
- The three type of hair are: (A) Lanugo or fine soft hair, (B) Long hairs. (C) Short, heavy and stiff hairs.
- The part of the hair lies within the follicle is known as the root, the portion projects beyond the surface of the skin is called as shaft.
- The hair follicle is made up of connective tissue and contains arteries, veins and nerves.
- The hair itself has no blood vessels but receives its nourishment from the blood vessels of the papilla.
- The hair follicle is placed obliquely in arrectores pilorum muscles.
- The color of the hair is due to a deposit of pigment during the growth of the hair in the intercellular spaces of the cortex.
- The hair normally is kept soft and pliable by the secretion of the sebaceous glands of the body.
- The general health affects the growth of hair, and when the vitality of the body is lowered the hair suffers in proportion.
- The hair needs light and air.

- Fever, worry and grief, affects state of hair.
- Endocrine abnormalities and imbalances greatly influence the growth of hair.

Microbiology
- An unclean scalp cannot function normally.
- Staphylococci grow at all times in the hair follicles and sweat ducts.
- While shampooing the hair, do not scrape or scratch the scalp with fingernail because infection may develop.
- Combs must be clean and separate for everyone because diseases may be transmitted by combs used in common.
- Dandruff is a non-inflammatory desquamation of the scalp without redness or edema and represents a disease of its own.
- Brushing and shampooing the hair well is important to remove the dandruff.
- Pediculosis capitis is infestation of the scalp by the head louse.
- Due to irritation patient may get infection of the scalp

Physics and Chemistry
- The power of forming an impulsion with the hair depends upon the low surface tension of the soap solution.
- The unit in which the hair wash is being given should be free from drafts and warm throughout the procedure. This will prevent chilling the patient by rapid evaporation of the moisture. Because evaporation is cooling process.
- In combing and shampooing the patient's hair the nurse must stand upright with her feet slightly separated to provide a wide base of support which gives a good balance.
- The patient should be drawn close to the edge of the bed to avoid the straining on the part of the nurse.
- Hair contains keratin which is a soluble nitrogenous substance
- Liquid soap are used for washing the hair because a liquid soap is more easily removed from the hair
- Soap emulsifies the oil of the hair and permits it to be washed out easily
- Shampoo which contain high alcohol make the hair dry and brittle
- A vinegar or lemon rinse softens the water, helps to remove all soap, and gives luster to the hair
- Soap should be well rinsed out of the hair to keep it from being sticky.

Pharmacology
- To remove the tangles an alcohol is applied to hair.
- Kerosene is used as parasiticide for pediculosis. To avoid its irritation it may be diluted one half with sweet oil.
- Tincture of larkspur kills pediculi but it does not loosen nits
- The acetic and in vinegar is used to dissolve gummy substance which attaches nits to the hair.
- DDT is also used to destroy pediculi.

Psychology
- When a person needs to remain in bed for a long time without a hair wash, the hair becomes sticky and heavy and acquires a sour, unpleasant odor This condition is disturbing the patient. Hair wash gives great improvement in patient's appearance.
- When the patient is bought to the edge of the bed for hair wash, she must be placed securely so she does not fear falling out of bed.
- Neat and tidy arrangement of hair gives a sense of well-being to the patient
- The hair may create a sympathetic reaction.

THE EYES, EARS AND NOSE

When nurses provide hygienic care, the eyes, ear and nose require careful attention. Cleansing of the sensitive sensory tissues should be done in a way that prevents injury and discomfort for the client, such as using care not to get soap in the client's eyes. In addition, the time a nurse spends with a client during the hygiene provides an excellent opportunity to ask if there have been any changes in vision, hearing or sense of smell.

Performing an Eye Care
Definition
Process of cleaning one/both eyes using prescribed solution for removing and preventing infection.

Purposes
- To prevent infection
- To relieve pain and discomfort
- To prevent any further injury to the eye
- To provide instillation of an eye-drop or application of an eye ointment.

Articles
- A clean tray containing
- **Sterile eye dressing pack containing:**
  - Gallipot
  - Cotton balls
  - Disposable towel
  - Sterile swabbing solution, e.g., normal saline
  - K-basin
  - Sterile glove (if eye is infected)
  - Mackintosh
  - Pillow.

Procedures
- Check the physician's order progress notes and nursing care plan.
- Identity the patient.
- Explain to patient what will be done and how he may cooperative. Allow patient to ask question.
- Ensure privacy.
- Collect and prepare articles.
- Position the patient comfortably. Preferably in the supine position or seated with head incline backwards.
- Ensure adequate light source taking care not to dazzle the patient.
- Wash and dry hands.
- Always bathe the lids first, with the eyes closed.
- Always treat the uninfected eye first.

- Lightly moisten swab in the prescribed solution.
- Gently swab from the inner canthus of the eye to the outer canthus using each swab only once until all discharge has been removed.
- Gently dry the patient's eyelids to remove excess moisture.
- Ensure that the patient is comfortable.
- Replace the equipment safely.
- Wash hands and dry.
- Document the procedure appropriately and report any abnormal findings.

Scientific Principles

Anatomy and Physiology

- In orbital cavity, the extrinsic muscles, the eye lids, the lacrimal glands and the conjunctiva are associated with the eye.
- The eyeball is spherical in shape and is about one inch in diameter.
- Six extrinsic muscles move the eyeball in the orbit.
- There are three coats in the eyeball.
  1. *Outer coat:* It is made by the sclera and the cornea.
  2. *Vascular coat:* The middle coat is vascular and is made up of iris, the ciliary body and the choroid It provides rich blood supply to the eye.
  3. *Inner coat:* It is made by retina. The retina is a thin, transparent membrane and contains the visual receptors, extensions of the optic nerve.
- Cavities of the eye—anterior and posterior.
- The anterior cavity is divided into anterior and posterior chambers.
- The anterior chamber lies between the iris and the cornea.
- The posterior chamber lies between the iris and the lens. Both chambers of the anterior cavity contain clear, colorless lymph like fluid called aqueous humor.
- The posterior cavity is large and occupies the space between the lens and retina. It contains gelatinous substance called vitreous humor.
- The eyeball is covered with conjunctiva, which is sensitive mucous membrane.
- Any type of stimulation of the cornea gives rise to pain.
- Constriction and dilatation of the pupil are reflex acts stimulated by light
- The optic nerve conveys sight impressions.
- The retina is supplied by a branch of the ophthalmic artery, it enters through the optic disc
- Images falling on the retina stimulate the nerve cells contained in it to send appropriate message to the brain.
- Blood vessels dilate with the application of heat
- The warm irrigation solution relaxes the of e eyes and gives comfort.

Microbiology

- The eyelashes protect the eyes from dust
- Tears contain a bactericidal substance called lysozyme. It protects the eyes from infection.
- *Staphylococcus, Gonococcus* causes serious infections to the eyes which may result into the corneal ulcers and impair the sight

- Wash hands before and after the procedure.
- Use gown, mask to prevent cross infection.
- Use sterile drugs or solutions and articles for eye treatment.
- Infected dressings should be burned.

Physics and Chemistry

- Light is the stimulus to the optic nerve.
- If images on the retina are not distinct due to impaired refractive power of the eye, glass lenses are used to retract rays of light and to aid in seeing.
- Normal tension in the eye ball is between 13 to 29 mm of mercury. In Glaucoma, pressure may rise to 35 mm or above
- The eyeball is a closed cavity, a pressure applied to its surface will be transmitted undiminished to the retina. so while irrigation the pressure is kept as low as possible in order to secure a steady flow of solution yet not cause pain or injury to the delicate issues.
- The temperature of the solution for an eye irrigation is about 98–100°F. to avoid the injury to the
- Tears lubricate the surfaces of the eyelids. So there is no friction while moving them. In trachoma, the roughness of the lids breaks down the comes into ulcers.
- The pH of normal tears is 7.0–7.4. Irrigating solution should be neutral in reaction. At pH 9.0 a slight feeling of imitation is produced.
- Vishal purple and visual yellow are substances that influence adjustment from light to darkness and from darkness to light respectively.
- The Adjustment of visual purple is dependent upon an adequate supply of vitamin A in the retina, which comes from vitamin A of food.

Pharmacology

- Solutions used for eye irrigations are made from sodium il-carbonate, boric acid, or sodium chloride,
- Weak solutions are used so that they will not irritate to the eye.
- Antiseptic, astringent, mydriatic, miotic or anesthetic drugs are used in the treatment of eye.
  - *Antiseptics:* These are silver salts. Silver nitrate is used in the eye of a newborn infant to prevent gonorrheal ophthalmia
  - *Astringent:* Zinc sulfate drops are put into the eye to reduce inflammation.
  - *Mydriatic:* Are used to dilate the pupil for eye examinations. It is prepared from atropine.
  - *Miotic:* It is used to reduce the size of the pupil, e.g., eserine or physostigmine.
- Penicilline is used in treating some infectious conditions of the eye.
- Vitamin A prevents night blindness.
- Vitamin B is useful in some conditions of the cornea, the retina and the optic nerve.
- Vitamin C is useful in the metabolism of normal lens.
- Vitamin D is used in some ocular conditions.

Psychology

- Patient must be treated with more kindness and more patience than usual, because eye is a very sensitive part of the body.

- Nurse must be very gentle in handling and treating the eye.
- Explain each and everything when you go to the patient, especially when patient is unable to see. and the confidence.
- Explain the procedure to the patient to get his cooperation win 5.
- Try to clear all doubts of the patient, so that he will be relaxed during the procedure.

Care of the Ears

- The ears are mostly cleaned during the bed bath. A clean moistened washcloth rotated gently into the ear is used for cleaning. a cotton-tipped applicator is useful for cleansing the pinna.
- The care of the hearing aid involves routine cleaning, battery care and proper insertion techniques. The nurse must assess the client's knowledge and routines for cleaning and caring for his/her hearing aid.
- The nurse will also determine whether the client can hear clearly with the use of the aid by talking slowly and clearly in a normal tone of voice.
- Have the client's suggest any additional tips for care of the hearing aid. When not in use, the hearing aid should be stored where it will not become damaged.
- The hearing aid should be turned off when not in use. The outside of the hearing aid should be cleaned with a clean, dry cloth. Hearing loss is a common health problem with the elderly and the aid assists in the ability to communicate and react appropriately in the environment.

Scientific Principles of Ear Care

Anatomy and Physiology

- Hearing and balance are the two physiological functions of the ear.
- Hearing depends upon the sound conduction apparatus and the sound perception apparatus.
- The ear drum, the ossicles, the Eustachian tube, and the cochlea are the sound conduction structures.
- The organ of Corti, nerve filaments of the eighth cranial nerve and the hearing center within the brain are the sound perception apparatus.
- The external ear consists with pinna and external auditory canal. The pinna collect sound waves and direct them into the bony ear canal.
- The ear canal is not straight, so it is lifted upward and backward in order to straighten the external canal to provide efficient irrigation. In children, ear canal is straighten by drawing the pinna downward and backward
- The ear drum is a cartilaginous ring, receives sound waves entering the auditory canal, vibrates them, and passes the vibration on to the middle ear.
- The middle ear or tympanic cavity is situated within the petrous bone.
- The malleus, the incus and the stapes are joined together and forms a chain. These are loosely attached to the ear drum. They convey sound vibrations to the membrane of the oval window, which in turn conveys them to the inner ear.
- The Eustachian tubes extends downward to the posterior wall of the throat.
- The Eustachian tube keeps the air pressure inside the eardrum the same as on the outside. The Eustachian tubes are opened during, swallowing, yawning, and while blowing the nose.
- The stapes transmits the sound vibrations to the endolymph within the cochlea. Vibrations carried by the air change into fluid vibrations. These are picked up by the receptors of hearing cells of the organ of Corti.
- The sound vibration is conducted by the eighth cranial nerve to the auditory center in the temporal lobe of the brain.
- The semicircular canals are located in the internal ear. These are concerned with balance. The semicircular canals may be affected if the temperature of the irrigating solution is too high or too low and patient may have dizziness, vomiting.

Microbiology

- Various forms of fungi or mold grow in the outer canal.
- Infection in the middle ear is called otitis media. The middle ear may get infection by way of Eustachian tube from the nose and throat.
- Infection may spread to the mastoid area because of continuity of the mucous membrane. It may spread to the meanings and cause fatal results.
- The middle ear provides a warm, moist and dark environment for the development of microorganism— *Spirochaeta pallida*, the *Pneumococcus*, and the *Streptococcus* are destructive organisms which attack middle ear.
- Toxins of infectious diseases may produce complications in the ear.
- Infection from diseased teeth, tonsils and adenoids may affect the ear.
- Wash hands before and after the procedure to avoid cross infection.
- Use sterile articles and solutions for ear irrigation.

Physics and Chemistry

- Sound waves are alternate condensation and rarefaction of air.
- Vibrations in the air cause ear drum to vibrate. The vibration is transferred through air to the stapes and beyond it through fluid endolymph, to the auditory nerve, and the sensation of sound is produced.
- The intensity or loudness is measured by the decibel. The voice in ordinary conversation produces 50–60 decibels.
- Mechanical hearing aids increase the intensity of sound and helps the hard of hearing person to hear better.
- Air in the middle ear cavity maintains an air pressure equal to that outside, so that vibrations can take place.
- The Eustachian tube. Keeps the air pressure against the inside surface of the drum equal to the air pressure against the outside surface of the drum.
- The three ossicles serve as a lever with two arms.
- Temperature changes affect the fluids in the internal ear. The drum is protected from drafts and changes in temperature by the length of the external canal.

- The temperature of irrigating solutions and liquid medication should be near body temperature (about 100°F). So that it will not affect in the ear.
- The pressure of flow should be low to avoid damage to the ear drum.
- The perilymph, and endolymph are alkaline fluids.

Pharmacology
- Solutions used for ear irrigations are mild and usually made from boric acid or salt.
- For removing the foreign body (beans, peas) alcohol is used, because, alcohol causes foreign body to shrink and be expelled easily.
- Hydrogen peroxide is sometimes used to soften impacted wax and it helps in removing it.
- Powders and ointments may be instilled in the outer canal to stop the growth of the fungus,
- Vitamin A and B is given in some ear conditions to improve the nutrition in general.

Psychology
- Explain the procedure to get the co-operation.
- Nurse must be gentle while caring the patient.

Care of the Nose

Purposes
- To clean allergens and irritants.
- To decrease swelling in the nose and increases airflow.
- To clean the mucus from the nose.

Procedure
- Secretions can usually be removed from the nose by having the client blow into a soft tissue paper and discard it into kidney tray with disinfectant or yellow garbage bag.
- The nurse must teach the client that harsh blowing could causes pressure capable of injuring the eardrum, nasal mucosa and even sensitive eye structures.
- If the client is not able to clean his nose, the nurse will assist using a moistened washcloth or cotton tipped applicator with saline. Do not insert the applicator beyond the cotton tip.
- Suctioning will be necessary in case of excessive secretions.
- When client receive oxygen per nasal cannula or have a nasogastric tube, you should cleanse the nares every 8 hours, use a cotton-tipped applicator moistened with saline.
- Secretions are likely to collect and dry around the tube; therefore, you will need to cleanse the tube with soap and water.

■ PERINEAL CARE/MEATAL CARE

Definition
"Perineal care involves cleansing the vulva and perineum using sterile techniques". —**Immanuel MS**

Indications
Perineal care is important for:
- All patients who have had vaginal operations.
- Patients with retention catheters
- After delivery the post-partum period.
- After the removal of radium from the vagina and the uterus.

Purpose
- To prevent infection of the genital tract
- To give comfort to the patient
- Help in healing when there are stitches on the perineum

Articles Required
For pre and -post-perineal care catheter pack:
- Tumbler/mug/small jug
- 1 cup
- 1 forceps/thumb or artery
- 6 large cotton balls
- 1 perineal towel
- Bed pan
- kidney tray

For delivery or postpartum use:
- 1 obstetric and gynecological perineal care pack
- 1 tumbler/mug/small jug
- 1 cup
- 1 forceps thumb or artery
- 6 large cotton balls.
- 1 perineal towel
- 1 sterile pad
- 2 gauze pieces
- 1sterile k Basin.
- Zephiran Cetavlon
- Bed pan.

Procedure
- Explain the procedure to the patient
- Provide privacy
- Bring the prepared trolley to the bed side
- Place a Mackintosh under the buttocks
- Put the patient on a bed pan, if possible pour water.
- Using the pre-catheterization perineal care park, clean the pubic area, with soap and water.
- Pour water.
- Dry with perineal care towel
- Irrigate with warm sterile water.
- Dry with perineal towel.
- **For cleaning use the following solutions:**
  - Obstetrics and Gynecology—(etavalon/Zephiran)
  - Betadine for catheterized patients
- Clear the mons pubis.
- With the forceps, paint the labia majora and the outer surface of the labia minora.
- Discard the forceps.
- Separate the labia minora with a gloved hand.
- With the second pair of forceps, clean the meatus and sides with downward strokes.
- Dry the meatus with dry swabs.
- Where there is a catheter, paint around the catheter from the urethral orifice back towards the outlet for 2" with betadine.
- **For episiotomy patients**, proceed with suture line care.

- Dry the area.
- Remove and clean equipment.
- Make the patient comfortable.
- Wash hands.
- Record the procedure in patient's record.

HANDLING GLASSES

- For many people, glasses are essential to see clearly.
- It is important to take proper care of eyeglasses so that vision is the best that it can be, and one does not have to spend money fixing or replacing them.
- Clean glasses regularly, and when handling them, take precautions to prevent scratching.
- With proper maintenance, glasses can last for years

Methods

1. First Method
Cleaning Your Glasses
Step 1:
- Run the glasses under warm water.
- Run the tap so that the water is lukewarm.
- Hold the frames beneath the water.
- Avoid using hot water as this can damage the glasses.
- This removes dust and other particles that can scratch the lens if rubbed into it.

Step 2:
- Add a drop of dish detergent.
- If you do not have detergent, you may also use gentle hand soap or a special eyeglass lens cleaner.
- With the fingers, rub the detergent over the frames.
- Make sure to cover both sides of the lenses.
- Rinse.

Step 3:
- Dry with a clean cloth.
- Use a microfiber cloth or a smooth weave cotton cloth.
- Gently, rub circles over the glasses until they are dry.
- Avoid using paper towels, rough rags, or tissues, as these might scratch the lenses or leave lint on the glass.

Step 4:
- Wipe off smudges with a lens cloth. In between cleanings, use a microfiber lens cloth to wipe off any smudges.
- Gently move the cloth in circles over each lens.
- Avoid using the shirt or a paper towel as these can scratch the lens.
- Laundry treated with fabric softener and/or dryer sheets can leave streaks on the lens, so avoid using the shirt to wipe your lens, or using a cloth that has been laundered using these products.

2. Second Method
Handling your Glasses
Step 1:
- Remove glasses with both hands.
- When one take off their glasses, use both hands to remove each temple (or arm) of the glasses from behind your ears.
- This prevents the glasses from becoming misaligned.
- Do not push the glasses on top of the head when one is not wearing them.
- This could also cause them to become misaligned.

Step 2:
- Avoid touching the lenses.
- Touching the lenses can leave finger prints and smudges behind.
- When one handle the glasses, touch only the temples of the frames, not the bridge.
- This will prevent any accidental contact.

Step 3:
- Rest the glasses with the frames up.
- Even clean surfaces can leave scratches on lenses.
- When one set your glasses down, make sure that they are resting on the temples, not on the frames.
- The frames should be facing up.
- Do not leave the glasses on a cluttered, wet, or dirty surface such as a bathroom counter.
- Soft cases are often made of a microfiber cloth that can be used to clean off occasional smudges.

Step 4:
- Take off the glasses during certain activities.
- There are certain situations when one should not wear the glasses.
- Keep the glasses in their case until one's works is finished. These situations include:
  - Sports
  - Showering
  - Sleeping
  - Swimming

3. Third Method
Keeping the Glasses in Good Shape
Step 1:
- Have the glasses adjusted.
- Over time, the frames may start to feel loose on the head, or they may sit unbalanced on the nose.
- The glasses should be realigned.
- Take the glasses to the nearest optician, and they will refit the glasses to the client's head.
- Many opticians will realign them for free.

Step 2:
- Carry the glasses in a case.
- A hard shell case is ideal for protecting the glasses.
- Make sure that the glasses fit inside.
- The case should not have too much extra room, or the glasses might rattle and break.
- Never leave the glasses loose in a purse or in your pocket.
- This can scratch the glasses, and you might accidentally crush or break the frames.

Step 3:
- Avoid wearing glasses during sports.
- If one wears the normal glasses during sports, there is risk of breaking them.
- If the lenses break while one wears them, it may cause injury to the eye.

- One may want to consider investing in sports glasses.
- Look for polycarbonate lenses and padded frames that stay firmly on your face while one swim, run, or play sports.
- Some designs look more like sunglasses.
- These would be suitable for sports like baseball, basketball, or soccer.
- Other types function as prescription goggles.
- These are good for swimming and skiing.
- Let the optician know what activities you participate in.
- They may be able to recommend a certain design of sports goggles for particular hobbies.

Step 4:
- Use a strap to avoid misplacing the glasses.
- If one only use glasses for reading or certain tasks, one may not wear them constantly.
- Instead of accidentally misplacing the glasses, one can attach a special strap to them that will keep them around the neck.
- Straps can also help keep the glasses on the head.

Tips
- When buying glasses, note that spring-loaded frames do not bend easily.
- Make sure one set their glasses case where it would not fall or harm the glasses.
- Anti-glare coatings can be a good way to help keep glasses clean.
- Many of the anti-glare coatings have treatments that repel water, oil and dust.

CARE FOR CONTACT LENSES AND EYES

- Wash hands with soap before.
- Pat them dry using a lint-free towel before one handles the contact lenses.
- Keep the contact lenses away from water. Remove lenses before going to swimming or while bathing.
- Avoid using saline solution and rewetting drops for disinfecting the lenses.
- Wear lenses as per guideline. Replace them according to the schedule as prescribed by the eye specialist.
- NEVER put the contact lenses in your mouth to get them wet.
- When cleaning, rub the contact lenses using fingers first.
- After that, rinse the lenses with a solution and then soak them.
- As per the eye experts, this "rub and rinse" method is the best way of cleaning the contact lens.
- Even if the solution is a "no-rub" variety then also one can use it to rub the lenses.
- Follow proper guideline for cleaning and storing the lenses. Ask the eye specialist for the guidelines.
- NEVER rinse or wash the contact lenses with water. Do not even think of keeping them in water instead of the solution.
- If one is storing the lenses in the case for a longer period, follow the instructions to determine if one need to re-disinfect the lenses before wearing them again. In any case, avoid wearing a contact lens after storing it for at least 30 days without re-disinfecting the lenses.
- ALWAYS rinse the contact lens case using fresh solution.
- NEVER use water. Leave the empty case open and air-dry it.
- Never let the tip of the solution bottle to come in contact with any other surface. Tightly close the bottle after use or when not in use.
- Replace the contact lens case at least every three months. These can be a source of infection. NEVER use damaged lens cases.
- NEVER re-use old contact lens solution.
- Avoid transferring the contact lens solution into any other container. This affects the sterility of the solution, and this might cause an eye infection.

Take Care of Eyes
- If one wear lenses, then take proper care of eyes to avoid any kind of infection.
- Wear contacts as per the doctor recommends.
- Wear them as long as the doctor thinks it is necessary.
- In case one cannot keep track of the time when to change the lenses, ask the eye doctor to give a chart for tracking your schedule. Or else, make a chart for yourself.
- Never ever wear someone else's contact lenses, especially if its wearer already uses those lenses.
- Using other's contact lenses can get eye infections or other foreign bodies from their eyes to yours.
- Never sleep with the contact lenses in.
- Avoid doing it unless one have an extended-wear lens.
- When one close their eyelids, their tears do not get much oxygen to the eyes compared to when it is open. So, take the lenses off before going to sleep.
- When going out, wear sunglasses with complete UV protection. one can even wear a hat. Contact lenses make the eyes light-sensitive.
- Keep the eyes moist and use a rewetting solution (if only recommended by your doctor).
- Often people accidentally wear contact lenses inside out. Although this does not hurt it does not feel good even.
- In order to avoid this keep the lens on the tip of your finger so that it forms a cup. Now, look at the contact from the side.
- If the cup of the lens appears like it flares out at the top and has a lip that means the lens is inside out.
- And if it appears like the letter "U," then it is the right side out.
- If wearing contact lenses gets your eye irritated, take out the lenses. Talk to the doctor and do not wear them until as suggested by the doctor. If you continue wearing them, your eye will get infected.
- In case you have sudden vision loss or have a blurred vision that would not get better; if you experience light flashes, swelling and unusual redness in your eye, go to your eye doctor right away.
- If you smoke, then quit smoking.
- Contact lens wearers who smoke are more likely to get eye problems than non-smokers.
- Do not use any decorative lenses.
- Avoid buying lenses that are sold at the at costume shops. These lenses can damage your eyes permanently.
- Get your eyes regularly checked.

❖ If you wear contact lenses, you should visit an eye care specialist quarterly or annually as per your need and as suggested by the doctor.

You are suffering from a contact-lens related infection if you experience these following symptoms:
❖ Blurry vision
❖ Unusual redness of the eye
❖ Feeling like there is something in your eye
❖ Pain in the eye
❖ Light sensitivity
❖ Tearing or heavy discharge from the eye

Do not avoid these symptoms as contact lens-related eye infections can cause severe complications and even cause vision loss. Rush to an eye specialist if you wear a contact lens and experience all these symptoms.

CARE FOR REMOVABLE DENTURES

Removable partial or full dentures require proper care to keep them clean, free from stains and looking their best.

Good denture care:
❖ Remove and rinse dentures after eating.
❖ Run water over your dentures to remove food debris and other loose particles.
❖ You may want to place a towel on the counter or in the sink or put some water in the sink so the dentures would not break if you drop them.
❖ Handle your dentures carefully. Be sure you do not bend or damage the plastic or the clasps when cleaning.
❖ Clean your mouth after removing your dentures.
❖ Use a soft-bristled toothbrush on natural teeth and gauze or a soft toothbrush to clean your tongue, cheeks and roof of your mouth (palate). If used, remove any remaining denture adhesive from your gums.
❖ Brush your dentures at least daily.
❖ Remove and gently clean your dentures daily.
❖ Soak and brush them with a soft-bristled brush and nonabrasive denture cleanser to remove food, plaque and other deposits.
❖ If you use denture adhesive, clean the grooves that fit against your gums to remove any remaining adhesive. Do not use denture cleansers inside your mouth.
❖ Soak dentures overnight. Most types of dentures need to stay moist to keep their shape.
❖ Place the dentures in water or a mild denture-soaking solution overnight.
❖ Check with your dentist about properly storing your dentures overnight.
❖ Follow the manufacturer's instructions on cleaning and soaking solutions.
❖ Rinse dentures thoroughly before putting them back in your mouth, especially if using a denture-soaking solution.
❖ These solutions can contain harmful chemicals that cause vomiting, pain or burns if swallowed.
❖ Schedule regular dental checkups.
❖ Your dentist will recommend how often to visit to have your dentures examined and professionally cleaned.
❖ Your dentist can help ensure a proper fit to prevent slippage and discomfort, and also check the inside of your mouth to make sure it is healthy.
❖ See your dentist if you have a loose fit. See your dentist promptly if your dentures become loose. Loose dentures can cause irritation, sores and infection.

Things to be avoided:
❖ Abrasive cleaning materials.
❖ Avoid stiff-bristled brushes, strong cleansers and harsh toothpaste, as these are too abrasive and can damage your dentures.
❖ Whitening toothpastes.
❖ Toothpastes advertised as whitening pastes often contain peroxide, which does little to change the color of denture teeth.
❖ Bleach-containing products.
❖ Do not use any bleaching products because these can weaken dentures and change their color.
❖ Do not soak dentures with metal attachments in solutions that contain chlorine because it can tarnish and corrode the metal.
❖ **Hot water:** Avoid hot or boiling water that could warp your dentures.

CARE AND MAINTENANCE OF HEARING AID

❖ Prevent it from falling down
❖ Do not spill liquids on the hearing aid.
❖ It must fit well.
❖ Cords should not be twisted or knotted.
❖ Protect it from dust, dirt and heat.
❖ Remove the battery from hearing aid when it is not in use.
❖ Remember to detach the ear mould from the receiver before washing the mould.
❖ Receiver should not come in contact with the water.
❖ Do not expose the hearing aid to medicinal or hair sprays

CHAPTER 5

Elimination Needs

URINARY ELIMINATION

Introductions

- Elimination refers to the expelling of waste materials from the body.
- It takes place through the lungs, skin, urinary system and the intestinal tract.
- Elimination by all four routes are natural processes that must occur for the maintenance of good body function and health.
- While some fluid leaves the body through each route of elimination, the largest amount is excreted as urine through the urinary system.
- Small amounts of salts and other mineral compounds are excreted in the fluid waste, but most of the solid waste leaves through the intestinal tract.
- The elimination of wastes is a natural function, but between of cultural practices and personal habits, many people find it embarrassing to request help to care for normal elimination.
- Respectful assistance given in privacy is helpful in causing a patient to feel at ease.

Review of Physiology of Urine Elimination

- **The organs of the urinary system are (Fig. 5.1):**
  - Kidneys
  - Ureters
  - Urinary bladder
  - Urethra.
- After the kidneys filter blood and return most water are many solutes to the bloodstream, the remaining water and solutes constitute urine.
- **Nephrons perform three basic tasks (Fig. 5.2):**
  1. Glomerular filtration
  2. Secretion
  3. Tubular reabsorption.
- The ureters are retroperitoneal and consist of a mucosa, muscularis, and adventitia. They transport urine from the renal pelvis to the urinary bladder, primarily via peristalsis.
- The urinary bladder is located in the pelvic cavity posterior to the pubic symphysis; its function is to store urine before micturition.

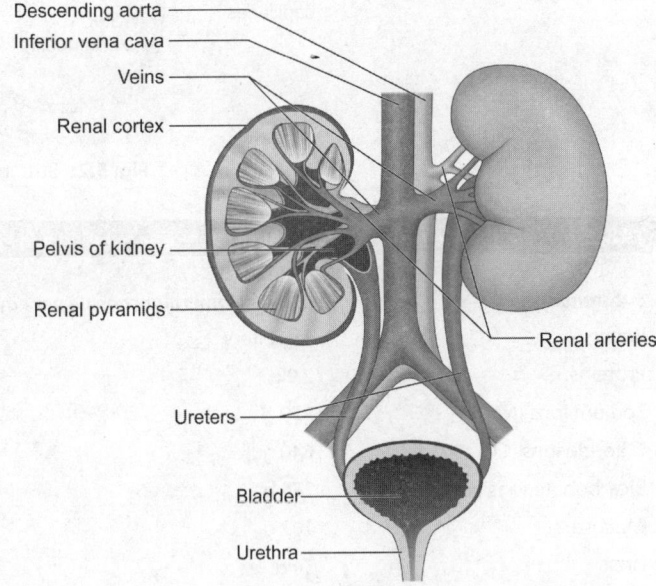

Fig. 5.1: Urinary system.

- The urinary bladder consists of a mucosa with rugae, a muscularis (detrusor muscle), and adventitious (serosa over the superior surface).
- The micturition reflex discharges urine from the urinary bladder via parasympathetic impulses that cause contraction of the detrusor muscle and relaxation of the internal urethral sphincter muscle and via inhibition of impulses in somatic motor neurons to the external urethral sphincter.
- The urethra is a tube leading from the floor of the urinary bladder to the exterior. Its anatomy and histology differ in females and males. In both sexes, the urethra functions to discharge urine from the body; in males, it discharges semen as well.

Composition of Urine

See **Table 5.1**.

Characteristics of Normal Urine

pH

Ranges between 4.5 and 8.0; average 6.0 (slightly acidic); varies considerably with diet. High-protein diets increase acidity.

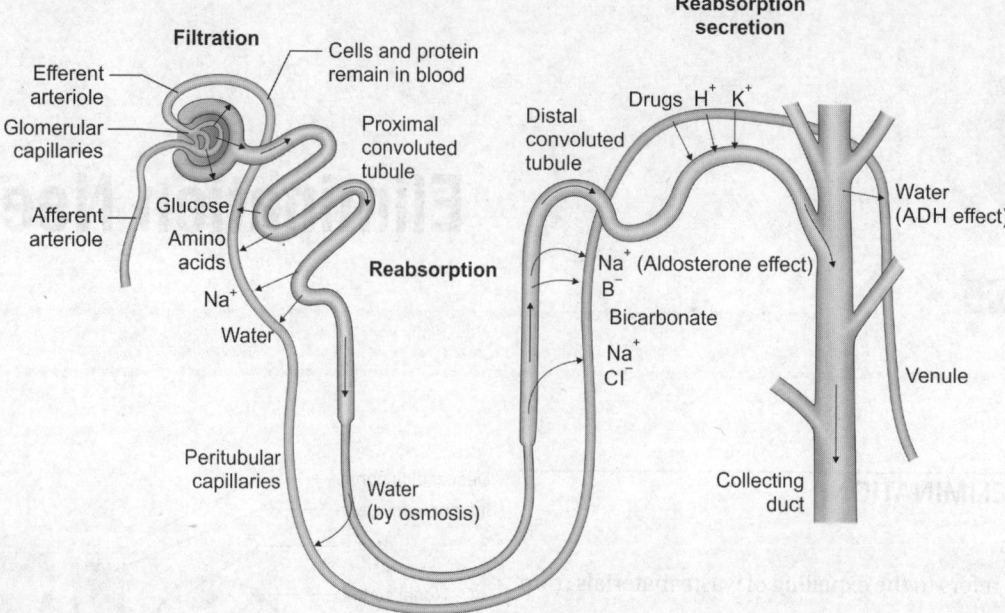

Fig. 5.2: Structure of nephron.

TABLE 5.1: Composition of urine—substance filtered, reabsorbed and excreted in urine.

Substance	Filtered (Enters glomerular capsule per day)	Reabsorbed (Returned to blood per day)	Urine (Excreted per day)
Water	180 Liters	178–179 Liters	1–2 Liters
Proteins	2.0 g	1.9 g	0.19 g
Sodium ions (Na^+)	579 g	575 g	4 g
Chloride ions (Cl^-)	640 g	633.7 g	6.3 g
Bicarbonate ions (HCO^-)	275 g	275 g	0.03 g
Glucose	162 g	162 g	0 g
Urea	54 g	24 g	30 g
Potassium ions (K^+)	29.6 g	29.6 g	2.0 g
Uric acid	8.5 g	7.7 g	0.8 g
Creatinine	1.69	0.9 g	1.7 g

Vegetarian diet, prolonged vomiting and bacterial infection of urinary tract increases alkalinity.

Volume
One to two litres in 24 hours but varies considerable.

Color
Yellow or amber but varies with urine concentration and diet. Color is due to urochrome (pigment produced from breakdown of hemoglobin). Concentrated urine is darker in color. Diet (reddish-colored urine from beets), medications, and certain diseases affect color. Kidney stones may produce blood in urine.

Turbidity
Transparent when freshly voided but becomes turbid (cloudy) upon standing.

Odor
Mildly aromatic but becomes ammonia like upon standing some people inherit the ability to form methyl mercaptan from digested asparagus that gives urine a characteristic odor. Urine of diabetics.

Factors in Influencing Urinary Elimination
Urinary elimination depends on the function of the kidneys, ureters, bladder and urethra. The kidneys remove wastes from the blood and urine. The ureters transport urine from the kidneys to the bladder. The bladder holds the urine until the urge to urinate develops. The urine leaves the body through the urethra. All these organs must be intact and functional for the successful removal of urinary wastes.

❖ **Growth and development:**
- Infants and young children cannot concentrate urine and reabsorb water effectively.
- Children cannot control urination voluntarily until 18–24 months.
- A child must be able recognize the feeling of bladder fullness, to hold urine for 1–2 hours, and to communicate the sense of urgency to a parent.

- With age, the ability, to concentrate urine declines and the frequency of urination increases.
- The process of aging may impair micturition.
- Problems of mobility sometimes make it difficult for older adults to reach the toilet or bedside commode on time.
- Chronic diseases, such as multiple sclerosis or stroke, alter urinary pattern.

❖ **Sociocultural factors:**
- Cultural and gender norms vary on the privacy or publicness of urination. Most individuals expect toilet facilities to be private, whereas few cultural accept communal toilet facilities.
- Social expectations (e.g., school recesses) influences the time of urination.

❖ **Psychological factors:**
- Anxiety and stress do not affect the characteristics of urine but may affect a sense of urgency and increase the frequency of urination.
- Anxiety may prevent complete urination because tension make it difficult to relax abdominal muscles.

❖ **Personal habit:** Privacy and adequate time to urinate are usually important to most people. Some people need distractions to relax.

❖ **Muscle tone:**
- Weak abdominal and pelvic floor muscles impair bladder contraction and control of the external sphincter.
- Decreased muscle tone may be cause by immobility childbirth or trauma.
- Muscle tone may also be lost with continuous drainage of urine through an indwelling catheter.

❖ **Fluid intake:**
- If fluids electrolytes and solutes are balanced, increased fluid intake increase urine production
- Alcohol stops the release of antidiuretic hormones, thus promoting urine production.
- Fluids containing caffeine increase urinary output frequency.
- Foods, with high fluid content, such as fruits and vegetables, may increase urine production.

❖ **Pathological conditions:**
- Diabetes mellitus and multiple sclerosis cause neuropathies that alter bladder function.
- Rheumatoid arthritis, degenerative joint disease, and parkinsonism slow or hinder physical activity and interfere with urination.
- Acute renal disease reduces urine volume; chronic renal disease initially increases volume of poorly concentrated urine.
- Febrile conditions reduce the amount of urine but increase its concentration.
- Spinal cord injuries interrupt voluntary bladder emptying.

❖ **Surgical procedures:**
- The stress response to surgery reduces the amount of urinary output to increase circulatory fluid volume.
- Anesthetics and pain-killing abdominal and pelvic surgery may obstruct flow, so indwelling catheters may be needed.
- Local trauma during lower abdominal and pelvic surgery may obstruct urine flow, so indwelling catheters may be needed.

❖ **Medications:**
- Diuretics prevent reabsorption of water and certain electrolytes, and urinary output disease.
- Some drugs also change the color of urine (e.g., amitriptyline turns it blue-green, and methyldopa turns it red, warfarin sodium turns it orange, and indomethacin turns it green).
- Medications may affect the ability to relax and empty the bladder.

❖ **Diagnostic examination:**
- Following intravenous pyelograms, monitor patient for complications such as hypersensitivity reactions and acute renal failure.
- Cystoscopy may cause localized edema of the urethral passage and bladder sphincter spasm, resulting in urinary retention and the passing of red or pink urine.

Alterations in Urinary Elimination

Clients with urinary problems most commonly have disturbances in the act of micturition that involve a failure to store urine or a failure to empty urine. These disturbances result from impaired bladder function, obstruction to urine outflow, or inability to voluntarily control micturition. Some clients may have permanent or temporary changes in the normal pathway of urinary excretion. The client with a urinary diversion has special problems because urine drains to the outside through a stoma.

❖ **Different terms that are most commonly used for passing urine:**
- Urination
- Micturition
- Voiding

❖ **Patients often use a term that has been used in the family of community:**
- *Oliguria:* A decreased amount of urine passed.
- *Anuria:* A complete lack of urine.
- *Suppression:* An anuria is due to the kidneys failing to produce urine.
- *Retention:* When urine is produced, but kept in the bladder.
- *Incontinence:* Uncontrolled urination is incontinence.
- *Frequency:* If a person must urinate often, is called frequency.
- *Dysuria:* It is painful urination.
- *Polyuria:* It is an abnormally large amount of urine.
- *Glycosuria:* Glycosuria is sugar (glucose) in the urine.
- *Albuminuria:* Albumin (protein) in the urine and is sometimes called *proteinuria*.
- *Pyuria:* It is pus in the urine.
- *Calculi:* These are stones, formed from minerals, in the urine.
- *Hematuria:* It is blood in the urine.
- *Chyluria:* It is the urine giving it a milky appearance.

Common Urinary Disorders

Urinary Retention
Urine flow is obstructed; urine accumulates in bladder, low fluid intake can lead to retention.

Lower Urinary Tract Infection
Microorganisms may be introduced resulting in bacterial spread, causing inflammation of bladder muscle.

Urinary Incontinence
Incontinence involves incompetent or weakened sphincter and loss of control of voiding.

Types of Urinary Incontinence

Total
Total uncontrollable and continuous loss of urine.

Functional
Involuntary unpredictable passage of urine in patient with intact urinary and nervous systems.

Stress
Increased intra-abdominal pressure causing leakage of small amount of urine.

Urge
Involuntary passage of urine after strong sense of urgency to void.

Reflex
Involuntary passage of urine occurring at somewhat predictable intervals when specific bladder volume is reached.

Managing Urinary Incontinence

- Independent nursing interventions for patients with urinary incontinence include
- A behaviour-oriented continence training program that may consist of bladder training, habit training, prompted voiding, pelvic muscle exercise, and positive reinforcement;
- Meticulous skin care;
- For males, application of an external drainage device (condom).
- The physician may order urinary catheterization for patients unable to control micturition.

Complications of Alteration in Urine Elimination
See **Table 5.2**.

TABLE 5.2: Complications of alteration in urine elimination.

Sl. No.	Complications	Causes	Interventions
1.	Sepsis	• High glucose content of fluid. • Venous access device contamination	• Monitor temperature, WBC count and Insertion site for signs and symptoms of infection • Maintain strict surgical asepsis when changing dressing and tubing. • Consider decreasing glucose content of fluid • Consider removal of venous access device with replacement in alternate site • If blood culture is positive consider institution of antibiotic therapy
2.	Electrolyte imbalance	• Iatrogenic • Effect of underlying diseases, i.e., fistula, diarrhea, vomiting	• Monitor for signs and symptoms of electrolyte imbalances • Treat underlying cause • Change concentration of electrolytes in TNA as necessary
3.	Hyperglycemia	High glucose content of fluid Insufficient insulin secretion	• Monitor blood glucose frequently • Decrease glucose content of fluid if possible • Administer exogenous insulin
4.	Hypoglycemia	Abrupt discontinuation of TNA administration through a central vein	After discontinuation of centrally administered TNA, start 10% dextrose at the same rate
5.	Hypervolemia	• Iatrogenic • Underlying disease such as congestive heart failure (CHF) and renal failure	• Monitor intake and output, daily weight, sounds and peripheral edema. • Consider administering more concentrated TNA solution
6.	Hyperosmolar diuresis	High osmolarity of parenteral nutritional fluid	Consider decreasing the concentration or amount of fluid administered
7.	Hepatic dysfunction	High concentration of carbohydrates/fats relative to protein	• Monitor liver function tests, triglyceride levels and presence of jaundice • Consider alteration in formula
8.	Hypercarbia	High carbohydrate content of fluid	Consider changing formula to increase the proportion of fat relative to carbohydrate
9.	Lipids intolerance	• Low birth weight or premature infant • History of liver disease • History of elevated triglycerides	• Monitor triglyceride levels and liver function test, hepatosplenomegaly, decreased coagulation, cyanosis, dyspnea • Monitor oxygen levels for impaired oxygenation • Monitor allergic reactions such as nausea, vomiting, headache, chest pain, back pain and fever • Administer lipid containing solution slowly • Monitor fat overload syndrome • Monitor for bleeding
10.	Lipid particulate aggregation	Unstable mixture of dextrose solution with lipid emulsion	Observe for cracking or creaming of fluid and avoid use of fluid with these characteristics

FACILITATING URINE ELIMINATION

For the patient who has difficulty in voiding, there are certain nursing measures that can be provided to assists him.
- Help the patient to assume a natural position of voiding.
- Provide a commode or preferably assist the patient to the bathroom if this is possible (male patients frequently find it easier to void when they are standing rather than sitting or lying down).
- Open tap for patient's to hear.
- Provide water in which he can dangle his fingers.
- Provide privacy and allow time for voiding.
- Provide a warm bedpan or urinal.
- Apply a hot water bottle to the patient's lower abdomen. (This may require doctors order).
- Pour warm water over the perineum (the water must be measured).
- Relieve pain.

PROVIDING URINAL

Urinal is used for male patients to void the urine the nurse should assist the bedridden to void into a urinal (a plastic or metal receptacle for urine in bed) **(Fig. 5.3)**.

In case of female patients, nurse should provide bedpan for bedridden to collect the urine.

Purposes
- To promote comfort
- To assist to void
- To prevent bed wetting
- To maintain the urinary output record
- To minimize the physical strain.

Factors Influences
- Normal urinary elimination habits
- Nature of disease condition
- Environment (privacy)
- The amount of intake (food and fluids)
- Availability of equipment and personal.

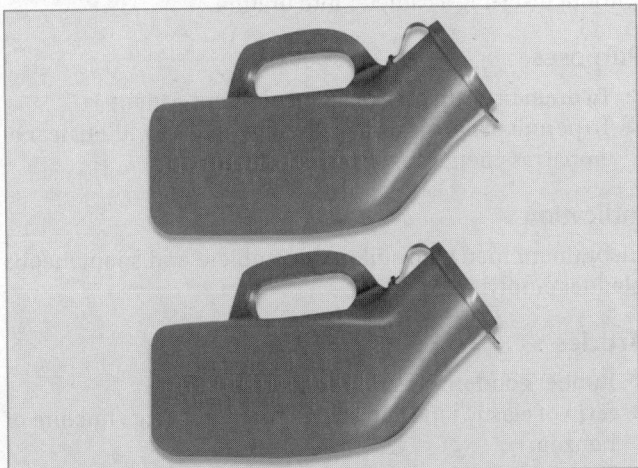

Fig. 5.3: Urinals.

Preliminary Assessment
Check
- Doctors order for specific precautions such as movements and position
- Level of consciousness
- Self-care ability of the patient
- Frequency of urination
- Articles available in the unit.

Preparations of the Patient and Environment
- Provide adequate privacy
- Arrange the article (urinal) ready at bedside
- Place the Mackintosh and draw sheet
- Place the patient in proper body alignment.

Equipment
- Clean urinal
- Disposable gloves
- Clean linen if required
- Hand washing basin, mug and water
- Soap with soap dish
- Measuring jar.

Procedures
- Wash hands thoroughly
- If the patient is conscious, allow him to place urinal or else position penis into urinal
- Prevent soiling of urine on bed or patients body
- Remain with helpless patient get assistance from relative if needed
- Remove urinal after patient has voided
- Measure and empty the urine in slice room.

Aftercare
- Assist the patient to wash perineal area and hands
- Place the patient in a proper body alignment
- Change the bed linen, if required
- Replace the articles used after cleaning
- Wash hands.
- Record the procedure in nurse's record sheet and the amount in intake-output chart.

PROVIDING BEDPAN
- Bedpan is made from steel or plastic device to meet elimination need of patient confined to bed.
- Bedpan may be used by a person who is unable to get out to bed.
- Bedpans used by females for elimination of urine and feces and by male for elimination of feces.

Purposes
- To provide comfort
- To facilitate bowel and bladder elimination
- To collect specimen for diagnostic purposes
- To promote continence during bowel and bladder training
- To give perineal wash.

Indications

- Patient with spinal injury
- Post operative patients
- Patients with fracture and traction
- Chronic bedridden patients
- Patients those who are strict bedrest.

Types of Bedpans

- The regular high bedpan (**Fig. 5.4**).
- The slipper pan or fracture pan (**Fig. 5.5**).

Preliminary Assessment

Check

- The doctors order for specific precautions such as movements and positions
- General condition of the patient
- Level of consciousness
- Mental healthy to follow instructions
- Self-care ability
- Articles available in the unit.

Preparation of Patient and Environment

- Explain to assist (hip to lift)
- Arrange the articles at the bedside
- Provide privacy
- Position the patient in comfortable position
- Place the Mackintosh under the buttocks to prevent soiling.

Equipments

- Bedpan with lid
- Clean gloves
- Draw Mackintosh if needed
- Water and mug
- Tissue paper
- Soap with soap dish
- K-Basin and towel.

Procedures

- Encourage patient to assume normal position for defecation, if possible
- Place the dry bedpan under patients buttocks.
- Assist patient to lift buttocks by supporting the back with left hand
- Instruct and assist patient to raise hips or turn patient to side and place bedpan firmly close to buttocks.
- Provide adequate time to pass motion/urine.
- Check the well-covered be pan to avoid embarrassment
- Once patient has passed, permit to clean self. Assist by pouring water
- If patient is unable to clean, pour water and clean using long artery clamp and cotton balls rag pieces
- Remove bedpan by lifting patient careful.

Aftercare

- Cover bedpan immediately and try Mackintosh of wet
- Secure draw sheet and position the patient comfortably
- Provide water and soap to wash hands
- Empty the articles to stop-hopper in sluice room
- Replace the articles after cleaning
- Wash hands thoroughly
- Record the procedure in the nurses' sheet.

CONDOM DRAINAGE

Definition

Applying a thin condom sheath to penis for drainage of urine without inserting a catheter into urethra.

Purposes

- To drain urine in case of an incontinent patient
- To permit patient's normal physical activity without fear of embarrassment caused by incontinence.

Indication

Incontinent men who still have complete and spontaneous bladder emptying.

Articles

- Rubber condom sheath (Proper size)
- Strip of elastic tape and skin preparation, (e.g., tincture of benzoin)
- Urinary collection bag with drainage tubing
- Basin with warm water and soap

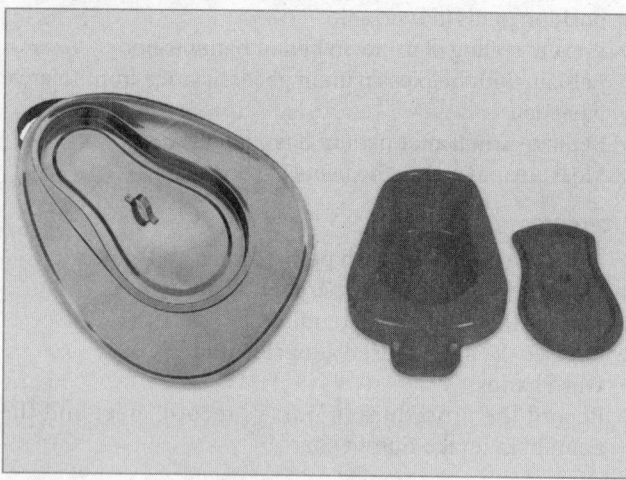

Fig. 5.4: Bedpan.

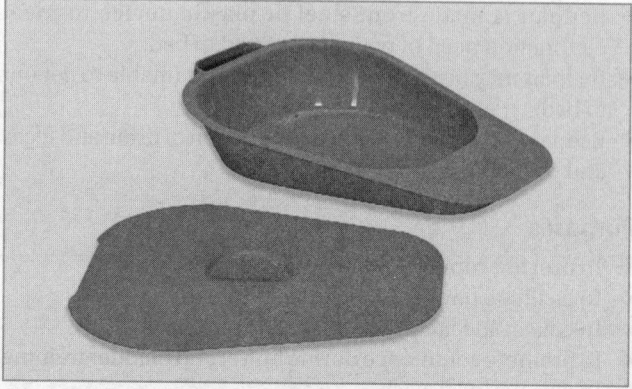

Fig. 5.5: Slipper pan.

- Towel and wash cloths
- Disposable gloves
- Sheets
- Razor (optional).

Procedure of Condom Drainage
See **Table 5.3**.

Special Considerations
- Remove the condom once a day to clean the area and assess the skin for signs of impaired skin integrity. This will promote hygiene and reduce the possibility of skin breakdown.
- Do not reattach the condom catheter if it falls off. It will not stick any better in second try. Apply a new catheter and strip.
- Clients may have latex allergy and may require latex-free condoms.

■ PROVIDING GENITAL CARE/HYGIENIC PERINEAL CARE

Definition
Genital involves thorough cleansing of external genitalia and surrounding skin.

Purposes
- To promote patient's comfort and cleanliness
- To prevent infection in high-risk patients.

TABLE 5.3: Steps of procedure for insertion of condom drainage catheter.

Nursing Interventions	Rationale
Explain procedure to patient and assess status of patient	Reduces anxiety and promotes cooperation
Wash hands	Reduces transmission of infection
Provide privacy	Maintains patient's self-esteem
Assist patient to supine position. Place bath blanket over upper torso. Fold sheets so that lower extremities are covered. Only genitalia should be exposed	Promotes patient comfort and prevents unnecessary exposure of body parts
Assess condition of penis for skin irritation, excoriation, swelling or discoloration	Provides baseline to compare changes in condition of skin after condom application. The patient may require an indwelling catheter if there is significant amount of skin breakdown
Apply disposable gloves. Provide perineal care and dry thoroughly. Clip hair at the base of penis, if required	Removes irritating secretions. Rubber sheath rolls onto dry skin more easily. Hair adheres to condom and pulls during adhesive tape removal causing discomfort
Prepare urinary collection bag and tubing or prepare leg bag for connection to condom, if necessary. Clamp off drainage exit ports. Secure collection bag to bed frame or patient's legs. Bring drainage tubing up through side rails on to bed	Provides easy access to drainage equipment after condom is in place
Apply skin preparation to penis and allow to dry for 30–60 seconds	Prepares penis for easy condom placement
With nondominant hand, grasp penis along shaft and with dominant hand roll condom sheath onto penis	
Allow 2.5-5 cm (1-2 inches) of space between root of penis and end of condom catheter. This space prevents a irritation of the tip of the penis	Allows free passage of urine into collecting tubing when patient passes urine
Encircle penile shaft with a strip of elastic adhesive. Strip should touch only condom sheath. The strip should be applied one inch from the proximal end of penis and do not completely encircle or tighten the penis	Condom must be secured so that it fits snugly and will stay on but not too tight to cause vasoconstriction
Connect drainage tubing to end of condom catheter. Be sure that condom is not twisted	Allows urine to be collected and measured. Keeps patient dry. Twisted condom obstructs urine flow
Coil the excess tubing on bed and secure to bottom sheet	Prevents looping of tubing and promotes free drainage of urine
Place the patient in safe and comfortable position (lying down/sitting)	Promotes patient's comfort
Remove gloves. Dispose off contaminated supplies and wash hands	Prevents spread of infection
Return in 30-60 minutes to observe for urinary drainage	Determines whether normal voiding is occurring
Regularly inspect skin on penile shaft for signs of breakdown/irritation	Indicates whether condom or urine is causing irritation or whether adhesive is too restrictive
Record and report, time of condom application, condition of skin and voiding pattern	Provides data to determine change in elimination status

Indications

- Patients who are unable to do self-care
- Patients with indwelling catheter
- Patients with incontinence of urine or stool
- Patients having excessive vaginal discharge
- Patients recovering from rectal or genital surgery
- Following childbirth.

Articles

- Wash basin
- Soap dish with soap
- Washcloths (2)
- Bath towel
- Bath blanket/bed sheet
- Bedpan
- Disposable gloves.
- Cotton swabs
- Kidney tray
- Toilet tissues or diaper wipes.

Procedures

- Explain procedure and its purpose to patient.
- Wash hand and Don clean gloves.
- Position patient with legs spread apart.
- Assess genitalia for signs of inflammation, skin breakdown, infection or contamination with fecal matter.
- If fecal material is present enclose in a fold of pad or toilet tissue and remove. With disposable wipes or tissue cleanse buttocks and anus, washing from front to back. Cleanse, rinse and dry area thoroughly. Remove and discard underpad and replace with clean one.
- Change gloves if they are soiled.
- Help patient to flex knees and spread legs apart.
- Fold top linen toward foot of bed and fold patient's gown above genital area.
- Diamond drape patient by placing bath blanket/top sheet with one corner between patient's legs, and another corner over patient's chest. The two side corners should hangover sides of bed. Truck corner around patient's legs and under hips.
- Place washbasin and toilet tissue on over bed table, place washclothes in basin.
- Raise side rails, fill basin with warm water.
- **Female genital care:**
  - Lower side rails and instruct patient to maintain dorsal recumbent position with knees flexed and legs apart. Note any restriction or limitation in positioning patient.
  - Fold lower corner of bath blanket/sheet up between patient's legs onto abdomen. Wash and dry patient's upper thighs.
  - Wash labia major a while using nondominant hand to retract labia form thigh. With dominant handwash carefully in skin folds and wipe in direction from perineum to rectum. Repeat on opposite side using separate section of wash cloth. Rinses and dry area thoroughly.
  - Separate labia with nondominant hand to expose urethral meatus and vaginal orifice. With dominant handwash downwards from public area towards rectum using separate quarters of washcloth for each stroke. Clean the vulva and labia minora on both sides and inside of labia majora on both sides.
  - If patient can use bedpan, place bedpan and pour water over perineal area. Dry perineal area thoroughly with bath towel from front to back.
  - Fold lower corner of bath blanket back between patient's legs and over perineum. Ask patient to lower legs and assume comfortable position.
- **Male genital care:**
  - Lower side rails and assist patient to supine position note restriction in mobility if any.
  - Fold top half of bath blanket/sheet down below the penis. Position gown to cover chest. Wash and dry patient's upper thighs.
  - Gently raise penis and place bath towel underneath. Firmly grasp shaft of penis, if patient is un-circumcized, retract foreskin. If patient has an erection, defer procedure until later.
  - Wash top of penis at urethral meatus first using circular motion. Cleanse from meatus outwards. Discard wash cloth and repeat with clean cloth until penis is clean. Rinse and dry gently.
  - Return foreskin to its original position.
  - Wash shaft of penis with gentle but firm downward strokes. Pay special attention to underlying surface of penis. Rinse and dry penis thoroughly. Instruct patient's to spread legs apart slightly.
  - Gently cleanse scrotum. Lift and wash underlying skinfold. Rinse and dry.
- Fold bath blanket over patient's perineum and assist patient in turning to side lying position.
- If patient has urinary or bowel incontinence, apply thin layer or skin barrier containing petroleum jelly over skin.
- Apply under-pads if required.
- Remove disposable gloves and dispose in proper receptacle.
- Assist patient to comfortable position and cover him or her with top sheet.
- Remove bath blanket, dispose of all soiled bed linen and return unused articles to storage area.
- Record procedure and presence of any abnormal finding. For example, character and amount of discharge and condition of genitalia.
- Report any abnormality observed to nurse in-charge and physician.

CATHETERIZATION OF THE URINARY BLADDER

- **Urinary catheterization:** It is the introduction of a tube (a catheter) through the urethra into the urinary bladder to drain the bladder.
- This is an aseptic method of introducing the catheter into the urinary bladder through the external urethra for withdrawal of urine.

Purposes

- To obtain a clear specimen for diagnostic purpose.
- To relieve distension on bladder caused by retention of urine.
- To determine whether the failure to void is due to retention or suppression.
- To determine the amount of residual urine present in the bladder.
- To empty the bladder prior to surgery, bladder, irrigation or before instillation of a drug.
- To avoid soiling and infection of the wound following operations on the genital region.
- To manage incontinency, when all other measures to prevent skin breakdown have failed.
- To provide for intermittent or continuous bladder drainage and irrigation.
- To prevent urine form passing over a wound, e.g., after repair of the perineum.

Principles Involved

- Pathogenic organisms are transmitted from the source to a new host directly on by contaminated articles.
- Urinary bladder is a sterile cavity and the urinary meatus acts as a portal of entry for pathogenic organisms.
- Cleaning an area minimizes the spread of organisms.
- A break in the integrity of the skin and mucous membrane provides ready entrance for microorganism.
- Lubrication reduces friction.
- Through knowledge of anatomy and physiology of the genitourinary system facilitates catheterization of the urinary bladder.
- Systematic ways of doing save time, energy and material.
- Unfamiliar situation produce anxiety.

General Instruction

- Apply all the nursing measures to induce urination before the catheterization of the bladder.
- Observe strict aseptic techniques to prevent the urinary tract infection.
- Catheterization should be done slowly and never use force.
- Always catheterize in a good light.
- Clean the perineum from the pubis downwards to the anal region.
- Use on cotton ball for one swabbing.
- Do not touch the portion of the catheter that is going into the urinary tract.
- Lubricate the catheter well before introducing into the urinary tract.
- Keep the patient relaxed by providing privacy and adequate explanations.

Preliminary Assessment

Check

- Doctors order for any specific precautions
- Identify the purpose of catheterization
- Level of consciousness
- Any contraindications
- General conditions of the patient
- Mental status to follow instructions
- Articles available in the unit.

Preparations of Patient and Environment

- Explain the sequences of the procedure
- Arrange the articles at the bed side locker
- Provide privacy
- Position the patient in dorsal recumbent
- Place the Mackintosh and towel under the buttocks
- Provide adequate light by placing extra spotlight.

Equipment

A sterile tray containing:

- Catheter of correct size
- Small bowl containing an antiseptic
- Cotton swabs
- Pair of gloves
- Thumb forceps and artery forceps one each
- Sterile kidney tray-1 prefilled syringe with sterile water
- Sterile towel, sterile drainage tubing and collection bag
- Test tube or specimen bottle (if needed)
- Small cup containing lubricant.

A clean tray containing:

- Mackintosh and towel
- Flashlight or spotlight
- Bath blanket
- Kidney tray
- Adhesive tape and scissors
- Bedpan to empty the urine from the kidney tray
- Measuring jar
- Urobag or collection bag.

Cleaning the Perineum in Female Patients

- Clean only in one direction
- Use one swab for one swabbing
- Clean labia major a on both sides
- Clean the inside of the labia major a on both sides
- Clean the labia minora on the both sides
- Clean the vulva.

Cleaning the Perineum for Male Patients

- Retract the foreskin during the cleaning process
- Draw the penis upward and forward at 90° angle to the patients leg in order to straighten the urethra before the catheter is introduced
- Foreskin is replaced as quickly as possible after the insertion of the catheter.

Types of Catheterizations

Intermittent Catheterization

An intermittent catheter is used to drain the bladder for short periods (5–10 minutes). It may be inserted by the patient.

Short-term/Long-term Indwelling Catheterization/ Retention Catheterization

This type of catheter is placed into the bladder and secured there for a period of time. It is used following surgery, bladder injury or in bladder infections. It may also be used for an incontinent or non-responsive patient.

- It provides continuous temporary or permanent drainage of urine.
- It is used for gradual decompression of an over distended bladder.
- It is used for intermittent drainage and irrigation.

Foley's Catheter (Figs. 5.6A to D)

- The most commonly used indwelling catheter is the Foley's catheter.
- A drainage tube and collection device are connected to the catheter.
- It has a balloon at the distal end, which is inflated with sterile water or saline to prevent the catheter from slipping out of the bladder.
- It is multi-lumened (having several passages within the catheter).
- One lumen provides a passage for fluid to inflate the balloon.
- This passage may be self-sealing or may require a clamp.
- The second lumen is the passage through which the urine drains.
- Some indwelling catheters have a third lumen for instilling irrigation fluid.

Figure 5.7 shows the parts of catheter.

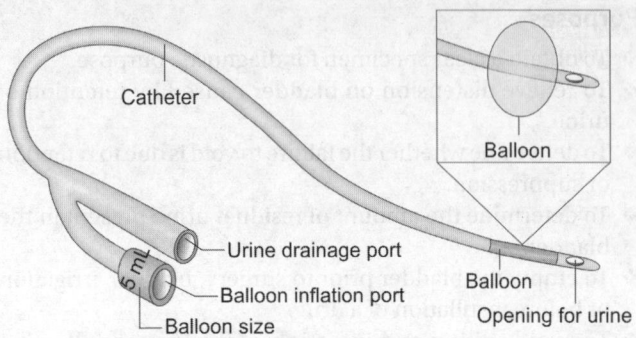

Fig. 5.7: Parts of catheter.

Urinary Catheter Sizes

The French scale (Fr.) is used to denote the size of catheters. Each unit is roughly equivalent to 0.33 mm in diameter, The smaller the number, the smaller the catheter. A larger sized catheter is used for a male because it is stiffer, thus easier to push the distance of the male urethra. Catheters come in several sizes **(Table 5.4)**:

- Number 8 Fr. and 10 Fr. are used for children.
- Number 14 Fr. and 16 Fr. are used for female adults.
- Number 20 Fr. and 22 Fr. are usually used for male adults

Suprapubic Catheter

This type of catheter is inserted into the bladder through a small incision above the pubic area. It is used for continuous drainage.

Procedure

Refer **Tables 5.5 and 5.6**.

Aftercare

- Wash and dry the perineum
- Remove the drapes, replace, the garments and bed covers
- Place the patient comfortably
- Take all the articles to the utility room, clean in and replace it
- Send specimen to the lab immediately
- Wash hands
- Record the procedure in the nurse's record sheet.

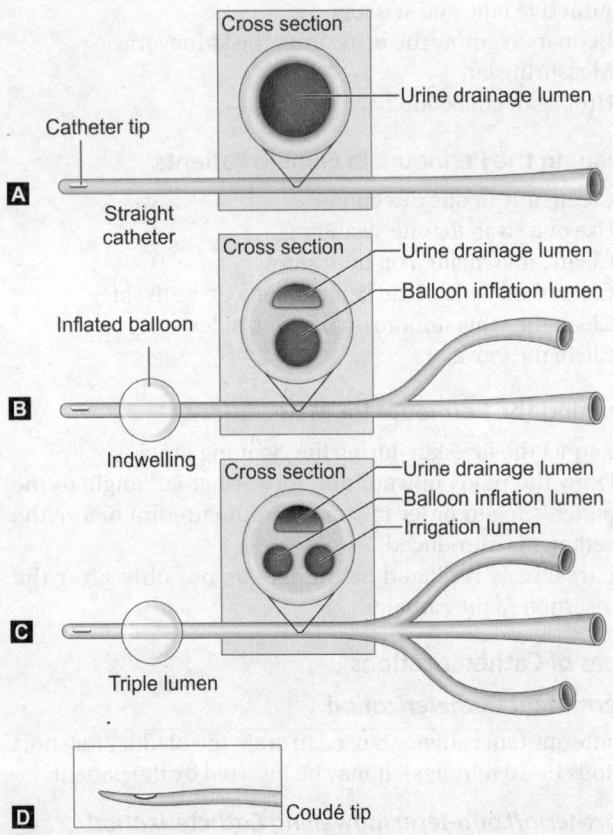

Figs. 5.6A to D: Types of catheters: (A) Straight catheter; (B) Indwelling (Foley) catheter; (C) Triple lumen indwelling catheter; (D) Coudé tip catheter.

TABLE 5.4: Color coding of catheter according to size.		
Color	Size (French)	Size (mm)
Light green	6	2.0
Light blue	8	2.7
Gray	10	3.3
White	12	4.0
Green	14	4.7
Orange	16	5.3
Red	18	6.0
Yellow	20	6.7
Purple	22	7.3
Blue	24	8.0
Black	26	8.7

TABLE 5.5: Steps of procedure for female catheterization.

Nursing action	Rationale
Identify the patient and explain the procedure to the patient	To get cooperation and to reduce anxiety
Provide privacy	To reduce the patient's hesitation
Move the patient to the edge of bed near to the nurse	For proper positioning
Place the patient in dorsal recumbent position	It helps in easy insertion of catheter
Wash the area around the meatus with soap and warm water. Rinse and dry	To clean the area
Wash your hands	To prevent infection
Open the sterile catheterization kit, using sterile technique	To start the procedure
Put on sterile gloves	To prevent the hands from contamination
Place the fenestrated drape on the patient with the hole over the female genitalia	To drape the patient
Apply sterile lubricant liberally to the catheter tip. Lubricate at least three inches of the catheter for the female. Leave the lubricated catheter over the cotton balls	For easy insertion of the catheter
Place the urine specimen collection container within reach	To collect the urine specimen, if needed
Place the thumb and forefinger of your non-dominant hand between the labia minora, spread and separate upward. The gloved hand that has touched the patient is now contaminated	To prevent the contamination of both hands
Using the forceps, pick up a cotton ball saturated with antiseptic solution. Use one cotton ball for each stroke. Swab from above the meatus downward towards the rectum	To clean from less to more contaminated area
Keeping the labia separated, cleanse each side of the meatus in the same downward manner. Do not go back over any previously cleansed area	To prevent the contamination of surrounding area
Deposit each cotton ball into the disposal bag. After the last cotton ball is used, deposit the forceps into the bag as well	To dispose the contaminated cotton balls
Continue to hold the labium apart after cleansing. Insert the lubricated catheter into the female patient's urinary meatus	To drain out the urine
Angle the catheter upward as it is advanced. If the catheter will not advance, instruct the patient to inhale and exhale slowly. This may relax the sphincter muscle. Do not force the catheter	To prevent any injury
When urine starts to flow, insert the catheter approximately one inch further. Place the cup under the stream of flowing urine to obtain a sterile specimen, if required	To ensure the correct placement of catheter
Hold the catheter in place while the urine drains into the collection container.	To collect the specimen
Attach the syringe to the balloon port of the catheter. Inject the water slowly to inflate the balloon. If the water will not inject easily or the patient complains of pain, deflate the balloon completely and advance the catheter further, then reinflate	To prevent the displacement of catheter
Remove the syringe. To position the balloon correctly, pull on the catheter gently until you feel resistance	To fix the catheter in place
Connect the drainage bag to the catheter. Secure the catheter to the inner aspect of the female patient's thigh	For regular drainage of urine
Attach the urinary drainage bag to the bed, below the level of the bladder but off the floor. Coil any extra tubing on the bed	To prevent any blockage or kinks

Irrigating an Indwelling Catheter

The purpose of irrigating a catheter is to remove particles that are interfering with the drainage of urine. A catheter that drains well does not need irrigating, except to instill medication. If the patient has a generous fluid intake (2500 cc to 3000 cc of fluid daily), the increase in urine production will dilute the particles that form and irrigate the catheter naturally, thus, invasive procedures may be avoided. Because the drainage system is opened when irrigation takes place, sterile technique is followed.

❖ Gather sterile supplies and equipments:
- Asepto syringe
- Basin
- Tubing protector
- Gauze moistened with antiseptic
- Sterile normal saline (or other irrigation solution).

Chapter 5: Elimination Needs

TABLE 5.6: Steps of procedure for male catheterization.

Nursing action	Rationale
Identify the patient and explain the procedure to the patient	To get cooperation and to reduce anxiety
Provide privacy	To reduce the patient's hesitation
Move the patient to the edge of bed near to the nurse	For proper positioning
Place the patient in supine position	It helps in easy insertion of catheter
Wash the perineal area with soap and warm water. Rinse and dry	To clean the area
Wash your hands	To prevent infection
Open the sterile catheterization kit, using sterile technique	To start the procedure
Put on sterile gloves	To prevent the hands from contamination
Open the sterile drape and place on the patient's thighs. Place fenestrated drape with opening on the penis	To drape the patient
Apply sterile lubricant liberally to the catheter tip. Lubricate at least six inches of the catheter for the female. Leave the lubricated catheter over the sterile field	For easy insertion of the catheter
Pour the antiseptic solution over the cotton balls	To clean
Place the urine specimen collection container within reach	To collect the urine specimen, if needed
Grasp the patient's penis between your thumb and forefinger of your non-dominant hand. Retract the foreskin of an uncircumcised male The gloved hand that has touched the patient is now contaminated	To prevent the contamination of both hands
Use the forceps to hold the cotton balls. This will maintain the sterility of other hand. Using the forceps, pick up one cotton ball and swab the center of the meatus outward in a circular manner	To clean from less to more contaminated area
Continue outward, using a new cotton ball for each progressively larger circle. Clean the entire gland. Deposit each cotton ball in the disposal bag. After the last cotton ball is used, drop the forceps into the disposal bag as well	To dispose the contaminated cotton balls
Hold the penis at a 90° angle. Advance the catheter into the patient's urinary meatus. You may encounter resistance at the prostatic sphincter Pause and allow the sphincter to relax Lower the penis and continue to advance the catheter	For easy insertion of the catheter
When the catheter has passed through the prostatic sphincter into the bladder, urine will start to flow into the collection bag if it is pre connected. If it is not pre connected, collect a specimen if required, then place the end of the catheter into the tubing of the sterile receptacle	To connect with continue drainage
Attach the syringe to the balloon port and inject the water slowly to inflate the balloon. Connect the urine collection bag if it is not preconnected	To prevent the displacement of the catheter
Anchor the catheter tubing to the lateral abdomen with tape	To fix the catheter in place
Secure the urinary collection bag below the level of the bladder and off the floor. Coil any extra tubing on the bed	To prevent any blockage

- Using gauze moistened with antiseptic solution, wipe the area where the catheter and tubing join.
- Place the sterile tubing protector on the end of the drainage tubing. An alternative is to cover the opening with sterile gauze moistened with antiseptic.
- Fill the syringe with 30 to 60 cc of solution and insert the syringe tip well into the end of the catheter.
- Gently compress the ball or end of the syringe to instill the irrigating solution. Do not apply force. Replace the catheter, if it cannot be irrigated.
- Allow the instilled solution to flow back into the basin by gravity.
- Connect the catheter and drainage tube.
- Note the total amount of solution used for irrigating and measure the amount of solution returned in the basin. In some cases, there is less solution returned than solution instilled. Both amounts must be recorded. The amount that remains will eventually drain into the collection bag.
- Discard the solution drained into the basin. Replace or protect the irrigating equipment.

❖ Record that the irrigation was done, by whom and the patient's response to the procedure.

CARE OF URINARY DRAINAGE

Definition
Cleansing the urethral meatus, the skin surrounding the catheter insertion site and perineum for patients with retention catheter who are bed ridden.

Purposes
❖ To promote patient comfort
❖ To reduce chances of developing urinary tract infection.

Articles
❖ **A sterile "catheter care kit" containing:**
  - Artery forceps
  - Thumb forceps
  - Cotton balls/swabs
  - Bowls for antiseptic lotion and sterile water.
❖ **A clean tray containing:**
  - Clean washcloth or towel—2 Nos.
  - Warm water and soap
  - Antiseptic lotion
  - Normal saline
  - Mackintosh/waterproof pads and draw sheets
  - Antibiotic ointment
  - Clean gloves
  - Sterile gloves
  - Drapes
  - Kidney tray
  - Adhesive tape and scissors.

Procedure Care of Urinary Drainage
See **Table 5.7**.

TABLE 5.7: Steps of procedure for care of urinary drainage.

Nursing action	Rationale
Prepare necessary equipment and supplies	Ensures efficiency and smooth functioning
Explain procedure to patient, offer opportunity for self-care if possible	Reduces anxiety and promotes cooperation
Provide privacy	Maintains patient's self-esteem
Wash hands	Reduces transmission of microorganisms
Position patient: • **Female:** Dorsal recumbent position with legs flexed • **Male:** Supine position	Ensures easy access to perineal area
Place waterproof pad/Mackintosh and draw sheet under patient	Protects bed linen from soiling
Drape sheet over patient exposing only perineal area	Prevents unnecessary exposure of body parts
Don clean gloves	
Remove anchor tapes to free catheter tubing	
Expose the urethral meatus (with nondominant hand): • **Female:** Gently retract labia to fully expose urethral meatus and catheter insertion site. Maintain position of hand throughout procedure • **Male:** Retract foreskin if patient is not circumcised and hold penis at shaft just below glans. Maintaining position of hand throughout procedure	Provides full visualization of urethral meatus. Retraction prevents foreskin contaminating the meatus, during cleansing. Accidentally letting go of penis requires that process be repeated
Assess urethral meatus and surrounding tissue for inflammation, swelling and discharge. Note amount, color, odor and consistency of discharge. Ask patient if burning or discomfort is felt	Determines presence of local infection and hygiene status
Cleanse perineal tissue: • **Female:** Use clean cloth, soap and water and clean towards anus. Cleanse catheter first and then meatus, labia minora and majora. Be sure to cleanse each side and dry area well • **Male:** Cleanse catheter first and then clean from urethral meatus till glans penis in circular motion	Cleansing reduces number of microorganisms at urethral meatus. Use of clean cloth prevents transfer of microorganisms. Moving from the most clean area decreases risk of recontamination
Reassess urethral meatus for any discharge	Determines whether cleaning is complete
Remove clean gloves and wash hands	
Don sterile gloves	
Clean the perineal area with disinfectant: • **Females:** Retract labia and wipe using sterile cotton swabs dipped in antiseptic solution from center to periphery in straight dipped in antiseptic solution from center to periphery in straight strokes from front to back, using one cotton ball for each stroke • **Male:** Retract foreskin and wipe using swabs from center to periphery in circular stokes	Moving from an area where there is less number of organisms to an area where there is more number of organisms will help in preventing spread of infection
Repeat previous step using cotton swabs soaked in sterile water/normal saline.	Antiseptic solution may act as an irritant to skin.
Apply antiseptic ointment at urethral meatus and along 2.5 cm (inch) of catheter. Anchor catheter	Reduces further growth of microorganisms at insertion site

After Care

- Place patient in safe and comfortable position.
- Remove gloves, dispose of contaminated supplies and wash hands.
- Record and report condition of perineal tissue, the time procedure was performed, patient's response and abnormalities noted.

Special Consideration

Catheter has to be changed periodically as per agency policy.

REMOVING AN INDWELLING URINARY CATHETER

Purposes

- To promote normal bladder function
- To prevent trauma to the urethra
- To prevent infection.

Articles

- Syringe without needle (10 mL)
- Clean gloves
- Protective pad
- Soap, towel and washcloth
- Container for waste disposal
- Urinal or bedpan
- Kidney tray.

Procedure Removing an Indwelling Urinary Catheter

See **Table 5.8**.

Special Consideration

- Instruct patient to inform the nurse, if experiencing any pain, or symptoms of bladder infection, after the catheter is removed.
- Check if physician has ordered bladder conditioning before removal of catheter.

TABLE 5.8: Steps of procedure for removing an indwelling urinary catheter.

Nursing action	Rationale
Wash hands and Don gloves	Reduces transmission of microorganisms
If bladder conditioning is to be performed: • 10 hours before removal, clamp indwelling catheter for 3 hours • Unclamp and drain urine for 5 minutes • Repeat clamping for 3 hours and draining for 5 minutes two more times	Volume of urine stretches bladder wall to stimulate muscle tone. Unclamping the catheter simulates voiding. Patients who receive bladder conditioning are able to feel urge to void sooner than those who have no conditioning
Wash hands	Decreases the transmission of microorganisms
Check the doctor's order	Ensures correct patient and treatment
Identify the patient and explain procedure	Elicits patient's cooperation
Provide privacy and position patient on back	Providing privacy demonstrates respect for patient's dignity
Remove covers and drape so as to expose catheter but do not overly expose perineal area	Protects patient's privacy and reduces embarrassment
Place protective pad under patient's thighs	Prevents bed from becoming soiled
Empty urine in tubing into urobag	Prevents leakage from catheter onto patient, and onto the bed when the catheter is removed
Remove any tape that may be holding the catheter to the leg	Allows for easy removal of catheter
Insert syringe end into the balloon port and remove all the air or fluid from the balloon, generally 5 to 10cc. Do not cut the port	Removal of fluid from balloon prevents damage to urethra, while removing the catheter
Ask the patient to take a deep breath if able and gently and smoothly remove the catheter on expiration. Stop if you meet resistance and recheck the balloon port	Damage to the urethra may occur if the balloon is not fully deflated
Note any sediment, mucus or blood that may be on the catheter. If needed, culture the tip of catheter by cutting it off with sterile scissors and placing in appropriate container	Assess for any indications of infection or trauma related to the catheter
Cleanse the patient's perineal area or provide a warm, moist cloth	Provides comfort and reduces transmission of microorganisms, with instructions for self-cleaning
Remove gloves and wash hands	Reduces transmission of microorganisms
Cover patient and position comfortably	Provides for privacy and comfort
Instruct the patient to drink oral fluids as tolerated and to call when he/she needs to void	Determines that patient has returned to usual voiding pattern
Record time and amount of first voiding. Offer bedpan/urinal every 24 hours	Allows assessment of the patient's voiding pattern
If the patient is unable to void within 8 hours, report to the physician	Allows assessment and intervention to determine the cause of the patient's inability to void after catheter is removed

- Keep record of intake and output for at least 24 hours after removal of catheter.
- If patient has not voided within 8 hours after catheter removal, the catheter (intermittent or indwelling, depending on order of physician) may have to be reinserted.

URINARY DIVERSIONS

A cystectomy is removal of the bladder, performed in urinary cancer. A bladder diversion may also be required for congenital defects. Permanent urinary diversion requires surgery to create an external pouch through an opening in the wall of the abdomen, called a stoma or to a surgically created internal reservoir. There are three types of surgeries (**Fig. 5.8**):
1. Conventional urostomy (ileal conduit)
2. Continent urinary reservoir (continent diversion)
3. Neobladder

Conventional Urostomy (Ileal Conduit)

In ileal conduit, a piece of small intestine or colon is removed and connected to ureters creating a passageway (bypass) known as ileal conduit. The ureters are attached to one end of the conduit. The other end of the conduit is connected to abdominal wall to create a stoma.

Continent Urinary Reservoir

In cutaneous ureterostomy, ureters are directly attached to a stoma. This procedure is performed when the bowel cannot be used to create a stoma because of disease conditions. In this procedure urinary bladder is removed and an internal reservoir is constructed from a segment of the small or large intestine. A valve is created in a pouch made from piece of small intestine.

Neobladder

In neobladder, there is substitution of urinary bladder with a piece of small bladder The ureters are connected to the neobladder. A urinary reservoir is made out of bowel and is attached to the urethra to allow voiding by the normal route. The patient voids by relaxing the urinary sphincter while contracting the abdominal muscles. In some cases, a catheter must be inserted through the urethra to completely empty the reservoir.

Possible Indications for Urinary Diversions

- **Cancer:**
  - Bladder
  - Prostate
  - Urethra
  - Ovary
  - Uterus
  - Cervix
  - Vagina
- Trauma
- Radiation injury to bladder
- Vesicovaginal fistula
- Urethrovaginal fistula
- Neurogenic bladder
- Chronic cystitis.

Care of Patient Before Urinary Diversion

- Assess knowledge of the patient regarding surgery.
- Explain about the procedure, postoperative tubes and drains, self-care of stoma.
- Assist the patient to identify the stoma site. The stoma site should be visible to patient, so that patient can cover and maintain seal to prevent leakage and effectively clean and maintain the site.
- Perform bowel preparation activities to prevent fecal contamination of the peritoneal cavity.

Care of Patient after Urinary Diversion

- Monitor intake output charts carefully, assessing urine output every hour for the first 24 hours, then every 4 hours or as ordered.
- Assess the color of urine. The pink or red color of urine fade to pink and then to clean by third postoperative day but brick red color of urine may indicate hemorrhage.
- Assess the condition of stoma and surrounding skin every 2 hourly for first 24 hours, the stoma is expected to appear red and edematous.

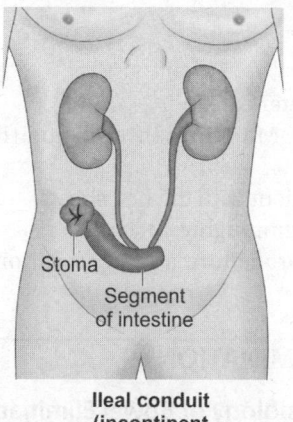
Ileal conduit (incontinent diversion to skin)

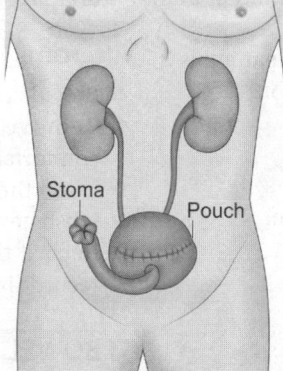
Continent cutaneous reservoir (Continent diversion to skin)

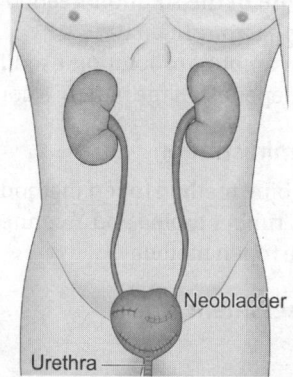
Orthotopic neobladder (Continent diversion to urethra)

Fig. 5.8: Surgical management for urinary diversions.

- Clean the ileal diversion with 30–60 mL of normal saline every 4 hourly as initially mucus produced by intestinal wall may accumulate and obstruct the catheter.
- Monitor renal function test to maintain the normal state of homeostasis.
- Assist and teach the patient and family about the stoma and urinary diversion care, skin care, pouch application and identify signs of infection.

■ BLADDER IRRIGATION

Bladder irrigation or wash is defined as washing of urinary bladder by directly a stream of solutions into the bladder through the urinary meatus by means of a catheter tubing and funnel.

Purposes

- To cleanse the bladder from decomposed urine, bacteria, excess mucus and pus.
- To medicate the lining of the bladder of antiseptic irrigation.
- To prepare the bladder for surgery as a preoperative measure.
- To promote healing.
- To relieve congestion and pain in case of inflammatory conditions of cystitis.
- To arrest bleeding and prevent clotting of blood.

Solutions Used

- Normal saline 0.9%
- Boric acid solution 2%
- Sterile water
- Acetic acid 1:4000 to pseudomonas infection
- Sodium nitrate 1:8000 to prevent clot formation
- $KMnO_4$ 1:5000 – 1:10,000
- Acriflavin 1:10,000
- Silver nitrate 1:5,000
- Mercury compounds in low concentrations.

General Instructions

- The temperature of the solution needed for cleaning purpose of body temperature.
- The temperature of the solution needed for therapeutic purposes ranging from 100–110°F.
- The maximum amount of solution used for cleaning is 2 pint and also depends on the patient's condition.

Methods of Administration

- Funnel and tubing method (open method).
- Irrigation can, rubber tubing and Y connection.
- Asepto syringe (open method).

Preliminary Assessment

Check

- Doctors order for specific precautions and instructions
- General condition of the patient
- Diagnosis of the patient
- Self-care ability of the patient
- Mental status to follow instructions
- Articles available in the unit.

Preparation of Patient and Environment

- Explain the sequences of the procedure
- Arrange the articles at the bedside
- Provide privacy
- Position the patient in comfortable position
- Place the mackintosh and towel under the buttocks.

Equipment

- **Sterile catheterization pack**
- **A sterile tray containing:**
  - Funnel, tubing 3 feet long which fits the connection screw clip and glass connection
  - A small mug of pint measures to pour solution
  - A Sterile pint jug with required solution
- **Clean tray:**
  - Solution thermometer kept in antiseptic solution in a bottle if available
  - Medication if ordered
  - Litmus paper.
- Bucket for emptying the return flow

Procedures

- Wash hands thoroughly.
- Wear gloves and empty the bladder keeping outlet of catheter uncontaminated.
- After urine withdrawal, attach glass, connection, tubing and funnel to the catheter.
- Place bucket or kidney tray conveniently near the meatus.
- Hold the funnel lowered with one hand and with other hand pour 75 to 100 mL of solutions along sides of the funnel.
- Raise the tube and keep the funnel 30 cm above the bed level.
- Never allow the funnel to be empty. Lower the funnel and slowly invert in cover the bucket.
- Repeat procedure until the return flow is clear.
- At the end of the procedure, clamp tubing disconnects glass connection, tubing and funnel, gently remove catheter and complete.
- In case of self-retaining catheter connect it into the drainage bag.

Aftercare

- Provide catheter care.
- Remove the Mackintosh and position the patient comfortably.
- Cover the patient with the bed sheets.
- Wash hands thoroughly.
- Record the procedure and observations in the nurses record sheet.

■ BOWEL ELIMINATION

Review of Physiology of Bowel Elimination

Waste from the intestines is composed mainly of indigestible food substances, secretions from the digestive tract (**Fig. 5.9**) material is called feces, excreta or stool.

Chapter 5: Elimination Needs

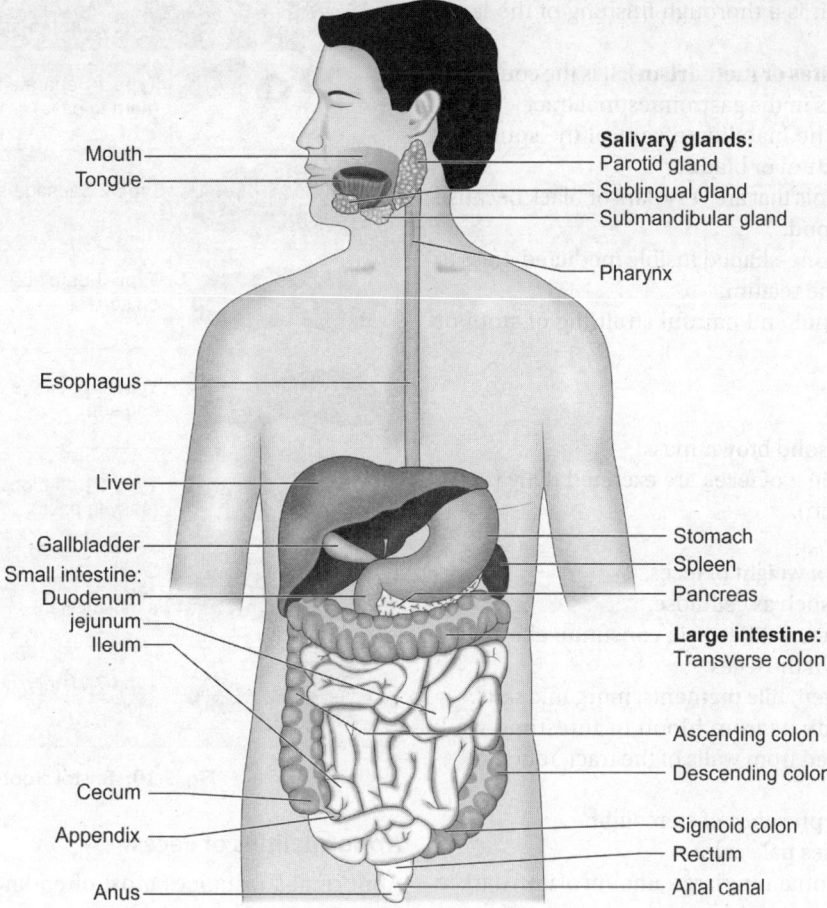

Fig. 5.9: Digestive system.

Anatomy of Digestive Tract and Formation of Feces

- The formation of fecal material and its passages from the body are natural functions resulting from the intake and digestive of food.
- Food taken into the mouth is chewed and broken into small particles that are swallowed and go into the stomach secretions by peristaltic and further liquefied before passing into the intestines.
- The first part is the small intestine which has three parts:
  1. The duodenum which is attached to the stomach
  2. The jejunum
  3. The ileum which is joined to the large intestine.
- The large intestine or colon has a number of sections:
  - The cecum,
  - Ascending colon
  - Transverse colon
  - Descending colon
  - Sigmoid colon
  - Rectum
- The anus is the opening to the outside of the body.
- The liquefied food (chime) passes from the stomach to the small intestine where it is mixed with still more digestive juices containing enzymes that react chemically with the food to separate the various food nutrients.
- The nutrients are absorbed into the blood through many blood vessels of the small intestine.
- The remaining indigestible fibrous material from the food along with water, passes through the ileocecal valve into the colon.
- They act upon the fibrous waste causing further breakdown and the formation of vitamins K, B1 and B12.
- The vitamins, electrolytes and water are absorbed from the colon.
- The remaining material continues moving through the colony until it reaches the rectum, usually as a soft, solid mass.
- It remains in the rectum until enough is present to produce pressure on the sphincter muscle of the anus causing the urge to defecate.

Key Words

- **Elimination:** It is the expulsion of the wastes for them body of way of lungs, skin, rectum and urinary bladder.
- **Defecation:** It is the act of expelling fecal material from the rectum.
- **Feces:** The content of the large bowel waste products.
- **Constipation:** It is infrequent or difficult evacuation of hard feces.
- **Diarrhea:** It is the passage of liquid feces more than normal frequency.
- **Enema (Clysis):** It is the introduction of the fluid into the rectum.

- **Colonic irrigation:** It is a thorough flushing of the large intestine.
- **Flatulence (tympanites or meteorism):** It is the condition of having flatus or gas in the gastrointestinal tract.
- **Incontinence:** It is the inability to control the sphincter which guards the rectum or bladder.
- **Melena:** Refers to stools that are very dark or black because of the presence of blood.
- **Suppository:** it is a cone-shaped fusible mediated mass to be introduced into the rectum.
- **Tenesmus:** Ineffectual and painful straining of stool or urine.

Composition of feces

Feces consist of a semi solid brown mass.
- **Amount:** Approx. 150 g of feces are excreted daily (100 g water and 50 g of solid).
- **Contents:**
  - *Water:* 60 to 70% of weight of feces.
  - Undigested food such as cellulose.
  - Dead and live bacteria: Bacteria constitute about 30% of the dry weight of the feces.
  - Fatty acids, nitrogen, bile pigments, inorganic salts.
  - Other waste products from blood or intestinal wall; epithelial cells shed from walls of the tract, mucus.
- **Color:**
  - Brown due to the presence of stercobilin.
  - Excessive fat causes pale color.
  - Blood and foods containing large amount of iron darken feces.
- **Odor:** Indole and skatole contributes to the odor of feces.
- Mucus helps to lubricate the feces and an adequate amount of roughage in diet ensures that contents of colon are sufficiently bulky to stimulate defecation.

Characteristics of Normal Stool

Color
- Color of stool varies from light to dark brown.
- Foods and medications may affect color.

Odor
Odor is aromatic, it is affected by ingested food and person's bacterial flora.

Consistency
Stool is formed, soft, semi-solid, moist due to the water content.

Frequency
Frequency is one to two per day.

Quantity
It varies with diet (about 100–400 g/day).

Constituents
- Stool contains a small amount of undigested roughage, sloughed dead bacteria and epithelial cells, fat, protein, dried constituents of digestive juices (bile pigments); inorganic matter (calcium, phosphates).
- Bristol stool chart is shown in **Figure 5.10**.

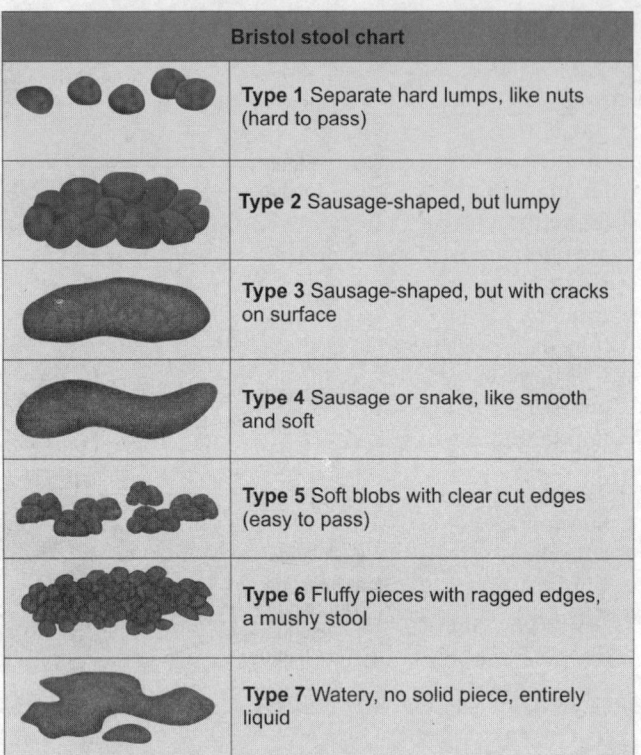

Fig. 5.10: Bristol stool chart.

Abnormalities of Feces

Abnormal substances most often knotted on feces include mucus, pus and parasites.

Appearance

Blood in Feces
- Blood from high in the digestive tract causes the feces to be a black color and is termed melena. It can be confused with the color change caused by iron medications. A laboratory test will clear questions of the problem.
- Blood from the colon, rectum and anus will be bright red. If there is blood in the stool, or even a suspicion of it, it must be reported to the doctor, he may wish to see the specimen. It is always best to save the entire specimen for him to examine.
- The blood may be due to a very serious problem or to a minor problem.

Other Colors that may be Observed
Though the normal color is brown, it will vary according to the food eaten.
- Babies taking only milk or adults receiving special feeding of a milk formula, will have a dark yellow stool.
- A very light or clay color is due to the absence of bile and may be indicate obstruction in the bile ducts.
- Undigested fat gives a light tan color to the feces.
- Starvation in babies cause green stools (hunger stool).

Mucus in Feces
- A small amount of mucus is normal in feces and gives it the smooth, shiny appearance.
- However, large amount of mucus especially in loose or watery stools indicate irritation or inflammation of the intestinal lining.

- The presence of pus means an inflamed ulcer is draining into the intestinal tract.

Parasites in Feces
- Parasites can be seen in feces, especially ascaris (roundworms) since they are 20 to 25 cm (8–10 inches) in length or longer.
- Sometimes hookworms or threadworms are seen, but they are often too small to be clearly identified.
- Laboratory examination shows worms are not present.
- Amoeba and tapeworm segments are seen as flat, white, moving objects under the microscope.
- If either is suspected, the specimen is kept warm and the entire specimen sent to the laboratory as quickly as possible for identification.

Other
- **Steatorrhea:** Bulky, greasy, foamy, gray (fat).
- **Diarrhea:** Digestive upsets—watery stools.
- **Cholera:** Rice water stools.
- **Chronic ulcerative colitis:** Mucus, dry, rock-hard masses passed with constipation and fecal impaction.

Factors Affecting Bowel Elimination

Age
- Infants have a smaller stomach capacity, less secretion of digestive enzymes, and more rapid intestinal peristalsis. The ability to control defecation does not occur until 2 to 3 years of age.
- Adolescents experience rapid growth of the large intestine and increased secretion of HCl.
- Older adults have decreased chewing ability. Partially chewed food is not digestive as easily. Peristalsis declines, and esophageal emptying slows. Absorption by the intestinal mucosa is impaired. Muscle tone in the perineal floor and anal sphincter weaken, causing difficulty in controlling defecation.

Diet
- Regular daily food intake promotes peristalsis.
- High fiber foods, raw fruits, cooked fruits, greens (cabbage and spinach), raw vegetables, and whole grains (cereals and breads) promote peristalsis and defecation by creating bulk.
- Low fiber foods (pasta, lean meats, and milky slow peristalsis).
- Gas-producing foods (broccoli, cauliflower, onions and dried beans) can stimulate peristalsis.
- Persons with lactose intolerance lack the enzyme lactose which is needed to digest the simple sugars in milk. Such intolerance can lead to diarrhea and cramping.

Position during Defecation
- Squatting allows a person to lean forward, exert intra-abdominal pressure, and contract thigh muscles to normally defecate.
- Older adults or those with arthritis may be unable to rise from a toilet seat.
- Immobilized patients, required to use a bedpan while lying, cannot contract muscles to defecate.

Pregnancy
As pregnancy advances and fetus enlarges, pressure is exerted on the rectum. Constipation commonly occurs.

Diagnostic Test
- Certain examinations involving visualization of GI structures requires the emptying of bowel contents, NPO status, bowel evacuants, and enema administration to cleanse the bowel before a test are factors that interference with normal elimination.
- Barium examination require ingestion of barium, a mixture that can harden and cause serious constipation unless eliminated soon after a test.

Fluid Intake
- Fluid liquefies intestinal contents for easier passage.
- Hot beverages and fruit juices soften stool and increased peristalsis.
- Large quantities of milk may slow peristalsis and cause constipation.

Activity
Immobilization depresses colon motility, and regular, physical exercise promotes peristalsis.

Psychological Factors
- Stress, anxiety, or fear can initiate parasympathetic impulses, causing acceleration of digestion and peristalsis.
- Diarrhea can decrease peristalsis and lead to constipation.
- Emotional depression can decrease peristalsis and lead to constipation.

Personal Habits
- Personal habits such as failing to respond to the need to defecate and lack of privacy interfere with normal elimination patterns and can lead to constipation.
- Hospitalized patients often share toilet facilities or use bedpans or beside commodes. The resulting embarrassment causes them to ignore the urge to defecate.

Medications
- Laxatives and cathartics soften stool and promote peristalsis.
- Antidiarrheal agents inhibit peristalsis.
- Narcotic analgesics, opiates, and anticholinergic, drugs depress peristalsis and can cause constipation.
- Antibiotics alter normal bowel flora and can produce diarrhea.
- Drugs that contain iron may cause a white discoloration anticoagulants may result in frank or occult blood in the stool.

Temperature
The fever will influence appetite which causes anorexia, muscle weakness, and decreased fluid intake as a result there will increased evaporation of body fluids due to increased metabolic needs that causes constipation.

Surgery and Anesthesia
- General anesthetics temporarily halt peristalsis.

- Surgery involving bowel manipulation temporarily stops peristalsis (paralytic ileus) for 24–48 hours.

ALTERATIONS IN BOWEL ELIMINATION

Diarrhea

- Diarrhea is defined as an increase in the number of stools and the passage of liquid, unformed feces. Diarrhea is loose, watery stools.
- A person with diarrhea typically passes stool more than three times a day.
- People with diarrhea may pass more than a quart of stool a day.
- Acute diarrhea is a common problem that usually lasts 1 or 2 days.
- Prolonged diarrhea persisting for more than 2 days may be a sign of a more serious problem and possess the risk of dehydration.
- Chronic diarrhea may be a feature of a chronic disease.
- Diarrhea can cause dehydration, which means the body lacks enough fluid to function properly.
- Dehydration is particularly dangerous in children and older people and it must be treated promptly to avoid serious health problems.

Causes

- Imitation or inflammation of the gastrointestinal tract, due to pathogenic
- Infection, highly spiced food or medication that increase intestinal mobility.
- Disorder of digestion or absorption.
- Disorders that affect secretion and utilization of bile or pancreatic juices.
- Emotional stress such as anxiety or stress.
- Food intolerance increases intestinal mobility.
- Medications like iron and antibiotics cause irritation of intestinal mucosa and suprainfection allowing over-growth of normal flora, inflammation and irritation of mucosa.
- Laxatives cause increased intestinal mobility leading to diarrhea.
- Surgical procedures like gastrectomy, colon resection, etc., leads to improper absorption and diarrhea.

Symptoms of Diarrhea

- Diarrhea may be accompanied by
- Loose stools with cramping
- Abdominal pain
- Bloating
- Nausea
- An urgent need to use the bathroom
- Depending on the cause, a person may have a fever or bloody stools

Nursing Management of Diarrhea

- Replacement of fluids and electrolytes. The fluid loss from the body should be replaced immediately to prevent shock and collapse of the patients. Intravenous fluids or oral intake of plenty of fluids or oral rehydration salt (ORS) fluids.
- Small and frequent feeding should be given to meet nutritional needs of the patients.
  - A bland diet should be given to meet nutritional needs of the patients.
  - Avoid foods that are excessively hot or cold, have spices as it stimulates peristalsis.
  - Replacement of potassium is important, as it lost in greater amount in diarrhea.
- Ensure easy or convenient access to bedpan or commode.
- Care of skin is essential as skin excoriation around the anal region is common in diarrhea. Ensure proper cleaning and drying of area after each defecation.
- Adequate rest is important for the patients, as reduced physical activity trends to reduce bowel
- Psychological support relieves anxiety of the patient and gives reassurance, as sustained anxiety is one of the causes of diarrhea.
- Medications: Certain drugs helps in relieving diarrhea like anti diarrheal drugs, intestinal antispasmodics.

Constipation

- Constipation is defined as a decrease in the frequency of bowel movements, accompanied by prolonged or difficult passage of hard, dry stools.
- Constipation may be a minor annoyance or uncommonly, a sign of a life-threatening disorder such as an acute intestinal obstruction.
- Untreated constipation can lead to headache, anorexia and abdominal discomfort and can adversely affect the patient's lifestyle and wellbeing.
- Constipation usually occurs when the urge to defecate is suppressed and the muscles associated with bowel movements remain contracted.
- Because the autonomic nervous system controls bowel movements by sensing rectal distention from fecal contents and by stimulating the external sphincter that may cause bowel dysfunction.

Causes

- Irregular bowel habit.
- Consuming a low fibre diet and lack of fluids leads to constipation. Dry stool are more compact and are difficult to pass through the colon.
- Lengthy bed rest or lack of regular exercise.
- Medication (anti-cholinergic, iron tablets and opioid analgesics, antacids patients may also experience constipation from excessive use of laxatives or enema.
- Older adults experience slower peristalsis, loss of abdominal elasticity and reduced intestinal mucosa secretions.
- Gastrointestinal abnormalities such as bowel obstruction, paralytic ileus.
- Neurological conditions that block nerve impulses to the colon.

Nursing Management in Constipation

- Privacy (while defecation).
- Posture (a squatting position is effective posture during defecation because it helps to increase abdominal pressure.

- Ensure an adequate intake of diet. Foods containing a high fibrous content should be included in the diet, e.g., raw and cooked vegetables, whole grains, fruits and salad.
- Establish a habit pattern-instruct or help the patient to establish a regular time pattern for defecation.
- Relaxation-relieve the patient from worry, anger, fear. That interfere with defecation reflex and reassure the patient to promote relaxation.
- **Exercise:** That improve muscle tone of abdominal and perineal muscles should encouraged.
- An adequate amount of fluids-2–3 L in a day.
- Postpone test if woman has menstrual periods, until three days after it has ceased.
- Consider that intake of folic acid, anticoagulant, barium, bismuth, mineral oil, vitamin C, and antibiotics may after the results.
- Use two bedpans for helpless patient—one for collecting specimen and the another for cleaning.

COLLECTING A STOOL SPECIMEN FOR ROUTINE EXAMINATION

Definition
Collection of a small quantity of stool sample in a container for testing in the laboratory.

Purposes
To test the stool for normalcy and presence of abnormalities.

Articles
- A clean specimen container.
- A spatula for putting the specimen into the container.
- Dry bedpan (for helpless patients). Additional bedpan for rinsing and cleaning.
- Laboratory requisition form.
- Clean gloves.
- Waste paper (for wrapping used spatula).
- Tissue/towel.

Procedures
- Check the physician's order and 'Nursing Care Plan'.
- Identify the patient.
- Explain to patient the procedure and make clear what is expected to him/her.
- **Give the labeled container and spatula to the patient with instructions:**
  - To defecate into clean dry bedpan.
  - Not to contaminate specimen with urine.
- Don gloves.
- For helpless patient, assist patient on to the clean bedpan.
- Leave him with instructions.
- When done, remove and keep aside the bedpan after appropriate requisition forms.
- Once the specimen is collected sent it to lab with the appropriate requisition forms.
- Wash and replace the reusable articles.
- Dispose off the spatula wrapped in waste paper.
- Wash and dry hands.
- Record information in the patient's chart.

Special Considerations
- Send specimen to be examined for parasites immediately, so that parasites may be observed under microscope while viable, fresh and warm.
- Inform if bleeding hemorrhoids or hematuria is present.

PASSING A FLATUS TUBE

Flatulence
- As gas accumulates in the lumen of the intestines. The bowel wall stretches and distends. This is called flatulence.
- It is a common cause of abdominal fullness, pain and cramping.
- Normally, intestinal gas escapes through the mouth (belching) or the anus (passing the flatus).
- If there is a reduction in intestinal motility resulting from opiates, general anesthetics, abdominal surgery, or immobilization, flatulence can become severe enough to cause abdominal distention and severe sharp pain.

Purpose of Passing Flatus Tube
To remove flatulence from the lower bowel.

Equipment
- Screen
- **A tray containing:**
  - One flatus tube in a kidney tray of water
  - Vaseline in a container
  - Wet swabs in a container
  - Mackintosh and towel or paper
  - Paper bag or kidney tray
  - Long artery forceps.

Procedures
- Prepare the patient as for enema.
- Position dorsal recumbent.
- Swab the anal region.
- Lubricate the flatus tube and introduce 12–15 cm.
- The free end being kept under water in the kidney tray, which is placed between two thighs
- A big piece of cotton is kept over the distal end of the rectal tube in water in the kidney tray, will act as a weight to keep it immersed under water. But care should be taken not to cover the outlet of the rectal tube.
- Water in the kidney tray will help to visualize the escape of gas from the tube and prevent the foul smell by dissolving the gas in water to a certain extent.
- Watch for expulsion of gas.
- Keep it for 10 to 20 minutes. Then the tube is removed and kept in the kidney tray after wiping off the Vaseline.
- Clean the anal region with swabs.
- Make the patient comfortable.
- Clean bowl and replace the tube and other articles, record the time, date and result of the treatment. If necessary repeat, it after half an hour.

ENEMA

- Enema (clysis) is defined as a introduction of the fluid into the rectum.
- An enema is an introduction of fluid into the bowl through the rectum for the purpose of cleansing or to introduce nourishment.

Purposes

- To remove fecal matter
- To relieve flatulence
- To relieve constipation
- To prevent involuntary defecation during surgery
- To reduce temperature, e.g., cold enema
- To check diarrhea, e.g., starch opium enema
- To stimulate peristalsis, e.g., purgative enema
- To make diagnosis, e.g., barium enema
- To cleanse the bowel before X-ray studies
- To induce anaesthesia, e.g., anaesthetic enema
- To administer medications
- To destroy intestinal parasites, e.g., anthelminthic enema
- To administer fluids and nutrients
- To establish regular bowel functions during bowel training program.

Contraindications

- Acute myocardial infarction and cardiac problems
- Acute renal failure
- Appendicitis
- Obstetrical and gynecological contraindications.

Classification of Enema

Evacuant Enemas

The most commonly used evacuant enemas are.
- Simple enema
- **Medicated enema:**
  - Oil enema
  - Purgative enema
  - Carminative enema
  - Astringent enema
  - Phosphate enemas
  - Microlax/Toilax
- Cold enema

Retention Enemas

The most commonly used retention enemas are:
- Stimulant enema
- Nutrient enema
- Sedative enema
- Emollient enema
- Anesthetic enema
- Prednisolone (steroid)—used for treatment of inflammatory bowel conditions
- Olive oil—used to soften stool

Description of some common enema are:

Soap Water Enema

- It is otherwise called saline enema. In this normal saline (Sodium chloride 1 teaspoon) to half litre of water.

- **The amount of solution used for:**
  - Adult 500–1000 mL
  - Children 250–300 mL
  - Infants 250 mL or less.
- **The temperature of the solution in:**
  - Adult 105–110°F
  - Children 100°F.

Oil Enema

- It is given to soften fecal matter in cases of severe constipation.
- The enema must be retained ½ or 1 hour to soften the feces.
- The solutions used are olive oil, gingelly oil, castor oil, 1:2, the amount of solution used is 115–175 mL the temperature of the solution is 100°F (37.7°C).

Carminative Enema

- It is called antispasmodic enema. It is given to relieve gaseous distension of abdomen by increasing peristalsis and expulsion of flatus.
- The solution used is 8–16 mL of turpentine mixed thoroughly with 600–1200 mL of soap solution.
- Milk and molasses 90–230 mL well mixed with equal quantity of warm milk.

Anthelminthic Enema

- It is given to destroy and expel worms from the intestine.
- Cleansing enema must be given prior to anthelminthic enema so that the drug comes in direct contact with worms and the lining of intestine.
- The solution used infusion of quassia 15 g of chips to 600 mL of water or hypertonic saline solution sodium chloride 60 mL of water.
- The amount of solution given is 250 mL.

Cold Enema

- Cold enema or ice-water enema is given to reduce body temperature in hyperpyrexia and heat stroke.
- It is given in the form of colonic irrigations.
- The temperature of the solution is 80–90°F (27–32°C).

Glycerine Enema

- Glycerine enema is given to children, to fever patients and postoperative patients.
- Pure glycerine and water 1:2 used.

Astringent Enema

- Astringent enema contracts the tissues and blood vessels checks bleeding and inflammation lessens the amount of mucus discharge and gives a temporary relief in the inflamed area.
- It is usually given in colitis and dysentery.
- The solution used are tannic acid 25 g to 600 mL water, alum 30 g to 600 mL of water and silver nitrate 2% (Silver nitrate is dissolved in the distilled water).

Sedative Enema

- Sedative enema contains an anaesthetic drug to produce anaesthesia in the patient.
- The commonly used drugs are paraldehyde. Dose is given as per doctor's order.

Stimulant Enema

- Stimulant enema is given in the treatment of shock and collapse.
- Coffee enema is given in case of opium poisoning.
- Solution used are black coffee- 1 tablespoon coffee powder to 300 mL of water and 15 mL of brandy added to 120–180 mL of glucose saline.
- The amount of solution used in 180–240 mL
- The temperature of solution is 108 to 110°F (42–43°C).

Emollient Enema

- Emollient enema or starch enema is given in case of diarrhea to relieve irritation in an inflamed mucous membrane.
- The solution used is starch and opium Tr.
- Opium 1–2 mL added to 120–180 mL of starch mucilage or rice water.
- The temperature of solution is 100–105°F (37.8–40.5°C).

Nutrient Enema

- Nutrient enema is given to supply food, fluids to the body.
- Selection of the fluids depends upon the ability of the colon to absorb it.
- Nutrient enema is particularly useful in conditions like hemophilia
- The solution used are normal saline. Glucose saline 250 mL; 5% peptonized milk 120 mL.
- The amount of solution used is 110–1700 mL in 24 hours or 180–270 mL at 4 hourly intervals.
- The temperature of solution is 100°F (37.8°C).

Methods of Giving Enemas

- Enema can and tube method—when large amounts of fluids are to be given, this method is used, e.g., soap and water enema.
- Funnel and catheter method—when a small quantity of fluids is to be given, this method is used, e.g., oil enema.
- Glycerine syringe and catheter method—a small quantity of fluids is to be given, this method is used, e.g., Purgative enema.
- Rectal drip method—when the fluid is to be administered very slowly in order to aid in this absorption, e.g., nutrient enema.

General Instructions

- **The appropriate size of rectal catheter or rectal tube of cleansing enema is:**
  - 22 French for adults,
  - 12 French for an infant
  - 14 to 18 French for school age child.
- The rectal tube needs to be smooth and flexible.
- The rectal tube is lubricated with a water-soluble lubricant or Vaseline to facilitate insertion and so decrease irritation of the rectal mucosa.
- The amount of the solution to be administered depends up on the type of enema and the age and size of the person.
- The temperature of the solution needs to be adjusted according to the purpose of the enema.
- The patient usually placed in left lateral position, when an enema is administered. In this position, sigmoid colon is below the rectum, thus facilitating installing of the fluid.
- **The distance to which the tube is inserted depend upon the age and size of the patient:**
  - For adult it is normally inserted 7.5 to 10 cm (3–4 inches)
  - For children It is 2.5–3.75 cm (1–½ inches).
- The height of the enema can should not be above 18 inches (20 cm) from the anus **(Fig. 5.11)**.
- The length of time that the enema solution is retained will depend upon the purpose of the enema, oil retention

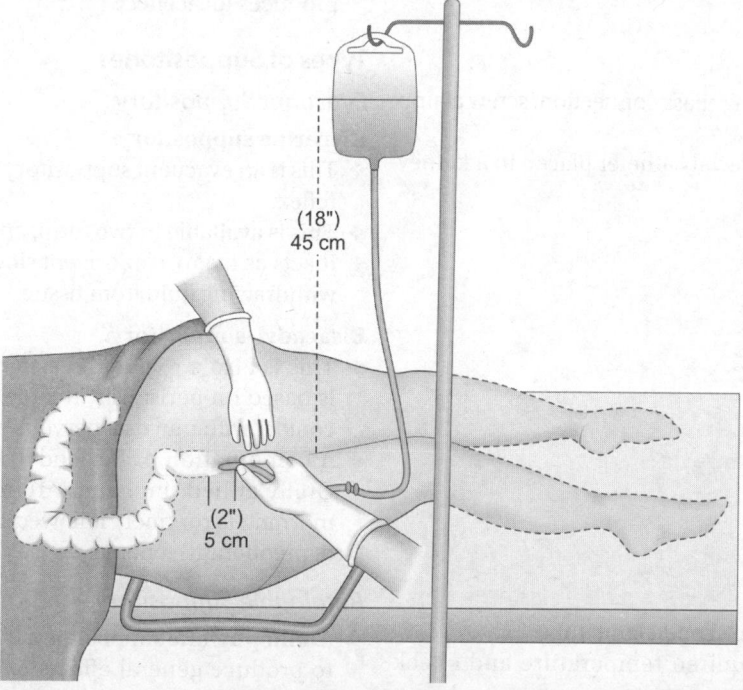

Fig. 5.11: Administration of enema.

enema is usually retained for 2–3 hours. Other cleansing enema are normally retained for 5–10 minutes.
- Prepacked enema will have their own instruction which need to be followed.
- Prevent air from entering into the rectum, by expelling air from the tube.
- If the rectum is impacted attempt to remove the fecal matter with a gloved finger.
- Make sure the whole apparatus used for the administration of enemas is in good working condition.
- Regulate the flow of fluid according to the type of enema.
- Listen to the complaints of the patient and should not ignore any discomfort however small they are.

Preliminary Assessment

Check
- Doctors order for any specific precautions
- Diagnosis of the patient
- Abilities and limitations concerning movements
- Level of consciousness to follow direction
- Availability for the articles
- Extra help needed
- Lesions on the rectal and perineal area
- Nature of enema ordered.

Preparations of the Patient and Environment
- Explain the sequence of the procedure
- Arrange the articles at the bedside
- Provide privacy
- Cover the patient in the left lateral position
- Place the Mackintosh and towel under the patient's buttocks.
- Place the patient in the left lateral position,
- Keep the bedpan under the bed, cover a stool.
- Adjust the IV pole to hold the enema can at the required height.

Equipment
- Enema cans, rubber tubing, glass connection, screw clamp
- Mackintosh and towel
- Rectal tube (adjusts) or rectal catheter placed in a kidney tray
- Vaseline
- Pint measure
- Soap jelly in a bottle
- IV stand
- Toilet tray
- Bedpan – 2
- Clean linen if needed
- Bath thermometer
- Rag pieces
- K-basin.

Procedures
- Wash hands thoroughly
- Attach tubing to enema can and clamp tube
- Prepare solution at required temperature and check temperature with bath thermometer.
- Attach rectal tube to tubing, expel air and clamp tube. Air entry into rectum may cause discomfort
- Hang enema can with solution on IV stand and adjust height to 18 inches for bed
- Lubricate tip of rectal tube
- Use rag pieces to separate patients' buttocks and visualize anus clearly, insert rectal tube gently to a distance of 2 to 4 inches
- Encourage patient to take a deep breath while inserting tube. Note level of fluid and make sure there is free flow
- Encourage patient to take a deep breath while breaths during administration of fluid
- Clamp or pinch the rectal tube if the fluid is about to get over
- Use rag pieces to remove the rectal tube.

Aftercare
- Instruct patient to hold solution for 10–15 minutes
- Discard rag pieces in K-basin, detach rectal tube and place in same K-basin
- Position the patient in supine and assist to toilet or provide a bedpan
- Assists patient to wash perineal area if not able to replace it
- Remove the articles to utility room, clean and replace it
- Keep the patient dry and comfortable
- Wash hands
- Record the procedure in the nurse's record.

SUPPOSITORY

Definition
- Suppository is a form of rectal medication mainly for local effects and sometimes for general effect.
- Usually, it is solid at room temperature.
- When introduced, it melts at body temperature and produces local effect.

Types of Suppositories

Evacuant Suppository

Glycerine suppository:
- This is an evacuant suppository use for starting defecation reflex.
- This is available in two form, adult and child.
- It acts as hygroscopic agent slowly causing evacuation by withdrawing fluid from tissue.

Bisacodyl/suppository:
- This is also a popular evacuant suppository procedure is based on peristalsis in large bowel by reflex action by contact with mucosal nervous plexus.
- A combination of Bisacodyl/two tablets (10 mg each) Orally at bed time and a 10 mg suppository following morning is routinely followed in many hospitals in place of preoperative enema.

Retainable Suppository
- **Aminophylline suppository:** It is given retention in rectum to produce general effects of aminophylline by way of absorption in case of bronchial asthma.

- **Anesthetic suppository:** Thiopentone is used sometimes as suppository to cause anaesthetic effect in children as alternate route to intravenous route.
- **Steroid suppository:** Hydrocortisone is used as suppository to produce desired effect in case of proctitis and ulcerative colitis.

Procedures

- Inform the procedure to the patient
- Put on sterile gloves
- Lubricate suppository with warm water or by lubricating solution
- Lubricate the anal area by inserting a lubricated gloved finger
- Bring the patient to left lateral position
- Insert the suppository gently into the rectum pass the internal sphincter one index finger, length in adults 5 cm (2 inches) and infants
- Ask the patient to take deep breath
- Apply pressure over area and hold buttocks together for short time If the suppository is for evacuation, put bed-pan under buttock as the patient may desire at any time to pass stool. If the suppository is retained instruct the patient to retain for 20 to 30 minutes till it completely melts to cause desired effect even if he feels to pass stool.
- Wash hands.
- Record the procedure in chart. Record drug name, dosage, route and time of administration on medication record.
- Observe for effects of suppository 30, minutes after administration like bowel movements, etc.

■ SITZ BATH

- Sitz bath is a bath in which only the pelvic area is immersed in warm fluid.
- The client sits in a special tub or chair or in a basin that fits on the toilet seat so that the legs and feet remain out of the water.
- Immersing the entire body causes widespread vasodilation and nullifies the effect of local heat application to the pelvic area.
- A disposable sitz basin contains an attachment resembling an enema bag that allows gradual introduction of warmer water.

Purposes

- To relieve pelvic congestion
- To relieve pain after rectal surgery
- For relieve pain from painful hemorrhoids
- To relieve pain from vaginal inflammation
- To relieve pain due to episiotomy during childbirth
- To treat dysmenorrhea
- To promote drainage of rectal abscess
- To relieve pain following cystoscopy.

General Instructions

- Take care to help prevent patient having chills, burns and fainting
- The temperature of the solution or water should be 110–115°F or 34–46°C.
- The temperature should be checked during procedure and on addition of hot water.
- The duration of bath is 15–20 minutes.
- Maintain sterile technique as far as possible to avoid transfer of microorganisms.

Solutions Used

- Betadine lotion
- Potassium permanganate 1:5000
- Basic acid 1 gram to 1 pint
- Eusol solution.

Contraindications

- Pregnancy
- Renal inflammation
- Increased irritability of genital organs.

Initial Assessment Check

- Correct orders
- Doctor's orders
- General condition and diagnosis of patient
- Type, duration, and medication to be used
- Patients self-care ability and ability to follow directions.

Preparations of Patient and Environment

- Explain the procedure to the patient
- Provide privacy if needed
- Arrange the articles at the patients' bed side
- Put off the fan and close the window
- Check the temperature of the water with the lotion thermometer
- Position the patient comfortably.

Equipments

- Basin/bath
- Bath blanker and safety pins
- Bath towel
- Lotion thermometer
- Mackintosh with cover
- Rubber rings.

Procedures

- Wash hands
- Spread Mackintosh with cover
- Place both towel and rubber ring in the bottom of tube
- Fill 1/3rd to ½ full of water
- Check the temperature with lotion thermometer
- Assist the patient into the bath tub
- The initial temperature should be 100°F and gradually increase to 115°F.
- Cover the patient with bath blanket.
- Leave the patient in the tube for 10 to 20 minutes.
- Observe patient's condition at least every 5 minutes.

Aftercare

- Observe for complications like burns and fainting

- Assist the patient in drying and putting on clothes to prevent chilling
- Care must be taken to help prevent falling
- Provide comfortable position in bed to the patient
- Wash and replace all articles
- Wash hands
- Record the procedure in the nurse's record sheet.

BOWEL WASH

- Bowel wash or colonic lavage or enteroclysis is defined as washing out colon with large quantities of solution.
- Bowel irrigation or enteroclysis is defined as washing out of the colon after the feces has been expelled by using large quantities of prescribed solution.

Purposes

- To prepare for diagnostic examination or before certain surgery
- To relieve inflammation
- To stimulate peristalsis
- To supply fluid and electrolyte those are absorbed from intestine
- To dilute and remove toxic agents
- To reduce temperature in hyperpyrexia
- To relieve fecal incontinence
- To supply medications locally
- To clean the colon of feces, gas and barium
- To treat infection and other pathological condition of colon.

Contraindications

- Rectal infection
- Fistula in anus
- Painful and bleeding hemorrhoids
- Painful skin lesions around the anus
- Massive carcinoma or tumors of the rectum
- Loose sphincter
- Polyps and diverticulosis of the intestine.

General Instructions

- A cleaning enema should be given one hour before the colon irrigation.
- The bladder should be emptied before colonic irrigations.
- The temperature of the solution is kept constant throughout the procedure.
- Allow only 200–300 mL of fluid to run into the rectum at a time.
- Make sure that the return flow is not blocked.
- Use a smooth and flexible rectal tube and lubricate it well.
- Prevent air entry into the intestines.
- Stop the procedure temporarily if the patient complaints of pain.
- Listen to the complaints of the patient and should not ignore any discomfort however small they may be.

Methods Used for Bowel Irrigation

- Funnel and catheter
- Y connection and a rectal tube
- Two tube method.

Solution Used

- Tap water
- Cold water
- Normal saline
- Sodium bicarbonate 1–2%
- Antiseptic solution $AgNO_3$ 500–1:1000
- $KMnO_4$ 1:5000
- Boric solution 1–2%
- Tannic acid 1:100
- Alum 1:100.

Temperature of the Solution

- Cleaning purpose 104°F (40°C)
- Thermal effect 110–150° (43.3–46°C)
- Reducing temperature 80–90°F (27–32°C) amount of solution used for bowl irrigation is 2–3 liters or till the return flow is clear.

Preliminary Assessment

Check

- Doctor's order for any specific precautions
- Diagnosis of the patient
- General condition of the patient
- Self-care ability of the patient
- Mental status to follow instructions
- Any contraindication
- Need for any extra help
- Articles available in the unit.

Preparations of the Patient and Environment

- Explain the sequence of the procedure
- Arrange the articles at the bedside
- Provide privacy
- Place the Mackintosh and towel under the patient
- Place the patient in left lateral position
- Keep the bucket on a low stool to receive the outflow of fluid
- Remove the back rest and extra pillows.

Equipments

A Clean Tray Containing

- Funnel and tubing with glass connection
- Mackintosh and towel
- Rectal tube placed in a kidney tray
- Vaseline
- Rag pieces in a container
- Hot and cold water in jugs
- Prescribed solution in jug
- Paper bag
- Bucket
- Toilet tray (if needed)
- Clean linen (if needed)
- Bath thermometer.

Procedures

- Wash hands thoroughly
- Prepare the solution at the required temperature.
- Attach the tubing and the rectal tube with the funnel, pour solution in it and check for any leakage.

- Lubricate the tip of the rectal tube about 4 inches
- Separate patient's buttocks to visualize anus clearly and insert tip of tube about 4–5 inches, while patient takes deep breath.
- Lower funnel below level of rectum and empty return flow into bucket.
- Fill funnel again. Pour 200–300 mL of fluid each time.
- Raise funnel and allow fluid to run continuously.
- When 200–300 mL of fluid has gone in pinch tube before funnel is completely lower and invert funnel over bucket and siphon fluid, noting characteristics of return flow
- Repeat this process, till return flow is clear.
- Remove the rectal tube by using rag pieces.

Aftercare
- Remove rectal tube by using rag pieces
- Discard rag piece into K-basin
- Place patient comfortably
- Provide bedpan, if needed
- Change linen, if soiled
- Replace equipment after cleaning
- Handwash
- Record the procedure in nurse's record sheet.

DIGITAL EVACUATION OF FECES

Definition
Digital evacuation or digital disimpaction is also known as manual disimpaction of feces. It is the removal of stool from the rectum using a finger in circular motion. It may be used in people with fecal impaction.

Etiologies of Fecal Impaction
- Chronic constipation
- Faulty dietary practices
- Neurogenic conditions
- Certain medication related side effects
- Anorectal stenosis
- Neoplasm of lower GI tract
- Anatomic and functional anorectal anomalies
- Abnormal rectal sensation

Symptoms Associated with Fecal Impaction
- Rectal discomfort
- Anorexia
- Nausea and vomiting
- Abdominal pain
- Paradoxical diarrhea
- Urinary frequency
- Urinary overflow incontinence
- Lower abdominal heaviness
- Heartburn

Indications for Digital Evacuation of Feces
Digital evacuation of feces is typically used:
- When laxatives or enemas are unable to resolve fecal impaction.
- For people who cannot pass stools due to a spinal cord injury, older adults with dehydration, obese persons in traction.
- For people who experience impaction as a result of a barium enema.

Procedure
- Check the vital signs of the patient to get baseline data. Determine the patient's history of any cardiac problem or contraindication.
- Check the order for administering retention, edema before the procedure.
- Provide comfortable position to the patient, i.e., left side with the right knee flexed towards his head. Cover the patient and expose only the rectal area.
- Place the mackintosh and draw sheet beneath the left hip.
- Wash hands and Don clean gloves.
- Expose the patient's buttocks; place a bedpan next to the buttocks.
- Place a wet wash cloth and moist towel nearby the rectal area to clean after the completion of the procedure.
- Lubricate the gloved forefinger and middle finger of dominant hand with lidocaine.
- Slowly slide one lubricated finger into the rectum and observe for perianal irritation.
- Gently rotate the finger and begin to break the stool into small pieces and place in the bedpan.
- Instruct the patient to take slow and deep breaths during the procedure. Allow the patient to take rest intervals.
- Reapply the lubricant each time fingers are re-inserted.
- Keep assessing the patient's condition during the procedure. If heart rate decreases or rhythm changes from initial assessment, stop the procedure.
- When the removal of stool is completed, cover the bedpan and clean the rectal area with the wet wash cloth
- Provide comfortable position to the patient.
- Dispose the stool and clean all the articles.
- Remove gloves and wash hands.
- Document the procedure and note the color, amount and consistency of stool.

Side Effects of Digital Evacuation
Digital evacuation should only be performed by a medical professional as there are risks associated with the procedure, including:
- Rectal bleeding
- Anal fissures
- Rectal perforation
- Anal sphincter damage
- Urinary tract obstruction
- In rare instances, fatal cardiac arrhythmias (typically in chronically ill older adults).

COLOSTOMY
Colostomy is named according to place where in the bowel is formed. It may be ascending, transverse, descending or sigmoid colostomy. The type of effluent is dependent on the location of the bowel used **(Table 5.9)**.

TABLE 5.9: Type of effluent in relation to location of stoma.

Location of stoma	Type of effluent
Ileostomy	Liquid to mushy
Cecostomy, ascending colostomy	Liquid to mushy, foul odor
Right transverse colostomy	Mushy to semi-formed
Left transverse colostomy	Semi-formed soft
Descending or sigmoid colostomy	Soft to hard formed

Indications

- Cancer of colon/rectum.
- Intestinal obstruction.
- Diverticular disease.
- Hirschsprung's disease (a condition that affects the large intestine and causes problem with passing stools)
- Crohn's disease.
- Ulcerative disease.
- Trauma to abdomen.

Types of Colostomies

According to Duration

- **Temporary colostomy** is made to allow colon to rest and heal for a period of time. It is kept for weeks, months or years. Once, definitive surgery is done, temporary colostomy is closed and bowel movements will return to normal.
- **Permanent colostomy** is made when part of colon is removed as cannot be used again. According to disease/abnormality of intestine, stoma is made. It may be ileostomy, jejunostomy, cecostomy, etc.

According to Anatomic Location

- **Ascending colostomy:** Stoma is made on right side of abdomen. Fecal matter will be of liquid form.
- **Transverse colostomy:** Stoma is located in upper abdomen towards middle or right side. Fecal content may be loose or soft.
- **Descending colostomy:** Stoma is present on lower left side of abdomen. The fecal content is firm, and drain can be controlled.
- **Sigmoid colostomy:** Stoma is made in sigmoid colon, few inches lower than descending colostomy. Fecal matter is like normal stool. Frequency of fecal discharge may be regulated.

According to Construction of Stoma (Fig. 5.12)

- **End stoma:** An end stoma is formed when the proximal end of the bowel is brought to the outside of abdominal wall. If an abdominal perineal resection is done, the rectum is removed, and the proximal sigmoid or descending colon is brought out as a stoma. Another procedure may be done, involves. removing the segment of diseased bowel and using the proximal portion for the stoma. The remaining limb of bowel is sutured closed and left in the peritoneal cavity, so that the rectum is intact. This is called a Hartmann's pouch or mucus fistulas and it may be temporary or permanent depending on the diagnosis.

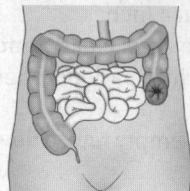 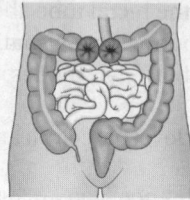 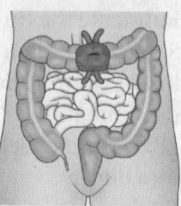

Signal barrel or end stoma only one end is taken out

Double barrel two end are taken out but not connected

Loop stoma two ends are taken out and are connected

Fig. 5.12: Construction of stomas.

- **Double-barrel stoma:** With a bowel barrel stoma the bowel is completely dissected and both ends of the colon are brought to the outside of abdominal wall to form two separate stomas. The proximal stoma is the functioning stoma that expels stool. A double-barrel stoma is often temporary, allowing the bowel to rest during healing after trauma or surgery.
- **Loop stoma:** To create a loop stoma, a loop of bowel, usually the transverse colon, is pulled outside the abdominal wall and a bridge is slipped under the loop to hold it in place. An incisional slit is made on the top of the exposed colon to allow stool to exit.

Nursing Management

- **Assessment:**
  - Assess patient's knowledge about self-care.
  - Recognize patient readiness and ability to learn and perform self-care is of primary importance.
  - The patient experiencing pain, nausea or vomiting is less likely to be ready to look at the ostomy or learn about care.
- Encourage patient to verbalize feelings about the stoma.
- Demonstrate stoma care, daily care and encourage patient participation.
- **Appliance change:**
  - Depending on the type of stoma, the appliance will need to be changed as often as every 3rd day. If leakage occurs, the appliance should be changed as soon as possible to avoid peristomal skin irritation.
  - The skin barrier that is placed over the stoma on the skin should fit within 1/6th to 1/8th inch of the base of the stoma to prevent skin contact with stool.
  - An open-ended or drainable pouch should be used for all colostomies, during the first 8 weeks after surgery.
- **Daily care and hygiene:**
  - The amount of effluent and the frequency of emptying depends on the location of the stoma in the bowel. If the pouch is allowed to get more than half full of stool, the weight of the effluent will pull on the pouch, and weaken the seal of the skin barrier. The patient is instructed to empty the pouch when it is one-third to one-half full.
  - Patient can bath or shower with the appliance in place but needs to check the seal and retape or change it if it is loosening.
- **Dietary consideration:** Eat at regular intervals.
  - Chew food well to avoid blockage at the stoma site.

- The patient needs to be aware of foods that contribute to odor and gas. Drink adequate amount of fluids.
- It is important that the patient know the foods that contribute to and control diarrhea and what to do for constipation
- A list of food that may contribute to blockage should be avoided, e.g., spinach, green leafy vegetable, corn, popcorn, apple, grape, potatoes, mushroom, coconut, nuts, apricots, meats with casings and Chinese vegetables.
- **Colostomy irrigation:** Colostomy irrigation is rarely done to regulate an ostomy. Irrigation is performed in a manner similar to an enema, except that special equipment is used to instill fluid into the bowel via the stoma because the stoma does not have a sphincter.
- **Disturbed body image:** Altered body image, fear of the uncertainty, and concerns regarding acceptance by significant others can take control of the patient with an ostomy.
  - The idea of feces being expelled from the abdomen can make the patient feel dirty and abnormal.
  - One of the most common fears expressed by patients with ostomies is the fear of gas and odor. Because the stoma does not have a sphincter, flatus is expelled unexpectedly.
  - Encourage the patient to always carry an extra appliance to determine the cause of the leakage.
- **Sexual dysfunction:** Change in body image can also lead to sexual dysfunction. If the male patient had an abdominal perineal resection for cancer of the rectum, there is a chance that he will be impotent. The impotent may be transient, depending on the severity of nerve damage or edema associated with the surgery.

CARE OF OSTOMIES

Definition
Maintenance of hygiene by regular emptying of colostomy bag and cleaning colostomy site.

Purposes
- To prevent leakage
- To prevent excoriation of skin and stoma
- To observe stoma and surrounding skin
- To teach patient and relatives about care of colostomy and collection bag.

Articles
Tray containing:
- Rubber sheet
- Long sheet
- Towel
- Clean gloves
- Cotton swabs and gauze pieces
- Wash cloth
- Water in basin
- Soap in dish
- Disposable colostomy bag with clamp (**Figs. 5.13 and 5.14**)
- Stoma measuring guide
- Zinc oxide ointment
- Skin barrier
- Bedpan with cover.

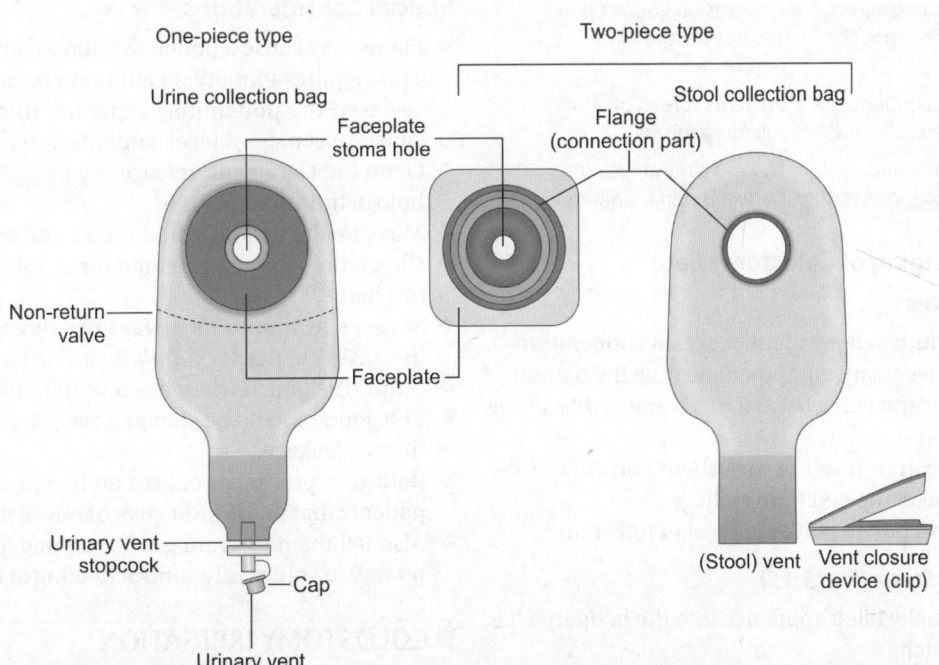

Fig. 5.13: Colostomy bag.

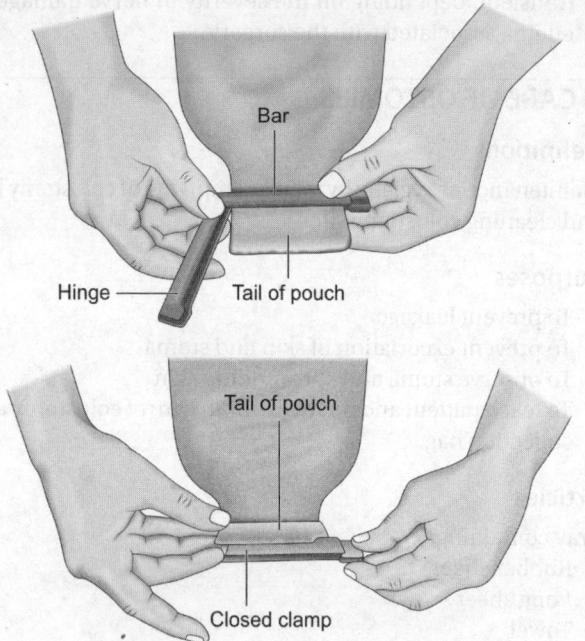

Fig. 5.14: Colostomy bag with clamp.

Emptying Colostomy Bag Without Changing (Table 5.10)

TABLE 5.10: Steps of procedure for emptying colostomy bag.

Nursing action	Rationale
Empty contents into bedpan or toilet. Rinse pouch with tepid water	Rinsing provides clean appearance and minimizes odor
Empty contents into bedpan or toilet. Rinse pouch with tepid water	Drying the lower section of the pouch removes additional fecal material
Instill deodorant in bag and uncuff the edge of the pouch and apply the clamp	Prevents bad odor. Clamp secures closure of the appliance
Dispose of used equipment, discard gloves and wash hand	Prevents spread of microorganisms
Document procedure and patient's reaction to procedure	Ensures communication between staff members

Procedure (Changing of Colostomy Bag)

Preprocedural Steps

- Explain procedure to the patient to obtain cooperation
- Assemble the necessary equipment near by the patient
- Provide privacy and assist patient to a comfortable sitting or lying position
- Place mackintosh or towel or absorbent pads under the patient: To protect the bed from spillage
- Wash hands and put on gloves to prevent infection.

Intraprocedural Steps (Fig. 5.15)

- Empty the partially filled appliance into the bedpan if it is a drainable pouch.
- Then remove the appliance slowly. Stretch the abdominal skin tight beginning at the top of the appliance. If any resistance is felt, use warm water or adhesive solvent to facilitate removal.
- Use tissue paper or gauze pad to remove any excess stool from the stoma
- Clean skin around stoma with cleansing agent (normal saline) or soap and water.
- Gently pat dry the peristomal skin. Make sure that the skin around the stoma is thoroughly dry.
- Assess the appearance of peristomal skin and stoma. A moist-reddish-pink stoma is considered normal.
- Apply the skin barrier cream on the dry skin. Let it get dry.
- Select size of stoma opening by using the measurement guide. Cover the stoma with a gauze pad
- Trace same size circle on the back at the center of the appliance. Use scissors to cut an opening 1/4 or 1/8 inch larger than stoma.
- Remove the backing to expose sticky side. Fill in irregular stoma borders with skin paste applied around the opening in the wafer before applying it to the skin.
- Remove gauze pad covering stoma. Apply barrier and pouch over the stoma and gently press onto skin while smoothing out creases or wrinkles. Hold the pouch in place for 3–5 minutes.
- Micropore may be used to stick on the edges of the pouch on the skin
- Close the pouch if it is drainable by folding the end upward and using a clamp or clip according to manufacturer's direction.

Postprocedural Steps

- Remove and discard the gloves
- Make the patient comfortable
- Assess the patient's response to the procedure
- Dispose off the disposable equipment appropriately.

Special Considerations

- Flatus may cause a pouch to balloon out.
- This requires immediate attention because if flatus is not released the pouch may separate from the skin barrier causing seepage of fecal contents or release of fecal odor.
- Open the clamp and release the flatus (never puncture a hole in the appliance).
- Measure the patient's fluid intake and output.
- Check the stoma appliance for quality and quantity of discharge.
- Stoma site should be always dry. Presence of moisture increases chance for *Candida* or yeast infection.
- Empty the pouch when it is one-third filled.
- The pouch should be changed every 4–5 days or whenever there is leakage.
- Return of peristalsis causes an increase in flatus. Advice patients that this is indicative of bowel functioning.
- Also tell them to avoid gas containing food since there is no way to voluntarily control passing of flatus.

■ COLOSTOMY IRRIGATION

- Irrigation should be done at the same time each day in order to establish regularity of bowel evacuation.

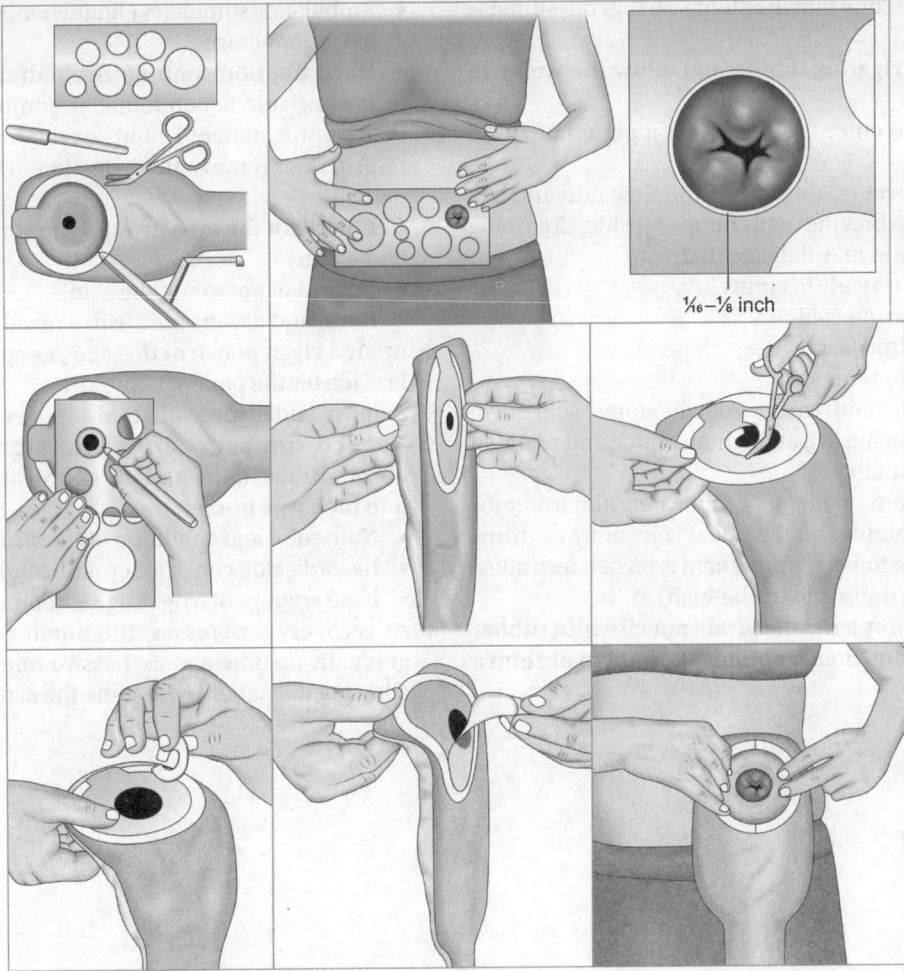

Fig. 5.15: Steps of procedure for changing colostomy bag.

- Unless contraindicated or otherwise ordered by the physician, it is best to establish a routine of daily irrigation in accordance with the patient's former bowel habits.
- For example, if the patient has always moved his/her bowels after breakfast, establish the irrigation routine for that time, rather than some other arbitrary schedule.

Articles Required

- Irrigation kit (irrigation bag with clamp and tubing, cone tip irrigation catheter, irrigation drain pouch).
- Water soluble lubricant.
- IV pole (or other suspending hook).
- Soap and water.
- Washcloth and towel.
- Ostomy appliance.
- Waste receptacle.
- Prescribed irrigating solution, usually 500–1000 cc warm (100–105°F) tap water.
- Clean gloves.

Procedure

- Review the procedure with the patient, if necessary.
- Wash hands and don gloves.
- Provide privacy to patient.
- If the patient is ambulatory, have the patient sit on the toilet or on a chair facing the toilet. If the patient is bedridden, elevate the head of the bed 45–90° and position rubber sheet around the patient.
- Fill the irrigation bag with the prescribed solution and hang it on the IV pole or hook.
    - The bottom of the bag should be at the patient's shoulder level when he/she is seated to prevent fluid from entering the bowel too rapidly.
    - The bottom of the bag should be placed 18 to 20 inches above the stoma when the patient is in bed.
- Open the clamp on the irrigation tubing and allow the solution to fill the tubing. Reclamp (This prevents the administration of air into the intestines).
- **As necessary, prepare to begin the colostomy irrigation:**
    - Remove the Ostomy pouch, if applicable and place the irrigation drain pouch over the stoma. (Attach stoma belt, if required).
    - Place the bottom, open end of the irrigation drain pouch in the toilet (or bedpan) to facilitate drainage by gravity.
    - Connect the cone tip catheter to the tubing and flush with solution.
- Lubricate the cone with the water soluble lubricant to avoid irritating the mucous membranes.

- Gently insert the cone into the stoma, so that the stoma is occluded.
- **Unclamp the irrigating tubing and allow the water to flow in slowly:**
  - Allow water to enter the colon over a period of 10–15 minutes.
  - If cramping occurs, slow down the flow rate and ask patient to deep breathe until cramps subside. Cramping during irrigation may indicate that:
    - The bowel is ready to empty.
    - The water is too cold.
    - The flow is too fast.
    - The tube contains air.
- Clamp the catheter and remove from the stoma. Fold down the top opening of the irrigation drain pouch and secure it in the closed position.
- Have the colostomy patient sit on or near the toilet for about 15 to 20 minutes so the initial colostomy re- turns can drain into the toilet. (If the patient is on bed rest, allow the colostomy to drain into the bedpan).
- **Close the colostomy irrigation drain pouch with a rubber band or pouch clip, then ambulate the patient or return him/her to bed:**
  - Ambulating stimulates elimination, producing improved irrigation return.
  - Have the non-ambulatory patient lean forward or massage his/her abdomen to stimulate return.
- Wait approximately 1 hour for the rest of the colostomy return, then remove the irrigation drain pouch from the patient.
- **Gently clean the area around the stoma with mild soap and water:**
  - Be careful not to rub the skin.
  - Rinse and dry the area with a towel.
- Apply a clean pouch or dressing, as applicable.
- Provide for the patient's comfort.
- Remove and dispose off used supplies.
- **Record the procedure and significant nursing observations in the patient's clinical record and report it to incharge nurse:**
  - Note color and condition of stoma and peristomal skin.
  - Record color, consistency and amount of drainage.
  - Note amount of irrigating solution used.
- As recovery progresses, the nursing personnel should gradually assume a more passive role in colostomy care, allowing the patient to assume the active role.

CHAPTER 6

Diagnostic Testing

DIAGNOSTIC TEST

Introduction

- A diagnostic test is an examination that helps to identify an individual's specific areas of strength and weakness in order to determine a condition, disease or illness.
- These are designed to help investigate or diagnose a disease condition, identify its causes and symptoms, or to measure for the presence of a particular factor that contributes to occurrence of some specific disorder or disease that could affect the normal individual profile.
- These diagnostic tests are approaches used in clinical practice that helps a physician to understand with high accuracy the disease of a particular patient and thus, provide early and proper treatment or interventional therapy as per the current condition of the patient(s) so as to allow patient(s) to recover as quickly as possible with the least amount of complications.
- A diagnostic test could be used in clinical settings for disease confirmation, triage, monitoring, prognosis, or screening.
- Medical diagnostic tests encompass a wide variety of physical examinations-both invasive and non-invasive by medical professionals to confirm the presence or absence of illness/disease in patients.

Definition

- A diagnostic test is defined as a procedure which is performed to confirm or determine the presence of disease or deviation from normal health parameters, in an individual suspected of having a disease, deficiency or abnormality usually following the report of symptoms, or based on other medical test results.
- These are performed by professionally competent and skilled medical professionals to detect, identify, and diagnose for the presence of any disease or infirmity in various body systems of body and plan treatment and interventions accordingly to prevent occurrence of any further complexity in patient's health condition.

Phases of Testing

Diagnostic testing in the laboratory testing is a cyclic process divided into three phases:

1. Pre-test (pre-analytical) phase
2. Intra-test (analytical) phase
3. Post-test (post-analytical) phase

Pre-test Phase

- The pre-test phase also known as pre analytical phase is the first phase that occurs in the laboratory process.
- This phase may include specimen handling issues that occur even prior to the time the specimen is received in the laboratory.
- Important errors can occur during the pre-test phase with specimen handling and identification.
- Therefore, the pre-test phase must have rigorous control measures to avoid unintentional impediment or errors.

Nurse's Responsibilities

- Assessment of patient to assist in determining precaution
- Preparation of consent form, if required.
- Preparation of equipment.
- Providing information about the procedure to patient and family.
- Appropriate handling and labeling of the collected specimen(s).

Intra-test Phase

- Also known as analytical phase is the second phase in the cyclic process of diagnostic testing
- This phase is considered as the "actual phase" in the process of laboratory testing or the diagnostic procedures, processes, and ultimately ends to provide the results after the diagnostic evaluations.

Nurse's Responsibilities

- Use of standard precautions, if necessary.
- Rechecking and ensuring the correct labeling storage and transportation of specimen.
- Monitoring patient's response during the procedure.
- Providing emotional support to patient and family

Post-test Phase

- The post-test or post-analytical phase is the final phase of laboratory testing.
- The process of diagnostic testing concludes with the generation of a final lab value; result of the laboratory

investigations conducted, or in the case of histology/biopsy studies, a diagnostic pathology report.
❖ These testing results are then transmitted to the concerned medical practitioner (physician/surgeon) for outlining plan of action, i.e., implementing further treatment and interventional therapies for the patient, set for routine check up and plan for re-testing to evaluate for the condition of the patient and effect of therapeutic intervention.

Nurse's Responsibilities
❖ Compare the patient's previous and current test results.
❖ Reporting of the results to the appropriate member of the health care team.

List of Diagnostic Tests

Laboratory diagnosis: Diagnostic tests are performed through the collection of specimen and diagnosis is made on the basis of laboratory reports.

Radiology diagnosis: Diagnosis is made by a specialized imaging procedure which provides the images of inside of the body. The images are interpreted to diagnose a disease or injury

Prenatal diagnosis: These are the diagnostic tests which are done before the birth.

COMPLETE BLOOD COUNTS (CBC) (HEMOGRAM) (CELL COUNTER)

Complete blood counts include the following:
❖ Hb
❖ RBC count
❖ DLC
❖ Reticulocyte count
❖ TLC
❖ Plt. count
❖ PCV/hematocrit
❖ Peripheral smear examination for red cell morphology, platelet morphology, parasites and any atypical cell.

All the above tests can be carried out on a 2 mL EDTA sample along with 2 peripheral smears.

Automated cell counters:
❖ These are single button switch equipments and aspirate the blood sample with an autoprobe wiping facility.
❖ The screen displays the parameters along with 3 histograms for WBCs, RBCs and platelets
❖ The various parameters obtained in the cell counter report are:
- Hb
- MPV
- MCH
- TLC
- Platelet count
- MCV
- Hematocrit
- RDW
- MCHC
- PDW
- Differential count 3 part or 5 part
- Reticulocyte count

• The report also demonstrates histograms of WBCs, red cells and platelets.

Hemoglobin and Hematocrit
❖ Hb is obtained using a cyanide free reagent (Sodium Lauryl Sulfate).
❖ The counter calculates the mean MCV which gets multiplied by red cell count to give the hematocrit (Hct).
❖ Though packed cell volume (PCV) and Hct are used interchangeably, PCV is obtained by centrifuging the blood sample.

Red Cell Parameters and Histogram
❖ The red cell parameters are hemoglobin, red cell count and MCV.
❖ MCH and MCHC are also displayed indicating the hemoglobin content of the red cells
❖ Red cell histogram displays red cell distribution width (RDW) in the form of standard deviation (SD) or coefficient of variation (CV).
❖ The bell-shaped curve indicates the degree of variation in the cell size, i.e., anisocytosis.
❖ RDW CV is normally between 10.4–15.2% (RDW-SD is 35.5–49.5 11).
❖ RDW >16 indicates anisocytosis of red cells and evaluation of the peripheral blood film is essential to look for spherocytes, fragmented red cells, tear drop cells, target cells and polychromatophils.

WBC Histogram
❖ The WBC histogram is based on the size of cells in femtolitres on the x-axis and the relative frequency of the cells on the y-axis.
❖ It displays 3 peaks the first one of lymphocytes (30–60), the second one of middle cells and the third one of large cells (115–150 fl) corresponding to neutrophils.
❖ Absolute counts of lymphocytes, middle cells and neutrophils are also displayed.
❖ The middle cell count (78–114 11) includes eosinophils, monocytes, blasts, promyelocytes, myelocytes and metamyelocytes.
❖ 5-part differential count is obtained in the present day hematology analyzers.
❖ The count includes % of neutrophils, lymphocytes, monocytes, eosinophils and basophils and also absolute counts.

Platelet Histogram
❖ This depicts the platelet distribution width (PDW) indicating the variation in the size of platelets.
❖ P-LCR, platelet large cell ratio gives an idea of the percentage of mega thrombocytes, with platelets having a size of >12 ft.
❖ MPV indicates the mean platelet volume.

Flags
❖ The cell counters have a system of depicting abnormal values above/below the normal range on y-axis in the form of flags.

- These can be appreciated on the histogram and the report, e.g., when the same contains nucleated red cells, unlysed red cells and platelet clumps, the WL flag appears when these cells constitute >20% of the nucleated cells.
- Similarly, flags appear when there is abnormality of size of red cells, e.g., fragmented red cells or agglutinated red cells.
- In acute leukemia, there is a peak in the middle cell area since the size of blast cells is between lymphocytes and neutrophils.

Automated Differential Count

- Cell counters are now available that give 3 or 5-7 part differential count.
- These differential counts are more precise than a manual count.
- However, for abnormal counts, examination of a peripheral smear by a pathologist is essential.
- 3 part differential analyzer is equipped with impedance based volumetric analysis alone.
- 5 part differential equipment is more accurate since it has laser optics, cell specific reagents and in-built artificial intelligence to differentiate white cells equally well.

Quality Management

- Most of the cell counters have in built control quality control (QC) programs.
- Besides, external quality assurance program is being run in India and many of the laboratories are participating in this program.

Complete blood count- meaning

- A complete blood count (CBC) is a group of tests used for basic screening purposes.
- It is probably the most widely ordered laboratory test.
- Results provide the enumeration of the cellular elements of the blood, measurement of RBC indices and determination of cell morphology by automation and evaluation of stained smears.
- The results can provide valuable diagnostic information regarding the overall health of the patient and the patient's response to disease and treatment.

Indications

- Detect hematologic disorder, neoplasm, leukemia, or immunologic abnormality.
- Determine the presence of hereditary or congenital hematologic abnormality.
- Evaluate known or suspected anemia and related treatment.
- Monitor the effects of physical or emotional stress.
- Monitor blood loss and the response to blood replacement.
- Monitor fluid imbalances or treatment for fluid imbalances.
- Monitor hematologic status during pregnancy.
- Monitor progression of non hematologic disorders, such as chronic obstructive pulmonary disease, malabsorption syndromes, cancer, and renal disease.
- Monitor response to chemotherapy and evaluate undesired reactions to drugs that may cause blood dyscrasias.
- Provide screening as part of a general physical examination, especially on admission to a health care facility or before surgery.
- Regular CBCs are necessary for people taking some psychiatric drugs, such as clozapine and carbamazepine, which in rare cases can cause a life-threatening drop in the number of white blood cells (agranulocytosis).

Purposes of CBC

- To monitor for any variations or deviations in the hematological profile of an individual.
- CBC also can help determine, if one has any immune system related disorder.
- To screen for diseases as part of a medical assessment.
- To diagnose a wide range of conditions, disorders, diseases and infections and help confirm that diagnosis.
- To rule out the cause of signs and symptoms such as weakness, fatigue, fever, inflammation, bruising or bleeding, etc.

VARIOUS BLOOD COMPONENTS MEASURED UNDER COMPLETE BLOOD COUNT

Red Blood Cells (RBCs) or Erythrocytes

- The name "Erythrocytes is from Greek word "Erythros" means "red" and "Cyte" means "cell"
- Red blood cells are the most numerous blood cells.
- They comprise about 99% of all blood cells.
- They are circular, bi concave non-nucleated discs about 7 micrometers (um) in diameter and is about 2 um thick at periphery and 1 um in center.
- RBCs are shaped like a disc or dumbbell and are slightly concave on top and bottom like a doughnut (without the hole).
- This shape provides a larger surface area for gas diffusion than a flat disc or a sphere.
- Number of red cells per liter or cubic millimeter of whole blood ($1 \text{ mm}^3 = 10^{-3}/L$):
  - No. of RBC = 4.8-5.4 million/mm^3 of blood (approximately 4-6 million/mm^3 of blood)
  - In males: 5-5.5 million/mm^3
  - In females: 4.5-5 million/mm^3
- Erythrocytes are 700 times more numerous than WBCs and 17 times more numerous than platelets.
- People living at high altitudes have greater number of RBCs.

White Blood Cells (Leukocytes)

- Leukocytes are the largest blood cells (range from slightly larger to much larger than erythrocytes).
- These are clear or white colored cells.
- Leukocytes have nuclei.
- Cells are able to move about independently and pass through blood vessel walls into the tissues.
- Leukocytes leave the circulation and enter tissues by diapedesis, a process in which they become thin and elongated and squeeze through the pores of capillary walls.
- Most leukocytes are motile, having amoeboid movements, which is the ability to move like an amoeba by putting out irregular cytoplasmic projections.

- WBCs are attracted to inflamed tissue areas by chemotaxis.
- This is the phenomenon in which many chemicals produced by inflamed tissue cause WBCs to move towards them.

Leukocytes Count

- Total leukocyte count (TLC)-4000–11000/mm³.
- **Leukocytosis versus leukopenia:** Leukocytosis is an elevation in the absolute WBC count whereas leukopenia is a reduction in the WBC count.

Medical conditions which cause increased production of WBC count:
- Burns
- Inflammation
- Thyroid problems
- Excessive physical or emotional stress

Medical conditions which causes decreased production of WBCs includes the following:
- Bone marrow disorders
- Lymphoma
- Vitamin B12 deficiencies
- Systemic lupus erythematosus (SLE)
- Human immunodeficiency virus (HIV)

Classification of Leukocytes

Two basic types of leukocytes (based on presence or absence of granules):
1. **Granulocytes:**
   a. *Neutrophils:* 60–70% of total leukocytes.
   b. *Eosinophils:* 1–49% of total leukocytes.
   c. *Basophils:* 0.5–1% of total leukocytes.
2. **Agranulocytes (20–30%):**
   a. *Monocytes:* 3–8% of total leukocytes.
   b. *Lymphocytes:* 20–25% of total leukocytes.

Hemoglobin (Hb)

- Hemoglobin is an O_2 carrying globular protein.
- Plasma membrane of RBCS encloses hemoglobin, which was synthesized before the loss of nucleus.
- More than 90% of the weight of erythrocyte consists of Hb and it occupies about 1/3rd of the total cell volume.
- Each RBC contains about 280 million Hb molecules.

Normal Values of Hemoglobin

- **Adult males:** 14–16.5 g/dL of blood.
- **Adult females:** 12–15 g/dl mL of blood.
- **Infants:** 14–20 g/dL of blood.

Composition of Hemoglobin

- 1.5% heme (iron containing pigment).
- 295% globin (polypeptide protein).

Functions of Hemoglobin

- Hemoglobin transports O_2 from lungs to body tissues.
- Function of Hb depends on its ability to combine with O_2 where O_2 concentration is high (in the lungs) and to release O_2 where about the 98.5% of O_2 is transported in blood in combination with Hb in RBCs and the remaining 1.5% is dissolved in water part of plasma.
- When Hb is exposed to O_2, one O_2 molecule can be come associated with each heme group. This oxygenated form of Hb is called oxyhemoglobin (it is bright red). Hb containing no O_2 is called deoxyhemoglobin (darker red color).
- Hb also carries waste CO, from the tissues to the lungs, where the CO_2 is exhaled. CO_2 does not combine with iron atoms but is attached to amino group of globin molecules. This Hb is carbaminohemoglobin.
- By removing CO_2, Hb also helps to maintain a stable acid-base balance in the blood.

Hematocrit

- Blood consists of a fluid portion (plasma) and a solid portion that includes red blood cells (RBCs), white blood cells, and platelets.
- The hematocrit, or packed cell volume, is the percentage of RBCs in a volume of whole blood.
- For example, a hematocrit (Hct) of 45% means that a 100-mL sample of blood contains 45 mL of packed RBCs.
- Although Hct depends primarily on the number of RBCs, the average size of the RBCs plays a role.
- Conditions that cause the RBCs to swell, such as when the serum sodium concentration is elevated, may increase the Hct level.
- Hct level is included in the complete blood count (CBC) and is generally tested together with hemoglobin (Hgb).
- These levels parallel each other and are the best determinant of the degree of anemia or polycythemia.
- Polycythemia is a term used in conjunction with conditions resulting from an abnormal increase in Hgb, Hct, and RBC count.
- Anemia is a term associated with conditions resulting from an abnormal decrease in Hgb, Hct, and RBC count should be evaluated simultaneously because the same under lying conditions affect this traid of test similarly.
- The RBC count multiplied by three should approximate the Hgb concentration.
- The Hct should be within three times the Hgb if the RBC population is normal in size and shape.
- The Hct plus six should approximate the first two figures of the RBC count within three (e.g., Hct is 40%; therefore 40 + 6 = 46, and the RBC count should be (4.3–4.9). There are some culture variations in Hgb and Hct (H and H) values.
- After the first decade of life, the mean Hgb in African-Americans is 0.5–1.0 g lower than in Caucasians.
- Mexican-Americans and Asian Americans have higher H and H values than Caucasians.

Indications

- Detect hematologic disorder, neoplasm, or immunological abnormality.
- Determine the presence of hereditary hematologic abnormality.
- Evaluate known or suspected anemia and related treatment, in combination with Hgb.
- Monitor blood loss and response to blood replacement, in combination with Hgb
- Monitor the effects of physical or emotional stress

- Monitor fluid imbalances or their treatment.
- Monitor hematologic status during pregnancy, in combination with Hgb
- Monitor the progression of non hematologic disorders, such as chronic obstructive pulmonary disease, malabsorption syndromes, cancer, and renal disease.
- Monitor response to drugs or chemotherapy, and evaluate undesired reactions to drugs that may cause blood dyscrasias.
- Provide screening as part of CBC count in a general physical examination, especially upon admission to a healthcare facility or before surgery.

Platelets (Thrombocytes)

- Platelets are so named because of their plate like flatness.
- They are very small non-nucleated discs and are about one quarter the size of the RBCs (2–4 um is diameter).
- Platelets exhibit many granules.
- As they have no nucleus, so they are incapable of cell division, but they have a complex metabolism and internal structure.

Platelets Count

Platelets are much more numerous than leukocytes. Normal value of platelets—1.50,000–4,00,000/mm³ of blood (average 2,50,000/mm³).

Functions of Platelets

Their main function is to prevent blood loss by:
1. **Forming platelet plug:**
   - Platelet plug seals holes in small vessels
   - After entering the bloodstream, platelets begins to pick up and store chemical substances that can be released later to help seal vessel breaks (so help to repair slightly damaged blood vessels).
2. **Forming clot:**
   - Main function of platelets is to start the intricate process of blood clotting.
   - The granules in platelets contain chemicals that release to promote blood clotting.

SERUM ELECTROLYTES

- Electrolytes, charged ions capable of conducting electricity are present in all body fluids and fluid compartments
- Although the concentration of specific electrolytes differs between fluid compartments, a balance of cations (positively charged ions) and anions (negatively charged ions) always exists.
- Electrolytes are minerals in human body that are the electrically charged particles and are found in blood, sweat and urine.
- When these minerals dissolve in a fluid, they form electrolytes positive or negative ions used in metabolic processes.
- If the levels of electrolyte are too low or too high, cell and organ functions will decline, which could give rise to life-threatening conditions.
- These are essential for regulating the pH levels and hydration in body cells, help rebuild damaged tissue.
- Our muscle cells and neurons are sometimes referred to as the "electric tissues of the body as they rely on the movement of electrolytes through the fluid inside, outside, or between cells, thus, it is said that electrolytes play an essential role in maintaining the function of muscle contraction and nerve impulse generation and conduction.
- The serum electrolyte test is performed—to assess problems in the water and pH balance of the body and as a part of routine health check-up.
- **The serum electrolyte test includes a group of tests to measure the following electrolytes that are required for various bodily processes:**
  - Sodium
  - Potassium
  - Chloride
  - Calcium
  - Magnesium
  - Phosphate
  - Bicarbonate
- Most electrolytes enter the body through dietary intake and are excreted in the urine.
- Some electrolyte, such as sodium and chloride, are not stored by the body and must be consumed daily to maintain normal levels.
- Potassium and calcium, on the other hand, are stored in the cells and bone, respectively.
- When serum levels drop, ions can shift out of the storage "pool" into the blood to maintain adequate serum levels for normal functioning
- Electrolytes are important for—maintaining fluid balance, contributing to acid-base regulation, facilitating enzyme reactions, and transmitting neuromuscular reactions

Serum Sodium (Na⁺)

- Chief electrolyte of ECF that moves easily between interstitial spaces and moves across cell membranes by active transport; influential in many chemical reactions in the body, particularly in nervous tissue cells and muscle tissue cells.
- Sodium is found in many foods, such as bacon, ham, processed cheese and table salt.
- Sodium is the most abundant cation in the extracellular fluid and, together with the accompanying chloride and bicarbonate anions, accounts for 92% of serum osmolality.
- Hypernatremia (elevated sodium level) occurs when there is excessive water loss or abnormal retention of sodium.
- Hyponatremia (low sodium level) occurs when there is inadequate sodium retention or inadequate intake.
- Normal serum sodium levels are 135–145 mEq/L

Regulation

- Renal reabsorption and or excretion
- Aldosterone increase Na reabsorption in collecting ducts of nephrons.

Functions
- Sodium functions largely in controlling and regulating water balance.
- Regulating ECF volume and distribution
- When sodium is reabsorbed from the kidney tubules, chloride and water are reabsorbed with it, thus maintaining ECF volume.
- Maintaining blood volume
- Transmitting nerve impulses and contracting muscles
- Sodium plays a major role in maintaining homeostasis in a variety of ways, including maintaining the osmotic pressure of extracellular fluid, regulating renal retention and excretion of water, maintaining acid-base balance, regulating potassium and chloride levels, stimulating neuromuscular reactions, and maintaining systemic blood pressure.

Serum Potassium (K^+)
- Potassium is the major cation in intracellular fluids, with only a small amount found in plasma and interstitial fluid.
- Cations, including potassium, carry a positive charge.
- Potassium is the most abundant intracellular cation.
- Electrolytes dissociate into electrically charged ions when dissolved.
- Body fluids contain approximately equal number of anions and cations, although the nature of the ions and their mobility differs between the intracellular and extracellular compartments.
- Both types of ions affect the electrical and osmolar functions of the body.
- Electrolyte quantities and the balance among them are controlled by oxygen and carbon dioxide exchange in the lungs absorption, secretion, and excretions of many substances by the kidneys; and secretion of regulatory hormones by the endocrine glands.
- ICF levels of potassium are usually 125–140 mEq/L while normal serum potassium levels are 3.5–5.0 mEq/L.
- The ratio of intracellular to extracellular potassium must be maintained for neuromuscular response to stimuli.
- Potassium is a vital electrolyte for skeletal, cardiac and smooth muscle activity.
- Potassium must be ingested daily because the body can't conserve it.
- Many fruits and vegetables, meat, fish, and other foods contain potassium

Potassium-rich Foods
- **Vegetables:** Avocado, Raw carrot, Baked potatoes, Raw tomato, Spinach
- **Fruits:** dried fruits (e.g., raisins and dates), Banana, Apricot, Cantaloupe, Orange,
- **Meat and fish:** Beef, Cod, Pork, Veal
- **Beverages:** Milk, Orange juice, Apricot nectar

Abnormal potassium can be caused by a number of contributing factors, which can be categorized as follows:
- Altered renal excretion: Normally, 80–90% of the body's potassium is filtered out through the kidneys each day (the remainder is excreted in sweat and stool); renal disease can result in abnormally high potassium levels.
- **Altered dietary intake:** A severe potassium deficiency can be caused by an inadequate intake of dietary potassium.
- **Altered cellular metabolism:** Damaged red blood cells (RBCs) release potassium into the circulating fluid, resulting in increased potassium levels.
- Normal value: 3.5–5 mEq/L.

Indications
- Assess a known or suspected disorder associated with renal disease, glucose metabolism, trauma, or burns
- Assist in the evaluation of electrolyte imbalances, this test is especially indicated in elderly patients, patients receiving hyperalimentation supplements, patients on hemodialysis, and patients with hypertension.
- Evaluate cardiac arrhythmia to determine whether altered potassium levels are contributing to the problem, especially during digitalis therapy, which leads to ventricular irritability.
- Evaluate the effects of drug therapy, especially diuretics
- Evaluate the response to treatment for abnormal potassium levels.
- Monitor known or suspected acidosis, because potassium moves from RBCs into the extracellular fluid in acidic states.
- Routine screen of electrolytes in acute and chronic illness.

Regulation
- Renal excretion and conservation Aldosterone increases K^+ excretion
- Movement into and out of cells
- Insulin helps move K into cells; tissue damage and acidosis shift K' out of cells into ECF

Functions
- Maintaining ICF osmolality
- Transmitting nerve and other electrical impulses
- Regulating cardiac impulses transmission and muscle contraction
- It is essential for the transmission of electrical impulses in cardiac and skeletal muscle thus help in Skeletal and smooth muscle function
- **Regulating acid-base balance:** Potassium helps maintain acid-base equilibrium, and it has a significant and inverse relationship to pH: A decrease in pH of 0.1 increases the potassium level by 0,6 mEq/L.
- It is involved in maintaining acid base balance as well, and it contributes to intracellular enzyme reactions.
- It functions in enzyme reactions that transform glucose into energy and amino acids into proteins.

Serum Calcium (Ca^{2+})
- The vast majority, 99%, of calcium in the body is in the skeletal system, with a relatively small amount in ECF
- Although this calcium outside the bones and teeth amounts to only about 1% of the total calcium in the body, it is vital in regulating muscle contraction and relaxation, neuromuscular function, and cardiac function.

- ECF calcium is regulated by a complex interaction of parathyroid hormone, calcitonin, and calcitriol, a metabolite of vitamin D.
- When calcium levels in the EC fall, parathyroid hormone and calcitriol cause calcium to be released from bones into ECF and increase the absorption of calcium in the intestine, thus raising serum calcium levels.
- Conversely, calcitonin stimulates the deposition of calcium in bone, reducing the concentration of calcium ions in the blood.
- With aging, the intestine absorbs calcium less effectively and more calcium is excreted via the kidneys.
- Calcium shift out of the bone to replace this ECF loss increasing the risk of osteoporosis and fractures of the wrist, vertebrae, and hips. Lack of weight bearing exercise (which helps keep calcium in the bones) and a vitamin D deficiency because of inadequate exposure to sunlight contribute to this risk.
- Milk and milk products are the richest sources of calcium with other foods such as dark green leafy vegetables and canned salmon containing smaller amounts.
- Many clients benefit from calcium supplements.
- Calcium, the most abundant cation in the body, participates in almost all of the vital process.
- Calcium concentration is largely regulated by the parathyroid glands and by the action of vitamin D.
- Of the body's calcium reserves, 98–99% is stored in the teeth and skeleton.
- Calcium values are higher in children because of growth and active bone formation.
- About 45% of the total amount of blood calcium circulates as free ions that participate in coagulation, neuromuscular conduction, intracellular regulation, glandular secretion, and control of skeletal and cardiac muscle contractility.
- The remaining calcium is bound to circulating proteins (40% bound mostly to albumin) and anions (15% bound to anions, such as bicarbonate, citrate, phosphate, and lactate) and plays no physiologic role.
- Calcium values can be adjusted up or down by 0.8 g/dL for every 1 g/dL that albumin is greater than or less than 4 g/dL.
- Calcium and phosphorus levels are inversely proportional.
- Normal value: 8.6–10.3 mg/dL.
- Fluid and electrolyte imbalances are often seen in patients with serious illness or injury, in these clinical situations, the normal homeostatic balance of the body is altered.
- During surgery or in the case of a critical illness, bicarbonate, phosphate, and lactate concentrations can change dramatically.
- Treatments may also cause or contribute to electrolyte imbalance. This is why total calcium values can sometimes be misleading.
- Abnormal calcium levels are used to indicate general malfunctions in various body systems.
- Ionized calcium is used in more specific conditions.

    Calcium values should be interpreted in conjunction with results of other tests:
    - Normal calcium with an abnormal phosphorus value indicates impaired calcium absorption (possibly because of altered parathyroid hormone level or activity).
- Normal calcium with an elevated urea nitrogen value indicates possible hyperparathyroidism (primary or secondary).
- Normal calcium with decreased albumin value is an indication of hypercalcemia.
- The most common causes of hypercalcemia (higher calcium levels) are hyperparathyroidism and cancer.
- The most common cause of hypocalcemia (low calcium levels) is hypoalbuminemia.

Indications
- Detect parathyroid gland loss after or other neck surgery, as indicated by decreased levels.
- Evaluate cardiac arrhythmias and coagulation disorders to determine, if altered serum calcium level is contributing to the problem.
- Evaluate the effects of various disorders on calcium metabolism, especially diseases involving drugs on calcium levels.
- Monitor the effectiveness of therapy being administered to correct abnormal calcium levels, especially calcium deficiencies.

Regulation
- Redistribution between bones and ECF
- Parathyroid hormone and calcitriol increases serum Ca' levels; calcitonin decreases serum levels

Functions
- Forming bones and teeth) Transmitting nerve impulses
- Regulating muscle contraction
- Maintaining cardiac pacemaker (automaticity)
- Blood clotting
- Activating enzymes, such as pancreatic lipase and phospholipase

Serum Magnesium (Mg^{2+})
- It is the second most abundant intracellular cation with normal serum levels of 1.5–2.5 mEq/L.
- It is important for intracellular metabolism, being particularly involved in the production and use of adenosine triphosphate (ATP).
- Magnesium also is necessary for protein and deoxyribonucleic acid (DNA) synthesis within the cells.
- Only about 1% of the body's magnesium is in ECF; here it is involved in regulating neuromuscular and cardiac functions.
- Urine magnesium levels reflect magnesium deficiency before serum levels.
- Magnesium deficiency severe enough to cause hypocalcemia and cardiac arrhythmias can exist despite normal serum magnesium levels.
- Normal value: 1.7–2.2 mg/dL.
- Cereal grains, nuts, dried fruits, legumes, and green leafy vegetables are good sources of magnesium in the diet, as are dairy products, meat, and fish.

Regulation
- Conservation and excretion by kidney

- Intestinal absorption increased by vitamin D and parathyroid hormone

Functions
- Intracellular metabolism
- Operating sodium-potassium pump
- Relaxing muscle contraction
- Transmitting nerve impulses
- Regulating cardiac functions
- Magnesium is required as a cofactor in numerous crucial enzymatic processes such as protein synthesis, nucleic acid synthesis, and muscle contraction
- Magnesium is also required for the use of adenosine diphosphate as a source of energy.
- Magnesium is needed for the transmission of nerve impulses and muscle relaxation.
- It controls absorption of sodium, potassium, calcium, and phosphorus utilization of carbohydrate, lipid, and protein; and activation of enzyme systems that enable the B vitamins to function.
- Magnesium is also essential for oxidative phosphorylation, nucleic acid synthesis, and blood clotting

Indications
- Determine electrolyte balance in renal failure and chronic alcoholism.
- Evaluate cardiac arrhythmias (decreased magnesium levels can lead to excessive ventricular irritability).
- Evaluate known or suspected disorders associated with altered magnesium levels.
- Monitor the effects of various drugs on magnesium levels.

Serum Chloride (Cl⁻)
- Chloride is the most abundant anion in the extracellular fluid.
- Chloride is the major anion of ECF.
- Chloride functions with sodium to regulate serum osmolality and blood volume.
- The concentration of chloride in ECF is regulated secondarily to sodium—when sodium is reabsorbed in the kidney, chloride usually follows.
- Chloride is a major component of gastric juice as hydrochloric acid and is involved in regulating acid-base balance.
- It also acts as a buffer in the exchange of oxygen and carbon dioxide in red blood cells (RBCs).
- Chloride is found in the same foods as sodium.
- Chloride levels generally increase and decrease proportional to sodium levels and inversely proportional to bicarbonate levels.
- The chloride content of venous blood is slightly higher than that of arterial blood because chloride ion enter red blood cell in response to absorption of carbon dioxide into the cell.
- As carbon dioxide enters the blood cell, bicarbonate leaves and chloride is absorbed in exchange to maintain electrical neutrality within the cell.
- Chloride is provided by dietary intake, mostly in the form of sodium chloride.
- It is absorbed by the gastrointestinal system, filtered out by the glomeruli, and reabsorbed by the renal tubules.
- Excess chloride is excreted in the urine.
- Serum values normally remain fairly stable.
- A slight decrease may be detectable after meals because chloride is used to produce hydrochloric acid as part of the digestive process.
- The patient's clinical picture needs to be considered in the evaluation of electrolytes.
- Fluid and electrolyte imbalances are often seen in patients with serious illness or injury because in these cases the clinical situation has affected the normal homeostatic balance of the body.
- It is also possible that therapeutic treatments being administered are causing or contributing to the electrolyte imbalance.
- Children and adults are at high risk for fluid and electrolyte imbalances when chloride levels are depleted.
- Children are considered to be at high risk during chloride imbalance because a positive serum chloride balance is important for expansion of the extracellular fluid compartment.
- Anemia, the result of decreased hemoglobin levels, is a frequent issue for elderly patients.
- Elderly patients are also at high risk because their renal response to change in pH is slower, in more rapid development of electrolyte imbalance.
- **Normal value:** 97–105 mEq/L

Indications
- Assist in confirming a diagnosis of disorders associated with abnormal chloride values, as seen in acid-base and fluid
- Differentiate between types of acidosis (hyperchloremic versus anion gap).
- Monitor effectiveness of drug therapy to increase or decrease serum chloride levels.

Regulation
- Excreted and reabsorbed along with sodium in the kidney
- Aldosterone increases chloride reabsorption with sodium

Functions
- Buffer in oxygen-carbon dioxide exchange in RBCs
- Regulating acid-base balance: Its most important function is in the maintenance of acid-base balance, in which it competes with bicarbonate for sodium.
- Since hemoglobin participates in a major buffer system in the body, depleted hemoglobin levels affect the efficiency of chloride ion exchange for bicarbonate in red blood cells which in turn affects acid-base balance.
- **Regulating ECF balance and vascular volume:** Chloride also participates with sodium in the maintenance of water balance and aids in the regulation of osmotic pressure.
- **HCl production:** Chloride contributes to gastric acid (hydrochloric acid) for digestion and activation of enzymes.

Serum Phosphate (PO₄⁻)
- Phosphate is the major anion of intracellular fluid.

- It is also found in ECF, bone, skeletal muscle, and nerve tissue.
- Children must have higher phosphate level than adult, with that of newborn nearly twice that of an adult.
- Higher levels of growth hormone and a faster rate of skeletal growth probably account for this difference.
- Phosphate is involved in many chemical actions of the cell; it is essential for functioning of muscles, nerves, and RBCs.
- It is also involved in the metabolism of proteins fats and carbohydrates.
- Phosphate is absorbed from the intestine and is found in many foods, such as meat, fish, poultry, milk products, and legumes.
- Phosphorus, in the form of phosphate, is distributed throughout the body, approximately 85% of the body's phosphorus is stored in bones; the remainder is found in cells and body fluids.
- It is the major intracellular anion and plays a crucial role in cellular metabolism, maintenance of cellular membranes and formation of bones and teeth.
- Phosphorus also indirectly affects the release of oxygen from hemoglobin by affecting the formation of 2,3 bisphosphoglycerate.
- Levels of phosphorus are dependent on dietary intake.
- Phosphorus excretion is regulated by the kidneys.
- Calcium and phosphorus are interrelated with respect to absorption and metabolic function.
- They have an inverse relationship with respect to concentration—serum phosphorus is increased when serum calcium is decreased.
- Hyperphosphatemia can result in an infant fed only cow's milk during the first few week of life because of the combination of a high phosphorus content in cow's milk and the inability of infants' kidney to clear the excess phosphorus.
- **Normal value:** 2.5–4.5 mg/dL

Indications
- Assist in establishing a diagnosis of hyperparathyroidism.
- Assist in the evaluation of renal failure.

Regulation
- Excretion and reabsorption by the kidney
- Parathyroid hormone decreases serum levels by increasing renal excretion
- Reciprocal relationship with calcium; increasing serum calcium levels decrease phosphate levels; decreasing serum calcium increases phosphate

Functions
- Forming bones and teeth
- Metabolizing carbohydrate, protein and fat
- Cellular metabolism; producing ATP and DNA
- Muscle, nerve and RBC function
- Regulating acid-base balance
- Regulating calcium levels

Serum Bicarbonate (HCO_3^-)
- Bicarbonate is present in both intracellular and extracellular fluids.
- Its primary function is regulating acid-base balance as an essential component of the carbonic acid-bicarbonate buffering system.
- Extracellular bicarbonate levels are regulated by the kidneys.
- Bicarbonate is excreted when it present in excessive amount; if more is needed; the kidneys both regenerate and reabsorb bicarbonate ions.
- Unlike other electrolytes that must be consumed in the diet, adequate amounts of bicarbonate are produced through metabolic processes to meet the body's needs.
- The bicarbonate ion acts as a buffer so maintain the normal levels of acidity (pH) in blood and other fluids in the body.
- Bicarbonate levels are measured to monitor the acidity of the blood and body fluids
- Alteration in the bicarbonate indicates a number of conditions such as diarrhea, liver failure, kidney disease and anorexia.
- **Normal value:** 22–30 mmol/L
- Bicarbonate level more than 30 mEq/L can be caused by compensated respiratory acidocis, metabolic alkalosis.

Indications
- Heart burn
- Sour stomach

Regulation
- Excretion and reabsorption by the Kidney
- Regeneration by the kidney

Functions
- Major body buffer involved in acid-base regulation.
- Bicarbonate is an electrolyte that helps to keep our body hydrated and maintains the right amount acidity of the blood
- Bicarbonate helps to maintain a normal acid-base balance which prevents the body from becoming too acidic, which can cause many health problems.

LIVER FUNCTION TESTS (LFTs)

Liver function tests are the laboratory studies or tests, which describes if the liver functions are disturbed by a disease process and the diagnosis of a disease.

The following are the LFT:
- Serum bilirubin
- Dye excretion tests
- Protein metabolism
- Lipid metabolism
- Serum enzyme tests
- Hemostatic functions (prothrombin and Vitamin K).

Uses:
- Liver function tests assess the functional damage of the liver.
- LFTs provide the information of progress in a liver disease.
- LFTS help in diagnosing the hepatic insufficiency.

1. **LFTs help to assess the functions of the liver:**
   - *Total plasma protein concentration:* 6.4–8.3 g%
   - *S. albumin:* 3–5 g%

- S. globulin: 2–3 g%
- S. fibrinogen: 0.3 g%
- S. prothrombin: 40 mg%

2. **Thyroid turbidity test:** Thyroid turbidity in liver insufficiency.
3. **Test for coagulability of blood increases:**
   - S. fibrinogen and S. prothrombin decreases in liver insufficiency.
   - Prothrombin time (normal 11–16 sec.) increases in liver insufficiency.
4. **Liver enzymes estimation:**
   - Increased SGOT indicate liver insufficiency.
   - Increased S. alkaline indicates liver cell damage.
5. **Blood urea:** Normal value—20–40% blood urea level decreases in insufficiency of liver.
6. **Blood ammonia:** Normal value—20–80% pg blood ammonia increases in insufficiency of liver.
7. **Urine ammonia:** Normal value—350–1200 mg/day urine ammonia increases in insufficiency of liver.

LFTS TO ASSESSMENT OF METABOLIC

Functions of Liver

1. **For glucose metabolism:**
   - *Galactose tolerance test:* Galactose Index (GI normal valve is 68–160 mg) in liver damage condition is markedly increasing
   - *Blood glucose test:* Normal value is 50–90 mg% Blood glucose decreases in liver inefficiency.
2. **For protein metabolism:**
   - *Blood amino acid level:* Normal value-30–65 mg%. Blood amino acid level increases in insufficiency of liver.
   - *Urine test for amino acid:* Amino acids appear in urine (amino acid urea) which indicates liver insufficiency.
3. **Fat metabolism (Table 6.1):**

TABLE 6.1: Fat metabolism.

	In liver in sufficiency	Normal
S. cholesterol	Decrease	150–240 mg%
S. Triglycerides	Decrease	30–150 mg%
S. phospholipids	Decrease	150–300 mg%
Total lipids	Decrease	350–800 mg%
S. ketone bodies	Increase	0.7–1.5 mg%

Indications

- Assess liver malfunction, detect alcohol-induced liver disease, hemolytic anemia, and hyperbilirubinemia in newborns.
- Evaluate progress of liver and pancreatic disease and response to treatment.
- Measure GGT in differential diagnosis of liver disease in children and pregnant women and to detect alcohol induced liver disease.

Liver Function Tests (Table 6.2)

TABLE 6.2: Components of liver function tests.

Parameter name	Normal value
Aspartate aminotransferase (AST/SGOT)	8–331U/L
Alanine transaminase (ALT/SGPT)	4–36 IU/L
Alkaline phosphatase (ALP)	44–147 IU/L
Serum bilirubin	
Direct	0.3 mg/dL
Indirect	0.2–1.2 mg/dL
Total	0.2–1.2 mg/dL
Gamma-glutamyl transferase (GGT)	0–30 IU/L
Protein (Total)	6–83 g/dL
Serum albumin	3.4–54 g/dL
Serum globulin	2.0–3.5 g/dL
A/G ratio (Albumin/Globulin)	1.1–2.5

Alanine Aminotransferase

- Alanine aminotransferase (ALT), formerly known as serum glutamic pyruvic transaminase (SGPT), is an enzyme produced by the liver.
- It acts as a catalyst in the reversible transfer of an amino group between alanine and alpha ketoglutarate.
- The highest concentration of ALT is found in liver cells, moderate amounts are found in kidney cells, and smaller amounts are found in heart and skeletal muscle.
- When liver damage occurs, serum levels of ALT rise to 50 times normal, making this a useful test in evaluating liver injury.
- ALT is also used to screen donated blood before transfusion because the enzyme may be elevated in the absence of detectable serologic markers of hepatitis.
- Normal value: 7-55 IU/L

Indications

- Compare serially with aspartate aminotransferase (AST) levels to track the course of liver disease.
- Monitor liver damage resulting from hepatotoxic drugs.
- Monitor response to treatment of liver disease, with tissue repair indicated by gradually declining levels.
- In blood banks, use as a routine screen for hepatitis in donor blood samples. Samples are rejected, if levels are greater than 1.5 times the upper limits of normal.

Aspartate Aminotransferase

- Aspartate aminotransferase (AST) is an enzyme that catalyzes the reversible transfer of an amino between aspartate and ketoglutaric acid.
- It was formerly known as serum glutamic oxaloacetic transaminase (SGOT).
- AST exits in large amounts in liver and myocardial cells and in smaller but significant amounts in skeletal muscle, kidneys, pancreas, and the brain.
- Serum AST rises when there is cellular damage to the tissues where the enzyme is found.

- AST values greater than too U/L are usually associated with hepatitis and other hepatocellular diseases in an acute phase.
- AST levels are very elevated at birth and decrease with age.
- Measurement of AST in evaluation of myocardial infarction has been replaced by more sensitive tests, such as creatine kinase MB fraction (CK-MB) and troponin
- **Normal value:** 5–40 IU/L

Indications

- Assist in the diagnosis of disorders of injuries involving the tissues where AST is normally found.
- Assist (formerly) in the diagnosis of myocardial infarction (note: AST rises within 6–8 hours, peaks at 24–48 hours, and declines to normal within 72–96 hours).
- Compare serially with alanine aminotransferase levels. to track the course of hepatitis.
- Monitor response to therapy with potentially hepatotoxic or nephrotoxic drugs.
- Monitor response to treatment for various disorders in which AST may be elevated, with tissue repair indicated by declining levels.

Alkaline Phosphatase

- ALP is an enzyme found in the liver in Kupffer cells lining the biliary tract, and in bones, intestines, and placenta.
- Additional sources of ALP include the proximal tubules of the kidneys, pulmonary alveolar cells, germ cells, vascular bed, lactating mammary glands, and granulocytes of circulating blood.
- ALP is referred to as alkaline because if functions optimally at a pH of 9.0.
- This test is most useful for determining the presence of liver or bone disease.
- Isoelectric focusing methods can identify 12 isoenzymes of ALP.
- Certain cancers produce small amounts of distinctive Regan and Nagao ALP isoenzymes.
- Four main ALP isoenzymes, however, are of clinical significance: ALP1 of liver origin, ALP2 of bone origin, ALP3 of intestinal origin (occasionally present in individuals with blood type O and B) and ALP4 of placental origin (third trimester). ALP levels vary by age and gender.
- Values in children are higher than in adults because of the level of bone growth and development.
- An immunoassay method is available for measuring bone specific ALP as an indicator of increased bone turnover and estrogen deficiency in post-menopausal women.
- **Normal value:** 20–140 IU/L

Indications

- Evaluate signs and symptoms of various disorders associated with elevated ALP levels, such as biliary obstruction, hepatobiliary disease, and bone disease including malignant processes
- Differentiate obstructive hepatobiliary tract disorder from hepatocellular disease; greater elevations of ALP are seen in the former
- Determine effects of renal disease on bone metabolism.
- Determine bone growth or destruction in children with abnormal growth patterns.

Albumin

- Albumin is the most abundant protein (about 60% of all plasma proteins) which is synthesized in the liver.
- It maintains plasma osmotic pressure at its normal level of about 25 mm Hg 80% of osmotic pressure of blood is due to albumin.
- It promotes water retention in the blood which in turn maintains normal blood volume and pressure.
- If the amount of albumin in the plasma decreases, fluid leaves the blood stream and accumulates in the surrounding tissue causing a swelling known as edema.
- **Normal level:** 3.5–5 g/100 mL.

Indications

- Hypovolemia
- Hypoalbuminemia
- Acute respiratory distress syndrome (ARDS)
- Nephrotic syndrome

Bilirubin and Bilirubin Fractions

- Bilirubin is a byproduct of heme catabolism from aged red blood cells.
- Bilirubin is primarily produced in the liver, spleen, and bone marrow.
- Total bilirubin is the sum of us conjugated bilirubin, monoglucuronide and diglucuronide conjugated bilirubin.
- Unconjugated bilirubin is carried to the liver by albumin, where it becomes conjugated.
- In the small intestine, conjugated bilirubin converts to urobilinogen and then to urobilin.
- Urobilin is then excreted in the feces. Increases in bilirubin levels can result from prehepatic and/or post-hepatic conditions, making fractionation useful in determining the cause of the increase in total bilirubin levels.
- Delta bilirubin has a longer half-life than the other bilirubin concentration increases the yellowish pigment deposits in skin and sclera.
- This increase in yellow pigmentation is termed as jaundice or icterus.
- **Normal value:** 0.1–1.2 mg/dL

Indications

- Assist in the differential diagnosis of obstructive Jaundice.
- Assist in the evaluation of liver and biliary disease
- Monitor the effects of drug reactions on liver function
- Monitor jaundice in newborn patients Monitor the effects of phototherapy on jaundiced newborns.

Gamma-Glutamyl Transferase (GGT)

GGT is an enzyme present in the blood. Its higher level may indicate liver or bile duct damage.

Indications

- Identifying the nature of liver diseases.
- Screen for liver disease.

TABLE 6.3: Normal range of PT-INR.

Test	Normal range
PT 1	0–12 seconds
PTT	30–45 seconds
INR	1:2 ratio

- Assess severity and prognosis of liver disease
- **Normal value:** In adults, GGT level in the range of 0–30

Prothrombin Time (PT)

- Increased PT may indicate liver damage but it can also be elevated, if a person is taking certain blood thinning drugs, such as Warfarin.
- Normal values of coagulation tests.
- Prothrombin time (Table 6.3)
- PT-Prothrombin time
- PTT-Partial thromboplastin time
- INR-International normalized ratio

LIPIDS/LIPOPROTEIN PROFILE

- Lipid is a fat or fat-like substance which is essential for the proper functioning of our body. It is a source of energy for our normally stored both in our blood and tissues.
- However, too much lipid to diseases that are even life-threatening, for instance, coronary artery disease, stroke or heart attack.
- Both triglycerides and cholesterol are lipids.
- A lipid profile or lipid panel is a group of blood tests used to rule out abnormalities in serum lipid levels.
- It comprise of combination of blood tests, namely—total cholesterol, very low density lipoproteins (VLDL), low density lipoproteins (LDL or bad cholesterol).
- High density lipoproteins (HDL or good cholesterol) and Triglycerides.
- The results of this test can identify certain genetic diseases and can also assess the health of the heart and approximate risk of developing cardiovascular diseases in a patient.

Normal Lipid Profile

- Total cholesterol normal range-lower than 200 mg/dL.
- Low density lipoproteins (LDL)—between 70–130 mg/dL.
- High density lipoproteins (HDL)—between 40–60 mg/dL.
- Triglycerides—between 10–150 mg/dL

Human Plasma Contains Four Types of Lipids

1. Cholesterol
2. Triglycerides
3. Phospholipids
4. Non-esterified fatty acids (NCIA)
   Lipids are transported in blood as a complex with proteins. This complex is called lipoprotein and the protein part of the lipoprotein is called apoproteins.

There are five major classes of lipoproteins:

1. Very low density lipoprotein (VSDL)
2. Intermediate density lipoprotein (ID)
3. Low density lipoprotein (LDL). Also known as bad cholesterol
4. High density lipoprotein. Also known as good cholesterol
5. Chylomicrons

Cholesterol

- Cholesterol is a soft, white, waxy substance found widely in the body. Our body needs cholesterol for proper functioning.
- However, high cholesterol level can block coronary anterior and cause heart disease and stroke.
- Cholesterol and its esters are first hydrolyzed and then oxidized to liberate hydrogen peroxide which converts a color-producing substance to a colored substance.
- The intensity of the colored substance depends on the concentration of cholesterol which is measured by a calorimeter.
- High-density lipoprotein cholesterol (HDLC) and low density lipoprotein cholesterol (LDLC) are the major transport proteins for cholesterol in the body.
- It is believed that HDLC may have protective properties in that its role includes transporting cholesterol from the arteries to the liver.
- LDLC is the major transport protein for cholesterol to the arteries from the liver.
- LDLC can be calculated using total cholesterol, total triglycerides, and HDLC levels.
- HDLC levels less than 40 mg/dL in men and women represent a coronary risk factor.
- There is an inverse relationship between HDLC and risk or coronary artery disease (CAD) (i.e., lower HDLC levels represent a higher risk of CAD).
- Levels of LDLC in terms of risk for CAD are directly proportional to risk and vary by age group.
- The LDLC can be estimated using the following Friedewald formula:

    LDLC (Total cholesterol) − (HDLC) − (VLDLC)
- Very-low-density lipoprotein cholesterol (VLDLC) is estimated by dividing the triglycerides (conventional units) by 5. Triglycerides in SI units would be divided by 2.18 to estimate VLDLC.
- It is important to note that the formula is valid only if the triglycerides are less than 400 mg/dL or 4.52 mmol/L.

Indications

- Determine the risk of cardiovascular disease.
- Evaluate the response to dietary and drug therapy for hypercholesterolemia.
- Investigate hypercholesterolemia in light of family history of cardiovascular disease.

Sources

- Animal fat
- Egg yolk
- **Endogenous source:** Liver synthesizes cholesterol estimation. Cholesterol is estimated by enzymatic method.

Cholesterol Levels

* <200 mg/dL. Normal
* 200–239 mg/dL. Borderline high
* >/=240 mg/dL High

Triglycerides

* Triglycerides are neutral fat.
* 95% of the stored fat is triglyceride.
* These are stored in the adipose cells.
* **Estimation.** Triglyceride estimation is done by enzymatic method using a kit.
* Serum triglycerides are converted to glycerol-3 phosphate oxidase (GPO) through multiple steps involving multiple enzymes.
* GPO liberates hydrogen peroxide which changes chromogenic substance (color-producing substance) to a colored complex.
* The intensity of the color is proportional to the concentration of triglyceride which is measured by a calorimeter.
* Triglycerides are a combination of three fatty acids and one glycerol molecule.
* They are necessary to provide energy for various metabolic processes.
* Excess triglycerides are stored in adipose tissue, and the fatty acids provide the raw material needed for conversion to glycose (gluconeogenesis) or for direct use as an energy source.
* Although fatty acids originate in the diet, many are also derived from unused glucose and amino acids that the liver converts into stored energy.
* Triglyceride levels vary by age, sex, weight and race.
* **Normal levels:** 53–150 mg/100 mL. Lower value is desirable. According to the American Heart Association a level of 100 mg/dL or less is optimal.
* 150–199 mg/dL. Borderline high
* 200–499 mg/dL. High
* 500 mg/dL. and above Very high

Indications

* Evaluate known or suspected disorders associated with altered triglyceride levels. Identify hyperlipoproteinemia (hyperlipidemia) in patients with a family history of the disorder.
* Monitor the response to drugs known to alter triglyceride levels.
* Screen adults who are either over 40 years of age or obese to estimate the risk for atherosclerotic cardiovascular disease.

Levels Increase with Age

* Levels are higher in men than in women (among women, those who take oral contraceptives have levels that are 20–40 mg/dL higher compared to those who do not.
* Levels are higher in overweight and obese populations compared to those with normal weight.
* Levels in African-Americans are approximately 10–20 mg/dL. lower compared to Caucasians.

Phospholipids

* Phospholipids are esters of glycerol.
* These are present in cell membranes, parts of cells, brain and nerve cells. Phospholipids are estimated calorimetrically.
* Phospholipid estimation is generally not important except in some rare diseases, such as a beta or hypobetalipoproteinemia.

Non-esterified Fatty Acids (NEFA)

* Non-esterified fatty acids are free fatty acids which circulate in plasma in bound form (bound to albumin).
* These are very small fractions of the total plasma lipids,

LIPOPROTEINS

Very Low Density Lipoproteins (VLDL)

Sources

* Liver and intestines. Major component is triglycerides.
* In the liver get converted to triglycerides
* Triglycerides are then released in blood in complex with a protein (apoprotein)
* This complex is called very low density lipoprotein or VLDL
* Normal value 2–38 mg/dL.

Intermediate Density Lipoprotein (IDL)

* These are present in minor quantity and originate from VLDL
* Its major components are triglyceride and cholesterol esters. IDL is further changed to low density lipoproteins.

Low Density Lipoproteins (LDL) (Table 6.4)

Source: It is synthesized from IDL

* LDL constitutes 50% of the blood lipoprotein.
* Its major constituent is cholesterol esters.

Function: LDL provides cholesterol to cells of different organs, such as adrenal cortex, kidneys and lymphocytes.

The cholesterol of the LDL is utilized by these cells to synthesize the following:

* Cell membrane
* Steroid hormone
* Vitamin D synthesis
* Synthesis of bile acids

TABLE 6.4: Interpretation of LDL according to level of LDL.

Level of LDL	Interpretation
<70 mg/dL	Ideal for people at very high risk of heart disease
<100 mg/dL	Ideal for people who are at risk of heart disease
130–159 mg/dL	Borderline high value
160–189 mg/dL	High value
>190 mg/dL	Very high level

Normal value: Lower than 130 mg/dL. Lower value is desirable. However, since LDL is a major risk factor for heart disease, the desired safe level can vary depending on the underlying risk of heart disease as shown below.

High Density Lipoproteins (HDL)

Source
- Synthesized in liver and intestine.
- The major lipid component of HDL is cholesterol esters and small amount is triglycerides.

Normal Value
- >40–60 mg/dL.
- Higher value is better.

Poor Level of HDL
<40 mg/dL, in men
<50 mg/dL, in women

Tests for Lipid Profile

Lipid profile is group of blood tests measured to estimate the risk of heart disease.

These tests include the estimation of levels of the following lipids:
- Total cholesterol
- Triglycerides
- LDL (called bad lipoproteins)
- VLDL
- HDL (called good lipoproteins)

Collection of blood: Blood is collected after 9–12 hours of fasting during which the person should not eat or drink anything except water.

Indications
- **High-risk individuals:** A lipid profile is indicated in persons with the following risk factors—diabetic (both adults and children):
  - High blood pressure
  - Heart disease
  - Previous history of stroke
  - High cholesterol and other lipids
  - Family history of high cholesterol
  - Family history of heart attack in male members before the age of 55 years and female members before the age of 65 years
- On medications with statin group of drugs to lower lipid
- Men should have their first screening test before the age of 35 years and women before the age of 45 years.

Significance
When the serum cholesterol level or triglyceride level is higher than their normal level, it is called hyperlipidemia.

Different conditions that are indicated by hyperlipidemia are discussed briefly:

Atherosclerosis
- In a hyperlipidemic state, the cholesterol starts getting deposited in the intima of blood vessels.
- This is called atherosclerosis
- Some of the important sites are aorta and coronary arteries.
- The depositing cholesterol raises the intima (atherosclerotic plaque formation), sometimes partially or completely obstructing the lumen of the vessel, e.g., blocking of the coronary artery causes myocardial infarction.
- The risk of such heart diseases can be monitored by investigating the lipid profile. Increased level of VLDL increases the risk of heart diseases.
- In contrast, higher the level of HDL (good lipoprotein), lower the risk of heart diseases
- The treatment of decreasing this risk of heart disease is to decrease the level of cholesterol by reducing the intake of dairy products and meat; and increasing the intake of fruits and vegetables, losing excess weight and quitting the risk factors, such as smoking, drinking alcohol, etc.
- Medication by statin group of drugs is also advisable.

Hyperlipoproteinemia

Hyperlipoproteinemia is due to abnormal elevation of triglycerides and cholesterol.

This is of two types:
1. Primary hyperlipoproteinemia → due to genetic defect in lipid metabolism.
2. Secondary hyperlipoproteinemia → due to underlying disorders, such as:
   - Nephrotic syndrome
   - Diabetes mellitus
   - Chronic renal failure
   - Alcoholism
   - Hypothyroidism
   - Obstructive liver disease

BLOOD GLUCOSE TECHNOLOGIES

Alternative Site Testing (AST)
- AST means using parts of the body other than fingertips to check blood glucose levels.
- The system allows us to test from the palm, forearm, calf, or thigh, with equivalent results to fingertip testing.
- With the Microlife GlucoTeq blood glucose monitor system the fingertips feel less pain.
- At other body sites, nerve endings are not so numerous, and one will not feel as much pain as one will experience at the fingertip.

AC/PC Setting
- AC (Ante Cibum) and PC (Post Cibum) meal markers provide more details on the test results of your blood glucose before and after meals.
- Testing the blood glucose both before and after meals, allows one to see how that meal affects the blood glucose levels and helps us to understand which meals may be best for our blood glucose control.
- During the day, levels tend to be at their lowest just before meals.
- A normal blood sugar level is less than 100 mg/dL after not eating (fasting) for at least 8 hours. And less than 140 mg/dL, 2 hours after eating.

- The most powerful influence on blood glucose levels comes from food.
- Whether you have type 1 or type 2 diabetes, the peak blood glucose levels are often likely to occur around two hours after a meal.
- The advantage of testing in so called "pairs" of before and after meals, is that you can see how much the sugar levels have gone up (or even down) between meals.

A1C Test

- The A1C test is a blood test that provides information about your average levels of blood glucose, also called blood sugar, over the past 3 months.
- The A1C test can be used to diagnose type 2 diabetes and prediabetes
- The A1C test is also the primary test used for diabetes management.
- The A1C test is sometimes called the hemoglobin A1C, HbA1c, glycated hemoglobin, or glycohemoglobin test.
- Hemoglobin is the part of a red blood cell that carries oxygen to the cells.
- Glucose attaches to or binds with hemoglobin in your blood cells, and the A1C test is based on this attachment of glucose to hemoglobin.
- The higher the glucose level in your bloodstream, the more glucose will attach to the hemoglobin.
- The A1C test measures the amount of hemoglobin with attached glucose and reflects your average blood glucose levels over the past 3 months.
- The A1C test result is reported as a percentage.
- The higher the percentage, the higher your blood glucose levels have been.
- A normal A1C level is below 5.7%.

Indications for A1C Test

Testing can help health care professionals find prediabetes and counsel clients about lifestyle changes to help you delay or prevent type 2 diabetes, find type 2 diabetes, work with clients to monitor the disease and help make treatment decisions to prevent complications

A1C Test is used to Diagnose Type 2 Diabetes and Prediabetes (Table 6.5)

- Healthcare professionals can use the A1C test alone or in combination with other diabetes tests to diagnose type 2 diabetes and prediabetes.
- Clients do not have to fast before having their blood drawn for an A1C test, which means that blood can be drawn for the test at any time of the day.
- If clients do not have symptoms but the A1C test shows that they have diabetes or prediabetes, clients should have a repeat test on a different day using the A1C test or one of the other diabetes tests to confirm the diagnosis.
- A1C results and what the numbers mean
- The A1C test should not be used to diagnose type 1 diabetes, gestational diabetes, or cystic fibrosis
- The A1C test may give false results in people with certain conditions.

TABLE 6.5: Diagnosis according to A1C level.

Diagnosis	A1C level
Normal	Below 5.7%
Prediabetes	5.7–6.4%
Diabetes	6.5% or above

- Having prediabetes is a risk factor for developing type 2 diabetes.
- Within the prediabetes A1C range of 5.7–6.4%, the higher the A1C, the greater the risk of diabetes.

Capillary Blood Glucose Monitoring and its Role in Diabetes Management

- Capillary blood glucose monitoring (CBGM) plays an important part in achieving levels of diabetes control which are associated with reduction in the risk of developing diabetes complications.
- It is vital that the results of CBGM are used to adjust treatment to achieve the recommended blood glucose targets.
- Equipment used for CBGM, whether by health professionals or people with diabetes, needs to be properly maintained so that the results are accurate and reliable.

Capillary Blood Glucose Test

- A blood drop sample is usually collected from a fingertip prick.
- Blood samples can also be sourced from alternate sites such as the earlobe, heel, forearm, palm.
- Alternate site testing provides similar results to finger-prick testing, especially in the fasting and two-hour post meal times.
- Using alternate sites may be less painful but may need a deeper lance.
- Check with the manufacturer of the glucometer if the machine may be used for alternate site testing.
- Equipment used includes a lancet used to prick the skin, a glucometer, and test strips.
- Glucometer have a range of features with modern smart machines requiring a very small sample of blood (from 0.3–1 µL), have Bluetooth capabilities that synchronize data with paired applications (apps) on smart phones.
- These machines and apps record data and provide trends in glucose measurements undertaken.
- Further, some apps also provide options to record diet and medications used, type of physical activity undertaken, which may be useful to the health care practitioner when managing the care plan for the client with diabetes.

Advantages

Small blood sample, range of alternate sites capable of testing, short testing time, large display on glucometer, less painful than venipuncture.

Disadvantages

- Manufactures often provide low cost or subsidized glucometer but sell testing strips and accessories at a significant profit margin.

- The test strips are expensive, time-limited (short expiry dates), and are affected by a range of variables including temperature, humidity, size, and quality of blood sample.
- Accuracy of the results is dependent on the clinical presentation of the client and may not be very reliable in clients with hypoglycemia, anemia, altered hematocrit, hypotension, or those who are critically ill.
- Older machines may need calibration with test strips, and results could be compromised if the calibration is not undertaken appropriately.

Venous (Plasma) Blood Sample

Venous blood is collected via venipuncture, and the sample processed in a commercial-grade laboratory with appropriate sophisticated quality control checks.

Advantages

Accurate measurement of blood glucose is superior to the capillary blood glucose test. However, this is dependent on the laboratory meeting established industry standards.

Disadvantages

Painful procedure, risk of local tissue damage, unsuitable for frequent specimen collection.

Continuous Glucose Monitoring (CGM)

- **Flash blood glucose monitoring (continuous interstitial fluid glucose monitoring):** This test involves applying a water-resistant disposable sensor on the back of the upper arm or abdomen.
- The sensor can remain on the patient for 3–14 days, depending on the product.
- The sensor can be scanned with a reader, which displays the patient's current and trends in the last 8 hours of interstitial fluid glucose levels.
- CGM machines can store 90 days of glucose data.
- Data from the CGM device could be shared with (family and care provider) via a smartphone device application, and these devices are often capable of sending alarms or messages of alerts, including hypoglycemia.
- Some CGM's can work with compatible insulin delivery devices and can stop insulin delivery if the machine predicts and or recognizes a drop in BSL.
- Some older CGM machines do require up to 2 finger-prick tests each day for purposes of calibration, however, the more recently introduced devices do not require this calibration.

Advantages

- In patients requiring insulin therapy (both type 1 diabetes and in patients with type 2 diabetes requiring intensive insulin therapy and or sulfonylureas, flash monitoring has been demonstrated to be cost-effective when compared to CBG self-monitoring of blood glucose (SMBG).
- Interstitial glucose measurements are recorded as frequently as every 5 minutes every hour, which has the benefit of monitoring for hypoglycemia during sleep at night.

Disadvantages

- Glucose is first seen in blood before it is seen in the interstitial fluid, which the CGM measures hence may not always be a reliable indicator in rapidly changing blood glucose levels.
- The high cost of sensors and machines may not make this a viable option in economically less advantaged clients and communities where health care is not subsidized by insurance or the government.

■ TESTING PROCEDURES

Capillary Blood Glucose (CBG) Testing

Preparation of Procedure

- Wash and dry hands and site (if the site is other than the hand) are to be tested.
- Skin or site preparation, if required.
- The recommended site on palm: Side of distal ends of fingertips to minimize injury to the bone.
- Avoid the little finger as the tissue may not be deep enough to prevent injury to the bone.
- Avoid the index finger and thumb as these are highly sensitive areas compared to other fingers.
- Avoid the arm if an intravenous infusion is underway or is the side of the body where a recent mastectomy, if any, was performed.
- Heel stick stab, if done, can be more painful and may require resampling.
- Consider pain management in the neonate.
- The preferred site on the heel is the lateral or medial plantar surface for babies up to one year of age.

Steps of Procedure

- Prime the lancet to no more than 2.0 mm to minimize the risk of bone injury.
- Remove the glucose testing strip without touching the sensor tip from the container. Insert glucose testing strip into the glucometer; this often leads to the glucometer turning itself on.
- Firmly apply lancet to the site of sample collection.
- Release the trigger on the lancet to pierce the skin.
- Recommendations are to wipe away the first drop of blood with clean gauze or tissue as this drop of blood may contain intracellular or interstitial fluid, or is hemolyzed, both of which could affect the blood sample.
- Gentle downward pressure applied close to the puncture site may facilitate blood flow and collection of the second drop of blood.
- Collect the second drop of blood as it forms by touching the tip of the glucose testing strip.
- Place glucometer down and cover the site of skin puncture with a clean tissue. Pressure may need to be applied to stop further bleeding from the puncture site.
- The machine normally provides a result at this stage unless there have been errors in collection; for example, insufficient sample, low battery, wrong code, or the machine times itself out. If an error displays on the glucometer, troubleshoot as appropriate.

- ❖ Wash hands and replace equipment in storage bag container.
- ❖ Make a note of test results relative to diet, exercise, and/or medication use as appropriate.

Results, Reporting, Critical Findings
- ❖ Blood glucose is measured in mmol/L (millimoles per liter) or mg/dL (milligrams per deciliter)
- ❖ **Normal range:** 4–6 mmol or about 72–108 mg/dL.

Lab-based Blood Glucose Testing
Lab-based testing is required for the appropriate diagnosis of diabetes.

Prediabetes
- ❖ Impaired fasting glucose range: 5.6–6.9 mmol per L, or 100–125 mg/dL
- ❖ Impaired (oral glucose tolerance test) glucose tolerance range at two hours post 75 g oral glucose ingestion: 7.8–11.0 mmol, or 140–199 mg/dL.

Diabetes
- ❖ Further testing may involve an oral glucose tolerance test to confirm the diagnosis.
- ❖ Advice the client to eat and drink over 150 grams per day of carbohydrate foods for three days.
- ❖ The client will need to fast overnight for at least 8–16 hours before the test.
- ❖ A fasting blood sample is collected, and a sweet drink containing 75 g of glucose is given to the client after the fasting blood sample collection.
- ❖ A further blood sample is collected at two hours following the consumption of the glucose drink.

Oral Glucose Tolerance Test
- ❖ Glucose tolerance range at two hours post 75 g oral glucose ingestion: ≥11.1 mmol, or ≥200 mg/dL.
- ❖ Random venous blood glucose of at or above 11.1 mmol/L (≥200 mg/dL), or fasting blood glucose at or above 7 mmol/L (≥126 mg/dL) on two or more separate occasions indicates the client is likely to have diabetes.

Other Tests
- ❖ **HBA1c:**
  - Glucose molecules tend to attach to hemoglobin.
  - This test interprets the percentage of glucose molecules that combine with hemoglobin to form glycated hemoglobin.
  - Once glucose molecules combine with the hemoglobin, the merger (glycated hemoglobin) remains for the life of the red blood cell, which is, on average, around 60–120 days.
  - Analyses of the red blood cell and its attached glycated hemoglobin reveals the average blood glucose levels in the client over those 2–4 months.
  - **Normal HBA1c:** 3.5–6% (15–42 mmol/mol).
  - A result of glycosylated hemoglobin (HbA1c) >6.5% confirms the presence of diabetes.
  - Pharmacological intervention is required in clients with HBA1c levels greater than 7.0%.
  - This test is currently recommended to be undertaken to diagnose and provide appropriate ongoing management of the diabetic client.

Note: There is a small but significant difference between capillary blood glucose measurements undertaken at home and the venous or arterial blood sampling done in clinical facilities.

Care must be taken when using the results from capillary tests and venous tests either exclusively or together.

Clinical Significance
- ❖ Blood glucose monitoring is an essential part of case management in clients with diabetes.
- ❖ Having very high or very low levels of blood glucose could impair cellular function and may be lethal if not managed appropriately.
- ❖ Stress-related hyperglycemia may also be seen in clients who have experienced an acute medical and or surgical event.

Hyperglycemia
Etiology of hyperglycemia includes:
- ❖ Inadequate insulin administration in clients with type 1 diabetes, insulin resistance with type 2 diabetes which inhibits glucose metabolism
- ❖ Stress-related experiences (such as critical illness) inducing glycogenolysis and gluconeogenesis)
- ❖ Client experiences of the dawn phenomena where there is a surge in hormones between 0400 and 0500 that cause a spike in blood glucose levels.
- ❖ Symptoms of hyperglycemia include polyuria (increased and frequent urination), polydipsia (increased thirst), blurred vision, headache and fatigue, and glucosuria. Acute symptoms of hyperglycemia are not usually seen at levels below 14 mmol/L or 250 mg/dL.
- ❖ Episodes of hyperglycemia for an extended period leads to either diabetic ketoacidosis or hyperglycemic hyperosmolar state.
- ❖ If left untreated hyperglycemia may cause the client to go into a state of ketoacidosis where the body begins to process fats (gluconeogenesis) to produce the energy required for cellular function.
- ❖ This could be as a result of a lack of insulin produced by the pancreas (as seen in type 1 diabetes).
- ❖ **Diabetic ketoacidosis** is a life-threatening scenario where a client could potentially go into a state of coma from a lack of insulin production and clients may have symptoms of fruity odor (from the ketones being produced in the body as a result of fat metabolism), ketonuria, tachypnea and or shortness of breath, nausea, and vomiting.
- ❖ In the hyperosmolar state, a rare condition is seen in clients with type 2 diabetes, the body in its attempt to get rid of the high glucose levels in the blood produces large amounts of urine causing life-threatening dehydration and potentially coma.

- Both diabetic ketoacidosis and hyperosmolar state require emergent management to reduce elevated blood glucose levels with insulin therapy.
- Long-term high blood glucose levels could potentially delay wound healing, damage nerves (peripheral neuropathy) and end-organs, such as the eyes (diabetic retinopathy), kidneys (renal failure), the brain (stroke), and the heart (myocardial infarction).

Hypoglycemia

- Symptoms of hypoglycemia are seen when low blood glucose levels deprive the body of essential fuel to sustain life.
- Causes of hypoglycemia include taking too much insulin, and or not enough carbohydrates or inappropriate exercise in relation to diet and or insulin intake.
- Clients present with symptoms of confusion, sweating, tachycardia, blurred vision, feeling lightheaded, being clumsy, or may have seizures.
- Often clients do not recognize the onset of symptoms of hypoglycemia which may put them at high risk of injury either while undertaking regular activity (such as driving) or while asleep.
- Emergent treatment to restore normal blood glucose levels is imperative as certain organs (e.g., brain) do not store glucose and need a constant supply of blood glucose to sustain life.
- Antidiabetic therapy needs re-evaluation when BSL falls below 5.6 mmol/liter (100 mg/dL) and modification of antidiabetic therapy is essential if BSL drops below 3.9 mmol/liter (70 mg/dL).
- Clients across the life span with diabetes have varying clinical presentations (and underlying clinical pathologies linked to diabetes).
- They may not always report the effects of hypoglycemia or hyperglycemia which should involve monitoring for other signs and symptoms.
- Clients with renal insufficiency are at risk of hypoglycemia as the kidneys are primarily responsible for metabolizing exogenous insulin.

Glycemic Care in the Clinical Setting

- For appropriate glycemic control in clients with diabetes in non-critical care settings, capillary blood glucose testing is the recommended method of testing.
- In clients who are capable of eating, blood glucose testing is recommended before meals and at bedtime, and every 4–6 hours in clients receiving enteral feeds and or are nil by oris (NPO).
- All hospitalized patients will benefit from an initial screen for blood glucose irrespective of a history of diabetes.
- The use of glucose management protocols, with nurse-initiated treatment protocols, is ideal for the management of hypoglycemia in the hospital setting.

STOOL EXAMINATION

Introduction

- Stool is the digestive waste product excreted from the bowel.
- Its excretion is very important to maintain normal health.
- Digestion and absorption of the essential components of food occurs in the stomach and intestines.
- The undigested food and secretions from the stomach, liver, pancreas and intestines, which are not absorbed, appear in the stool. Stool examination is performed to evaluate various gastrointestinal (GI) diseases.
- These help in detection of GI bleeding, obstruction, obstructive jaundice, parasitic diseases, inflammatory bowel diseases, dysentery and increased fat excretion.
- The frequency of defecation in an average healthy adult ranges from 3 times a day to once in 3 days.
- An adult excretes 100–200 g (wet weight, or <66 g dry weight) of fecal matter daily, comprising about 75% water.
- Everyday 8–10 L of digested fluid-like material enters the gastrointestinal tract (GIT) comprising of foods, fluids as well as saliva, gastric and intestinal juices, pancreatic juice and bile. Out of this, only a small amount is excreted as stool.

Composition of Feces

The general composition of feces is as follows:
- Waste residue of indigestible material, for example, cellulose from food eaten during the previous 4 days
- Bile salts and pigments—bile pigments are altered by bacterial action providing color to the normal stool
- Intestinal secretions
- Water and electrolytes
- Shed epithelial cells
- Numerous bacteria
- Inorganic substances (10–20%) mainly calcium and phosphates. Undigested and unabsorbed food (comprising very small quantity)
- The amount of feces excreted depends on the balance between absorption, secretion and fermentation in the intestine by bacteria.

Stool Analysis

- The most frequently performed tests in stool examination are the tests for occult blood, fat, parasites, leucocytes and pathogens.
- Stool examination also helps in screening for colon cancer and asymptomatic ulceration and GI masses.
- Fat excretion is very important in the diagnosis of malabsorption syndromes.
- Stool testing for parasites is very essential in immune compromised patients

Problems in stool analysis are as follows:
- Feces cannot be collected on demand
- Patients usually do not like collecting and providing the specimen to the lab for examination

- The nursing and lab staff are averse to stool handling owing to its foul odor.
- However, the preceding problems should be overcome keeping in mind the importance of stool test in various GI disorders.

Collection and Transport of Stool Specimens

- Universal precautions must be followed while procuring and handling stool specimens to void infectious agents.
- Feces should be collected in a dry, clean and urine-free container with lid.
- Specimen should not be contaminated with urine, other body secretions or menstrual blood, possible, the patient should be instructed to urinate first and then collect the specimen.
- Stool can be collected from the diaper in case of infants and patients with incontinence and from colostomy bags.
- Specimen should be delivered to the lab as soon as possible.
- A morning specimen of stool, prior to breakfast is preferred and should be processed by the lab within 2–3 hours (warm stool)
- The specimen must be labeled properly bearing the name of patient, sex, age, hospital registration number, and ward number and so on. It should be accompanied by a requisition form bearing the corresponding patient's details along with provisional diagnosis and any specific test to be performed on stool

Collection and Transport of specimens for Ova and Parasites

Remember the following points:
- Warm stools are the best for detection of ova and parasites.
- Sample should never be refrigerated if testing for ova or parasites is desired
- Special vials containing 10% formalin and polyvinyl alcohol (PVA) fixative may be used for sample collection
- Random stool specimens should be analyzed owing to the cyclic life cycles of parasites

Collection and Transport of Specimens for Enteric Pathogens

Remember the following points:
- Some coli form bacilli produce antibiotic substances, which destroy enteric pathogens.
- To prevent this the specimen should be refrigerated
- A diarrheal stool usually gives good results Specimen of choice is a freshly passed stool
- Stool examination should be performed before antibiotic therapy is started
- If mucus or blood is present, it should be collected as it is more likely to have pathogens
- For best preservation and transport of pathogens, a Cary Blair solution may be used.

Considerations

Consider the following facts for stool test:
- The patient should not be receiving iron or other metallic components for 4–6 days before specimen collection
- Stool specimen from patient on tetracycline or antidiarrheal medication may not give accurate results
- The patient must be instructed not to collect the specimen in waxed paper/toilet paper as it may contain bismuth which interferes with accurate results
- Specimen from toilet bowl/bed pan should be avoided as it may be contaminated with urine, water and so on
- If the sample is not is not collected properly inaccurate results may be obtained
- Personal habits, lifestyle, travel and bathroom facility are certain factors, which may interfere with proper sample procurement
- Specimen should be transported and examined promptly as some parasites may disintegrate rapidly

Pretest Patient Care

- Explain the collection procedure and various factors interfering with the accurate results to the patient in his/her language
- Patient should be provided proper containers
- He should be instructed not to urinate in the container
- Toilet paper should not be put in the container
- If the patient has diarrhea, the sample should be collected in a large plastic bag
- Tests for ova and parasites and cultures for enteric pathogens may be ordered together.
- In such cases, the sample may be divided into two with one portion refrigerated for culture testing and one portion kept at room temperature for ova and parasites

PHYSICAL EXAMINATION

It includes inspection of feces to assess the following characteristics:
- Amount
- Frequency of defecation
- **Consistency:** Formed/semisolid/liquid/general

Color

- The large amounts of frothy and foul smelling stool are the characteristics of steatorrhea.
- Constipation is characterized by firm, spherical masses of stool. The consistency of the stool may be formed, soft, frothy or watery.
- The odor of the feces varies with the diet and the pH of the stool.
- The odor of the stool is caused by indole and skatole, which are formed by bacteria fermentation.
- Certain parasites, such as pinworms and tapeworm segments may be observed on macroscopic examination.

Normal Values

- 100–200 g/24 hours
- Characteristic odor
- Plastic, soft and formed-soft and bulky on a high fiber diet, small and dry on a high protein diet

Clinical Importance

Stool test is important as it can be used to diagnose various intestinal infections.

The features of stool and related diseases have been listed as follows:

Alterations in Fecal Consistency

Diarrhea can be caused by the following disorders:
- Infection by *Salmonella, Shigella, Yersinia*, HIV enteropathy and *Campylobacter*.
- Inflammatory bowel disease (Crohn's disease and ulcerative colitis)
- Steatorrhea—sprue, celiac disease
- Malabsorption of carbohydrates—lactase/sucrose deficiency
- Endocrine disorder, such as diabetes mellitus, hyperthyroidism, adrenal insufficiency
- Hormone producing tumors—gastrinoma, villous adenoma and so on
- Cancer of colon
- Drugs, antibiotics and chemotherapy
- Osmotically active substance, such as sorbitol, caffeine, ethanol
- GI-surgery—gastrectomy, intestinal resection
- Self-induced laxative abuse

Pasty stool with high fat content may be seen in the following disorder:
- Common bile duct obstruction
- Celiac disease
- Cystic fibrosis
- Bulky/frothy stool owing to steatorrhea and celiac disease

Alterations in Stool Size or Shape

- These indicate alterations in mobility or abnormalities of colonic wall
- Narrow, ribbon like stool indicates rectal narrowing or stricture, spastic bowel or partial obstruction
- Excessively hard stools can be seen in constipation owing to increased fluid absorption caused by increased transit time in intestine
- Stool with large circumference comply dilation of the intestine
- Small, round hard stools are seen in patients with chronic constipation

Fecal Odor Alterations

- A foul odor may be caused by undigested protein and excessive carbohydrate ingestion.
- Excessively sweet odor can be caused by volatile fatty acids and undigested lactose.

Mucus in Stools

Normally, a small amount of mucus is present in the stool. It is increased in constipation, malignancy and colitis.

Assessment of Diarrhea and Constipation

Factors to be noted are as follows:
- Volume and frequency of stool
- Consistency of stool
- Presence of blood, pus, mucus, oiliness and bad odor
- Painful defecation
- Assess dietary habits and food allergies
- Stool color
- Normal feces is brown in color owing to stercobilin (urobilin) derived from bile pigments.

A change in color can provide information about certain pathologic conditions or drug intake as follows:
- Severe diarrhea—yellow/yellow green
- Bleeding in upper GIT-black, tarry stool
- Bleeding in lower GIT from hemorrhoids, tumor, fissures—maroon, red
- Bile obstruction—clay colored
- Pancreatic deficiency causing fat mal-absorption—pale greasy

Factors interfering with color of stool are as follows:
- Stools darken on standing
- Color of feces is influenced by certain foods, drugs and so on
- Breast fed infants may have a yellow green color of feces due to lack of normal intestinal flora
- Barium chloride can produce pale yellow, white stools
- Diet containing excess of green leafy vegetables can produce green colored stools
- Foods, such as cherries, high proportion of meat, drugs, such as iron, charcoal can lead to black colored stools
- Diet high in beetroot and tomatoes can lead to red colored stool

Stool Test for Occult Blood

- In the early stages of GI disease, small amount of blood is excreted in feces; therefore no visible signs of bleeding may be present.
- Thus in early course of diabetes, the chemical detection of occult blood is necessary for identification and treatment of such diseases.
- However this is compounded by many false-positive and false-negative results.

Principle

This test is based on peroxidase like activity of hemoglobin, which reacts with hydrogen peroxide to oxidize colorless compound to colored one (blue).

Method

- Obtain random stool sample
- Apply thin smear of stool using wooden application to the indicated area and allow it to dry
- Do not refrigerate the sample The test should be repeated 3–5 times at intervals as some lesions may produce intermittent bleeding.

Clinical Considerations

Stool that appears dark red to very black indicates blood loss of 50–75 mL.

The causes may be:
- Cancer of colon, rectum
- Inflammatory bowel disease
- Cancer of stomach
- Peptic ulcer
- Gastritis

Factors Interfering in Tests

- Certain drugs, such as non-steroidal anti-inflammatory drugs (NSAIDS) are associated with an increased GI blood loss
- False-positive results may be obtained with boric acid, betadine and so on
- Certain foods may give false-positive test such as meat including processed meat and liver (contains hemoglobin), vegetables and fruits with peroxidase like activity (e.g., turnips, mushrooms, broccoli, apples, bananas)
- False-negative results may be caused by excess intake of ascorbic acid (vitamin C)
- Hematuria and menstrual blood may produce erroneous interpretations
- **Mucus in stool:** Mucus is normally secreted in the colon. However recognizable mucus in stool specimen w considered abnormal and should be reported.

Clinical Importance

- Gelatinous mucus adhering to the surface of formed stool may occur spastic constipation, emotionally disturbed patients and excess straining at stools
- Bloody mucus clinging to the stool suggests neoplasm and inflammation of rectal canal. Copious amounts of mucus may be passed in villous adenoma
- Mucus and diarrhea with presence of leukocytes and RBC may be seen in ulcerative colitis, bacillary dysentery and amoebiasis

Test for Stercobilin (Schlesinger Test)

- Take small amount of feces in a test tube
- Add 5 mL of 5% HCl in alcohol to emulsify
- Neutralize the acid with sodium hydroxide or ammonium hydroxide
- Add equal amount of 10% zinc acetate in alcohol
- Filter the mixture and observe the filtrate.
- If stercobilin is present, a green florescence can be seen.

Test for Reducing Substances (Lactose) Benedict's Test

- Take 5 mL of Benedict's solution and add 8 drops of stool specimen
- Boil for 5 minutes
- Change in color from green to brick red is indication of presence of reducing substance in stool
- This is only a qualitative test and not a semi quantitative test

Microscopic Examination of Stool

- A simple microscopic examination of stool can give important information regarding many diseases.
- Normally stool contains lot of undigested food particles, bacteria and many epithelial cells.
- **Epithelial cells:** Few desquamated epithelial cells can be seen.
- **Pus cells:** occasional puss cell may be seen in normal stool.
- **Red blood cell:** Sometimes RBC can be seen and if the test for occult blood is negative
- **Macrophages:** These are generally seen when there is some kind of bacterial infection Undigested food material: is normally seen.
- **Crystals:** Charcot Leyden crystals can be seen in amoebic colitis. In order to visualize cells and microorganisms/parasites and their ova different preparation are required to be made this can be unstained and stained.
- Various techniques are used to detect various types of protozoas, cyst and helminthic eggs. However a single technique does not yield satisfactory results, therefore a combination of two or more techniques is used for optimum results.

Direct Wet Film

- Direct wet film is the most useful techniques to detect trophozoites of amoeba and flagellates.
- Motility is the characteristic features of the forms, which can be appreciated in the wet film.
- Wet films are also valuable for immediate examination of the bloody mucus recovering during the colonoscopy
- A small portion of feces is mixed with a drop of normal saline and placed on a clean slide.
- A cover-slip is placed on a sample and examine without staining. In case of a watery stool, dilution with saline is not required.
- The film should not be very thick as it will make visualization of various structures difficult.
- The film just should be very thin enough so that newsprint can be read through it.
- The film should be screened thoroughly for trophozoites of amoeba and flagellates under low power and low illumination.
- An iodine stain can also be prepared for a wet film test.
- Iodine stains the cysts of amoebae and other protozoa revealing some details that are not seen in unstained films.
- However, trophozoites remain unstained in iodine film.
- Therefore, it is necessary to examine an unstained film first.
- Lugol's solution or gram iodine gives the satisfactory results.
- An iodine stained smear may be prepared by adding a small drop of iodine solution to the wet film. A concentrated stool sample may also be stained with iodine and will reveal large number of any organisms which may be mixed on direct wet film.

Concentration Techniques

The aim of the concentration techniques is to separate the protozoa cyst and helminthic eggs from the fecal matter by examine the difference in specific gravity.

This technique involves the following two types of method:
1. **Sedimentation:** It involves the sedimentation of the eggs and cysts, which are heavier than the suspending liquid at the bottom of the tube. The disadvantage of this method is that in addition to the eggs cysts of parasites excess fecal debris also sediment making the examination and detection of parasite is difficult.
2. **Floatation:** It involves use of heavy liquids to make the lighter parasites to float on the surface. The basic problem of floatation techniques is that all the eggs and cysts do not float in this technique.

The concentrated specimen may be examined directly for protozoan cysts (as trophozoites are not identified after concentrations) and helminth eggs. Addition of iodine stained may yield more information.

Sedimentation Techniques

The two sedimentation techniques for stool test are as follows:
* Formalin ether (formalin ethyl acetate) techniques
* Simple gravity sedimentation techniques

Formal-ether Sedimentation Techniques

* Put around half tea spoonful of feces in 10 mL of water in a container and mix well
* In a funnel put two layers of gauze and filter the content in to a 15 mL centrifuge tube
* Centrifuge at 500 rpm for two minutes
* Discard the supernatant and re-suspend the sediment in 10 mL of normal saline
* Again centrifuge at 500 rpm and discard the supernatant
* Re-suspend the sediment in 7 mL of 10% formaldehyde (40% formalin and saline in ratio of 1:3). Add 3 mL ether
* Close the tube and vigorously mix the contents. Removing the cover, again centrifuge at 500 rpm for 2 min.
* Place the tube in a stand.
* The following 4 layers become visible:
  1. The top layer of ether
  2. The second layer comprising a plug of debris
  3. The third layer of a clear layer of formalin
  4. The fourth layer of sediment
* Dislodge the debris plug from the side of tube with a glass rod and decant the liquid. leaving a small amount of formalin to suspend the sediment
* Remove the sediment using a pipette and put a drop of iodine.
* Examine the slide under microscope

Simple Gravity Sedimentation Technique

* An adequate quantity of stool specimen is mixed thoroughly with 15–20 mL of tap water and allowed to settle in a conical flask for 1–2 hours.
* This process is repeated several times till the supernatant becomes clear.
* Then the sediment is examined microscopically. If 0.5% solution of glycerin is made in tap water, it increases the sedimentation rate of parasites.

Floatation Techniques

Zinc Sulfate Floatation Technique

* Mix 1–1.5 g of stool sample in 2–3 mL of water. Pour the mixture into conical centrifuge tube (15 mL) and add distilled water to bring the level of fluid to within several millimeters of brim of tube.
* Centrifuge at 500 rpm for 2 min and discard the supernatant
* Add 1–2 mL Zinc sulfate solution to sediment and re-suspend the sediment by mixing the sediment well. Bring the level of fluid to few millimeters of rim by adding Zinc sulfate.
* Filter the suspension through 2 layers of wet gauze and return the filtrate to the tube. Add more Zinc sulfate.
* Centrifuge at 500 rpm for 2 min
* Without moving the centrifuge tubes lift 1–2 drops from the surface using freshly flamed wire loop and place them on a slide
* Examine without cover-slip.
* Then add a drop of iodine, put cover-slip and examine microscopically

Saturated Salt Floatation Technique

* Put 1 mL of stool in a 15–20 mL flat bottom container
* Add few drops of saturated salt solution (with specific gravity 1200) and mix properly
* Add more salt solution, stirring it thoroughly
* Remove any floating coarse matter
* Place the container on a level surface.
* Do the final filling using a dropper till a convex measure is obtained
* A glass slide is now placed on the container, just touching the fluid
* This is allowed to stand for 30 min. then glass slide is removed, turned quickly to avoid spilling and examined after putting a cover-slip.

Permanent Stained Slides

* In some cases, it is not possible to correctly identify certain protozoans.
* The permanent staining methods become essential for accurate identification as they reveal better cytological details.
* A small quantity of feces is transferred to a clean slide using an applicator slide.
* The material is spread out in a thin uniform film.
* Formed stools have a proper consistency for making films but if the specimen is hard, it should be mixed with saline to prepare a smear.
* To prepare film from liquid stools, a slide coated with serum/egg albumin should be used as liquid stool does not adhere to the slides.
* The film should be placed in a fixative immediately after it is prepared.
* Substances that interfere with stool examination for parasite are castor oil; mineral oil should not be administered prior to sample collection.
* Antibiotics that alter the intestinal flora during the previous month decrease the chances of finding intestinal protozoa as well as antimalarials-like chloroquine.
* Barium studies should not be done at 1 week before testing.
* Compounds containing muth, antacids also interfere with examination for parasites stains for direct smear
* **Lugol's solution:** DW 100 mL, potassium iodide—10 g, iodine crystals: 5 g
* **Gram's iodine:** Lugol's solution—1 part, DW 14 parts
* **Preservative solutions:** When delay in expected in transporting feces to the lab, these should be preserved in fixative

- The PVA fixative consists of mixture of polyvinyl alcohol, glycerin, glacial acetic acid and Schaudinn's solution. It is a very good fixative for preservation of morphology of intestinal protozoa, especially trophozoite stage. It can be used to fix small quantity of feces on a slide or a vial can be used for larger quantities. The solution preserves both trophozoite and cysts of protozoa, most eggs can be identified after PVA preservation.
- However, it is better to use a second vial containing 10% formalin for concentration of eggs from another aliquot of feces
- Merthiolate Iodine formalin (MIF) preservative is used with the preservative. Its composition is—DW: 250 mL, tincture of merthiolate: 200 mL, formaldehyde: 25 mL, glycerin: 5 mL.
- It is responsible for staining as well as fixation of protozoa. It is very useful in situations where immediate stool examination is not feasible and delay is anticipated.
- It is prepared from stock merthiolate formaldehyde (MF) and stock iodine solution. Before use 2.35 mL of stock MF is mixed with 0.15 mL of Lugol's iodine. Small sample stool is added to this solution and mixed well. Samples can be kept for several months in this solution. MIF preserved sample can be concentrated by MIF ether technique.

Special Methods for Recovering Parasites

- **Scotch tape method:** This is meant for detection of eggs or female worms of thread worm and occasionally eggs of *Taenia solium, Taenia saginata* and *Schistosoma mansoni*. A piece of scotch tape is looped over a tongue depressor adhesive surface being exposed. This then pressed against the perianal skin at different places. The tape is now removed from the stick and attached to slide with adhesive surface touching glass slide and examine microscopically. The specimen is best collected at night or early morning as the female thread worm crawls out of anus at night to lay eggs.
- **Entero test:** This is used for obtaining duodenal contents without incubation. It comprises a weighted gelatin capsule that contains a corded nylon line. One end of nylon line is fixed of the patient's face and then the capsule is swallowed with water. After 3–4 hours, the nylon thread is retracted and duodenal contents adherent to the distal end of line are squeezed onto a glass slide and examined. It is used for detecting trophozoites of Giardia lamblia, larvae of strongyloides and eggs of liver flukes.

Stained Smears

- **Iron hematoxylin:** It provides excellent contrast between nucleus and cytoplasm.
- **Trichrome staining:** It colors cytoplasm blue green and nucleus red.
  However, the chromatin dots not as well appreciated as with iron hematoxylin staining.
  However, trichrome staining has replaced iron hematoxylin in most labs as the details obtained is sufficient for diagnosis and the stain is easier to use.

It is not suitable for identifying the eggs and larvae of helminthes as they are dislocated and stained dark.

The method involves:
- Place the fresh fecal smears in Schaudinn solution for 1 hour.
- But over night fixation is preferred
- Immerse the smears in iodine alcohol working solution for 1 min
- Wash the smear in 2 changes of 70% ethyl alcohol, I min each
- Place the smear in trichrome stain for 8–10 min
- Use 1% acetic acid in 90% alcohol to acidify the smears for 10 sections
- Rinse the smears in 2 changes of 95% alcohol
- Remove alcohol with 2 changes of xylene, 2–5 min each
- Mount and examine under oil immersion Modified acid fast staining is used for cryptosporidium, cyclospora and isospora. This is especially important in suspected HIV infected patients.

Stool cultures: Culture methods should never be used as a substitute for routine and thorough microscopic examination by various methods.

Culture of *Entamoeba histolytica*: A wide variety of media may be used.

Some of these methods are as follows:
- **Jones medium:** It is monophasic medium which contain horse serum, yeast autolysate in phosphate buffered saline
- **Modified Boeck and Dr Habolov's medium:** It is a biphasic medium and supports the growth of *E. histolytica* and other intestinal amoebae.
- **Diamond's medium:** It consists of a basal medium and rice supplement

URINE TEST FOR ALBUMIN

- The test for protein is far more sensitive to albumin than to globulin.
- Albumin is important in determining the presence of glomerular damage.
- Albuminuria occurs when the glomerular membrane is damaged, a condition called glomerulonephritis.

Articles Required

- Test tube with test tube stand-1
- Test tube holder
- Dropper
- Acetic acid
- Spirit lamp
- Match box
- Kidney tray
- Urine specimen container

Procedure

- Explain the procedure to the patient
- Collect a urine specimen from the patient
- Take a test tube and fix it in the holder.
- Fill 2/3 of the test tube with urine.

- Heat the upper third of the test tube over the spirit lamp by keeping the mouth of test tube away from yourself.
- If there is cloudy appearance it denotes the presence of either albumin or phosphate.
- Add 2–3 drops of acetic acid with the help of dropper.
- If cloudiness disappears, it is due to the presence of phosphates.
- **If cloudiness does not disappear, then note its strength:**
  - Mild cloudiness—1+ albumin
  - Moderate cloudiness—2+ albumin
  - Thick cloudiness—3+ albumin
- Record the result in the urine chart.
- Discard urine specimen.
- Clean and replace all articles.
- Wash your hands.

TEST FOR SUGAR IN URINE

Intraprocedural Steps

- Explain to the patient about the test to be done and method of collecting specimen of urine.
- Provide container for collecting urine.
- Wear gloves and collect urine specimen from patient.
- Take test tube and fix in holder. Pour 5 mL of Benedict's solution into test tube.
- Light spirit lamp and heat Benedict's solution for 2 minutes.
- Add eight drops of urine using dropper, through the sides and allow it to boil for another few seconds and let it cool after flame is put off
- Watch for color change and compare with standard color code.
- Blue-nil (No sugar)
- Green liquid without deposit (+/1% sugar)
- Green liquid with yellow deposit (++/2% sugar),
- Colorless liquid with orange deposit (+++/3% sugar),
- Brick red (++++/5% sugar or above).

Post-procedural Steps

- Discard the urine and rinse the test tube.
- Replace articles.
- Discard gloves and wash hands.

URINE TEST FOR ACETONE

- At alkaline pH, sodium nitroprusside or ferricyanide forms a violet-colored complex with acetoacetic acid and acetone.
- These ketones are produced in excess in disorders of carbohydrate metabolism, especially in Type 1 diabetes mellitus
- These ketoacids and their salts spill into the urine causing ketonuria.
- Ketones are also found in the urine in several other conditions including fever, pregnancy, glycogen storage diseases and in persons on a carbohydrate restricted diet.

Articles

- 1 test tube in test tube stand
- Test tube holder
- Dropper
- Ammonium sulfate crystal
- Sodium nitroprusside
- Concentrated ammonia
- Match box
- Kidney tray
- Urine specimen container

Procedure

- Explain the procedure to the patient.
- Collect urine specimen from the patient.
- Take a test tube and fix it in the holder.
- Place 2–3 crystals of ammonium sulfate in the tube.
- Add 10–15 drops of urine in it.
- Put one crystal of sodium nitroprusside in it.
- Shake well.
- Add 5–6 drops of concentrated ammonia.
- Let it stand for 10 minutes.
- If acetone is present, the content will be permanganate color.
- Record the result in the urine chart.
- Discard urine specimen.
- Clean and replace all articles.
- Wash your hands.

URINE pH

- The pH of urine depends on the concentrating ability of kidneys to maintain hydrogen ion (H) concentration.
- Normal adult excretes about 50–100 mg hydrogen ions in 24 hours.
- The normal urine pH varies from 4.6–8.

Methods

1. **Reagent strip:**
   - Strips are available which have indicators, such as methyl red and bromothymol blue.
   - These reagents change color to various shades of orange, green and blue according to pH.
   - Thus, it is useful to estimate the varying range of pH.
2. **pH meter:** pH measured using pH meter containing glass electrode is more accurate than reagent strip method.

Causes of Alkaline Urine

- Diet rich in citrus fruits and certain vegetables
- Urine becomes less acidic following a meal.
- Infections
- Severe vomiting
- Renal tubular acidosis
- Glomerular filtration is normal but formation of ammonia and exchange of hydrogen ion and cations in the distal tubules are defective.
- As a result urine pH is between 6 and 6.5.
- Metabolic alkalosis. Alkaline urine is produced which has a higher amount of bicarbonate and lesser amount of ammonia.
- Respiratory alkalosis. Alkaline urine is produced because of increased excretion of bicarbonate.

Causes of Acidic Urine
- Diet high in proteins
- Ammonium chloride, methionine and methenamine are used to make urine acidic for the treatment of stones which dissolves in acidic urine.
- Respiratory acidosis or metabolic acidosis
- Diabetic ketoacidosis
- Fever
- Vomiting

SPECIFIC GRAVITY
- The specific gravity of normal urine depends on solutes, such as urea, sodium chloride, sulfate and phosphates.
- It varies with intake of water and solute, the state of tubular epithelium and effect of antidiuretic hormones on distal tubules.
- Normal specific gravity varies from 1.016–1.022

Methods of Measuring Specific Gravity Urinometer
- Urinometer is a hydrometer which directly measures the specific gravity at room temperature.
- Urinometer cylinder is filled three-fourths with urine (minimum volume required is 15 mL).
- The urinometer is then floated in it in a slow spinning motion to make sure that it is floating freely.
- The level to which the urinometer sinks depends on the specific gravity of urine (Archimedes' principle-law of buoyancy).
- This level on the urinometer is the specific gravity.

Precautions
- The urinometer should not touch the sides of the cylinder or the vessel.
- Bubbles should be avoided. It obscures the exact reading.

Disadvantages
- At least 15 mL urine is required.
- Urinometer is used at room temperature.
- Correction must be made for rise and fall in temperature.
- Proteinuria increases specific gravity.
- Glycosuria increases specific gravity.
- The accuracy of the urinometer is checked by distilled water or solutions of known specific gravity.
- With distilled water the urinometer should give a reading of 1.000.

Refractometer
- Specific gravity of a solution also depends on the amount of dissolved substance, i.e., refractiveness of the solution
- This is measured by refractometer.
- Advantage is that only a few drops of urine is required.

Reagent Strips
Reagent strips have a polyelectrolyte indicator and a buffer which measures the specific gravity.

Causes of Low Specific Gravity Urine
- Low specific gravity urine is also known as hypsthenuric urine.
- Specific gravity is less than 1.007.
- Diabetes insipidus
- Pyelonephritis
- Glomerulonephritis

Causes of High Specific Gravity Urine
- Diabetes mellitus
- Loss of water/Dehydration
- Adrenal insufficiency
- Hepatic diseases
- Congestive heart failure

Causes of Isosthenuric Specific Gravity
- The specific gravity is fixed at 1.010.
- This is because of loss of concentrating and diluting abilities of kidneys, e.g., late stages of chronic renal failure.

URINE CULTURE
- A culture is a test done in a laboratory to see whether urine has presence of microorganisms.
- A sample of mid-stream urine is put into a container.
- Then small plates with a growth medium that the germs can grow on are put into the sample and the container is closed tightly.
- The urine culture is then placed in an incubator for one to two days.
- If there are bacteria or fungi in the urine, visible colonies can grow.

Purposes of Urine Culture
- Urine cultures are usually done to detect bacteria and fungi in urine when testing for a urinary tract infection.
- This laboratory testing helps to identify antibiotic sensitivity.
- The type of antibiotic needed is usually determined at the same time.

Steps of Procedure
This method helps protect the urine sample from micro-organisms that are normally found on the peas or vagina.

The steps of the procedure are:
- Wash your hands before you collect the urine
- If the collection cup has a lid, remove it carefully
- Set the lid down with the inner surface up.
- Do not touch the inside of the cup with your fingers
- **Clean the area around your genitals:**
  - A man should retract his foreskin, if he has one, and clean the head of his penis with medicated towelettes or swabs
  - A woman should spread open the genital folds of skin with one hand. Then she can use her other hand to clean the area around the urethra with medicated towelettes or swabs. She should wipe the area from front to back so bacteria from the anus is not wiped across the urethra.

- Start to urinate into the toilet or urinal.
- A woman should hold apart the genital folds of skin while she urinates.
- After the urine has flowed for several seconds, place the collection cup into the urine stream.
- Collect urine in sample container without stopping the flow of urine.
- Move the cup out the urine stream. Do not touch the rim of the cup to your genital area
- Finish urinating into the toilet or urinal.
- Carefully replace and tighten the lid on the cup.

Result Findings

Normal: No bacteria or other germs (such as fungus) grow in the culture. The culture result is negative

Abnormal: Organisms (usually bacteria) grow in the culture The culture result is positive

COLLECTION OF URINE SPECIMEN

Midstream Urine Specimen

Midstream (clean catch) urine collection is the most common method of obtaining urine specimens from adults, particularly men. This method allows a specimen, which is not contaminated from external sources to be obtained without catheterization.

The specimen must be:
- Appropriate to the patient's clinical presentation.
- Collected at the right time.
- Collected in a way that minimizes contamination.
- Stored/transported appropriately.

Procedure

- Instruct the patient to clean the urethral area thoroughly.
- This will prevent external bacteria from entering the specimen.
- The female should wipe from front to back to avoid contaminating the vaginal and urethral area from the anal area.
- She should clean each side with a separate cotton ball, then use the last one for the urethral area itself.
- The male should cleanse the penis, using the first cotton ball for the urethral meatus, the next cotton ball to clean the end of the penis and the last to cleanse the urethral opening.
- Instruct the patient to void a small amount of urine into the toilet to rinse out the urethra, void the midstream urine into the specimen cup and the last of the stream into the toilet.
- The midstream urine is considered to be bladder and kidney washings, the portion that the physician wants tested.
- Complete the laboratory request form, label the specimen container with patient identifying information and send to the lab immediately.
- A delay in examining the specimen may cause a false result when bacterial determinations are to be made.
- Wash your hands and instruct the patient to do likewise
- Record that the specimen was collected.
- Note any difficulty the patient had or if the urine had an abnormal appearance.

24 Hours Urine Specimen

Definition

Collection of 24 hours urine without any wastage it begins with an empty bladder.

Purposes

- To detect any kidney or liver conditions.
- To detect and measure the total amount of waste the kidneys are eliminating, e.g., total protein, creatinine, electrolytes, etc.

Articles Required

- Clean container with cap (capacity of 3 liters).
- Bedpan or urinal.
- Recording sheet.
- Gloves.

Procedure

- Check the physician's order
- Explain the procedure to the patient.
- Instruct the patient to empty bladder before the time set to begin the procedure.
- Measure and pour specimen of urine in the container Collect the final specimen at the same time the patient voided 24 hours earlier, e.g., if started at 7:00 AM, it will be collected till 7:00 AM of following day
- Send the container to laboratory with label and reporting sheet
- Record the procedure in detail.

Collecting a Urine Specimen from Catheter

Equipment Required

- Container with label as required
- Disposable gloves (1)
- Spirit swabs or disinfectant swabs
- 10–20 mL syringe with 21–25 gauge needle.
- Clamp (1)
- Pen and laboratory form

Procedure

- Assemble equipment.
- Label the container.
- Explain the procedure to the patient and provide privacy.
- Perform hand hygiene and put on gloves, if available.
- **Clamp the tubing:**
  - Clamp the drainage tubing or bend the tubing
  - Allow adequate time for urine collection.
- You should not clamp longer than 15 minutes. Long time clamp can lead back flow of urine and is able to cause urinary tract infection.
- Cleanse the aspiration port with a spirit swab or another disinfectant swab (e.g., Betadine swab).

- **Withdrawing the urine:**
  - Insert the needle into the aspiration port.
  - Withdraw sufficient amount of urine gently into the syringe. This technique is used for non-contaminated urine specimen, preventing contamination of the patient's bladder.
- Transfer the urine to the labeled specimen container. Careful labeling and transfer prevents contamination or confusion of the urine specimen.
- The container should be clean for a routine urinalysis and be sterile for a culture. Appropriate container brings accurate results of urinalysis.
- Unclamp the catheter. The catheter must be unclamped to allow free urinary flow and to prevent urinary stasis.
- Prepare and pour urine to the container for transport Proper packaging ensures that the specimen is not on infection risk.
- Dispose of used equipment and disinfect, if needed.
- Send the container to the laboratory immediately because organisms grow quickly at room temperature.
- Remove gloves and perform hand hygiene.
- Document the procedure in the designated place and mark it off on the Kardex to avoid duplication.
- Documentation provides coordination of care.

NURSE'S RESPONSIBILITY IN COLLECTING URINE SPECIMEN

- Label specimen containers or bottles before the patient voids (Rationale: Reduce handling, after the container or bottle is contaminated).
- Note on the specimen label if the female patient is menstruating at that time. (Rationale: One of the tests routinely performed is a test for blood in the urine. If the female patient is menstruating at the time of urine specimen, a false positive reading for blood will be obtained).
- To avoid contamination and necessity of collecting another specimen, soap and water cleansing of the genitals immediately preceding the collection of the specimen is supported. (Rationale: Bacteria are normally present on the labia or penis and the perineum and in the anal area).
- Maintain body substances precautions when collecting all types of urine specimen. (Rationale: To maintain safety).
- Wake a patient in the morning to obtain a routine specimen. (Rationale: If all specimens are collected at the same time, the laboratory can establish a baseline. And also this voided specimen usually represents that was collecting in the bladder all night).
- Be sure to document the procedure in the designated place and mark it off on the Kardex. (Rationale: To avoid duplication).

SPUTUM CULTURE

Observation and Collection of Sputum

- Sputum is the mucous secretion from the lungs, and trachea.
- It is important to differentiate it from saliva, the clear liquid secreted by the salivary glands in the mouth.
- Thirty ounces of mucus produced/day.
- Healthy Individuals do not produce sputum.
- Clients need to cough to bring sputum up from the lungs, bronchi, and trachea into the mouth to expectorate into a collecting container.
- Document amount of sputum collected, color, odor, consistency (thick, tenacious, watery), and presence of blood.

Collection of Sputum Specimen
Purposes
- For culture and sensitivity to identify a specific microorganism and its drug sensitivities.
- For cytology to identify the origin, structure, and pathology of cells.
- For acid-fast bacillus (AFB) requires serial collection for three consecutive days to identify the organism.
- Sputum specimens are collected in the morning.
- Upon awakening, the client can cough up the secretions that have accumulated during the night. When a client cannot cough the nurse must use pharyngeal suctioning to obtain the specimen.

Steps of Procedure
- Explain client the method and purposes of sputum collection.
- Instruct client to rinse mouth with plain water and not with antiseptic mouthwashes.
- Ask the client to breathe deeply and then cough up 15–30 mL of sputum,
- Wear gloves and a mask to avoid direct contact with the sputum.
- Ask the client to expectorate or spit out the sputum into the container.
- Make sure that sputum does not contact the outside of the container
- Following sputum collection, offer mouth wash to remove any unpleasant taste.
- Label and transport the specimen to the laboratory with requisition immediately or it should be refrigerated because microorganisms may grow and multiply and produce false results.
- Document the collection of sputum specimens on the client's chart.
- Include the amount, color, consistency, odor and presence of blood, and any discomfort experienced by the client.

Characteristics of Sputum
- **Amount:** Normally, no sputum or very little is expectorated.
  Abnormal or disease condition: The amount may vary according to the diseases, e.g., asthma, bronchitis
- **Color:** It is color less and translucent.
  Abnormal or disease condition:
  - The yellowish color indicates a bacterial infection.
  - The blackish color indicates carbon pigment, e.g., smoking
  - Bright red/Dark red, tarry color indicates blood.
  - The greenish color indicates bronchiectasis.
  - Brown color indicates gangrenous condition of the lung.
  - Unpleasant odor indicates lung abscess, lung cancer.

- **Odor**: Odorless normally
  Abnormal or disease condition: Unpleasant odor indicates lung abscess, lung cancer.
- **Consistency:** Abnormal or disease condition—Frothy, watery tenacious, and thick depending on the type of condition.

RADIOLOGICAL PROCEDURES

Radiology is the medical discipline that deals with the use X-rays and other high-energy radiation, and medical sing for the diagnosis and treatment of disease within the bodies of animals and human beings. It can be categorized into two branches:
1. Diagnostic Radiology
2. Interventional Radiology

Diagnostic Radiology

Diagnostic radiology refers to the field of medicine that uses imaging scans to diagnose a patient.

Interventional Radiology

Interventional radiology (IR) is a medical subspecialty that performs various minimally-invasive procedures using medical imaging guidance, such as X-ray fluoroscopy, computed tomography, magnetic resonance imaging, or ultrasound.

Few examples of interventional radiology procedures are as follows:
- Angiography and peripheral venography.
- Percutaneous transluminal angioplasty (PTCA) or Stenting.
- Percutaneous tumor ablation suing radiofrequency of microwaves or cryotherapy.
- Venous access catheter placement such as CVP line, JVP catheter placement
- Transarterial chemoembolization, such as uterine artery embolization, tumor embolization.
- Pleural aspiration/Thoracentesis.
- Peritoneal (Ascitic) tap.
- Needle biopsy and FNAC of different organs, such as liver, breast biopsy under ultrasound guidance.
- Placement of Enteral feeding tubes.

DIAGNOSTIC RADIOLOGY

Computed Tomography (CT) Scan

In CT scanning, a computer translates the action of multiple X-ray beams into three dimensional oscilloscope images of the biliary tract, liver and pancreas. This test can be done with/without a contrast medium, but contrast is preferred (unless the patient is allergic to contrast medium).

Purposes
- Helps to distinguish between obstructive and non-obstructive jaundice.
- Detects occult malignancy.
- Identify abscess, cysts, hematomas, tumors and pseudocysts.
- Helps to diagnose disease of liver, spleen, kidney, pancreas and pelvic organs.

Indications
- Ureteric calculus
- Suspected subarachnoid hemorrhage
- Post-traumatic seizure
- Focal neurologic deficit
- Coagulopathies
- Suspected open or depressed fracture

Magnetic Resonance Imaging (MRI)
- MRI is a non-invasive technique that uses magnetic fields and radio waves to produce an image of the area being studied.
- MRI generates an image by energizing protons into strong magnetic field.
- Radio waves emitted as protons return to their former equilibrium state and are recorded
- MRI transmits non-ionizing radiation during the scan
- One limitation of MRI is the closed tube like space, i.e., required for the scanned patient lies in this space.
- Patient with metal or implanted devices cannot undergo this test, because of the strong magnetic field, it generates.
- MRI is useful in evaluating disorders of liver and other organs in order to identify tumors, masses or cysts.

Indications
- For patients who have lumbar spinal stenosis.
- If back pain is accompanied by constitutional symptoms that may indicate that the pain is due to a tumor or an infection.

Mammography

A mammogram is an X-ray of the breast. Mammograms are commonly used to screen for breast cancer. If an abnormality is detected on a screening mammogram, diagnostic mammogram is used to further evaluate that abnormality.

Nuclear Medicine

Nuclear medicine is a specialized area of radiology that uses very small amounts of radioactive materials to examine organ function and structure.

Indications
- Evaluation of chest pain
- Evaluation of pulmonary perfusion
- Evaluation of shortness of breath.

X-Ray

It is the radiographic study of body organs according to presence of symptoms, e.g., bones, joints, skull, face, spine, etc. The most common view used for chest X-ray is anterior posterior or lateral view.

Positron Emission Tomography (PET)

It determines the amount of blood flowing into specific body tissues and also measures blood flow, glucose metabolism and oxygen extraction

Ultrasound

High frequency sound waves are used to make images of organs and structures inside the body. Patient's preparation will depend on the part of the body being examined. For example, ultrasound of urinary bladder need to keep bladder full, while doing abdomen ultrasound, full bladder is not required

ENDOSCOPIC PROCEDURES

Endoscopic procedures are the non-surgical procedures used to visualize and examine inside the body cavity or hollow organs by inserting a flexible tube with a light and camera attached to it (called as endoscope). These procedures mostly involve visualization of organs of respiratory system, gastrointestinal system and genitourinary system.

Endoscopy

It is direct visualization of body system by inserting a light emitting flexible tube. It is used for diagnosis, biopsy, specimen collection or assessing changes in body part bronchoscopy, colonoscopy are examples of endoscopy.

Indications

- Esophageal reflux symptoms that persist or recur despite appropriate therapy.
- Persistent vomiting of unknown cause.
- Removal of foreign bodies.

Sigmoidoscopy

Sigmoidoscopy is a diagnostic test that looks at the rectum and lower part of the large intestine by using a flexible tube with a light on it. It is also known as flexible sigmoidoscopy.

Indications

- Rectal bleeding
- Unexplained anemia, weight loss or fever.
- Colorectal cancer screening.
- Abdominal pain.

Enteroscopy

Enterscopy is a procedure used to examine the small intestine (small bowel). During this test, a thin, flexible tube with an attached camera is inserted into the body. This is called an endoscope. There are usually one or two balloons attached to the endoscope.

- **Percutaneous endoscopic gastrotomy**: A procedure in which a flexible feeding tube is placed through the abdominal wall and into the stomach. Patients who have difficulty swallowing, problems with their appetite or an inability to take adequate nutrition through the mouth can benefit from this procedure.
- **Upper endoscopy:** An upper endoscopy is a procedure used to visually examine the upper digestive system with a tiny on the end of a long, flexible tube. The medical term for an upper endoscopy is esophagogastroduodenoscopy.

CHAPTER 7

Oxygenation Needs

REVIEW OF CARDIOVASCULAR AND RESPIRATORY PHYSIOLOGY

- The cardiovascular system consists of the heart and the blood vessels.
- The major function of the cardiovascular system is to deliver oxygen and nutrients to all tissues of the body through the blood and to remove carbon dioxide and other waste products of cellular metabolism from the tissues.
- The cardiovascular system is the link between external respiration (gas exchange between the atmosphere and lungs) and cellular respiration (use of oxygen for energy production by the mitochondria).

Other vital functions of the cardiovascular system include:
- Transport of heat to maintain body temperature,
- Delivery of white blood cells to sites where they defend against foreign material
- Transport of hormones from the site of release to their target organs.

Thus, the cardiovascular system is a key contributor to maintain the homeostasis of the body.

These tasks are accomplished by two components of the cardiovascular system—the pulmonary circulation and the systemic circulation. Each component is made up of:

- A pump (right ventricle for the pulmonary circulation, left ventricle for the systemic circulation) that provides energy to propel the blood.
- A system of arteries and arterioles that distributes blood throughout the region each pump supplies,
- A network of capillaries through which gases and nutrients are exchanged with the tissues supplied
- A system of venules and veins that returns the distributed blood to the pump.
- Pulmonary and systemic circulations are connected in series so that the blood flows through the chambers of the right heart and the lungs, then to the chambers of the left heart, and the rest of the body. (RA: right atrium; RV: right ventricle; LA: left atrium; LV: left ventricle; pa- pulmonary artery; PV: portal vein.)

RESPIRATORY SYSTEM (PHYSIOLOGY)

- Respiration is the interchange of gases between an organism and the medium in which it lives.
- In the human body, respiration takes place by external and internal processes.
- The external process of respiration involves the transfer of oxygen (O_2) and carbon dioxide (CO_2) that occurs in the lungs between the atmosphere and the pulmonary circulation.
- The internal process of respiration is the similar process that occurs at the cellular level.
- Both aspects of respiration are essential to life.
- The ultimate function of the respiratory system is gas exchange.
- This gas exchange consists of obtaining O_2 from the atmosphere and removing CO_2, from the blood.
- It is important to consider that O_2 is necessary for normal metabolism and CO_2, is a waste product of this metabolism.
- CO_2, is only inhaled in negligible quantity and thus the CO_2, we exhale is created within the body.
- While CO_2 plays a role in acid-base balance, it must be cleared from the body in appropriate levels through ventilation.
- Although gas exchange takes place in the lungs, the respiratory system is controlled by the central nervous system (CNS).
- The portions of the CNS that control respiration are located within the brain stem-specifically within the pons and the medulla.
- Three primary components of external respiration are:
  1. Ventilation
  2. Perfusion
  3. Diffusion.
- These components are responsible for the nerve impulses, which are transmitted via the phrenic and other motor nerves to the diaphragm and intercostal muscles, controlling our basic breathing rhythm.

Ventilation

- The most readily observable component of respiration involves the act of breathing, during which the lungs are provided with air through inhaling and CO_2, is removed through exhalation.
- This process of moving air into and out of the lungs is known as ventilation.

- The ability of air to flow into and out of the alveoli is dependent on a number of factors including integrity and compliance of the lung tissue and resistance to airflow within the airways.

Perfusion
- The second component of respiration is perfusion.
- This process involves the circulation of blood through the capillaries, which facilitates nutrient exchange.
- External respiration requires adequate delivery of blood to the capillary beds of the lungs via the pulmonary circulation.
- In the absence of this blood supply, there will be no transport mechanism for O_2.

Diffusion
- Diffusion is another important method of transport within the body and is the third component of respiration.
- Diffusion involves the movement of a substance in a solution (liquid or air) from higher concentration areas to lower concentration areas.
- In the case of respiration, diffusion involves the distribution of O_2 from the atmosphere through the pulmonary capillary walls and into the bloodstream.
- At the same time, CO_2 diffuses from the bloodstream into the alveoli.
- This process of diffusion is dependent on the characteristics of each individual gas, the rate of perfusion and the integrity of the alveolar-capillary membrane.

FACTORS AFFECTING RESPIRATORY FUNCTIONING

Levels of Health
- Acute and chronic illnesses can affect a person's respiratory function drastically.
- People with cardiac or renal disorders often have compromised respiratory functioning because of fluid overload and impaired tissue perfusion.
- People with chronic illnesses often have muscle wasting and poor muscle tone.
- These problems affect all the muscles, including those of respiratory system.
- Alterations in muscle functions contributes to inadequate pulmonary ventilation and respiration.
- Anemia can result in impaired respiratory function due to inadequate supply of oxygen to the tissues of the body.
- Hemoglobin also carries carbon dioxide to the lungs, anemia results in diminished carbon dioxide exchange.
- Myocardial infarction causes a lack of blood supply to the heart muscle.
- Damage to the heart muscle interfere with effective contraction of the heart muscle, leading to decreased perfusion of tissues and decreased gas exchange.

Developmental Considerations
There are many age-related developmental considerations affecting respiratory function

Neonates and Infants
- Many changes occur in the lungs of a newborn.
- In infants, chest is small and the airways are short therefore aspiration is a potential problem.
- The respiratory rate is 30–60 breaths per minute.
- As the alveoli increase in number and size, adequate oxygenation is accomplished at lower respiratory rates
- Surfactant is formed in utero between 34 and 36 weeks.
- An infant born before 34 weeks, may not have produced sufficient surfactant, leading to collapse of the alveoli and poor alveolar exchange.
- Respiratory pattern is primarily abdominal in infants.

Toddlers, Preschoolers, School-aged Children and Adolescents
- In pre-school children, Eustachian tubes, bronchi and bronchioles are elongated and less angular.
- Therefore the average incidence routine colds and infections decreases until the child enters daycare or school where he/she is exposed more frequently to pathogens.
- Most children at this age have colds or upper respiratory infections, but some have more serious problems of otitis media, bronchitis and pneumonia.
- At this stage, it is important to encourage good hand hygiene practices.
- By the end of late childhood and during adulthood, the immune system is prepared to protect the person from most infections.

Older Adults
- Specific physical changes occur in older adults, such as decreased elastic recoil of the lungs, expiration requiring use of accessory muscles, fewer functional capillaries and more fibrous tissue in alveoli, and reduction in vital capacity and increase in residual volume, all these lead to decreased gas exchange and increased work of breathing.
- There is decreased ventilation and ineffective cough due to less air exchange; more secretions remain in lungs, drier mucous membranes, altered pain sensation, greater risk of aspiration due to slower gastric motility.
- Airways collapse more easily. These alterations increase the risk for disease, especially pneumonia and other chest infections.

Medications
Many medications affect the function of the respiratory system. For example, opioids are chemical agents that depress the medullary respiratory center. As a result, the rate and depth of respirations decrease.

Lifestyle
- Activity levels and habits can affect a person's respiratory status. For example, sedentary activity patterns do no encourage the expansion of alveoli and the development of pulmonary exercise patterns.
- People who exercise (aerobics, walking, swimming) three to six times per week can better respond to stressors to respiratory health.

- Cigarette smoking, active or passive is a major contributor to lung disease and respiratory distress.

Environment

- There is a high correlation between air pollution cancer and lung disease.
- Occupational exposure asbestos, silica, or coal dust, as well as environment pollution, can lead to chronic pulmonary disease.

Psychological Health

- Many psychological factors and conditions can affected respiratory system.
- Individuals responding to stress ma sigh excessively or exhibit hyperventilation (increased rate and depth of ventilation, above the body's norm metabolic requirements).
- Hyperventilation can lead to lowered level of arterial carbon dioxide.
- Generalized anxiety has been shown to cause enough bronchospasm to produce an episode of bronchial asthma.

Some Common Factors that Affect Respiratory Functions

- **Pain:** Pain alters rate and rhythm of respiration. Patient inhibits chest wall movement while experiencing pain in chest or abdomen.
- **Exercise:** Exercise increases rate and depth of respiration to meet the body's need for additional oxygen.
- **Emotions:** Some strong emotions, such as fear, anger and nervousness can stimulate respiratory center, resulting in respiration pause or increased rate of respirations. Anxiety increases rate and depth as a result of sympathetic stimulation.
- **Body posture:** A straight, erect posture promotes full chest expansion and lying flat prevents full chest expansion.
- **Neurological injury:** Injury to brainstem impairs respiratory center and inhibits respiratory rate and rhythm
- **Medication:** Narcotic analgesics and sedatives depress rate and depth. Amphetamines and cocaine may increase rate and depth of respiration.
- **Blood pressure:** Blood pressure can influence respiration when it fluctuates in a large range. If the blood pressure increases, the respiration will decrease in rate and depth.

ALTERATIONS IN RESPIRATORY FUNCTIONING

Conditions Affecting Airway

- **Allergies:** It occurs when immune system responds to foreign particle like pollen, dust, any food, etc.
- **Asthma:** It is characterized by inflammation, bronchospasm and edema of the airway.
- **Common cold:** It is the infection of the upper respiratory tract which leads to the narrowing of the airway.
- **Cough:**
  - It is the forceful expulsion of respiratory content.
  - It is explosive expiration that provides a protective mechanism that arising the secretions and foreign body material from tracheobronchial tree.
  - It is the body's response when something imitates in or airways.
  - An irritant stimulate the nerves that send a message to brain.
  - The brain then send message to muscles of chest and abdomen to push air out of lungs to force out the irritant.
  - Hardly cough is normal and healthy.
  - A cough that persists for several weeks or one that brings up discolored or bloody mucus may indicate a condition that needs medical attention.
- **Types of cough:** There are two types of cough:
  1. **According to severity:**
     - *Acute cough:* It occurs due to irritation of trachea and it has sudden onset.
     - *Chronic cough:* It occurs in any disease condition like TB, asthma, COPD, etc.
  2. **According to presentation:**
     - *Dry cough:* It is cough without sputum production.
     - *Productive cough:* It is the cough accompanied with sputum, blood, secretions, etc.

Conditions Affecting Movement of Airway

Dyspnea

- **Definition:**
  - It is defined as the sensation of breathlessness or in adequate breathing. It is the abnormal uncomfortable awareness of breathing
  - Dyspnea, also called shortness of breath, is a tight feeling in chest in which person may not be able to take a deep breath. This is a symptom that can be connected to many different conditions, like asthma, heart failure and lung disease.
- **Grading:**
  - *Grade 1:* Dyspnea occurs while doing strenuous activities.
  - *Grade 2:* Person is restricted to some activities like climbing stairs.
  - *Grade 3:* Dyspnea occurs during usual activities but person can manage.
  - *Grade 4:* Person requires assistance while performing activities of daily living.
  - *Grade 5:* Dyspnea occurs at rest.

Tachypnea

It is defined as when respiratory rate is more than 20 breaths per minute.

Orthopnea

It is defined as shortness of breath when the patient is lying down.

Apnea

❖ **Definition:**
- It is the cessation of breathing in which there is no movement of respiratory muscles for inhalation and expiration and the volume of the lungs remain unchanged.
- Person is able to take breath.

Sleep Apnea

❖ **Definition:** It is the cessation of breathing during sleep.
❖ **Types:**
- *Central sleep apnea:* In this apnea brain is unable to send signals to respiratory muscles for breathing during sleep.
- *Obstructive sleep apnea:* It is characterized by collapse of airway during deep sleep.
- *Mixed sleep apnea:* It is the mixture of both central sleep apnea and obstructive sleep apnea.

Conditions Affecting Diffusion

❖ **Pulmonary edema:**
- *Definition*
- It is defined as an abnormal accumulation or collection of fluid in lung, lung tissue or alveolar space. It is a severe and life threatening condition.

❖ **Chronic obstructive pulmonary disease (COPD):**
- It is a respiratory disease in which airflow is obstructed by emphysema, chronic bronchitis or both.
- The air flow obstruction is progressive and irreversible and also associated with airway hyperactivity.
- Asthma is also considered within this disease group but asthma is reversible.

❖ **Atelectasis:**
- It is a respiratory disorder characterized by collapsed lung
- It may be chronic or acute.
- Most common atelectasis is acute one.
- Atelectasis is the collapse of part or (much less commonly) all of a lung.

Conditions Affecting Oxygen Transport

❖ **Heart failure:** Heart failure is the inability of heart to pump the sufficient.
❖ **Hypovolemia:** Loss of extracellular fluid volume and decreased circulating blood volume.
❖ **Dehydration:** Dehydration occurs when there is not enough fluid in the body, especially in the blood (intravascular area). Although, there are several types of dehydration.

ALTERATIONS OF OXYGENATION

The alterations of oxygenation includes:
❖ Hypoventilation
❖ Hyperventilation
❖ Hypoxia

Hypoventilation

❖ It is the condition when the level of carbon dioxide in body gets higher than oxygen level.
❖ It is defined as an increase in partial pressure of carbon dioxide (more than 45 mm Hg).

Hyperventilation

It is defined as when the partial pressure of oxygen is more than the partial pressure of carbon dioxide. The amount of carbon dioxide is less in blood.

Hypoxia

Hypoxia condition in which the body or a region of the body is deprived of adequate oxygen supply.

Types of Hypoxia

Hypoxic Hypoxia

❖ Low PaO_2 (arterial oxygen tension) which is secondary to $FiO_2 < 21\%$ or decreased barometric pressure (high altitude).
❖ Impaired ventilation secondary to neuromuscular weakness or narcotic overdose.
❖ Impaired oxygenation secondary to pulmonary fibrosis.

Circulatory Hypoxia

❖ Inadequate pumping of the blood from the lungs to tissues may be secondary to disorders causing decreased cardiac output, such as MI, low fluid volume, hypotension, poor supply of arteries.
❖ If the patient has myocardial ischemia supplemental O_2 is definitely indicated.
❖ A decrease in cardiac output results in a low BP and a prolonged systemic transit time.
❖ The PaO_2 can be high, but because of the time it takes to get to the tissues, the patient is hypoxic, cardiovascular instability or failure, shock, arrhythmias, treatment include increasing cardiac output with use of cardiovascular drugs and therapy.

Hemic Hypoxia

❖ Decreased oxygen carrying capacity as in anemia or carbon monoxide poisoning
❖ Having a decreased carrying capacity for oxygen, the patient with decreased or abnormal hemoglobin.
❖ Anemia.
❖ Carbon monoxide poisoning (Methemoglobinemia).
❖ Sickle cell anemia.
❖ Treatment involves blood transfusions, hyperbaric chamber, and bone marrow transplant.

Demand Hypoxia

Increased tissue consumption of oxygen in hypermetabolic states like fever, malignant hyperthermia.

Histotoxic Hypoxia

❖ Utilization of oxygen is abnormal, such as in cyanide poisoning there is inability for tissues to utilize oxygen available.
❖ Cyanide poisoning will inhibit cellular metabolism from occurring the cells cannot process the O_2.

NURSING INTERVENTIONS TO PROMOTE OXYGENATION

Inhalations

Inhalation means breathing air or vapor into the lung through the nose or mouth. Inhalation is of two types:
1. Dry inhalation
2. Moist inhalation

Dry Inhalation

- A substance such as ammonia may be inhaled in the treatment of fainting.
- Amyl nitrate may be inhaled to relieve angina (pain in the heart).
- Oxygen inhalation.
- Inhalation of general anesthetic drugs.
- Aerosol spray.

Moist Inhalation

Steam inhalation.

NEBULIZATION THERAPY

Definition

- The principle of nebulizer therapy is to liquefy and remove retained secretions from the respiratory tract.
- A nebulizer is a device that produces a stable aerosol of fluid and/or drug particles.
- The patient could do these procedures if instructed,
- Nebulization is the process of medication administration via inhalation.
- It utilizes a nebulizer which transports medications to the lungs by means of mist inhalation.

Purposes

- To relieve respiratory insufficiency due to bronchospasm.
- To correct the underlying respiratory disorders responsible for bronchospasm.
- To liquefy and remove retained thick secretions from the lower respiratory tract.
- To reduce inflammatory and allergic responses in the upper respiratory tract.
- To correct humidity deficit resulting from inspired air by passing the upper airway during the use of mechanical ventilation in critically-ill and post-surgical patients.

Types

1. Metered-dose nebulizer (**Figs. 7.1 and 7.2**)
2. Jet nebulizer
3. Ultrasonic nebulizer

Metered-dose Nebulizer

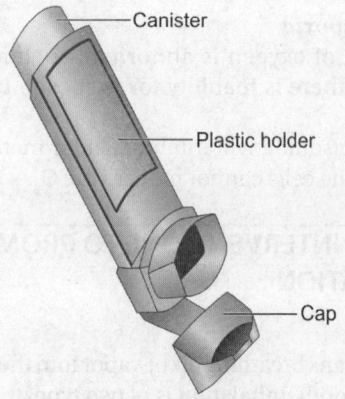

Fig. 7.1: Metered dose nebulizer.

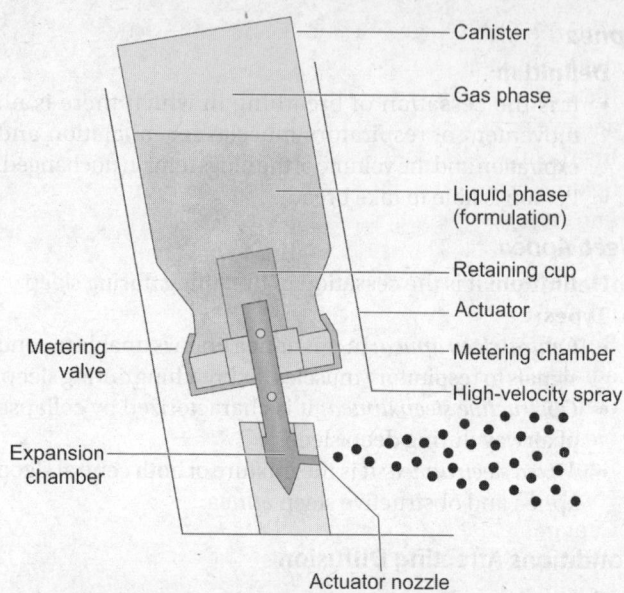

Fig. 7.2: Parts of metered dose nebulizer.

Equipment

- Metered dose nebulizer
- Physician's order
- Medication (if applicable)
- Sputum cup/disposable

General Instructions

Monitor the heart rate before and after the treatment, for patients using bronchodilator drugs as it may produce tachycardia and palpitations.

Procedure

- Check the physician's order and nursing care plans to obtain specific instructions and/or information.
- Identify the patient to perform the night procedure on the right patient
- Explain the procedure to the patient to allay fears and gain patient's confidence and cooperation and check the patient identification wristband against physician's written orders
- Encourage the patient to participate in the procedure as possible to promote patient education.
- Ensure privacy to avoid unnecessary embarrassment to the patient during the procedure
- Wash and dry hands to prevent cross infection.
- Assist the patient to a comfortable sitting or semi-Fowler's position. The diaphragmatic excursion and lung compliance is greater in this position. This ensures madmal distribution and deposition of aerosolized particles to the basilar area of the lung.
- Shake the inhaler well to ensure the mixing of medication
- Instruct patient to remove the cap from the mouthpiece to educate the patient to facilitate ready access to medication
- Instruct the patient to hold the canister with the index finger on top and the thumb on the bottom of the canister to ensure effective and safe handling of equipment.
- Instruct the patient to place the mouthpiece in the mouth and to inhale slowly while depressing the top of the canister

with the index finger. Breath carries the particles of the medications as far down into the lungs as possible.
- Instruct the patient to take a deep breath and exhale to achieve optimum lung expansion and medicinal effect
- Instruct the patient to hold the breath as long as possible before exhaling to achieve optimum penetration of the drug into the lower respiratory tract of the prescribed medication
- Release the index finger from the canister and remove the inhaler from the mouth to prevent overdose of the drug inhaled
- Repeat the procedure until the prescribed dose is administered to allow for effective perfusion of medication
- Settle patient in a comfortable position to assist in effective perfusion of medication.
- Replace canister cap after wiping dry and disposing off contaminated tissues.
- Contaminated equipment may cause nosocomial infection
- Wash and dry hands to prevent cross infection
- Document the procedure in the appropriate charts
- Evaluate the effects of the procedure and report abnormal findings.

Jet Medication Nebulizer (Fig. 7.3)

Definition
The jet medication nebulizer utilizes a high velocity gas flow to generate particles from the prescribed solution. Either oxygen or compressed air powers the nebulizer.

General Instructions
- Safety and hazards of oxygen administration should be observed.
- Recording of peak flow meter reading to be maintained pre and post procedure if indicated.

Equipment
- Oxygen cylinder/wall oxygen outlet with flow meter
- **A clean tray with:** Oxygen nipple adapter to fit to the connection tubing.
- **Nebulizer kit consisting of:**
  - Face mask/mouth piece
  - Nebulizer jar and nebulizer cap
  - Oxygen supply tubing
- Physician's written order.
- **Prescribed nebulizer solution:** 0.9% NaCl ampoules as diluent, if prescribed.
- 5 mL syringe with needle.
- Disposable sputum cup.
- Box of disposable tissues or gauze pieces.

Procedure
- Check the physician's order and nursing care plan to obtain specific instructions and/or information.
- Identify the patient to perform the right procedure on the right patient.
- Explain the procedure to the patient to allay fears and gain patient's confidence and cooperation and check the patient identification wristband against physician's written orders.
- Encourage the patient to participate in the procedure as possible to promote patient education
- Ensure privacy to avoid unnecessary embarrassment to the patient during the procedure.
- Wash and dry hands to prevent cross infection
- Unscrew the nebulizer jar and instill the prescribed dose of solution (dilute with prescribed solution)
- Rescrew cap on nebulizer jar to prevent any leakage of the medication.
- Connect one end of the oxygen tubing to the nebulizer and attach the other end of the supply tubing to the oxygen flow meter to ensure effective functioning of the system.
- Place the patient in a comfortable sitting or semi-Fowler's position to ensure maximal distribution and deposition of aerosolized particles to basilar areas of lung.
- Adjust the oxygen to a flow rate of 6–8 liters per minute or until a fine mist appears to ensure adequate and effective flow of aerosol.
- Place the mask snugly over the patient's face to cover the nose, mouth and chin and adjust the elastic strap around the patient's head to ensure an airtight seal between the mask and the patient's face for effective Nebulization.
- Instruct the patient to take a deep breath, repeat hold breath briefly, then exhale until all the medication is nebulized to encourage optimal dispersion of the medication into the lower respiratory tract.
- Observe expansion of the patient's chest during therapy to ensure that medication is deposited below the level of the oropharynx by taking deep breaths. Do not leave the patient unattended to allay fear and anxiety.

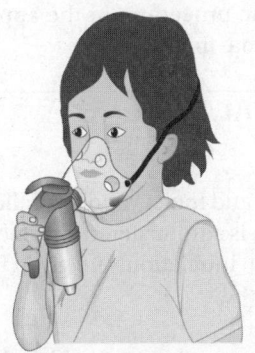
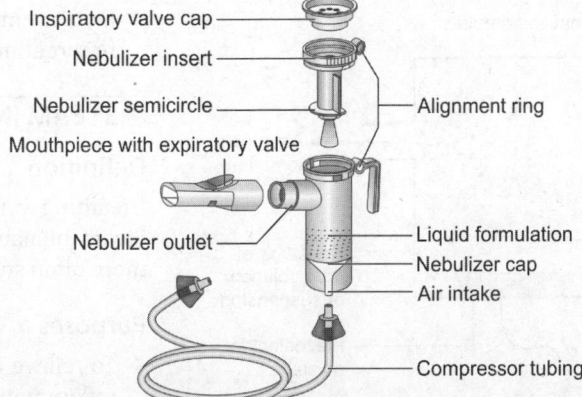

Fig. 7.3: Jet medication nebulizer.

- Observe the patient throughout the procedure and give constant reassurance to determine the patient's comfort and also to observe for any side effects of the medication
- Turn off the oxygen when all the solution has vaporized and remove the facemask. Medication usually will be nebulized within 10–15 min at a gas flow rate of 5–6 min.
- Encourage the patient to cough after several deep breaths. The deep lung inflation will encourage forceful coughing and facilitate the expectoration of secretions.
- Assist the patient to a comfortable position and wipe off the moisture from the face with face towel or disposable tissues. Change jacket/gown if necessary to maintain patient's comfort, hygiene and dignity.
- Dismantle the nebulizer kit and decontaminate in hot soapy water. Dry and store in dry plastic bag between treatments to prevent spread of nosocomial infections
- Wash and dry hands to prevent cross infection
- Document the procedure in the appropriate charts.
- Evaluate the effects of the procedure and report abnormal findings.

Ultrasonic Nebulizer (Fig. 7.4)

Definition

The ultrasonic nebulizer utilizes fluid contained in a chamber, which is rapidly vibrated, causing the fluid to break into small particles. It works on the principle that high frequency sound waves can break up water into aerosol particles by means of a transducer.

Equipment

- Ultrasonic nebulizer with manufacturer's instructions
- Circuit set up (according to manufacturer's instructions)
- Disposable aerosol mask
- Sterile water
- Physician's written order
- Prescribed solution
- Disposable sputum cup
- Box of disposable tissues or gauze pieces

Procedure

- Check the physician's order and nursing care plan to obtain specific instructions and/or information
- Identify the patient to perform the right procedure on the right patient.
- Explain the procedure to the patient to allay fears and gain patient's confidence and cooperation and check the patient identification wristband against physician's written orders. Encourage the patient to participate in the procedure as possible to promote patient education.
- Ensure privacy to avoid unnecessary embarrassment to the patient during the procedure
- Wash and dry hands to prevent cross infection.
- Fill the ultrasonic chamber with the prescribed solution to the appropriate level with sterile water.
- Transducer needs a constant water level for effective functioning.
- Assemble circuit according to manufacturer's instructions and plug the cord into an electrical outlet.
- Turn on the machine and adjust the setting the desired amount of mist is obtained to facilitate deeper penetration of particles into the tracheobronchial tree.
- Position the patient in a comfortable sitting or semi-Fowler's position to ensure maximal distribution and deposition of aerosolized particles to basilar area of the lung.
- Place the mask snugly over the patient's face to cover the nose Instruct the patient to breathe in slowly through his mouth and to exhale and repeat several times to allow for maximal particle deposition in the lower respiratory tract.
- Observe the patient for any adverse reaction to the treatment. Patient may develop bronchospasm due to the inhalation of aerosol particles. The fluid may also cause dried retained secretions resulting in airway narrowing. Continuous aerosol therapy may lead to fluid overload in infants. Do not leave the patient unattended to allay fear and anxiety.
- Encourage the patient to periodically cough and expectorate any secretion loosened during the treatment to facilitate a clear airway and to prevent further lung consolidation.
- Turn off the machine and discontinue the procedure.
- Remove face mask and decontaminate in hot soapy water.
- Dry and store in dry plastic bag at patient's bedside. Replace mask and tubing after 24 hours.
- Empty any residual water in containers and follow through with a disinfectant.
- Dispatch couplant to CSSD for terminal sterilization to prevent contamination with microorganisms
- Wash and dry hands to prevent cross infection.
- Document the procedure in the appropriate charts and report abnormal findings.

STEAM INHALATION

Definition

Breathing warm and moist vapors is called steam inhalation. Steam inhalation is administered for general (systemic) effect; more often steam inhalations are given for local effect.

Purposes

- To relieve the symptoms of cold and sinusitis caused by inflammation and congestion of mucous membrane
- To lose mucus and relieve coughing

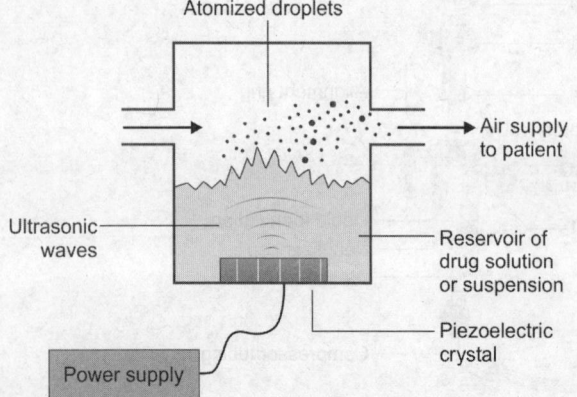

Fig. 7.4: Ultrasonic nebulizer.

- To warm and moisten the air to relieve dyspnea and irritation in air passages.
- To provide antiseptic effect.
- To prevent excessive dryness of the mucous membranes.
- To relieve spastic conditions of the larynx and bronchi.

Articles
- Nelson inhaler
- Jug with hot water
- Towel
- Face towel
- Sputum cup
- Small basin
- Cotton swabs
- Gauze pieces

General Instructions
- The water level in the inhaler should be just below the spout
- The temperature of the water should be maintained between 120–140°F or 60–76°C.
- The mouth of spout must be kept away from the patient to prevent scalding.
- Protect the patient from cold air. The windows and doors are closed and the fan is put off during the treatment.
- Ask the patient to empty the bladder before starting the therapy.
- Watch the patient closely throughout the procedure.
- Place a sputum cup in reach of the patient.

Nelson's Inhaler Method (Fig. 7.5)
- The inhaler has a glass mouthpiece passing through the cork of the inhaler and an air inlet at the side.
- Prepare the patient and get his cooperation.
- Protect him from cold air.
- Have him comfortably seated with a bed table in front.
- Keep sputum cup in easy reach of patient.
- Warm the inhaler with a little hot water and pour the water out
- Pour the boiled water below the air inlet.
- Add the drug ordered.
- Cork the inhaler.

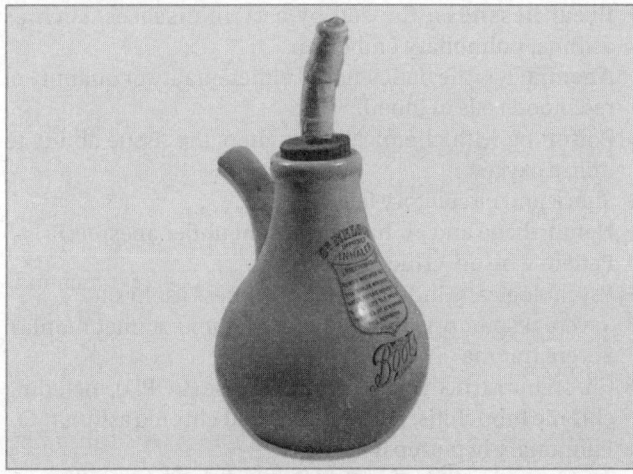

Fig. 7.5: Nelson's inhaler.

- Turn the mouthpiece away from the air inlet.
- Wrap the inhaler in flannel or a towel and place it in a small tray or basin.
- Take it to the bedside together with a towel and gauze piece.
- Wrap the piece of gauze around the mouthpiece of the inhaler.
- Cover the patient with a sheet or bath towel. Place the Inhaler in front of the patient and ask him to keep his mouth in the mouthpiece and breathe in by mouth to receive the steam and breathe out through nose removing his lips from the mouthpiece.
- Continue the treatment for 15-20 minutes.
- Perform chest physical therapy. The purpose of chest physical therapy, also called chest physiotherapy, help the patients to breathe more freely and to get more oxygen into the body.
- Wipe the patients face and keep him warm and in the same room for at least an hour.
- Wash the mouthpiece and boil it. Wash the inhaler and replace all the articles.
- Record the procedure and effect on the patient.
- Any waste should be disposed off in the garbage or in a biohazard container.

Steam Tent Method

Articles
- Boiling water in a kettle with spout
- Hot plate
- Tincture of Benzoin
- Old newspaper
- Screen
- Sheets
- Paper Bag

Procedure
- Fill kettle with water just below the level of the spout and bring the water to boiling point.
- Add 1 tsp of medication into the boiling water.
- Carry the hot plate and the kettle with caution near the bedside of the patient, if the patient is unable to stand or sit on the chair.
- If tent is indicated, open screen over the head of the patient and cover it with a sheet to form a tent.
- With the newspaper make a cylindrical tube to direct the steam into the tent away from the patient's face.
- If the patient is able to sit on the chair, he may sit near the hot plate. With the cylindrical tube of paper, the steam is directed into the patient's face for inhalation.
- **Treatment time:** 30 minutes to one hour, morning and evening, as tolerated.

Precautions
- Avoid all risks of burning
- Avoid drought during time of treatment.
- Close windows near the patient.
- Extra care must be observed when giving treatment to children and restless patients to avoid scalding.

MAINTENANCE OF PATENT AIRWAY

- Patent airway is the ability of a person to breathe, with airflow passing to and from the respiratory system through the oral and nasal passages.
- Airway is called patent whenever there is an open pathway between a patient's lungs and the outside world.
- An airway obstruction is a blockage in the airway.
- It may partially or totally prevent air from getting into your lungs.

Causes of Airway Obstruction

- Foreign body inhalations
- Allergic/anaphylactic reactions
- **Respiratory tract infections:** Diphtheria, tracheitis, epiglottitis
- **Trauma:** Burns, steam inhalations, penetrating injuries
- **Altered consciousness:** Head injuries, alcohol and drug overdose, cardiorespiratory arrest.

The Airway is Maintained Patent by Following Measures

- Coughing is the main mechanism for clearing the airway.
- The cough may be ineffective in disease states, such as pain from surgical incisions/trauma, respiratory muscle fatigue, or neuromuscular weakness.
- Other mechanisms that exist in the lower bronchioles and alveoli to maintain the airway include the mucociliary system and macrophages.

Signs of Airway Obstruction

- Abnormal breath sounds
- Changes in respiratory rate or depth
- Cough
- Hypoxemia
- Cyanosis
- Dyspnea
- Chest wheezing
- Tachycardia

Interventions to Maintain Patent Airway

- Ambulation and frequent position changes
- Use of Incentive Spirometry
- Use of abdominal muscles for more forceful cough
- Use of pillow or hand splints when coughing
- Optimal positioning (sitting position)
- Assist patient in performing deep breathing and coughing exercises.

Instruct Patient in the Following

- If cough is ineffective use suctioning as needed to remove sputum and mucus plugs.
- Encourage adequate intake of fluids to prevent dehydration.
- Administer medications (e.g., antibiotics, mucolytic agents, bronchodilators, expectorants) as ordered
- Consult respiratory therapist for chest physiotherapy
- Instruct patient how to use prescribed inhalers
- Provide steam inhalation to clear the secretions
- If the obstruction is not resolved insert artificial airway.
- Artificial airways

Most common invasive air ways are:
- Oropharyngeal airway
- Nasopharyngeal airway
- Tracheal intubation.

Surgical Management

Tracheotomy—is a surgically created opening from the skin of the neck down to the trachea.

OXYGEN ADMINISTRATION

Introduction

- Oxygen is a colorless, odorless, tasteless gas that is essential for the body to function properly and to survive.
- The air that we breathe in contains approximately 21% oxygen, and the heart relies on oxygen to pump blood.
- If not enough oxygen is circulating in the blood, it is difficult for the tissues of the heart to keep pumping.
- Supplemental oxygen is used to treat medical conditions in which the tissues of body do not have enough oxygen.
- Oxygen is a gas, but when administered as a supplement to normal atmospheric air, may also be considered as a medication (or drug).

Definition

- Oxygenation is the process that includes both the inspiratory and expiratory activities
- It is defined as when patients with respiratory dysfunctions are treated with oxygen inhalations to relieve anoxemia or hypoxemia
- Oxygen therapy is the administration of oxygen at a concentration of pressure greater than that found in the environmental atmosphere.

Indications

- **Cyanosis:** Bluish color of the skin, nail beds and mucus membranes, resulting from decreased amount of O_2
- **Breathlessness:** Caused by certain diseases, such as asthma, pulmonary embolism.
- **Anemia:** It is the deficiency of either quality or quantity of red blood cells in blood.
- Poisoning with chemicals that alters the tissue ability to utilize oxygen
- Shock and circulatory failure
- Hemorrhage and air hunger patient under anesthesia
- Patient who are critically ill
- Psychologically induced breathlessness asphyxia
- Severe respiratory distress (acute asthma or pneumonia)
- Severe trauma
- Chronic obstructive pulmonary disease (COPD), including chronic bronchitis, emphysema, and chronic asthma
- Pulmonary hypertension
- Acute myocardial infarction (heart attack).

Methods of Dispensing Oxygen

Piped in Cylinder

Oxygen is moistened by passing it through a humidification system to prevent the mucous membranes of the respiratory tree from becoming dry.

Using Oxygen Cylinders

- ❖ The oxygen cylinder is delivered with a protective cap to prevent accidental force against the cylinder outlet
- ❖ To release oxygen safety and at a desirable rate, a regulator is used. It consists of two parts:
  1. A reduction gauge that reduces the pressure to a working level and shows the amount of oxygen in the tank
  2. A flow meter that regulates the control of oxygen in liters perminutes.

Wall Outlet Oxygen

- ❖ The oxygen is supplied from a central source through a pipeline.
- ❖ Only a flow meter and a humidifier are required.

Classification Method of Oxygen Delivery Systems

Low Flow Systems

- ❖ Contribute partially to inspired gas patient breathes
- ❖ Do not provide constant FiO_2
- ❖ For example, nasal cannula, simple mask, non-rebreather mask, partial-rebreather mask.

High Flow Systems

- ❖ Deliver specific and constant percent of oxygen independent of patient's breathing
- ❖ For example, venturi mask, trach collar, T-piece.

■ METHODS OF OXYGEN ADMINISTRATION

Nasal Cannula (Prongs) (Fig. 7.6)

- ❖ It is a disposable
- ❖ Plastic devise with two protruding prongs for insertion into the nostrils, connected to an oxygen source.

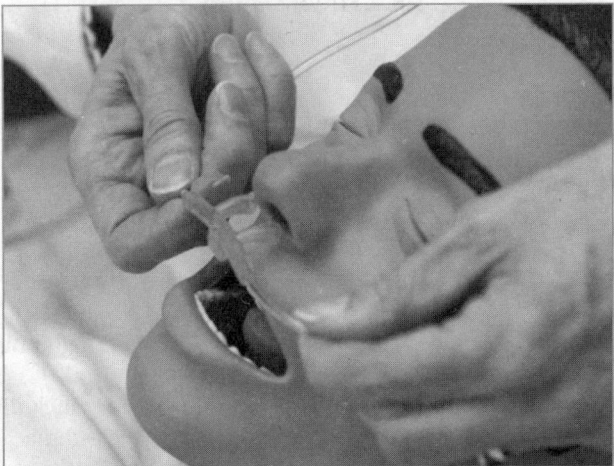

Fig. 7.6: Nasal cannula.

- ❖ Used for low-medium concentrations device of oxygen (24–44%).
  - 1 L/min = 24%
  - 2 L/min = 28%
  - 3 L/min = 32%
  - 4 L/min = 36%
  - 5 L/min = 40%
  - 6 L/min = 44%

Face Mask

- ❖ The simple oxygen mask
- ❖ The non-rebreather mask
- ❖ The partial rebreather mask
- ❖ The venturi mask.

The Simple Oxygen Mask (Fig. 7.7)

- ❖ Simple mask is made of clear, flexible, plastic or rubber that can be molded to fit the face.
- ❖ It is held to the head with elastic bands. Some have a metal clip that can be bent over the bridge of the nose for a comfortable fit.
- ❖ It delivers 35–60% oxygen. A flow rate of 6–10 L/minute.
- ❖ It has vents on its sides which allow room air to leak in at many places, thereby diluting the source oxygen.
- ❖ Often it is used when an increased delivery of oxygen is needed for short periods (i.e., less than 12 hours).

Partial Rebreather Mask (Fig. 7.8)

- ❖ The mask is have with a reservoir bag must romaine inflated during both inspiration and expiration.
- ❖ It collection of the first parts of the patients' exhaled air.
- ❖ It is used to deliver oxygen concentrations up to 80%.
- ❖ The oxygen flow rate must be maintained at a minimum of 6 L/min to ensure that the patient does not rebreathe large amounts of exhaled air.
- ❖ The remaining exhaled air exits through vents.

Nonrebreather Mask (Fig. 7.9)

- ❖ This mask provides the highest concentration of oxygen (95–100%) at a flow rate 6–15 L/min
- ❖ It is similar to the partial rebreather mask except one-way valves prevent conservation of exhaled air.

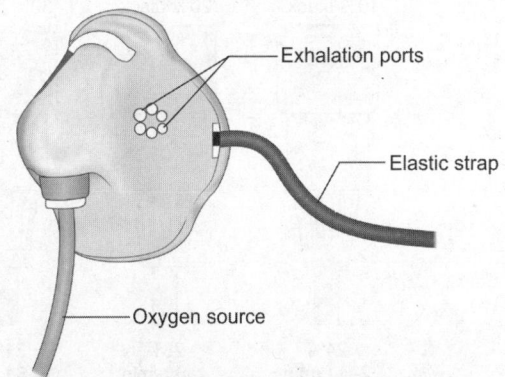

Fig. 7.7: Simple oxygen mask.

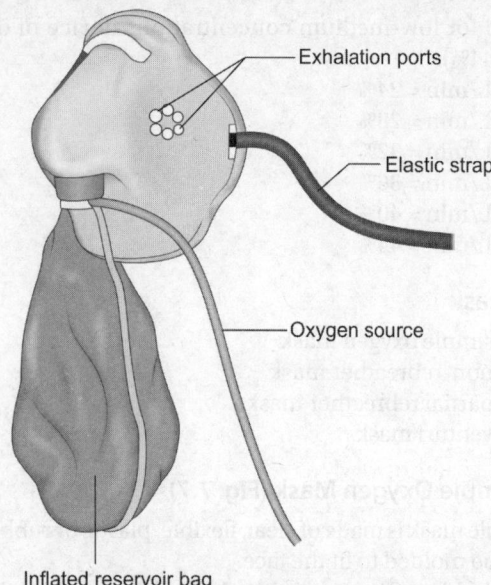

Fig. 7.8: Partial rebreather mask.

- When the patient exhales air the one-way valve closes and all of the expired air is deposited into the atmosphere
- The bag is an oxygen reservoir bag.

Venturi Mask (Figs. 7.10 and 7.11)

- It is high flow concentration of oxygen.
- Oxygen from 40% to 50%
- At liters flow of 4–15 L/min
- The mask is so constructed that there is a constant flow of room air blended with a fixed concentration of oxygen.
- It is designed with wide-bore tubing and various color coded jet adapters.
- Each color code corresponds to a precise
- Oxygen concentration and a specific liter flow.

The Venturi System

- Room air dilutes the oxygen entering the tubing to a certain concentration
- The amount of air drawn in is determined by the size of the orifice (jet adapter).

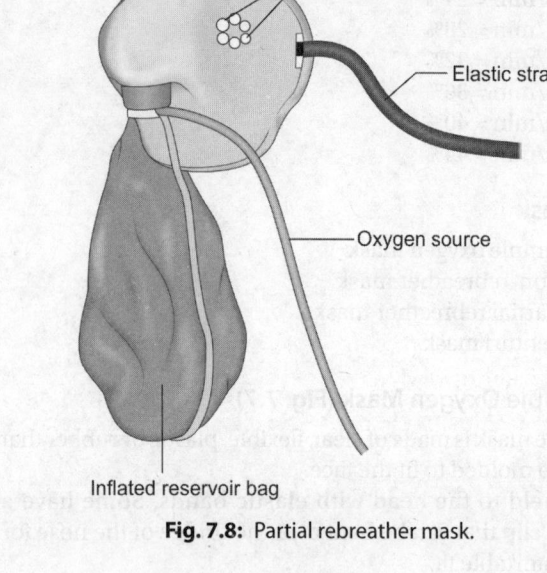

Fig. 7.9: Nonrebreather mask.

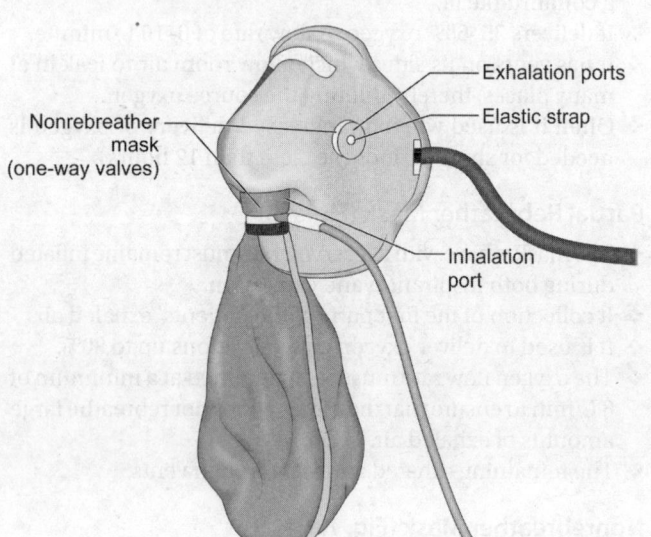

Fig. 7.11: Venturi mask.

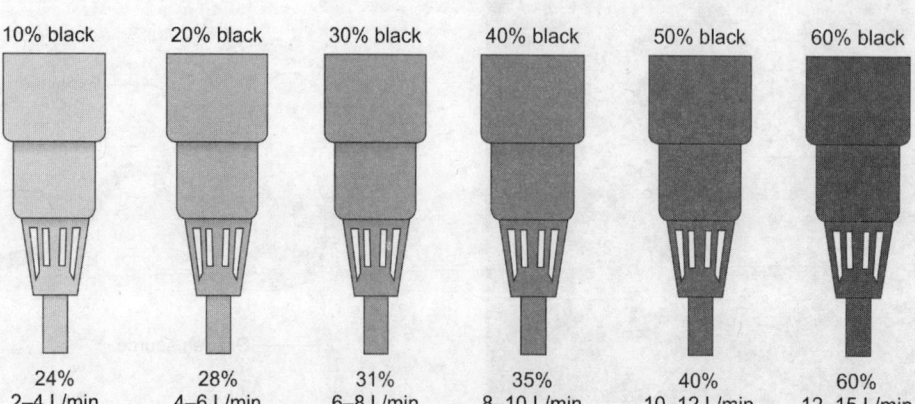

Fig. 7.10: Color coding of venturi mask adapter valves.

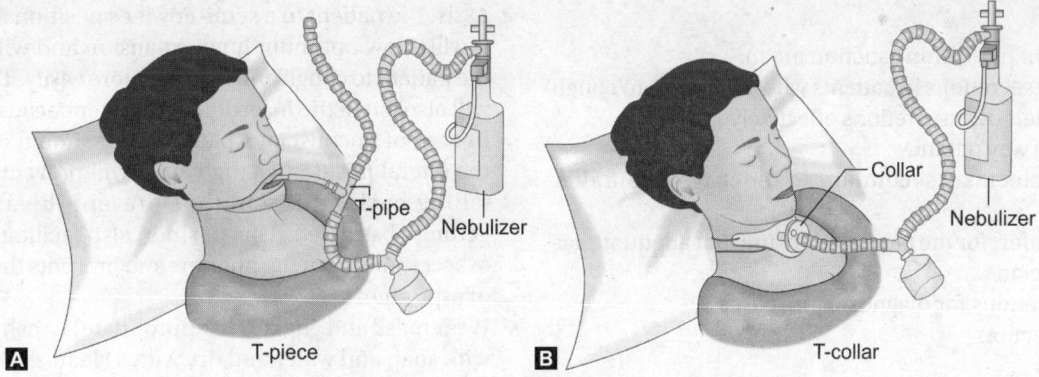

Figs. 7.12A and B: Tracheostomy.

Tracheostomy Collar/Mask (Figs. 7.12A and B)

- Inserted directed into trachea
- It is indicated for chronic O_2 therapy need
- O_2 flow rate 8–10 L
- Provides accurate FiO_2
- Provides good humidity
- Comfortable, more efficient
- Less expensive.

Hazards of Oxygen Administration

- Infection
- Drying of the mucus membranes
- Combustion
- O_2 toxicity
- Atelectasis
- Retrolental fibroplasias
- Asphyxia.

Articles

A tray containing:
- Nasal catheter/Cannula/O, mask
- A bowl with water
- Gauze pieces (wet and dry)
- No smoking indication
- Swab sticks and normal saline.

Steps of Procedure Preprocedural Steps

- Check the name and other identification of patient
- Check the diagnosis and need for oxygen
- Check the doctors order for initiation of the therapy
- Check the doctors order for specific positioning of the patient
- Check the patients vital signs
- Arrange the articles and select the most appropriate and comfortable oxygen delivery device.

Intraprocedural Steps

- Wash hands
- Clean the cannula/catheter mask firstly with wet gauze then with dry gauze.
- Attach the cannula/catheter mask to O, tubing and humidified 0, source adjusted to prescribe flow rate
- Check the flow of O_2 by dipping the tip of cannula into bowl of water.
- Place tips of cannula into patient's nares, if mask is applied snuggly to face.
- Check cannula/equipment every 8 hour.
- Keep humidification jar filled at all times
- Observe the patients nares and superior surface of both ears and skin.
- Check the O, flow rate Inspect the patient for relief of symptoms associated with hypoxia.
- Record procedure in the nurses record.

Postprocedural Steps

- Stay with the patient.
- Keep the patient warm and comfortable Evaluate the patient progress by observing the vital signs.
- Watch the patient for any deteriorating symptoms after the removal of O_2 inhalation.
- Record date and time.
- Take all the articles to utility room.
- Clean nasal catheter with wet and dry gauze piece and replace them back.

Special Considerations

- Safety precautions with oxygen therapy NO SMOKING sign should be placed on the patient's bedside.
- All electrical equipment's in the room must be functioning correctly and properly grounded (prevents fire hazards).
- Administer very low rate (2–3 L/min) of oxygen to patients with COPD Always check the oxygen level of portable cylinder before transporting the patient outside the unit.
- Since oxygen is a drug, it should be prescribed and administered in specific doses.
- Monitor saturation with a pulse oximeter when a patient is on oxygen therapy.

SUCTIONING

Introduction

Suctioning (endotracheal, oropharyngeal, nasopharyngeal and tracheostomy tube) is the method of clearing tracheal/oral/nasal secretions by the application of negative pressure using an appropriate size catheter. It could be required in an emergency or as a part of the patient's planned care.

Purposes

The purposes of performing suction are to:
- Remove the secretions in patients who are unable to cough and clear their own secretions effectively
- Maintain airway patency
- Prevent atelectasis secondary to blockage of smaller airways
- Provide comfort for the patient to ensure that adequate gas exchange occurs.
- Collect secretions for diagnostic purposes
- Prevent infection

Articles

Sterile Tray
- Sterile container for fluids
- Sterile drapes/towel

Clean Tray
- Mask
- Goggles and gown if necessary
- Kidney tray
- Sterile normal saline or water to flush and lubricate the suction catheter
- Stethoscope
- Sterile suction catheter (no. 8–10 Fr: children; and 12–16 Fr: adult)
- AMBU bag

Other
- Portable or wall suction with tubing and reservoir
- 100% oxygen source
- Resuscitation trolley

Procedure

Preprocedural
- Assess secretions in airway with or without the stethoscope and the rate and depth of respiration to determine the need for suctioning
- Check vital signs.
- Explain the procedure to the patient and the relatives regarding the need for suctioning.
- Gather all the articles at bedside
- Check the functioning of the suction machine
- If patient is on mechanical ventilator put patient on 100% oxygen
- Assess the condition of stoma for redness and swelling
- Ask the patient to blink eyes or raise a finger to indicate pain or distress during the procedure
- Keep extra tracheostomy tube and obturator at bedside
- Provide privacy
- Perform chest physiotherapy
- To dislodge the secretions
- Wash hands thoroughly and wear mask and gown (optional)

Intraprocedural
- Explain the purpose of the procedure to the patient and family/caregivers and offer them reassurance. Explain that the procedure is likely to be little uncomfortable.
- Assist the patient to a semi-Fowler's position if conscious. It will allow optimum lung expansion and will also allow the patient to cough and breathe more easily. This position will also aid in the insertion of catheter because of gravity.
- In case of unconscious patient, they should be placed in the lateral position facing you. It will prevent the tongue falling backwards and thus prevent the airway from getting obstructed. This position also facilitates drainage of secretions from the pharynx and prevents the possibility of aspiration
- Wear mask and goggles (if appropriate). Wash your hands with soap and water and dry with a clean cloth/towel
- Open the sterile tracheostomy set. Take out the towel and place on the patient's chest. Pour sterile normal saline in the container
- Open the sterile supplies, i.e., sterile catheter from the catheter pack and sterile gauze pieces into the sterile tray. Don sterile gloves
- Preoxygenate the patient with 100% oxygen to prevent hypoxemia
- Keep the dominant hand sterile and the nondominant hand clean. Pick up catheter with dominant hand (sterile hand) and the connecting tube with non-dominant hand (clean hand). Attach catheter to tubing using sterile technique
- Place catheter end into sterile saline. Test equipment by applying thumb of nondominant hand over open port to create suction
- Check the pressure by placing a tip of the finger over the end of the tube.
- Using clean hand, disconnect the patient from ventilator or any other oxygen source on which the patient is and place these tubings on the sterile towel
- Lubricate the catheter by dipping it into the container of sterile saline for easy insertion
- Turn on the suction source with clean hand
- Pinch the catheter if there is no 'Y' port and insert it into the tracheal/endotracheal tube (during inspiration when glottis is open) without applying suction. Using suction while inserting catheter can cause trauma to mucosa and removes oxygen from the respiratory tract
- Advance catheter about 6–8 inches or until you feel resistance. This usually means the catheter tip has reached the bifurcation of the trachea. Withdraw the catheter 1–2 cm before applying suction.
- Apply suction by releasing thumb from 'Y' port or by releasing the pinch on the catheter while withdrawing the catheter. Gently rotate the catheter with the thumb and index finger of the sterile gloved hand. It will help in properly cleaning the surface of respiratory tract and preventing injury to the mucosa.
- Limit suctioning time to 10 seconds per suction episode to prevent hypoxemia
- Clean the catheter in between each suction by dipping the catheter into the normal saline.
- Allow the patient to take 3–4 deep breaths between suction or encourage for coughing (if possible). Replace the oxygen delivery system

- Repeat the suctioning until the airway is clean. The patient should be re-assessed after each pass of the catheter to assess hypoxia and distress. Suctioning should not be more than four times per suction episode to prevent complications
- Return the patient to the ventilator or any other oxygen delivery system on which the patient was when the airway becomes clean
- Suction the oral secretions from the oropharynx after removing the oxygen mask if present.
- Move the catheter to oral cavity, until secretions are cleared
- Without applying suction, insert the catheter gently along the side of the mouth. Advance to oropharynx. Suction the oropharynx
- Replace the oxygen mask
- Rinse the catheter with normal saline/water until the tubings are cleared off secretions
- Turn off the suction machine. Disconnect the catheter from the suction tubings.

Postprocedural

- Remove gloves properly (inside out) and dispose off all the disposable supplies in the appropriate receptacles. Replace the articles.
- Clean AMBU bag with alcohol swab
- Assist the patient to a comfortable position. Auscultate over lung area.
- Wash hands
- Oral hygiene may be performed as per requirement.
- Documentation

TRACHEOSTOMY SUCTIONING

Definition

Tracheostomy is an artificial opening which requires being maintained secretion free, thereby insuring adequate ventilation for the patient.

Purposes

- To clear secretions from the artificial airway or tracheo-bronchial tree
- To maintain the patency of tracheostomy tube
- To ensure maximum ventilation of the patient
- To reduce the risk of respiratory infection.

Equipments

- A clean tray
- Sterile suction catheters size 14, 16 adult 10, 12 pediatric with thumb control
- Sterile gloves
- Sterile towel
- Sterile container and water or normal saline or flushing the catheter and tubing
- Normal saline for installation
- Sterile syringe 2 mL, 5 mL
- Resuscitation bag with reservoir connected to 100% oxygen source. Add positive end expiratory pressure valve to exhalation valve on resuscitation bag in an amount equal to that on the ventilator or (PAP, CPAP device)
- Receptacle for disposables
- Suction apparatus, e.g., portable machine or wall suction set at 80–120 mm Hg.

Preliminary Assessment

- Check physician's order, progress notes and nursing care plan.
- Explain the procedure to the patient. Include instructions on how to splint the surgical incision as coughing will be induced during the procedure.
- Ensure the patient's privacy.
- Position the patient in suitable position.
- Monitor heart rate, respiration rate and type, and arterial blood pressure. If blood gases are ordered, know baseline values.
- Collect and assemble equipment. Check function of suction and resuscitation bag connected to 100% oxygen source.
- Wash and dry hands.

Procedures

- Open sterile towel and place in bib-like fashion on patient's chest.
- Open sterile gloves and place on sterile field.
- If the patient is attached to ventilator test to ensure that disconnection of ventilator may be with one hand.
- Fill the sterile container with sterile water.
- Open the end of the pack containing the suction catheter and connect it to the tubing of the suction machine.
- Don sterile gloves, designation dominant hand for aseptic technique. Other hand is used to disconnect the patient from ventilator.
- Using the contaminated hand disconnect the patient from the ventilator CPAP device or other oxygen source.
- Ventilate and oxygenate the patient with the resuscitator bag 5–6 times. In the spontaneously breathing patient coordinate ventilation with patients own inspiratory effort.
- Slide the cover off the catheter and rinse it through with sterile water/saline to lubricate it.
- Insert the catheter into the tracheostomy as for as possible without applying suction.
- Apply suction and quickly rotate the catheter while it is being withdrawn.
- Limit suction time 10–15 seconds. Discontinue if heart rate decreases by 20 beats per minute of if cardiac ectopy is observed.
- Ventilate the patient between suction with 4–5 manual ventilation.
- Sterile normal saline 2–3 mL may be instilled into the airway followed by manual ventilation then suction.
- Rinse catheter between suctioning. Procedure with sterile water/saline.
- Continue procedure as necessary to a maximum of 4 suction passes.
- Give the patient 6–8 'sigh' breathes with the bag.
- Return the patient to the ventilator or apply CPAP or other oxygen delivery device.

- Suck oral secretions from the oropharynx above the artificial cuff.
- Deliver tracheostomy care as required.
- If patient is not an respiratory assistance apply filter or humidifier as indicated.
- Check vital signs.
- Leave the patient as comfortable as possible.
- Clear and clean equipment.
- Wash and dry hands.
- Document the procedure including patient's response in appropriate nursing notes.

CHEST PHYSIOTHERAPY

Chest physiotherapy (CPT) is a group of therapies used in combination to mobilize pulmonary secretions. These therapies include postural drainage, chest percussion, and vibration. Chest physiotherapy should be followed by productive coughing and suctioning of the client who has a decreased ability to cough. Chest physiotherapy is recommended for clients who produce greater than 30 cc of sputum per day or have evidence of atelectasis by chest X-ray examination.

Guidelines for Chest Physiotherapy

Nursing care and selection of chest physiotherapy (CPT) skills are based on specific assessment findings. The following guidelines help the nurse in physical assessment and subsequent decision making:
- **Know the client's normal range of vital signs:** Conditions, such as atelectasis and pneumonia requiring CPT can affect vital signs. The degree of change is related to the level of hypoxia, overall cardiopulmonary status, and tolerance to activity.
- **Know the client's medications,** certain medications, particularly diuretics and antihypertensive cause fluid and hemodynamic changes. These may decrease the client's tolerance to the positional changes of postural drainage. Steriod medications increase the client's risk of pathological rib fractures and often contraindicate rib shaking.
- **Know the client's medical history:** Certain conditions, such as increased intracranial pressure, spinal cord injuries, and abdominal aneurysm resection contraindicate the positional changes of postural drainage. Thoracic trauma or surgery may also contraindicate percussion, vibration, and rib shaking.
- **Know the client's level of cognitive function:** Participation in controlled coughing techniques requires the client to follow instructions. Congenital or acquired cognitive limitations may later the client's ability to learn and participate in these techniques.
- **Be aware of the client's exercise tolerance:** CPT maneuvers are fatiguing. When the client is not used to physical activity, initial tolerance to the maneuvers may be decreased. However, with gradual increases in activity and planned CPT client tolerance for the procedure improves.

Chest Percussion

- Chest percussion involves striking the chest wall over the area being drained. The hand is positioned so that the fingers and thumb touch and the hand is cupped.
- Percussion on the surface of the chest wall sends wave of varying amplitude and frequency through the chest, changing the consistency and location of the sputum.
- Chest percussion is performed by alternating hand motion against the chest wall.
- Percussion is performed over a single layer of clothing, not over buttons, snaps, or zippers. The single layer of clothing prevents slapping the client's skin. Thicker or multiple layers of material dampen the vibrations.
- Percussion is contraindicated in clients with bleeding disorders, osteoporosis, or fractured ribs.
- Caution should be taken to percuss the lung fields and not the scapular regions, or trauma may occur to the skin and underlying musculoskeletal structure.

Vibration

- Vibration is a fine, shaking pressure applied to the chest wall only during exhalation.
- This technique thought to increase the velocity and turbulence of exhaled air, facilitating secretion removal.
- Vibration increases the exhalation of trapped air and may shake mucus loose and induce a cough.

Postural Drainage

Postural drainage is the procedure to drain pulmonary secretions by gravity into the major bronchi or trachea and is accomplished by sequential repositioning of the patient. Usually, secretions drain best with the patient positioned so that the bronchi are perpendicular to the floor. Example Lower and middle lobe bronchi empty best with the patient in the head-down position and upper lobe bronchi, in the head-up position.

Position of Patients for Postural Drainage

Lower Lobes Posterior Basal Segments

Provide prone position to the patient with head lowered by elevating the foot of the bed by 30°. Position pillows under his chest and abdomen. Percuss his lower ribs on both sides of his spine **(Fig. 7.13)**.

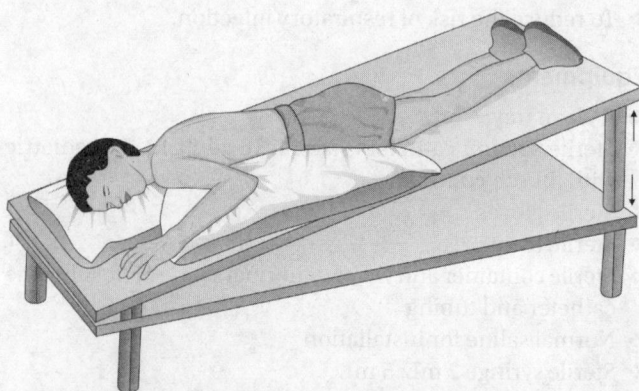

Fig. 7.13: Lower lobes posterior basal segments.

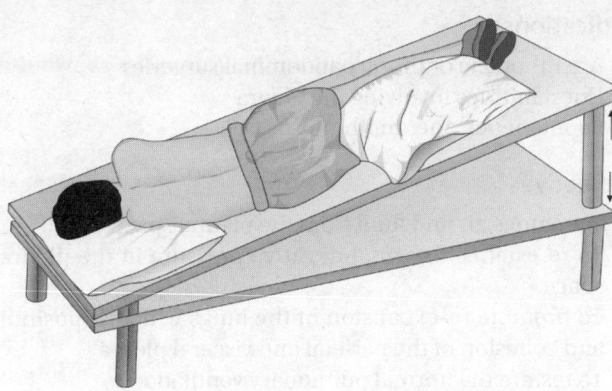

Fig. 7.14: Lower lobes lateral basal segments.

Lower Lobes: Lateral Basal Segments

Elevate the foot of the bed by 30° Instruct the patient to lie on his abdomen with his head lowered and his upper leg flexed over a pillow for support. Then make him rotate a quarter turn upward. Percuss his lower ribs on the uppermost portion of his lateral chest wall (**Fig. 7.14**)

Lower Lobes: Anterior Basal Segments

Elevate the foot of the bed by 30. Instruct the patient to be on his side with his head lowered. Then place pillows as Percuss with a slightly cupped hand over his lower ribs just beneath the axilla. If an acutely-ill patient has trouble breathing this position, adjust the bed to an angle he can tolerate. Then begin percussion (**Fig. 7.15**).

Lower Lobes: Superior Segments

With the bed flat, have the patient lie on his abdomen. Place two pillows under his hips. Percuss on both sides of his spine at the lower tip of his scapulae (**Fig. 7.16**).

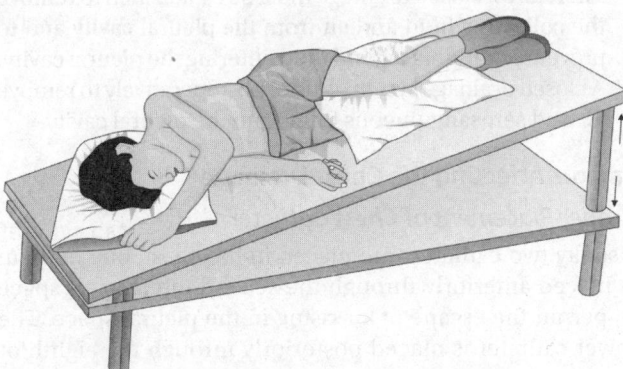

Fig. 7.15: Lower lobes anterior basal segments.

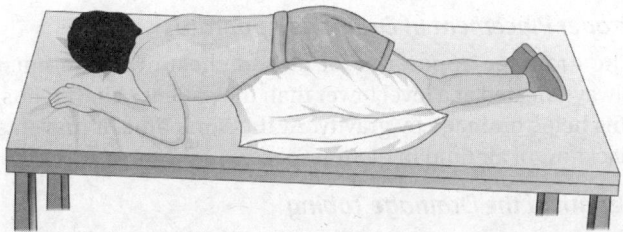

Fig. 7.16: Lower lobes: Superior segments.

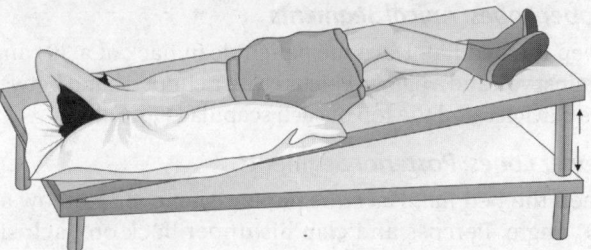

Fig. 7.17: Right middle lobe: Medial and lateral segments.

Right Middle Lobe: Medial and Lateral Segments

Elevate the foot of the bed by 15%. Have the patient lie on his left side with his head down and his knees flexed. Then have him a quarter turn backward. Place a pillow beneath him. Percuss with your hand moderately cupped under the right Apple. For a woman, cup your hand so that its heel is under the armpit and your fingers extend forward beneath the breast (**Fig. 7.17**).

Left Upper Lobes: Superior and Inferior Segments, Lingular Portion

Elevate the of the bed by 15" Have the patient lie on his right side with his head down and knees flexed. Then make mitate a quarter turn backward, place a pillow behind him, from shoulders to hips. Percuss with your hand moderately upped over his left nipple. For a woman, cup your hand so that its heel is beneath the armpit and your fingers extend forward beneath the breast (**Fig. 7.18**).

Upper Lobes: Anterior Segments

Make sure the bed is flat. Have the patient lie on his back with a pillow folded under his knees. Then make him rotate slightly away from the side being drained. Percuss between his clavicle and nipple (**Fig. 7.19**).

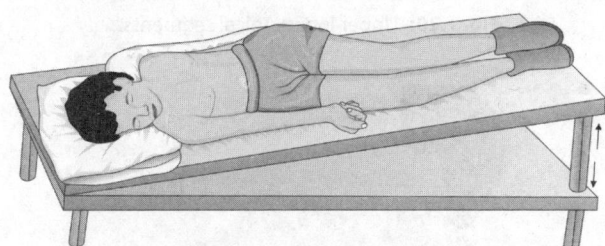

Fig. 7.18: Left upper lobes superior and inferior segments, lingular portion.

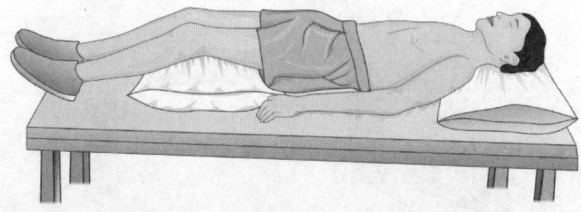

Fig. 7.19: Upper lobes: Anterior segments.

Upper Lobes: Apical Segments

Keep the bed flat. Have the patient lean back at a 30° angle against you and a pillow. Percuss with a cupped hand between his clavicles and the top of each scapula (**Fig. 7.20**).

Upper Lobes: Posterior Segments

Keep the bed flat. Have the patient lean over a pillow at a 30° angle. Percuss and clap his upper back on each side (**Fig. 7.21**).

Care of Water Seal Chest Drainage

- Water seal chest drainage means that a column of water in a bottle seals off the atmospheric air preventing from entering the chest drainage tube and thereby in the pleural space.
- Water seal drainage system are so called "closed chest drainage" is intended to allow air and flew to escape from the pleural space with each exhalation and to prevent that return flow with each inhalation.
- Water seal acts as an one way valve, permitting the unit–directional flow of air and fluid out of the pleural space, but permitting none to enter from the drainage system.

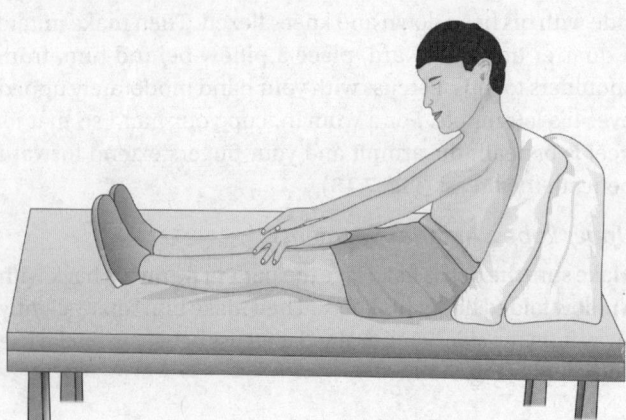

Fig. 7.20: Upper lobes: Apical segments.

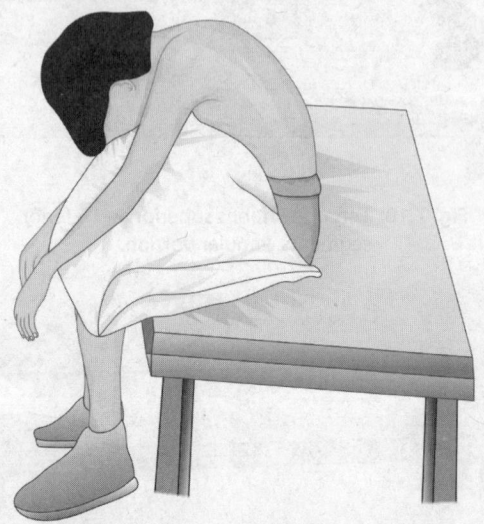

Fig. 7.21: Upper lobes: Posterior segments.

Indications

- After thoracic or thoracoabdominal surgeries
- Chest injuries involving the pleura
- Spontaneous pneumothorax.

Objectives

- To remove air and fluid from the pleural space
- To re-establish normal negative pressure in the pleural space
- To promote re-expansion of the lungs which apposition and cohesion of the parietal and visceral pleura
- To restore the normal pulmonary ventilation
- To prevent the reflex (Return flow) of air and fluid back into the pleural space from the drainage apparatus
- To prevent shifting of the mediastinum and collapse of the lung tissue by equalizing pressure on both sides.

Mechanisms

- In a thoracic surgery, the parietal pleura is incised and pleural space is opened.
- Atmospheric air rushes into the pleural space and the lungs collapse.
- When the chest wall is closed, the air is enclosed in the pleural space thus causing to have a pneumothorax in the operated site.
- Additional air may continue to leak into the pleural space through the openings in the pulmonary pleural incision.
- Trauma of surgery causes serosanguineous fluid to collect in the patient's chest until healing occurs.
- Negative pressure has been lost inside the space owing to pneumothorax.
- The body's ability to absorb air from the pleural cavity is limited.
- Therefore a closed drainage must be established to remove the collecting fluid and air from the pleural cavity and to prevent additional air and fluid entering the pleural cavity.
- A closed drainage system is used postoperatively to remove air and serosanguineous fluid from the pleural cavity.

Factors Affecting the Chest Drainage

Proper Placement of Chest Catheter

Usually two catheters are placed in the chest, one of them is placed anteriorly through the second intercostals space to permit the escape of air rising in the pleural space. The lower catheter is placed posteriorly through the eighth or ninth intercostals space in the maxillary line to drain off serosanguineous fluid accumulating in the lower portion of the pleural space.

Proper Placement of Drainage Apparatus

The drainage apparatus for closed chest drainage must always located at a level lower than the patient's chest. Thus, this helps drainage by gravity. At the same time, it prevents backflow of air fluid in pleural space.

Length of the Drainage Tubing

Drainage tubing which connect the chest catheters to the drainage apparatus should be neither too long nor too short.

It should fall in a straight line to the drainage apparatus with no dependent loops. Dependent loops of the tubing, that contain fluids obstruct the flow of air and water into the drainage bottle and create back pressure thus impairing the drainage of air or fluid.

Maintaining Patency of Tubings
Maintaining the patency of the drainage tubing and the chest catheter are checked frequently. Kinks and pressure on the tubing will cause obstruction in the flow of drainage. Observe the amount of drainage per hour to make sure that the tube is not internally plugged with pus or blood clots. Milking the tube helps to dislodge any clot that is formed in the drainage tubes.

Maintenance of an Air-tight Drainage System
Closed drainage system must be maintained air-tight. The bottles are sealed with tight stoppers and all connection of the tubes are taped to ensure its air tightness.

Position of the Patient
The patient is placed in a Fowler's position. This position helps to locate the fluid in the lower portion of the pleural space and drainage through the chest tubes, which are placed in the lower chest.

Activity of the Patient
The movement of the patient in bed helps to drain the chest. Coughing and deep breathing exercises help the patient to promote lung expansion and expulsion of air and fluid from the pleural space by increasing the intrapulmonic and intrapleural pressure.

Application of mechanical suction on the water seal drainage system:
- Continuous and gentle cough and respirations are too weak to force the air and fluid out of the pleural space through the chest catheters.
- In the treatment of empyema, thoracic drainage is too thick to drain.
- In those patients where air is leaking into the pleural space faster it can be removed by a water seal apparatus to speed up the removal of air or fluid out of the pleural space.

Types of Chest Drainage

The Single Bottle Water Seal System (Fig. 7.22)
- The end of the drainage tube from the patient's chest is covered by a layer of water which permits drainage and prevents lung collapse by sealing out the atmosphere.
- Functionally, drainage prevents lung collapse by sealing out the atmosphere.
- Functionally, drainage depends on gravity, on the mechanism of respiration and if desired on suction by the addition of controlled vacuum.
- The tube from the patient extends approximately 2.5 cm below the level of the water in the container. There is a vent for the escape of any air that might be leaking from the lung. The water level fluctuates as the patient exhales.
- At the end of the drainage tube bubbling may/may not be visible. Bubbling can mean either persistent leakage of air from the lung or other tissues or a leak in the system.

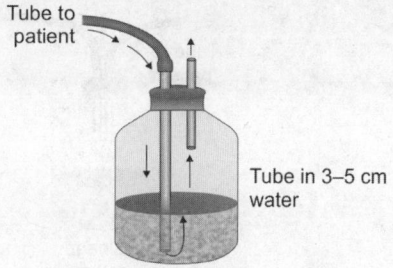

Fig. 7.22: Water seal system: Single bottle system.

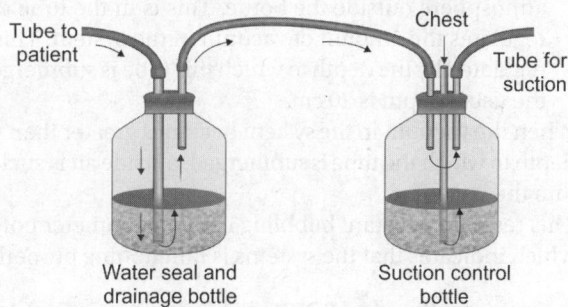

Fig. 7.23: Water seal system: Two bottle system.

The Two Bottle System (Fig. 7.23)
- The two bottle system consists of the same water seal chamber plus a fluid collection bottle.
- Drainage is similar to that of a single unit, except that when pleural fluid drains, the under water seal system in not effected by the volume of drainage.
- Effective drainage depends on gravity or on the amount of a suction added to the system.
- When vacuum is added to the system, from a vacuum source, such as wall suction, the connection is made at the vent stem of the underwater seal bottle.
- The amount of suction applied to the system is regulated to the wall gauge.

The Three Bottle System (Fig. 7.24)
- This system is similar in all respect to the two bottle system, except for the addition of a third bottle to control the amount of suction applied.
- The amount of suction is determined by the depth to which the tip of the venting glass tube is submerged.
- In the three bottles system drainage depends on gravity or the amount of suction applied.
- The amount of suction in the system is controlled by the manometer bottle. The mechanical suction motor or wall suction creates and maintains a negative pressure throughout the entire closed drainage system.
- The manometer bottle regulates the amount of the vacuum in the system. This bottle contains three tubes:
  • A short tube above the water level comes from the water seal bottle.
  • Another short tube leads to the vacuum or suction motor or wall suction.
  • The third tube is a long tube which extends below the water level in the bottle and which is open to the

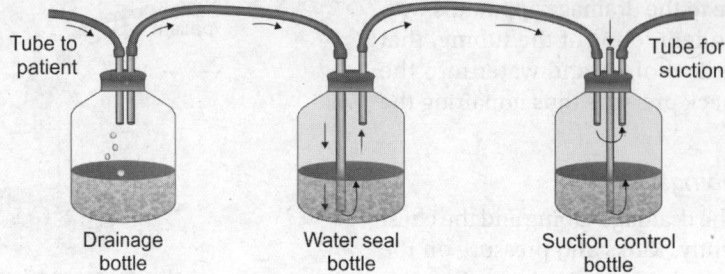

Fig. 7.24: Water seal system: Three bottle system.

atmosphere outside the bottle. This is in the tube that regulates the amount of vacuum in the system. This is regulated by the depth to which this tube is submerged. the usual depth is 20 cm.
- When the vacuum in the system becomes greater than the depth to which the tube is submerged, outside air is sucked into the system.
- This result in constant bubbling in the manometer bottle, which indicates that the systems is functioning properly.

Commercially Prepared Disposable Drainage Systems
- Combine drainage collection, water seal and suction control in one unit.
- These systems ensure patient safety with positive and negative pressure relief valves and have a prominent air leak indicator.
- Some systems produce no bubbling sound.
- System allows air and fluid to escape from the pleural cavity but does not allow the air to re-enter.
- The system may include one, two or three bottles to collect drainage, create a water seal, and control suction or it may be a self-contained disposable system.
- That combines the features of a multi-bottle system in a compact, one piece unit.

Equipment
- Thoracic drainage system which can function as gravity.
- Drainage systems to be connected to suction to enhance chest drainage.

Preparation of the Equipment
- Check the doctor's order to determine the type of drainage system to be used and specific procedural details, if appropriate, request the drainage system and suction system from the central supply department.
- Collect the appropriate equipment and take it to the patient's bedside.

Implementations
- Explain the procedure to the patient and wash your hands.
- Maintain sterile technique throughout the entire procedure and whenever you make changes in the system or alter any of the connections to avoid introducing pathogens into the pleural space.

Setting up a Commercially Prepared Disposable System
- Open the packaged system and placed it on the floor in the rack which is supplied by the manufacture to avoid accidental knocking it over or dislodging the components. After the system is prepared, it may be hung from the side of the patient's bed.
- Remove the plastic connector from the short tube that is attached to the water seal chamber. Using a 50 mL catheter tip syringe instill sterile distilled water into the water seal chamber.
- If suction is ordered, remove the cap on the suction control chamber to open the vent. Next instill sterile distilled water until it reaches the 0 cm mark on the ordered level and recap the suction control chamber.
- Using the long tube connect the patient's tube to the closed drainage system of suction source, and turn on the suction. Gentle bubbling should begin in the suction chamber, indicating that the correct suction level has been reached.

Managing Closed Chest Underwater Seal Drainage
- Repeatedly note the character, consistency and amount of drainage collection chamber.
- Mark the drainage level in the drainage collection chamber by noting the time and date at the drainage level on the chamber every 8 hours.
- Check the water level in the water seal chamber every 8 hours, if necessary; carefully add sterile distilled water until level reaches the 2 cm mark indicated on the water seal chamber of the commercial system.
- Check for fluctuation in the water seal chamber as the patient breathes. Check for fluctuation when a suction system is being used, momentary disconnect the suction system.
- Check the water level in the suction control chamber. Detach the chamber or bottle or bottle from the suction chamber when the bubbling ceases, observe the water level if necessary add sterile distilled water to bring the level to the 20 cm line or as ordered.
- Check for gentle bubbling in the suction of contra-chamber because it indicates that the proper suction level has been reached.
- Periodically check that the air vent in the system is working properly. Occlusion of the air vent results in a build up of pressure in the system that could cause the patient to develop a tension pneumothorax.
- Coil the systems tubing and secure it to the edge of the bed with a rubber band or tape and a safety pin. Avoid creating dependent loops, kinks or pressure on the tubing.
- Be sure to keep two rubbers tipped clamps at the bedside to clamp the chest tube if a bottle breaks or the commercially

prepared system cracks and to locate and air leak in the system.
- Encourage the patient to cough frequently and breathe deeply to help drain the pleural space and expand the lungs.
- Check the rate and quality of the patient's respirations and auscultate his lungs periodically to assess air exchange in the affected lung.
- Tell the patient to report any breathing difficulty immediately. Notify the doctor immediately if the patient develops cyanosis rapid or shallow breathing, subcutaneous emphysema, chest pain or excessive bleeding.
- When clots are visible you may be able to strip the tubing depending on your facility policy. This is a controversial procedure because it creates high negative pressure that could suck viable lung tissue into the drainage.
- Check the chest tube dressing at least every 8 hours. Palpate the area surrounding that dressing for crepitus or subcutaneous emphysema, which indicates that air is leaking into the subcutaneous tissue surrounding the insertion site.
- Encourage active or passive range of motion (ROM) exercises for the patient's arm or the affected side if he has been splints his arm to decrease his discomfort.
- Remind the ambulatory patient to keep the drainage system below chest level and to be careful not to disconnect the tubing to maintain the water seal.

Assessment of Proper Functioning

- Observing the oscillating movements of the fluid up and down in the water-sealed tube.
- Observing the intermittent bubbling in the water seal bottle.
- Observing the collection of drainage in the water seal or drainage bottles.
- Observing the periodic emptying of the suction control tube and bubbling in the suction control bottle when a mechanical suction is attached to the under water seal drainage system.
- Ascertain the status of the patient by assessing vital signs and the appearance frequently.

Precautions to be Taken While Replacing the Chest Drainage Bottles

- Assemble the bottle with tight stopper and tubes and check for there proper functioning.
- Double clamp to prevent entry of air into the pleural cavity.
- Clamps are applied at the end of a full inspiration to prevent the air being sucked into the pleural space.
- Disconnect the bottle to be replaced along with the drainage tubing and attach to the new set, taking care not to contaminate the end of the chest catheters.
- Be certain that the bottle is placed well before the chest level and is fixed safely to prevent falling or being kicked over accidentally.
- Unclamp the patient's chest catheter and make certain that the system is functioning properly before leaving the patient.

- Watch the patient's vital signs for few minutes to see any changes in the general conditions.

Chest Catheter Removal

- The chest catheter is removed only on the written order of the physician, and is removed by the physician.
- Usually the chest catheters are removed in two or three days, provided the remaining lung tissue is well expanded, the air leaks are absent and fluid drainage is less than 75 mL per day.
- A chest X-ray may be taken before the chest catheters are removed to make sure that the lungs are fully expanded.
- After removal of the chest catheters, the wound is covered with sterile petrolatum gauze and a firm dressing is applied over the wound which is secured with wide strips of adhesive tapes.
- After removal of the catheters the patient is observed closely for the development of respiratory distress.

Discharge Teaching

The following advice is given to these patients on discharge from the hospital.
- To have deep breathing and coughing exercise
- To maintain good nutrition
- To maintain good hygiene especially oral hygiene
- To avoid activities or environment that can cause irritation of tracheobronchial tree
- They are advised not to smoke, to avoid dusty place and to avoid exposure to the persons having respiratory infections.
- To consult the physician if symptoms of upper respiratory infections or other alignments develop
- To obtain a fitness certificate before they join their duty.

Common Problems and Suggested Actions

Lack of Drainage

Causes: Kinking, looping or pressure on the tubing may cause reflux of fluid into the intrapleural space or may impeded drainage, causing blocking of the intrapleural drain.
Nursing action: Check the system and straighten tubing as required. Secure the tubing to prevent a recurrence of the problem.

No Fluctuation of Fluid in Tubing from the Underwater Seal

Causes
- Re-expansion of the lung
- Tubing is obstructed by blood clots fibrin
- Failure of the suction apparatus.

Nursing Actions
- Ask medical staff if the drain may be removed following chest X-ray. The purpose of the drain has been fulfilled. Keeping the drain in any longer than necessary may lead to hazards from infection or air re-entry.
- "Milk" the tubing towards the drainage bottle to try to dislodge the obstruction and re-establish patency.
- Straighten tubing as required. Secure the tubing to prevent a re-occurrence. Disconnect the suction apparatus and ensure drain is patent.

Constant Bubbling of Fluid in the Drainage

Causes
An air leak in the system.

Nursing Actions
- Clamp the intrapleural drain momentarily close to the chest wall and establish whether there is a leak in the rest of the system.
- Clamping the tubing shows whether the leak is below the level of the clamp.

Patient Shows Signs of Rapid Shallow Breathing, Cyanosis, Pressure in the Chest, Subcutaneous Emphysema or Hemorrhage

Causes
Tension pneumothorax, mediastinal shift, postoperative hemorrhage, severe incision pain, pulmonary embolism or cardiac tamponade.

Nursing Actions
Observe record and report any of these signs to a doctor immediately.

Incision Pain

Nursing Actions
Provide analgesia as prescribed to reduce the patient's discomfort and to enable deep breathing exercises to be performed and mobilization to ensure adequate drainage and to avoid complications.

Accidental Disconnection of the Drainage Tubing from the Intrapleural Drain

Nursing Actions
- Apply an artery clamp to the drain immediately in order to avoid air entering the pleural space.
- Re-establish the connection as soon as possible in order to Re-establish drainage.
- If necessary use clean sterile drainage tube. Tubing may have been contaminated when it became disconnected.

Patient Needs to be Moved to Another Area

Nursing Actions
- Place the drainage bottle below the level of the intrapleural drain as close to the floor as possible in order to prevent reflux of fluid into the pleural space.
- Do not clamp the drain unless the doctor has ordered it.

Intrapleural Drain Falls Out

Nursing Actions
- Pull the purse-string suture immediately to close the wound.
- Cover the wound with an occlusive sterile dressing.
- Inform a doctor.
- The objective is to minimize the amount of air entering the pleural space.
- The drain will probably need reinserting.
- Reassure the patient with appropriate explanations.

CARE OF CLIENTS WITH CHEST TUBES

This skill requires problem solving and knowledge application unique to a professional nurse and should not be delegated. Assistive personnel may help with positioning.
- Inform and assist care provider in the proper positioning of a client with chest tubes to facilitate drainage.
- Explain to care provide what is the appropriate setup of drainage equipment for the type of system to be used.
- Instruct care provider to inform nurse of any changes in the vital sings, chest tube drainage, or excessive bubbling in water seal chamber.

Equipments
- Chest drainage system (bottles or disposable system)
- Suction source and setup (wall canister or portable)
- Nonsterile gloves
- Sterile irrigation saline or sterile water (500 mL bottle)
- Tape (2-inch width)

Steps
- Assess client for respiratory distress and chest pain, breath sounds over affected lung area, and stable vital signs.
- Observe for increased respiratory distress.
- **Observe:**
  - Chest tube dressing
  - Tubing for kinks, dependent loops, or clots
  - Chest drainage system, which should be upright and below level of tube insertion.
- Provide two hemostats for each chest tube, attached to top of the client's bed with adhesive tape. Chest tubes are only clamped under specific circumstances:
  - To assess air leak.
  - To quickly empty or change collection bottle or chamber, performed by nurse who has received training in procedure.
  - To change disposable system; have new system ready to be connected before clamping tube so that transfer can be rapid and drainage system re-established.
  - To change a broken water seal bottle in the event that no sterile solution container is available.
  - To assess if client is ready to have chest tube removed (which is done by physician's order); the nurse must monitor client for recreation of pneumothorax.
- **Position client:**
  - Semi-Flower's position to evacuate air (pneumothorax).
  - High-Flower's position to drain fluid (hemothorax).
  - Water-seal vent must be without occlusion.
  - Suction control chamber vent must be without occlusion when suction is used.
- Coil excess tubing on mattress next to client. Secure with rubber band and safety pin or system's clamp.
- Adjust tubing to hang in straight line from top of mattress to drainage chamber. If chest tube is draining fluid, indicate time (e.g., 0900) that drainage was begun on drainage

bottle's adhesive tape or one write-on surface of disposable commercial system.
- Strip or milk chest tube only if indicated:
  - Postoperative mediastinal chest tubes are manipulated if nursing assessment indicates obstruction of drainage secondary to clots or debris in rubbing.
  - Postoperative assessment is done every 15 minutes for the first 2 hours. This assessment interval then changes based on client's status.
- Wash hands.
- **Observe:**
  - Chest tube dressing, tubing, and chest tube drainage system which should be upright and below level of tube insertion.
  - Water seal for fluctuations with client's inspiration and expiration.
  - Bubbling in water seal bottle or chamber.
  - Type and amount of fluid drainage. Nurse should note colour and amount of drainage, client's vital signs, and skin color.
    - Less than 50–300 mL/hr immediately postoperative in mediastinal chest tube; approximately 500 mL in first 24 hours; dark red drainage is expected early in postoperative period, turning serous with time.
    - Between 100 and 300 mL of fluid may drain in posterior chest tube during first 2 hours, after insertion; rate will decrease after 2 hours, 500 – 1000 mL can be expected in first 24 hours; drainage will be grossly bloody during first several hours after surgery and then change to serous.
  - Bubbling in the suction-control chamber (when suction is being used).

Critical Decision Point
Review agency policy before milking or stripping chest tubes.

Recording and Reporting
Record in nurse's notes patency of chest tubes, presence of drainage, presence of fluctuations client's vital signs, chest dressing status, type of suction, and level of comfort.

Home Care Considerations
If client goes home with chest tube (i.e., empyema), teach client and family, to care tube and drainage bottle.

■ PULSE OXIMETRY

Introduction
- Pulse oximetry works on the principle that blood saturated with oxygen is of different color from blood depleted of oxygen.
- The probe for pulse oximetry contains red source and a detector.
- These shine through the tissues of the body and work together to measure the color difference between oxygenated and deoxygenated blood.
- The machine detects the pulse from an arterial blood source and is able to calculate the percentage of oxygen saturation by combining the detected color changes of the blood combined with the detected pulse of the artery.
- Because of the way the pulse oximeter works, it is susceptible to errors if, it is not able to accurately measure the transmission of light through the tissues or detect the pulse of the artery
- The oximeter consists of a light emitting diode (LED); a photodetector probe containing a permanent or disposable sensor; alarms for pulse rate and oxygen levels; a display screen and cables.
- The device works by emitting beams of red and infrared light that are passed through a pulsating arteriolar bed.
- Sensors detect the amount of light absorbed by oxyhemoglobin and deoxyhemoglobin in the red blood cells.
- The ratio of red to infrared light measured by the photo detector indicates the amount of oxygen present in the blood.
- The sensor is attached to the body over the arteriolar area in the ear, the finger tip, the big toe or across the bridge of the nose
- Clip sensors can be used on fingers and the ear lobe.

Purpose
- To measure the capillary blood oxygen saturation.
- To detect the presence of hypoxemia before visible signal develop.
- To assess the response of therapy.
- To assess the need to decrease the number of arterial blood gas specimen drawn.

Principles
- The light emitting diode emits light in wavelengths that are absorbed differently by the oxygenated and deoxygenated hemoglobin molecules.
- The amount of light transmitted through the tissues is then converted to a digital value representing the percentage of hemoglobin saturated with
- The more hemoglobin saturated by oxygen, the higher is the oxygen saturation.
- Normally oxygen saturation (SPO) is greater than 90%.

Factors Affecting Measurement of Oxygen Saturation

Insufficient Blood Flow
- The sensors in the probes, reach across to the blood to detect the saturation of oxygen.
- But in cases of poor perfusion where the blood flow is inadequate, readings will be affected greatly.
- It is a must for the blood pressure to be above 80.
- The low pressure of the blood can be caused by any of the following:
  - Cold, nerve blocker medications and fear.
  - Wrong placement of probes and compression.
  - Because of cardiac arrest.
  - Vascular impingement.
  - Tight clothing, pressure cuffs or restraints.

Increased Movement
- Patients with conditions that can lead to increased
- Moving and dislodging of the sensor, which may be caused by a rhythmic movement, such as the tremors of Parkinsonism, seizures or even shivering, may leads to inaccurate readings.
- Exercise and vibrations can also make it difficult for the pulse oximeter to determine correct reading

Nail polish
Fake fingernails might affect the readings in addition to nail polish colors as they are pigmentations and act as a hindrance for the probes and sensors.

Interference of Light
- Lights can also affect the readings of a pulse oximeter if it is too harsh.
- It can be tested by covering the light source and taking the readings again.
- The presence of any sort of radiated lights like infrared or ultraviolet have an impact on the reading.

Health Conditions
There are certain health conditions of the patient themselves that can lead to inaccurate reading for instance, patients with unreliable carboxyhemoglobin readings, methemoglobinemia, sickle cell anemia, thalassemias and anemia will always have wrong readings.

Types of Pulse Oximeters
Oximetry is a diagnostic procedure, and can be done using three devices, namely—pulse oximeter, handheld oximeter and fetal oximeter.
- Finger pulse oximeters.
- Hand-held pulse oximeters.
- Pediatric pulse oximeters.

Indications for Pulse Oximetry
- A sensor, attached to a device called a pulse oximeter, is clipped to your finger or ear, and then directs a beam of light through the tissue.
- The device is able to monitor oxygen saturation in the blood by measuring the amount of light absorbed by oxygenated hemoglobin (the oxygen-carrying pigment in red blood cells).

Pulse oximetry is indicated in following cases:
- Monitoring effectiveness of oxygen therapy.
- The need to monitor the adequacy of arterial oxyhemoglobin saturation.
- Endotracheal intubation.
- Cardiac arrest.
- Congestive heart failure (CHF).
- Procedural sedation or anesthesia.
- Hemodynamic instability (e.g., cardiac failure or myocardial infarction).
- Respiratory illnesses, e.g., asthma, chronic obstructive pulmonary disease, etc.
- Acute respiratory distress syndrome (ARDS).

Advantages/Disadvantages of Pulse Oximetry
Advantages
- Accurate/dependable.
- Fast response time.
- Non invasive.
- Multiple sensing sites.
- Continuous measurement.
- Monitors peripheral blood flow.

Disadvantages
- Poor function with poor perfusion.
- Delayed detection of hypoxic events.
- Erratic performance with irregular rhythms.
- Light interferences/deports on electricity.
- Measures functional saturation only (saturation may be falsely high when Hb is bound by carbon monoxide).
- Motion artifacts.

Steps to Procedure
- Refer to and follow care plan for the management of the patient's oxygen saturation level
- Explain the patient that oxygen saturation reading is needed and obtain consent to continue.
- Ensure the patient is comfortable and warm enough, especially if continuous monitoring is required.
- Check the probe and equipment is clean and in good working order
- Decontaminate hands. Use soap and water if hands are physically soiled, use alcohol gel, if hands appear clean
- Select a suitable area for the probe (usually fingertip).
- Other sites that may be considered includes ear lobes, bridge of nose and toes (Not all the probes are suitable for use on all sites)
- Place the probe as directed by the manufacturer's instructions assessing any barriers, such as nail varnish, nicotine staining, or dirt.
- Intravenous dyes, poor perfusion or skin pigmentation will also affect the reading
- Make sure that the probe sensor is detecting the pulse. Ensure that the patient's pulse is also checked manually
- Remove the probe and ensure that the patient is comfortable.
- Once oxygen saturation monitoring is complete, dean the reusable sensor and equipment with Tuffie wipe and return to storage as appropriate.
- Decontaminate hands. Use soap and water if hands are physically soiled, use alcohol gel if hands appear clean
- Make the patient comfortable.
- Document oxygen saturation in the patient's record and inform the patient.
- Also document the flow/concentration of any current oxygen therapy in liters/minute if the measurement was taken with patient at rest or walking
- **If the reading is outside the patient's parameters:** Check tracing strength.
- Reassure the patient and report immediately to the Case Manager or General Practitioner for further advice and guidance.

- Explain the results to patient and any necessary action needed to change current treatment plan and by when, if required
- Document all actions in patient's record

Special Considerations

Several steps can be taken to enhance accurate readings.
- If possible, the patient should be instructed not to smoke 24 hours prior to pulse oximetry.
- Fingernail polish should be removed, if the oximeter will be attached to the finger.
- For patients with poor circulation, hands should be slowly warmed with warm towels before attaching the oximeter.
- Abnormally high or low temperatures, as well as reduced hemoglobin, can influence the amount of oxygen adhering to the hemoglobin within the red blood cells, altering the reading
- Care should be taken while attaching the sensors and selecting the site for optimum reading levels.
- The sensor should be wrapped securely around the finger to prevent outside light from interfering with the reading and rendering it invalid.
- An appropriate site is chosen to monitor the oxygen levels by ensuring that there is strong arterial pulsation and that the capillary bed fills promptly, if squeezed.
- The device must not be used near flammable anesthetics.
- Older devices may be affected by motion.
- They should be checked regularly to ensure proper function.
- Explain to the patient that it is used for monitoring purposes.
- Monitor the site where the sensor has been applied every four hours for clip sensors and every six hours for wrapped sensors.
- Any loss of pulsation, swelling or change in color requires a change of site.

■ RESTORATIVE AND CONTINUING CARE

Hydration

- Normally, respiratory tract secretions are thin and are therefore, moved readily by ciliary action.
- However, when the client is dehydrated or when the environment has a low humidity, the respiratory secretions can become thick and tenacious.
- Adequate hydration maintains the moisture of the respiratory mucous membranes.
- Humidifiers are the devices that add water vapor to inspired air.
- Room humidifiers provide cool mist to room air.
- Nebulizers are used to deliver humidity and medications. They may be used with oxygen delivery systems to provide moistened air directly to the client.
- Their purposes are to prevent mucous membranes from drying and becoming irritated and to loosen secretions for easier expectoration.
- The basic function of the lung is to enable an efficient gas exchange between a complex inner aqueous body system and a dry outside atmosphere.
- Thus, the hydration status of bronchopulmonary structures contributes to the maintenance of an efficient function
- Adequate fluid intake Increased oral fluid intake as it is important to loosen secretions and also replace fluids lost through fever and increased respiratory rate.
- Drink plenty of fluids to reducing the viscosity of mucus and aids in easy expectoration.
- Steam inhalation is one of the most widely used hydration therapy and home remedy to soothe and open the nasal passages and get relief from the symptoms of both upper and lower respiratory tract infections.
- Also called steam therapy, it involves the inhalation of water vapors.
- The warm, moist air is thought to work by loosening the mucus in the nasal passages, throat, and lungs.
- Thus, may relieve symptoms due to narrowed, inflamed, swollen respiratory passages.
- **Breathing (by nose):** Encourage patient for nose breathing, in case of congestion apply a warm and moist cloth to face several times a day as it reduces nasal and sinus congestion by relieving swelling and inflammation of congested sinuses. It also helps to keep the mucous membranes moist by breathing in moist air.

Humidification

The human airway has an important role in heating and humidification of the inspired gas.

Physiological Concept

- The connective tissue of the nose is characterized by a rich vascular system of numerous and thin walled veins.
- This system is responsible for warming the inspired air to increase its humidity carrying capacity.
- As the inspired air goes down the respiratory tract, it reaches a point at which its temperature is 37°C and its relative humidity is 100%.
- The respiratory mucosa is lined by pseudostratified columnar ciliated epithelium and with numerous goblet cells.
- These cells, as well as sub-mucosal glands underneath the epithelium, are responsible for maintaining the mucous layer that serves as a trap for pathogens and as an interface for humidity exchange.
- When the upper airway is bypassed during invasive mechanical ventilation or after endotracheal intubation, as the upper airway loses its capacity to heat and moisture inhaled gas.
- This causes a burden on the lower respiratory tract, as it is not well prepared for the humidification process.
- Consequently, delivery of partially cold and dry medical gases brings about potential damage to the respiratory epithelium, manifested by increased work of breathing, atelectasis, thick and dehydrated secretions, and cough and/or bronchospasm.
- Humidifiers are devices that add molecules of water to gas.
- This is a method of artificially conditioning respiratory gas for the patient during therapy and involves humidification,

warming, and occasionally filtration of the gas being delivered.
- They are classified as active or passive based on the presence of external sources of heat and water (active humidifiers), or the utilization of patients' own temperature and hydration to achieve humidification in successive breaths (passive humidifiers).

Types of Humidifiers

Heat and Moisture Exchange Humidifiers
- Heat and Moisture Exchange humidifiers (HMEs) are devices used in mechanically ventilated patients intended to help prevent complications due to "drying of the respiratory mucosa, due to mucus plugging or/and endotracheal tube (ETT) occlusion.
- This type of humidifier use the patient's own humidity and moisture from exhalation, in order to humidify gases during inhalation.
- As soon as a patient is intubated, the upper airway is bypassed, which leads in a loss of humidification of inhaled air
- Dry air can have harmful effects for the patient, therefore to prevent causing trauma to the HME can be used as humidifier instead of the upper airway tract.

Heated Humidifiers
- Heated humidifiers typically use a hot plate beneath the water chamber to heat the water. It then sends the moisturized air through large-bore tubing to the mask (because this reduces amount of condensation in the heated wire circuit), delivering moisturized air for patient to breathe during CPAP therapy.
- Heated humidifiers operate actively to increase the heat and water vapor content of inspired gas.
- This help to alleviate dehydration, provide comfort to membranes of respiratory system, and prevent loss of body heat
- Heated humidifiers are capable of delivering gas at temperatures of 41°C (105.8°F) but a maximum gas (inspired) temperature of 37°C (98.6°F) and 100% relative humidity is recommended.

Coughing Techniques

Coughing is effective in maintaining a patent airway, Coughing permits the client to remove secretions from both the upper and lower airways.

The series of events in cough mechanism are:
- **Deep inhalation:** This increases lung volume and airway diameter. Thus air can pass to partially obstructing mucus plugs or other foreign matter.
- Closure of the glottis.
- Active contraction of the expiration muscles. When the expiratory muscles contract against the closed glottis, high intrathoracic pressure is developed.
- Opening of glottis.
  With high intrathoracic pressure, glottis is opened and a large flow of air is expelled at a high-speed providing momentum for mucus to move to the upper airway. After the cough, mucus can be expectorated or swallowed.

The various coughing techniques include cascade, huff, quad coughing, and controlled coughing:
- **Cascade cough:** Ask the client to take a slow deep breath and hold it for 2 seconds, while contracting expiratory muscles. Tell the client to open the mouth and perform a series of coughs throughout exhalation, thereby coughing at lowered lung volumes. This helps for airway clearance and maintains a patent airway in clients with large volumes of sputum.
- **Huff cough:** In this the client on exhalation opens the glottis by saying the word "huff". The huff cough stimulates a natural cough reflex. This method is useful for clearing central airway. Clients, who practice this regularly, inhale more air and may progress to cascade cough.
- **Quad cough:** This is used for client without abdominal muscle control, e.g., clients with spinal cord injuries. The client or nurse pushes inward and upward on the abdominal muscles to the diaphragm while the client breathes with maximal expiratory efforts, causing the cough.
- **Controlled coughing:** Ask the client to take two slow, deep breaths, inhaling through nose and exhaling through mouth. Inhale deeply third time and hold breath to count of 3. Cough for two or three consecutive coughs without inhaling between cough. Tell the client to push all air out of lungs. Client should be cautioned to cough properly and not just clearing the throat. Instruct the client to cough 2 or 3 times every 2 hours during walking hours.

The effectiveness of cough is determined by the amount of sputum expectorated and the client's report of swallowed sputum. Clients with upper and lower respiratory tract infections and chronic pulmonary disease should practice coughing exercise every 2 hours while they are awake and clients with copious amount of sputum must cough hourly while awake and expectorate out sputum till the acute phase of sputum production is over.

Controlled Coughing Technique Procedure
- To cough effectively
- Sit on a chair or on the edge of the bed, with both feet on the floor, lean slightly forward. Relax.
- Fold the arms across the abdomen and breathe in slowly through the nose. (The power of the cough comes from moving air)
- To exhale lean forward, pressing the arms against the abdomen. Cough 2–3 times through a slightly open mouth. Coughs should be short and sharp. The first loosens the mucus and moves it through the airways. The second and third cough enables the patient to cough the mucus up and out.
- Breathe in again by "sniffing" slowly and gently through the nose. This gentle breath helps prevent mucus from moving back down to airways.
- Rest
- Perform again, if needed.

Tips
- Avoid breathing in quickly and deeply through the mouth after coughing. Quick breaths can interfere with the

movement of mucus up and out of the lungs, and can cause uncontrolled coughing
- Drink 6–8 glasses of fluid per day unless the doctor has told to limit the fluid intake. When mucus is thin, coughing is easier.
- Use the controlled coughing technique after the use the bronchodilator medication or any time the patient feel mucus (congestion) in the airways.

Huffing Technique
- Huffing, also known as Huff coughing is a technique that helps move mucus from the lungs.
- It involves taking a breath in, holding it, and actively exhaling
- Breathing in and holding it enables air to get behind the mucus and separates it from the lung wall so it can be coughed out.
- Huffing is not as forceful as a cough, but it can work better and be less tiring, Huffing is like exhaling onto a mirror or window to steam it up.
- Huff coughing is an effective technique that the patient can be easily taught
- The goals of effective coughing are to conserve energy, reduce fatigue and facilitate the removal of secretions.

Procedure
- Sit up straight with chin tilted slightly up and mouth open.
- Take a slow deep breath to fill lungs about three quarters full.
- Hold breath for two or three seconds.
- Exhale forcefully, but slowly, in a continuous exhalation to move mucus from the smaller to the larger airways.
- Repeat this maneuver two more times and then follow with one strong cough to clear mucus from the larger airways.
- Do a cycle of four to five huff coughs as part of the airway clearance.

BREATHING EXERCISES
- Breathing exercises do not have to take a lot of time out of your day.
- It is just about setting aside time to pay attention to your breathing.
- Begin with just 5 minutes a day, and increase your time as the exercise becomes easier and more comfortable.
- If 5 minutes feels too long, start with just 2 minutes.
- Practice multiple times a day.
- Schedule set times or practice conscious breathing as you feel the need.

RESPIRATORY EXERCISES

Pursed Lip Breathing
- This simple breathing technique makes you slow down your breathing pace by having you apply deliberate effort in each breath.
- You can practice pursed lip breathing at any time.
- It may be especially useful during activities such as bending, lifting, or stair climbing.
- Practice using this breath 4–5 times a day when you begin so that you can correctly learn the breathing pattern.

To do it:
- Relax your neck and shoulders.
- Keeping your mouth closed, inhale slowly through your nose for 2 counts.
- Pucker or purse your lips as though you were going to whistle.
- Exhale slowly by blowing air through your pursed lips for a count of 4.

Diaphragmatic Breathing
- Diaphragmatic breathing (aka belly breathing) can help you use your diaphragm properly.
- Do belly breathing exercises when you are feeling relaxed and rested.
- It may also help reduce stress and help with challenges related to eating disorders, constipation, high blood pressure, migraine episodes, and other health conditions.
- Practice diaphragmatic breathing for 5–10 minutes 3–4 times daily.
- When you begin, you may feel tired, but over time the technique should become easier and should feel more natural.
- Lie on your back with your knees slightly bent and your head on a pillow.
- You may place a pillow under your knees for support.
- Place one hand on your upper chest and one hand below your rib cage, allowing you to feel the movement of your diaphragm.
- Slowly inhale through your nose, feeling your stomach pressing into your hand.
- Keep your other hand as still as possible.
- Exhale using pursed lips as you tighten your abdominal muscles, keeping your upper hand completely still.
- You can place a book on your abdomen to make the exercise more difficult.
- Once you learn how to do belly breathing lying down, you can increase the difficulty by trying it while sitting in a chair.
- You can then practice the technique while performing your daily activities.

Breath Focus Technique
- This deep breathing technique uses imagery or focus words and phrases.
- You can choose a focus word that makes you smile, feel relaxed, or is simply neutral.
- Examples include peace, let go, or relax, but it can be any word that suits you to focus on and repeat through your practice.
- As you build up your breath focus practice, you can start with a 10-minute session.
- Gradually increase the duration until your sessions are at least 20 minutes.

To do it:
- Sit or lie down in a comfortable place.
- Bring your awareness to your breaths without trying to change how you're breathing.

- Alternate between normal and deep breaths a few times.
- Notice any differences between normal breathing and deep breathing.
- Notice how your abdomen expands with deep inhalations.
- Note how shallow breathing feels compared to deep breathing.
- Practice your deep breathing for a few minutes.
- Place one hand below your belly button, keeping your belly relaxed, and notice how it rises with each inhale and falls with each exhale.
- Let out a loud sigh with each exhale.
- Begin the practice of breath focus by combining this deep breathing with imagery and a focus word or phrase that will support relaxation.
- You can imagine that the air you inhale brings waves of peace and calm throughout your body.
- Mentally say, "Inhaling peace and calm."
- Imagine that the air you exhale washes away tension and anxiety.
- You can say to yourself, "Exhaling tension and anxiety."

Lion's Breath

- Lion's breath is an energizing yoga breathing practice that is said to relieve tension in your chest and face.
- It's also known in yoga as Lion's Pose or Simhasana in Sanskrit.

To do this:

- Come into a comfortable seated position.
- You can sit back on your heels or cross your legs.
- Press your palms against your knees with your fingers spread wide.
- Inhale deeply through your nose and open your eyes wide.
- At the same time, open your mouth wide and stick out your tongue, bringing the tip down toward your chin.
- Contract the muscles at the front of your throat as you exhale out through your mouth by making a long "haaa" sound.
- You can turn your gaze to look at the space between your eyebrows or the tip of your nose.
- Do this breath 2–3 times.

Alternate Nostril Breathing

- Alternate nostril breathing, known as Nadi Shodhana Pranayama in Sanskrit, is a breathing practice for relaxation.
- Alternate nostril breathing has been shown to enhance cardiovascular function and lower heart rate.
- NadiShodhana is best practiced on an empty stomach. Avoid the practice if you are feeling sick or congested.
- Keep your breath smooth and even throughout the practice.

To do this:

- Choose a comfortable seated position.
- Lift your right hand toward your nose, pressing your first and middle fingers down toward your palm and leaving your other fingers extended.
- After an exhale, use your right thumb to gently close your right nostril.
- Inhale through your left nostril and then close your left nostril with your right pinky and ring fingers.
- Release your thumb and exhale out through your right nostril.
- Inhale through your right nostril and then close this nostril.
- Release your fingers to open your left nostril and exhale through this side.
- This is one cycle.
- Continue this breathing pattern for up to 5 minutes.
- Finish your session with an exhale on the left side.

Equal Breathing

- Equal breathing is known as SamaVritti in Sanskrit.
- This breathing technique focuses on making your inhales and exhales the same length.
- Making your breath smooth and steady can help bring about balance and equanimity.
- Research on older adults with high blood pressure showed that this technique may help improve mental well-being and increase the oxygen supply to the brain and lungs.
- You should find a breath length that is not too easy and not too difficult.
- You also do not want it to be too fast in order to maintain it throughout the practice.
- Usually, this is between 3 and 5 counts.
- Once you get used to equal breathing while seated, you can do it during your yoga practice or other daily activities.

To do it:

- Choose a comfortable seated position.
- Breathe in and out through your nose.
- Count during each inhale and exhale to make sure they are even in duration.
- Alternatively, choose a word or short phrase to repeat during each inhale and exhale.
- You can add a slight pause for breath retention after each inhale and exhale if you feel comfortable. (Normal breathing involves a natural pause.)
- Continue practicing this breath for at least 5 minutes.

Resonant or Coherent Breathing

- Resonant breathing, also known as coherent breathing, is when you breathe at a rate of 5 full breaths per minute.
- You can achieve this rate by inhaling and exhaling for a count of 5.
- Breathing at this rate maximizes your heart rate variability (HRV), reduces stress, and, can reduce symptoms of depression when combined with Iyengar yoga.

To do this:

- Inhale for a count of 5.
- Exhale for a count of 5.
- Continue this breathing pattern for at least a few minutes.

Sitali Breath

- This yoga breathing practice helps you lower your body temperature and relax your mind.
- Slightly extend your breath in length but do not force it.
- Since you inhale through your mouth during Sitali breath, you may want to choose a place to practice that's free of any allergens that affect you and air pollution.

To do this:
- Choose a comfortable seated position.
- Stick out your tongue and curl your tongue to bring the outer edges together.
- If your tongue does not do this, you can purse your lips.
- Inhale through your mouth.
- Exhale out through your nose.
- Continue breathing like this for up to 5 minutes.

Deep Breathing

Deep breathing helps to relieve shortness of breath by preventing air from getting trapped in your lungs and helping you to breathe in fresher air. It may help you to feel more relaxed and centered.

To do this:
- While standing or sitting, draw your elbows back slightly to allow your chest to expand.
- Take a deep inhalation through your nose.
- Retain your breath for a count of 5.
- Slowly release your breath by exhaling through your nose.

Humming Bee Breath (Bhramari)

- This yoga breathing practice's unique sensation helps create instant calm and is especially soothing around your forehead.
- Some people use humming bee breath to relieve frustration, anxiety, and anger.
- It may help reduce your heart rate, think more clearly, and feel less irritable or stressed.
- Of course, you will want to practice it in a place where you are free to make a humming sound.

To do this:
- Choose a comfortable seated position.
- Close your eyes and relax your face.
- Place your first fingers on the tragus cartilage that partially covers your ear canal.
- Inhale and gently press your fingers into the cartilage as you exhale.
- Keeping your mouth closed, make a loud humming sound.
- Continue for as long as is comfortable.

INCENTIVE SPIROMETRY

Introduction

- It is also referred to as a sustained maximal inspiration (SMI) device.
- Respiratory function is altered in patients who had any surgery, were on prolonged anesthesia, and were bedridden which may end up with respiratory complications.
- The incentive spirometer is given for these patients to improve air flow.

Definition

- Incentive spirometry is a procedure to improve the volume of air that is being breathed in and out of the lungs by initiating voluntary deep breathing using a specially designed incentive spirometer device.
- Assisting the patient for voluntary deep breathing by providing visual feedback about inspiratory volume by using a specially designed apparatus called spirometer.

Purposes

- To increase respiratory volume, maintain alveolar ventilation, and prevent atelectasis
- To counteract the effects of anesthesia or hypoventilation
- To reduce the chance of fluid accumulation in the lungs (e.g., rib fracture)
- To facilitate gas exchange
- To diagnose lung diseases, for example, asthma, bronchitis, or emphysema
- To improve pulmonary ventilation
- To counteract the effects of anesthesia or hypoventilation
- To loosen respiratory secretions
- To facilitate respiratory gaseous exchange
- To expand collapsed alveoli
- To prevent postoperative respiratory complications.

Indications

- Prolonged bedridden patient
- Surgery may alter respiratory functions
- Postoperative patient
- Patients recovering from
- Cardiac surgery Prolonged anesthesia
- Rib fracture
- Diseases involving respiratory muscles (chronic obstructive pulmonary disease (COPD), bronchial asthma, etc.)
- Patient's on medications that depress respiration

Contraindications

- Hemoptysis from unknown origin Pneumothorax
- Thoracic, abdominal or cerebral aneurysm (danger of rupture due to increase is thoracic pressure)
- Recent eye surgery, e.g., cataract Recent surgery of thorax, abdomen

Articles

- Incentive spirometer with appropriate mouthpiece (Fig. 7.25)
- Flow-oriented or Volume-oriented
- Sputum mug with disinfectant (1% Savlon)
- Cardiac table
- Stethoscope
- Tissue paper (towel)

A tray containing:
- Paper bag
- Kidney tray
- Weighing machine
- Wet and dry gauge pieces
- Pillow if needed.

Steps of Procedure

Preprocedural Steps

- Explain the reason and objectives to the patient for the therapy that the inspired air helps to inflate the lungs.

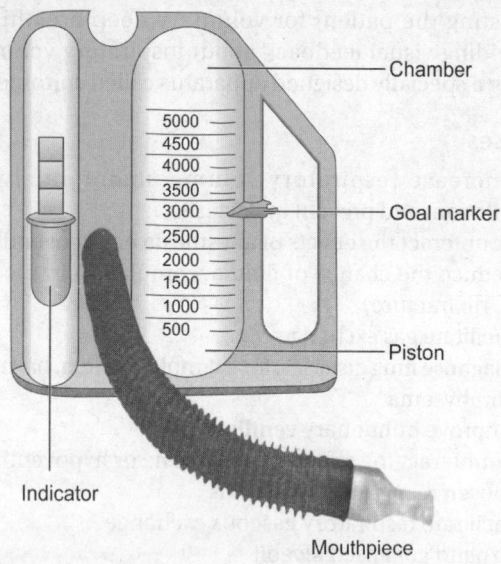

Fig. 7.25: Incentive spirometer.

- The halls weight in the spirometer will rise in response to the intensity of the intake of air.
- The higher the ball rises the deeper the breath. Helps in obtaining cooperation of patient
- Assess the patient's respiratory status by general observation and auscultation of breath sounds.
- Helps in comparison after procedure
- Review medical record for recent arterial blood gas.
- Determine need for using incentive spirometer Remove dentures Denture interfere with performance of procedure
- Wash hands. Reduces the transmission of microorganisms.

Intraprocedural Steps

- Instruct patient to assume a semi-Fowler's, high Fowler's position or sitting. Promotes optimal hung expansion
- Clean the mouth piece of the spirometer with wet gauze piece and then with dry gauze piece
- If the patient is preoperative then (weight x 10) and postoperative (weight x 8)
- Set pointer on incentive spirometer at appropriate level or point to level where disk or ball should reach.
- Encourage patient to reach appropriate goals
- For the postoperative patient, try as much as possible to avoid discomfort with the treatment.
- Coordinate treatment with administration of pain relief medications.
- Most likely to have best results in using incentive spirometer when patient has a little pain as possible
- Instruct and assist the patient with splinting of incision with pillow
- Hold or place the spirometer in an upright position

- A tilted flow-oriented device requires less effort to raise the balls or disc.
- A volume-oriented device will not function
- Demonstrate how to steady device with one hand and hold mouthpiece with the other hand
- Instruct the patient to exhale normally and then place lips securely around mouthpiece
- Instruct to take a slow deep breath to elevate the balls or cylinder and then hold the breath for 2 seconds initially to 6 seconds to keep the balls or cylinder elevated, if possible
- Instruct patient not to breathe through his/her nose.
- Use a nose clip, if necessary Tell patient to remove lips from mouthpiece and exhale normally
- Instruct patient to relax and repeat the procedure several times and then 4–5 times hourly.
- Practice to increase inspiratory volume maintains alveolar ventilation and prevents atelectasis
- Instruct patient to cough after the procedure and provide sputum mug.
- Deep ventilation can loosen secretions and coughing can facilitate their removal
- Clean the mouth piece with water and shake it dry.
- Change disposable mouth pieces every 24 hours.

Postprocedural Steps

Documentation
- Record lung volume in cubic centimeter, respiratory assessment (rate and depth of respiration, the amount of secretion expectorated).
- Act as a communication between staff members.

Termination
- Make the patient comfortable
- Take all the articles to the utility room and clean them
- Wash hands thoroughly
- Record and report observations and the care given to the patients with date, time and signature.

Complications
- Pneumothorax
- Increased ICP
- Bronchospasm
- Paroxysmal coughing

Activities that should be avoided Prior to Spirometry are as follows:

- Smoking within 1 hour of testing
- Consuming alcohol within 4 hours of testing
- Vigorous exercise within 30 minutes of testing
- Eating a large meal within 2 hours of testing
- Patient should take several normal breaths before attempting another one with the incentive spirometer usually one with the incentive breath per minute minimizes patient fatigue.
- No more than 4 or 5 maneuvers should performed per minute to minimize hypocarbia.

Fluid, Electrolyte, and Acid-Base Balances

CHAPTER 8

REVIEW OF PHYSIOLOGICAL REGULATION OF FLUID, ELECTROLYTE AND ACID-BASE BALANCES

Body Fluid Compartments and Exchange

Water is most abundant constituent of body comprising 60% of body weight in men and 50% in women. The body gains water primarily from eating and drinking, and a small amount is generated during metabolism. Water is lost from the body as urine, feces, sweat, tears and insensibly from respiration and skin surface. Sweat and saliva are hypotonic (dilute), while most other fluids are isotonic and have osmolarity similar to plasma. In all cases, water must cross an epithelial cell barrier (skin, respiratory mucosa, GI tract) to enter or exit the body.

Within the body, water is distributed into two compartments, i.e., intracellular and extracellular. Two-thirds of the body water lies within cells called intracellular fluid and one-third lies outside the cells called extracellular fluid. Water can freely cross the cell membrane and move from one compartment to the other. In contrast, ions cannot cross the cell membrane; they exert a pressure called osmotic pressure which determines the movement of water in or out of the cells. For example, if there is rise in osmolarity of extracellular fluid, water moves from intracellular compartment to extracellular fluid compartment to equalize each side and vice-versa is also true **(Fig. 8.1)**.

The most common extracellular ions are sodium (Na), chloride (Cl) and bicarbonate (HCO).

The extracellular fluid compartment is further subdivided into intravascular (plasma water) and extravascular compartments (interstitial spaces) in a ratio of 1:3. Plasma is a key medium through which compounds and water enter or exit the body before entering the cells. The exchanges of fluid between intravascular and extravascular compartments are determined by the balance of hydrostatic (fluid) pressure and osmotic pressure exerted by plasma proteins.

HOMEOSTASIS: MECHANISMS OF CONTROLLING FLUID AND ELECTROLYTE MOVEMENT

Fluid/Water Homeostasis

Homeostasis means constant internal environment of the body, naturally maintained by adaptive mechanisms that promote healthy survival. Fluid homeostasis means water intake equals the water lost from the body. An approximately daily water intake and output of an adult taking 2.500 mL/day **(Table 8.1)**.

TABLE 8.1: Normal water intake and water loss.

Intake		Output (loss)	
Route	Gain (mL)	Route	Loss (mL)
Water in food	1000	Skin	500
Water from oxidation	300	Lungs	350
Water as liquid	1200	Feces	150
		Kidney	1500

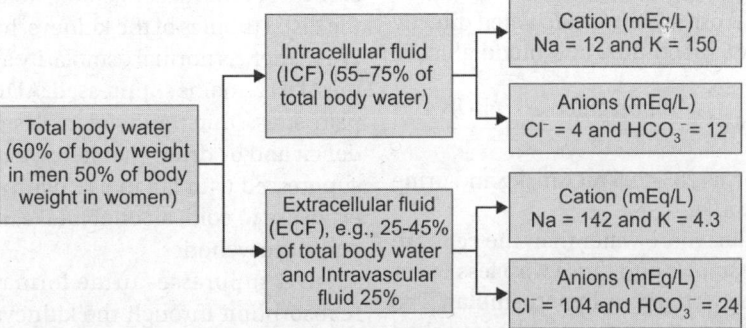

Fig. 8.1: Distribution of total body water and major cations and anion in different compartment.

Mechanisms of Controlling Fluid and Electrolyte Movements

Fluid and electrolyte movements between intracellular and extracellular fluid compartment is controlled by the following mechanisms:

Simple Diffusion

Diffusion is defined as movement of a substance or solute from an area of higher concentration to area of lower concentration. The membrane separating the two areas must be permeable to the diffusing substances. Energy is not required in this process. The example is exchange of O_2 and CO_2 through the alveolocapillary membrane.

Facilitated Diffusion

It is similar to simple diffusion, but molecules diffuse slowly into the cells, hence, required to be facilitated by some carrier molecule. Glucose transport into the cells under the action of insulin is an example of facilitated diffusion.

Active Transport

It is the movement of molecule against diffusion gradient. The fluid moves from lower concentration to higher concentration against concentration gradient with the help of energy provided by ATP. By active transport, sodium moves out and potassium moves into the cell through sodium-potassium pump.

Osmosis

It is defined as movement of water not of solute through a semi-permeable membrane between two compartments. Here, the water moves from the area of low solute concentration to high solute concentration across a semi-permeable membrane, the process stops itself when concentrations become equal on two sides. Osmosis is important to maintain the chemical stability of cells.

Fluid Pressures

Osmotic (Oncotic Pressure)

It is the pure exerted by colloids (proteins) in the food. Osmotic prior is driving force for movement of water by osmosis. Osmotic pressure thus is a force of pulling of water (retaining forces)

Osmolarity: It is defined as osmotic force of solutes per unit weight of solvent. It measures the total milliosmoles of solutes per unit of total volume of solution. It is expressed as mOsm/kg.

In clinical practice, serum osmolarity is calculated directly by measuring the serum Na, blood urea and blood glucose concentration as follows:

$$\text{Serum oamolarity} = 2[Na^+] + \frac{\text{Blood glucose}}{18} + \frac{\text{BUN}}{3}$$

Normal serum osmolarity is 285–295 mOsm/kg and urine osmolarity is 300–800 mOsm/kg.

The solutions that contains more water than the cells are called hypotonic or hypo-osmolar and those with less water than the cells are called hypertonic or hyperosmolar. The fluids having same amount of water as that of cells are called isotonic or normo-osmolar.

Hydrostatic Pressure

It is the force exerted by the fluid on the wall of the container/vessel. In the cardiovascular system, heart is the main pumping organ, generates high pressure (e.g., 120 mm Hg) and pushes the blood into the aorta and main vessels. As the blood moves from the arteries to arterioles, the pressure falls gradually and it reaches about 40 mm at the end of capillary. Because of the size of capillary and movement of fluid from the capillary into interstitial, the pressure falls to just 10 mm at the venous end of the capillary.

Hydrostatic pressure is the driving force that moves the fluid from the capillary into the interstitial, and oncotic (osmotic pressure) is the retaining force that does not allow this movement of fluid.

Filtration

It is the process of movement of fluids and electrolytes through the capillaries. The hydrostatic pressure moves the fluid from the capillaries to interstitial at the arterial end and oncotic pressure draws the fluid from interstitial into blood at the venous end. This filtration occurs through the capillaries throughout the body. Absorption means movement of substances from organs into the vascular system. Reabsorption means movement of water, electrolytes, vitamins, amino acids, glucose and other essential substances from one compartment, i.e., interstitial or renal tubules back into vascular system.

Regulation of Fluid and Electrolytes

There is homeostatic mechanism in the body which keeps the fluid and electrolytes within normal limits. The various mechanisms are:

Thirst

Hypothalamus contains a thirst center which regulates fluid ingestion. The thirst is stimulated by hypotension, fluid deficit and increased serum osmolarity (increased Na^+ intake, ingestion of hypertonic solutions or hypertonic IV fluids) and inhibited by excess fluid volume. During thirst, ADH and kidneys are functioning normally; water ingestion is equal to water excretion in an individual.

Anti-diuretic Hormone (ADH)

ADH is a hormone manufactured by hypothalamus. It is stored in the posterior pituitary gland and released, if needed, i.e., in case there is intracellular fluid deficit. It retains water through the distal tubules of the kidneys, hence, called "anti-diuretic". When there is normal osmolarity and normal plasma volume, the ADH remains suppressed. ADH is released in response to pain, stress, thirst, and rise in plasma osmolarity, fluid volume deficit and by drugs (narcotics, barbiturates, anesthetic). It is suppressed with fall in osmolarity, increased blood volume, exposure to cold, alcohol intake, intake of diuretics, lithium, and antipsychotics.

ADH suppresses urine formation and promotes water reabsorption through the kidneys, which is why thirst and ADH are stimulated simultaneously into fluid deficit.

Role of Corticosteroids

In addition to ADH, corticosteroids secreted by adrenal cortex regulate water and electrolytes. Two groups of corticosteroids, e.g., glucocorticosteroids increase blood glucose while mineralocorticosteroids (aldosterone) retain sodium and excretes potassium. Cortisol is the hormone water and which has properties of both glucocorticoids and mineralocorticosteroids. Aldosterone is secreted by the adrenal cortex under the influence of anterior pituitary. Hypovolemia is the main stimulus for aldosterone production.

Role of Kidneys

The kidneys being main filtering organs, maintain fluid volume and concentration of urine. The excretion of ECF and re-absorption of useful substances occur in the renal tubules under the effect of 3 hormones, i.e.,
1. ANP (atrial natriuretic peptide), which is secreted by cardiac atrial distension
2. ADH
3. Aldosterone.

The actions of these hormones have already been described. The main functions of kidneys in water and electrolyte balance are:
1. Regulation of ECF volume and plasma osmolarity by selective reabsorption and excretion of fluids.
2. Regulation of pH by retention of H+ ions.
3. Regulation of electrolytes in ECF by selective retention of useful substances and excretion of unneeded substances.
4. Act as the main excretory organs for metabolic wastes and toxic metabolites.

Role of GI Tract

Daily intake and output of water is about 2–3 liters and GI tract is the main organ for water intake. Water intake includes water or fluids taken by mouth, water released during food metabolism and water contents of the food items. Fruits and vegetables are rich in water content. Kidneys are the main organs for excretion of water, but a small amount of water is passed in stools.

Role of Lungs

Lungs are vital organs for maintaining water balance: Normal insensible loss of about 900 mL of fluids occurs daily through evaporation from the lungs and skin. Lungs also assist in regulating body temperature. During fever, water is lost through via sweating and lungs via exhalation. About 300 mL of water is excreted via exhalation through lungs in a normal adult.

Blood Circulation

The pumping action of heart and pressure within vessels, i.e., arterioles of glomeruli help in the formation of urine called glomerular filtration pressure. Failure of this action leads to fall in renal perfusion and urine formation and retention of electrolytes along with waste products.

Body Fluid Homeostasis

See **Flowchart 8.1**.

ACID AND BASE DISTURBANCE

The acid and base are maintained within a normal range by homeostatic mechanism its disturbance will lead to either acid or alkali burden leading to acidemia or alkalemia.

Definitions

- **Acid:** An acid is a chemical substance that can release or donate H+ ion in solution.
- **Base:** Base is a substance that would accept the H+ ion released by acid.
- **pH:** It is a negative (–) log of hydrogen ion concentration. Normal arterial pH varies from 7.36–7.42.
- **Acidemia/Acidosis:** It is a condition in which hydrogen ions concentration rises or would rise resulting in fall in pH. Acidosis results when there is too much acid in the blood or too little base.
- **Alkalemia/Alkalosis:** It is a pathological condition in which there is excess base in the body resulting in rise in pH. The blood becomes alkaline. It results either due to too much base or too little acid.

Regulation of Acid-base Balance

Normal pH of blood is constantly being maintained within normal range by three physiological systems that act interdependently.

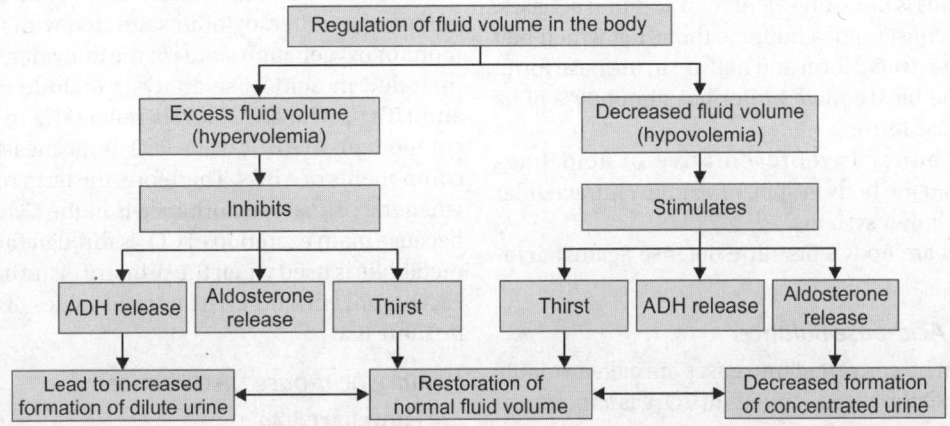

Flowchart 8.1: Body fluid homeostasis.

1. Chemical buffering of excess acid or base by buffer systems in the blood and in the cells.
2. Excretion of acid by the lungs.
3. Excretion of acid or regeneration of base by the kidneys.

Buffer Systems

A buffer system consists of a weak acid (one that does not readily release H⁺ into solution) and a salt of a base. For example, carbonic acid (H_2CO_3) is a weak acid and sodium bicarbonate ($NaHCO_3$), the salt of a base with which H⁺ ion can combine, makes up a buffer system called *bicarbonate buffer* in the blood. Strong acids produced during cellular metabolism contribute free H⁺ to body resulting in alterations of pH. These strong acids are buffered by buffer systems. The pH of buffered solutions tends to remain fairly stationary despite the addition of strong acids or bases because buffer systems convert these acids or bases into weaker forms. This is illustrated below with examples.

Strong Acid Buffered

$$\begin{pmatrix}HCl\\ \text{Strong}\\ \text{Acid}\end{pmatrix} + \begin{pmatrix}\frac{H_2CO_3}{NaHCO_3}\\ \text{(Bicarbonate Buffer)}\end{pmatrix} \rightarrow \begin{matrix}H_2CO_3\\ \text{(Weak acid)}\end{matrix} + \begin{pmatrix}NaCl\\ \text{Sodium}\\ \text{Cloride}\end{pmatrix}$$

Strong Base Buffered

$$(NaOH) + \begin{pmatrix}\frac{H_2CO_3}{NaNCO_3}\\ \text{Buffer}\end{pmatrix} \rightarrow \begin{matrix}NaHCO_3\\ \text{(Weak base}\\ \text{of sodium}\\ \text{bicarbonate)}\end{matrix} + H_2O$$

There are several buffer systems in the blood, both within the red blood cells and in the plasma. Numerous negative charges on proteins present in the blood such as hemoglobin and albumin permit the binding of large quantities of H² cations, hence called *blood buffers*. Negatively charged ions, such as phosphates within the body cells and carbonate within the bone, also act as intracellular buffers.

In clinical settings, the bicarbonate buffer is monitored because of its accessibility within plasma and acts as an open buffer system. In open buffer system, the end products of acid-buffering reactions are continuously eliminated from the body by lungs and kidneys in spite of accumulation of end products. The dissociation constant (pka) of this buffering system is ideal for buffering fluids such as plasma in which the addition of acids is more prevalent than addition of bases. The dissociation constant of a buffer is the pH at which half its components are in acid form and half are in the base form. At normal pH, the bicarbonate buffer has about 90% of its components in base form.

Bicarbonate buffer is representative of acid-base homeostasis within the body in spite of so many intracellular and extracellular buffer systems.

Buffer systems are body's first-line defense against acid-base disturbance.

Role of Lungs in Acid-base Balance

The acids that can be converted into gases are called volatile acids. The lungs exhale large quantities of CO_2 gas as potential volatile acids. CO_2 is produced during oxidative metabolism of nutrients in the tissues which diffuses into the blood and combines with H_2O to form carbonic acid (H_2CO_3) which dissociates into its components as H⁺ and HCO_3^-. This hydrolysis is reversible.

$$H_2O + CO_2 \rightarrow H_3CO_2 \rightarrow H^+ + HCO_3^-$$

From this equation, it is evident that rise in CO_2 concentration in the blood raises the H⁺ ion concentration (lower pH), hence produces acidosis. Conversely, lower CO_2 levels are associated with low H⁺ and rise in pH causing alkalosis.

Role of Kidneys in Acid base Homeostasis

The kidneys regulate blood pH by secreting H⁺ ion into urine and by regenerating HCO_3^- for reabsorption into the blood. The bicarbonate filtered at glomerulus from the blood is poorly absorbed from proximal tubules. H⁺ is actively secreted throughout the tubules. The HCO_3^- and H⁺ will be dealt with by bicarbonate buffer system. Any HCO_3^-, filtered in excess of H⁻ will be excreted into the urine. The H⁺ ion in tubules lowers the pH of tubular cells until pH of tubules fall to 4.5. At lower pH, significant amount of H⁺ leaks from the tubules into the blood. This would result in fall of further secretion of H⁺. Urinary bicarbonate buffer system deals with secretion of H⁺ and regeneration of HCO_3 their combination would result in CO_2 production by reversal of hydrolytic reaction. The CO_2 is reabsorbed into tubules where it combines with H_2O to form H_2CO_3 which is acted upon by tubular Carbonic Anhydrase (CA) and converted into H⁺ and HCO_3^-. This HCO_3 in tubules combines with Na⁺ and absorbed as $NaHCO_3$. Thus, for every H⁺ secreted, a molecule of HCO_3^- is returned to blood as $NaHCO_3$ to restore the plasma bicarbonate buffer system. Another system called *ammonia buffer* system operates in the renal tubules where NH_3 is generated from the amino acids in the renal tubules. This NH_3 diffuses into the tubular lumen, where it combines with H⁺ to form NH_4^+ (ammonium), which cannot be reabsorbed. NH_4^+ is excreted in the urine in combination with chloride (Cl) from NaCl. Na⁺ is actively reabsorbed along with tubular HCO_3^-.

Analysis of Arterial Blood Gases

Arterial blood gases (ABGs) are determined to know the oxygenation status and the acid-base status. The partial pressure of O_2 (PaO_2) means percentage of hemoglobin saturated with O_2 and partial pressure of CO_2 ($PaCO_2$) means percentage of hemoglobin saturated with CO_2. These gases monitor oxygenation status of the individual. The parameters included in acid-base analysis include pH, $PaCO_2$, PaO_2 and HCO_3^-. The HCO_3 levels reflect the metabolic or renal components of ABGs while PaO_2 is the measure of respiratory components of ABGs. Therefore, the term respiratory is used when the primary disturbance is in the CO_2 tension ($PaCO_2$) because main excretion of CO_2 is through the lungs. The term metabolic is used when the primary disturbance is in plasma HCO_3^- concentration. The normal values of ABG are enlisted in **Table 8.2**.

Primary Acid-base Disturbance

See **Flowchart 8.2**.

TABLE 8.2: Normal values of various components of arterial blood gas analysis.

Component	Values
pH	7.35–7.45
PaO_2	80–100 mm Hg
$PaCO_2$	35–45 mm Hg
HCO_3	22–26 mEq/L

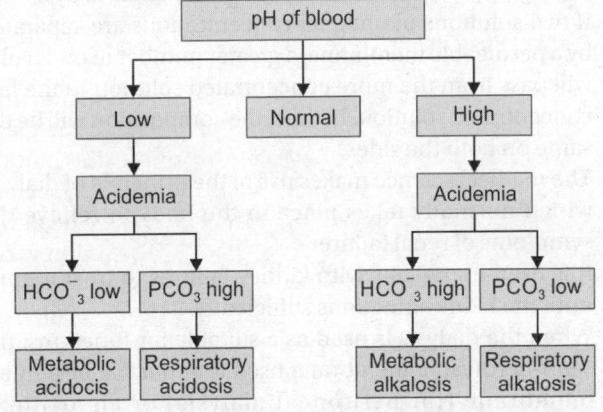

Flowchart 8.2: Primary acid base disturbance.

FACTORS AFFECTING FLUID, ELECTROLYTE AND ACID-BASE BALANCES

Factors Affecting the Fluid and Electrolyte Movements in the Body

- Body fluids are not static, but they shift from compartment to compartment to meet the metabolic needs such as tissue oxygenation, response to illness, acid base disturbance and response to drug therapies.
- The various factors which affect the movement of body fluid and electrolyte are diffusion, osmosis, osmotic pressure, filtration hydrostatic pressure, active transport, etc.

Diffusion

- Diffusion is the term applied to the spreading or scattering of molecules of gases or liquids
- When two gases or liquids are brought into contact, the continual movement of the molecules will soon produce a uniform mixture, irrespective of their density.
- The processes of diffusion occur even when two substances are separated by a thin membrane.
- In the body, diffusion of the body fluids, electrolytes and other substances takes place through the of capillary and cell membranes.
- The rate of diffusion varies according to the size of molecules, the concentration of the solution and the temperature of the solution.
- Smaller molecules move more quickly than the larger ones
- Molecules move from a solution of higher concentration to a solution of lower concentration. Increase in the temperature increases the rate of diffusion.

Osmosis

- The diffusion of water molecules (solvent) through a permeable membrane, from an area of lesser solute concentration to an area of greater solute concentration, is known as osmosis.
- If copper sulphate solution (colored) and water are separated by a permeable membrane, the water molecules will pass through the pores of the membrane to the copper sulphate solution, thereby raising its level.
- The copper sulphate in the solution exerts a pressure known as 'osmotic pressure'. It is due to this osmotic pressure that the water flows to the salt side rather than in the reverse direction.
- The concentration of a solution is measured in osmols, which reflect the amount of a substance in solution in the form of molecules, ions or both.
- Osmotic pressure is the drawing force of water exerted by the solute particles.
- The solute particles may be crystalloids (salts) or colloids (protein particles).
- When the concentration of the solute on one side of the membrane becomes greater than the other side, the osmotic pressure and the attraction for water will increase.
- Water will flow towards the solution of greater concentration until the concentration gradient disappears.
- The osmotic pressure of a solution is also called its osmolarity, which is expressed in osmols or milliosmoles per kilogram (MOsm/kg) of the solution.
- The normal serum osmolarity is 280–295 MOsm/kg.
- The principle of osmosis can be applied clinically in the administration of intravenous fluids.
- Usually, the solutions given as intravenous infusion are isotonic having the same concentration (osmolarity) as blood plasma.
- This prevents sudden shifts of fluids and electrolytes from the vascular bed to the interstitial fluids.
- In some cases, hypertonic solutions, which have a greater concentration of solutes than plasma, are advisable. (e.g., 50% glucose).
- This may be given to reduce cerebral edema.
- The high concentration of glucose temporarily draws fluid from the interstitial spaces of brain tissue into the blood compartment.
- The uses of hypotonic solutions are rare.
- They may be used in cases of subcutaneous infusions to help in the quick absorption of fluids.
- Both hypertonic and hypotonic solutions are to be used cautiously for the intravenous infusions.
- The hypertonic solutions can destroy the blood cells by shrinking them as they give off water and the hypotonic solution can hemolyze the blood cells as they take in more water than the cell membrane can support.
- The osmotic pressure of the blood is affected by plasma proteins, especially albumin, a serum protein naturally produced by the body.
- Osmotic pressure is greatest in the blood vessels due to the presence of plasma proteins.

- The protein concentration is greater than that of the interstitial fluid.
- Albumin exerts colloid osmotic or oncotic pressure, which tend to keep fluid in the capillaries.
- The proteins molecules are large and do not readily pass across the capillary membrane.
- This greater colloid osmotic pressure of plasma maintains the intravascular fluid volumes. The plasma proteins work somewhat like a sponge, holding the water within the blood vessels and sucking back that water which escapes from the blood vessels.
- At the venous end of the capillaries, the oncotic pressure and decreased venous hydrostatic pressure facilitates the movement of the water and waste products back into the capillaries.

Filtration

- It is the process by which water and diffusible substances move together in response to fluid pressure.
- This process is active in capillary beds, where pressure differences determine the movement of water, electrolytes and other dissolved substances between the capillaries and interstitial fluid.

Hydrostatic Pressure

- Hydrostatic pressure is the pressure exerted by a fluid within a closed system.
- Counterbalancing the osmotic pressure of the plasma, which attracts fluid into the vascular system, is the hydrostatic pressure of the blood flowing through the capillaries which pushes fluid out of the vascular system.
- Thus the hydrostatic pressure of the blood is the force exerted by the blood against the vascular walls. It is also referred to as filtration force.
- The principle involved in the hydrostatic pressure is that, fluids move, from the area of greater pressure to the area of lesser pressure.
- For this reason, the fluid moves out of the blood vessels. The net movement of fluids from the vascular space to the tissue spaces and vice versa depends upon two forces the hydrostatic pressure, which forces the fluids out of the blood vessels and the osmotic pressure which draws fluid into the blood vessels.
- Normally fluid moves of capillaries at the arterial end where the hydrostatic pressure exceeds the colloid osmotic pressure.
- At the venous end of capillaries, fluid is drawn from the interstitial compartment into the vascular compartment, where the osmotic pressure is greater of the two.

Active Transport

- It is the movement of materials across the cell membrane by chemical activity or energy expenditure that allows the cell to admit larger molecules than it would otherwise be able to admit or to move molecules from area of lesser concentration to areas of greater concentration.
- Unlike diffusion and osmosis, active transport requires metabolic activity and energy expenditure.
- Active transport in the body is found in sodium and potassium pumps.
- Sodium is pumped out of the cell.
- Potassium is pumped in against concentration gradient.
- Active transport is enhanced by carrier molecules within a cell that bind themselves to incoming molecules.
- Active transport is the mechanism by which the cell absorbs glucose and other substances to carry out metabolic activities.

Dialysis

- The diffusion of molecules of soluble constituents (solute) through a permeable membrane is known as dialysis.
- If two solutions of unequal concentrations are separated by a permeable membrane, a greater number of molecules will pass from the more concentrated solution to the less concentrated solution. In time, the composition will be the same on both the sides.
- The medical science makes use of the principle of dialysis which normally takes place in the body to relieve the symptoms of renal failure.
- It is used in persons with kidney failures to treat uremia until the kidney functions sufficiently.
- When the dialysis is used as a suitable for functions, the semi-permeable membrane used is either the peritoneal membrane (for peritoneal dialysis) or an artificial membrane (for hemodialysis).
- This membrane must have pores large enough to allow passage of electrolytes, urea and creatinine but too small to allow passage of blood cells and other protein molecules
- The two solutions used on the opposite sides of the membranes are:
  - Blood
  - A especially prepared electrolyte solution called dialysate.
- It must be remembered that the solute particles and water can move freely across the membrane in either direction between the blood and the dialysate.
- If the patient's blood has higher concentration of urea, creatinine and other electrobytes than the prepared dialysate solution, these particles will move into the dialysate solution, thus lowering their level in the blood.
- Likewise, if the blood is deficient in a substance, such as bicarbonate, a higher concentration of this sub- stance in the dialysate will cause it to move into the blood, raising the blood level.
- Excess fluid can be removed from the blood by increasing the particle concentration of the dialysate with a solution such as dextrose.
- This increased particle concentration will cause water to move into the dialysate, while at the same time the dextrose moves into the blood.
- The tendency is always to- wards an equalization of concentration of the two solutions.

Selective Permeability of Membranes

- In body, the capillary and the cell membranes are described as selectively permeable.
- This is because, not all substances move with the same ease across the cell membranes.

* The cellular membranes are selective in regard to the electrolytes of sodium and potassium.

Variables Affecting Fluid, Electrolyte and Balance

* Fluid, electrolyte and acid base status is neither a static nor single physiological entity.
* Many variables can change the distribution of body fluid and electrolytes.
* The major factors than can affect fluid, electrolyte and acid base states include age, body size, environmental temperature, lifestyle and level of health.
* **Age:** It affects distribution of body fluids and electrolytes. The major differences are observed in infants, older adults and pregnant women.
* **Body size:** It has an effect on total body water. Because fat contains no water, the obese client has proportionately less water. Women have more fat deposit than men. As a result the total body water in women is less than that of men.
* **Environmental temperature:** Fluid and electrolyte imbalances are associated with extremes in environmental temperature and relative humidity. The overall body response to environmental temperature exceeding 28" to 30°C is to increase the sensible water loss by sweating which cools the peripheral blood and help reduce the body temperature.
* **Lifestyle:** It can have an indirect effect on fluid, electrolyte, and acid base balance. Habits that can affect fluid balance include:
  * Diet
  * Stress
  * Exercise.
* **Level of health:** Generally a healthy person easily tolerates fluid and electrolyte changes than a sick person. Surgery, burns, cancer, cardiovascular diseases, respiratory and renal disorders, gastrointestinal diseases and endocrine disorders can upset the homeostasis.

Illness

* When a person is sick, especially if the illness involves vomiting, diarrhea, or fever, he is at greater risk for fluid and electrolyte imbalance.
* These factors cause body to lose water.
* If a large amount of water is lost from the body, the result is dehydration.
* This would obviously alter the fluid balance of the body, because electrolytes are dissolved in body fluids. It can also alter the electrolyte concentrations.
* Water can be replenished by drinking, but sometimes when the person is sick it can be difficult to drink enough water to replenish what is lost.
* Stress and alcohol consumption also affect fluid, electrolyte and acid-base balance as the person may not consume adequate fluids and electrolytes.
* Trauma causes release of intracellular potassium which is an extremely dangerous imbalance.

Medications

There are certain medications that could lead to electrolyte imbalances when taken against the physician's orders.

Environmental Factors

* Various environmental factors, such as temperature, humidity, radiation, and atmospheric pressure affect mainly sweating and urinary water loss, while physical exercise causes increased respiratory water loss from the increased expiratory volume and frequency of breathing
* Dehydration is also a concern for people who are engaged in heavy exercise.
* This risk is accentuated if the activity is performed in a hot environment.
* For example, if the atmospheric temperature is 90°F and a person runs quite a long distance it is certain that he will lose a lot of water and salt through sweat. This loss will decrease the level of water and electrolytes in the body.
* To correct this imbalance, the person needs to rehydrate properly.

Diet

* The fluid and electrolyte balance in the body is affected by the diet because the foods and beverages a person takes provide fluid and electrolytes.
* This explains why people with conditions like anorexia nervosa, which is an eating disorder characterized by self-starvation, or bulimia, which is an eating disorder characterized by self-induced vomiting, can develop an imbalance.
* Retention of sodium causes fluid retention and imbalance.
* Same way excessive loss of sodium is associated with decreased volume of body fluid.
* Fluid volume deficit results from loss of body fluids and occurs more rapidly with decreased fluid intake
* Fluid volume excess may be related to a simple fluid overload or diminished function of the homeostatic mechanisms responsible for regulating fluid balance.

Kidney Problems

* The kidneys are important regulators of fluid and electrolyte balance in the body.
* The kidneys have the ability to excrete excess water and electrolytes through the urine.
* They can also retain water or electrolytes if their levels drop too low.
* Thus, the kidneys help maintain a balance between daily consumption and excretion of electrolytes and water.
* If kidney problems develop due to infection, inflammation, or trauma, the kidneys' ability to maintain fluid and electrolyte balance can be thrown off.
* The Rennin-Angiotensin-Aldosterone System (RAAS) is a hormone system which is mainly comprised of three hormones rennin, Angiotensin II and aldosterone.
* Primarily it is regulated by the rate of renal blood flow.

Fluid Volume Deficit results from loss of body fluids and occurs more rapidly with decreased fluid intake

Fluid volume excess may be related to a simple fluid overload or diminished function of the homeostatic mechanisms responsible for regulating fluid balance.

Examples of Nursing Diagnoses Related to Fluid, Electrolyte and Acid-base Disturbance (NANDA-Approved Nursing Diagnoses)

- ❖ **Actual or potential fluid volume deficit related to:**
  - Loss of plasma associated with burns
  - Vomiting
  - Failure of regulatory mechanism
- ❖ **Actual or potential fluid volume excess related to:**
  - Sodium retention
  - Compromised regulatory mechanism
- ❖ **Impaired tissue integrity related to:** Edema
- ❖ **Impaired gas exchange related to:**
  - Altered oxygen supply
  - Alveolar capillary membrane changes
  - Altered blood flow
  - Altered oxygen carrying capacity of blood
- ❖ **Decreased cardiac output related to:** Dysrhythmias associated with electrolyte imbalance.

DISTURBANCES IN FLUID VOLUME

Fluid Volume Deficit (*Hypovolemia*)

Fluid volume deficit is a decrease in intravascular, interstitial or intracellular fluid in the body. It occurs when loss of ECF volume exceeds the intake of fluid. It is a relatively common problem that may exist alone or in combination with other electrolyte or acid base imbalances.

Causes of Fluid Volume Deficit

- ❖ The most common cause of fluid volume deficit is excessive loss of GI fluids from vomiting, diarrhea, GI suctioning, intestinal fistulas and intestinal drainage.
- ❖ Other causes may include:
  - Excessive renal losses of water and sodium from diuretic therapy or renal disorders.
  - Water and sodium losses during sweating from excessive exercise or increased environmental temperature.
  - Hemorrhage.
  - Chronic use of laxatives or enemas.
- ❖ Fluid volume deficit also takes place by inadequate fluid intake may results from:
  - Lack of access to fluids.
  - Inability to swallow.
  - Oral trauma.
  - Altered thirst mechanism.
- ❖ Fluid volume deficit can develop slowly or rapidly depending on the type of fluid loss.
  - *Hypovolemia:* Loss of extracellular fluid volume and decreased circulating blood volume.
  - *Isotonic fluid volume deficit:* Electrolytes are often lost along with fluid resulting in isotonic fluid volume deficit.
  - *Third spacing:* Third spacing is a shift of fluid from the vascular space into an area where it is not available to support normal physiologic processes. The third space is a space in the body where fluid does not normally collects in larger amount or where any significant fluid collection is physiologically non functional. For example, the peritoneal cavity and pleural cavity still small amount of fluid does exist normally in such spaces and function as a lubricant in case of pleural cavity.

Clinical Manifestations

- ❖ With a rapid fluid loss manifestations of hypovolemia occur rapidly.
- ❖ When loss of fluid occurs gradually, the patient's fluid volume may be very low before symptoms develop.
- ❖ **Mucous membranes:** Dry, may be sticky.
- ❖ **Neurologic:** Altered sensorium, anxiety, restlessness, diminished alertness, possible coma.
- ❖ **Integumentary system:** Diminished skin turgor, dry skin, pale, cool extremities.
- ❖ **Musculoskeletal system:** Fatigue, decreased urinary output, oliguria, increased specific gravity.
- ❖ **Cardiovascular system:** Tachycardia, orthostatic hypotension. Falling systolic/diastolic pressure (severe fvd), flat neck vein, decreased venous filling, decreased capillary refill, decreased hematocrit
- ❖ **Potential complication:** Hypovolemic shock.

Assessment

- ❖ Collect assessment data through the health history, interview and physical examination.
- ❖ **Health history:** Risk factors, such as medications, acute or chronic renal or endocrine disease, precipitating factor such as hot weather, extensive exercise, lack of access to fluids, recent illnesses (fever vomiting and diarrhea)
- ❖ **Physical assessment:** Weight vital signs, skin color, temperature, turgor, level of consciousness, urine output.

Diagnostic Tests

Serum osmolarity, electrolytes, hemoglobin and hematocrit urine specific gravity and osmolarity, CVP readings

Management of Fluid Volume Deficit

- ❖ The primary goal of care related to fluid volume deficit is to prevent deficits in patients at risk and to correct deficits and their underlying causes.
- ❖ Treatment may include replacement of fluids and electrolytes by IV, oral or enteral routes.

Fluid Management

- ❖ Oral rehydration the safest and most effective treatment in adult patients who are able to take oral fluids.
- ❖ For mild fluid deficits in which the loss of electrolyte has been minimal, water alone may be used for fluid replacement.
- ❖ Severe fluid deficits in which electrolytes have also been lost (e.g., vomiting, diarrhea) electrolytes solutions such as sports drinks, rehydrating solutions is more appropriate.
- ❖ When the fluid deficit is severe and patient is not able to ingest fluids, the IV route is used to administer replacement fluids.
- ❖ Isotonic electrolyte solutions are used to expand plasma volume in hypotensive patients or to replace abnormal losses.
- ❖ Normal saline (0.9% NaCl) tends to remain in the vascular compartment, increasing blood volume. When administer rapidly this solution can precipitate acid base imbalance

so balanced electrolyte solution such as ringer lactate solutions are preferred to expand plasma volume.

Nursing Management
- Assess for presence or worsening of fluid volume deficit.
- **Administer oral fluids, if indicated:**
  - Consider the patient's likes and dislikes when offering fluids.
  - If the patient is reluctant to drink provide frequent mouth care and offer fluids at frequent intervals.
  - Explain the need for fluid replacement to the patient
  - Administer medications, if nausea is present.
- **Interventions for patients with impaired swallowing:**
  - Assess gag reflex
  - Position the patient in an upright position with a head and neck flexed slightly forward during feeding
  - Provide thick fluids or semi-solid foods.
- Patient unable to eat and drink, discuss possibility of tube feeding or TPN with the physician.
- Monitor response to fluid intake, either orally or parenterally.
- Monitor patients with tendency for fluid retention for signs of overload.
- Turn patient frequently, apply moisturizing agents to skin.

Fluid Volume Deficit (Dehydration)
- Diarrhea can cause dehydration, which means the body has lost too much fluid and too many electrolytes and cannot function properly.
- Dehydration is particularly dangerous in children and in older people it must be treated promptly to avoid serious health problems.

Signs of Dehydration
- Thirst
- Less frequent urination
- Dry skin
- Fatigue
- Light headedness
- Dark colored urine

Signs of Dehydration in Children
- Dry mouth and tongue
- No tears when crying
- No wet diapers for 3 hours or more
- Sunken eyes
- High fever
- Listlessness or irritability
- Skin that does not flatten when pinched and released.

Prevention
- The fluid and electrolytes lost during diarrhea need to be replaced promptly because the body cannot function without them.
- Electrolytes are the salts and minerals that affect the amount of water in the body, muscle activity and other important functions.
- Although water is extremely important in preventing dehydration, it does not contain electrolytes.
- Broth and soups that contain sodium and fruit juices, soft fruits or vegetables that contain potassium, helps to restore electrolyte levels.
- Over-the-counter rehydration solutions such as Pedialyte, Ceralyte and Infalyte are also good electrolyte sources and are especially recommended for use in children.

Diagnostic Tests
Diagnostic tests to find the cause of diarrhea may include the following:
- Medical history and physical examination
- Stool culture
- Blood tests
- Fasting tests
- Sigmoidoscopy
- Colonoscopy
- Imaging tests

Treatment
- In most cases of diarrhea, replacing lost fluid to prevent dehydration is the only treatment necessary
- Medicines that stop diarrhea may be helpful, but they are not recommended for people where diarrhea is caused by a bacterial infection or parasite.
- Viral infections are either treated with medication or left to run their course, depending on the severity and type of virus

Nursing Considerations
- Administer an analgesic for pain and to decrease intestinal motility, unless the patient has a possible or confirmed stool infection.
- Ensure the patient's privacy during defecation and empty bedpans promptly.
- Clean the perineum thoroughly and apply ointment to prevent skin breakdown.
- Note the amount and characteristics of the patient's stool.
- Monitor intake and output.
- Obtain serum samples for electrolytes and treat imbalances.
- Provide fluid replacement orally or IV as appropriate.
- Ensure adequate rest.
- If oral diet is tolerated, then small frequent feedings of bland food may be helpful to meet the nutritional requirements of the patient.
- Provide psychological support to the patient.
- Avoid foods that cause allergy in patient.

Patient Teaching
- Stress the need for medical follow-up to patients with inflammatory bowel disease (particularly ulcerative colitis) who have an increased risk of developing colon cancer
- Emphasize the importance of maintaining adequate hydration.
- Explain food or fluids that should be avoided.
- Discuss stress reduction techniques.
- Explain the diagnosis and treatment plan.

FLUID VOLUME EXCESS

Fluid Overload

- Fluid volume excess results when both water and sodium are retained in the body. FVE may be caused by fluid overload (excess water and sodium intake) or by impairment of the mechanisms that maintain homeostasis. The excess fluid can lead to excess intravascular fluid (hypervolemia) and excess interstitial fluid (edema).
- Fluid volume excess usually results from conditions that cause retention of both sodium and water.

These conditions include:
- **Compromised regulatory mechanisms, such as:**
  - Renal failure.
  - Congestive heart failure.
  - Cirrhosis of liver.
  - Cushing's syndrome.
- Corticosteroid administration.
- Stress condition causing the release of ADH and aldosterone.
- Excessive intake of sodium containing foods.
- Drugs that cause sodium retention.
- The administration of excess amounts of sodium containing IV fluids.

Causes of Fluid Volume Overload

- **Excess fluid retention with decreased excretion:**
  - Cirrhosis of liver (ascites, edema)
  - Renal disorders (interstitial fluid retention)
  - Hypoproteinemia (edematous state)
  - Heart failure
  - Lymphatic and venous obstruction
- **Excess ingestion of fluids or food rich in sodium:**
  - Excess IV saline infusion
  - Ingestion of sodium rich foods and medications
- **Increased secretion of ADH and aldosterone:**
  - Barbiturates and narcotics (morphine)
  - Cushing syndrome, hyperaldosteronism (Conn's syndrome),
  - Excess use of corticosteroids
  - Syndrome of inappropriate secretion of ADH (SIADH)

Clinical Manifestations

- Excess extracellular fluid leads to hypervolemia and circulatory overload.
- Excess fluid in the interstitial space causes peripheral or generalized edema.

The following manifestations of fluid volume excess relate to both the excess fluid and its effects on circulation are:
- The increase in total body water causes weight gain over a short period of time.
- Peripheral edema.
- Excess of fluid in interstitial space.
- Distended neck veins and peripheral veins.
- Slow-emptying peripheral veins.
- CVP over 11 cm H_2O.
- Crackles and wheezes in lungs.
- Polyuria (if renal function normal).
- Ascites, pleural effusion (when FVE is severe, fluid transudes into body cavities).
- Decreased BUN (due to plasma dilution)
- Decreased hematocrit (due to plasma dilution).
- Bounding, full-pulse.
- Pulmonary edema, if severe.

Assessment

Collect assessment data through the health history, interview and physical examination.
- **Health history:** Risk factors, such as medications, heart failure, acute or chronic renal or endocrine disease, precipitating factor, such as recent illness, change in diet or change in medication, recent weight gain, complaints of persistent cough, shortness of breath, swelling of feet and ankles or difficulty sleeping when lying down.
- **Physical assessment:** Weight, vital signs, peripheral pulses, capillary refill, jugular neck vein distention, edema, lung sounds (crackles or wheezes), dyspnea, cough and sputum, urine output, mental status.

Diagnostic Tests

Monitor serum osmolarity, electrolytes, hemoglobin and hematocrit, urine specific gravity and osmolarity, CVP readings.
- Urine specific gravity and osmolarity are low.
- Plasma osmolarity less than normal (<295 mOsm/kg).
- Hematocrit is low <45%.
- Plasma sodium low (<135 mEq/L).
- Blood urea is lower than normal.
- X-ray chest shows cardiomegaly with lung congested and pulmonary edema.
- Pulse oximetry shows decreased tissue O_2 saturation.
- Arterial blood gas analysis may show hypoxia and hypercapnia.

Management

Managing fluid volume excess focuses on prevention in patients at risk, treating its manifestations and correcting the underlying cause. Management includes limiting sodium and water intake and administering diuretics
- **Fluid management:** Fluid intake may be restricted in patients who have fluid volume excess. The amount of fluid allowed per day is prescribed by primary care provider. All fluid intake must be calculated, including meals that used to administer medications orally or intravenous.
- **Dietary management:** Sodium restricted diet is prescribed. A mild sodium restriction can be achieved by instructing the patient and primary food preparer in the household to reduce the amount of salt in recipes by half, avoid using the table salt during meal.

Nursing Management

- Assess the presence or worsening of FVE
- Encourage adherence to sodium restrictions to avoid over the counter drugs

When indicated, encourage rest period.
- Monitor the patient's response to diuretics
- Monitor the rate of parenteral fluids and the patient response.

- Teach self monitoring of weight and intake and output measurements (such as in case of CCF, renal failure, cirrhosis of liver).
- If dyspnea or orthopnea is present position the patient in semi fowler's position.
- Turn and position the patient frequently.

Nursing Care in General

- Assess the presence of fluid overload by history and clinical examination (edema, raised JVP, crackles in the lungs).
- Perform investigations as discussed already. If there is fluid overload or hypervolemia, restrict sodium and fluids. Because sodium retains water, hence sodium must be restricted, especially in renal and cardiac failure. Low sodium diet (1–2 g sodium diet) may be given.
- Encourage to adhere to sodium-restricted diet and avoid food and medications containing sodium, ie. cereals, chips, meat, cheese, sausages, pickles, pizza, soups, etc. They should take low sodium food items, i.e., fruits, vegetables, low salt bread and pizza, unsalted popcorn, fresh meat, chicken and fish. Use of salt substitutes, i.e., potassium salts, instead of sodium, can be helpful in some patients.
- Collaborate with the dietician to formulate fluid restriction. Try to suppress the thirst by teaching the client to keep either the ice chips or hold water in the mouth for a while to hydrate the tongue and mucous membrane.
- **Mobilization of fluids:**
  - Instruct the client, if edema present, to avoid long period of standing and to sit with legs elevated.
  - In case of CHF, encourage rest period as lying down promotes diuresis and relieves edema.
  - Mild diuretics, a combination of potassium sparing and potassium losing may be used to promote diuresis and prevent hypokalemia.
- **Reduction of complications:**
  - If pulmonary edema (dyspnea, orthopnea) present, position the patient in semi-Fowler's position.
  - Give O_2 to keep saturation around 90%.
  - Turn the client frequently to prevent breakdown of edematous skin under the pressure of weight of the client.
  - Lubricate the skin to prevent cracks and fissures. Keep the heels elevated.
  - Monitor the rate of parenteral fluids and the client response. Discuss the findings with the physician.
- **Monitoring:**
  - Check the vital signs every 2 hourly in the beginning, then 4 hourly and so on.
  - Each morning, assess the skin of sacrum for pressure sores and palpate for edema.
  - Examine the legs simultaneously for pitting edema.
  - Have a look at JVP after positioning the patient at 45°.
  - Raised JVP and full veins over the hands, which do not empty or flatten within 3–5 seconds when hand is raised above the heart, suggest still fluid overload.
  - Compare intake and output after every 4 hours.
  - Observe the level of consciousness.
  - Weigh the client daily. Weight loss is good response to treatment.
  - Monitor plasma osmolarity, sodium level, hematocrit, urine output daily.

Edema

- Edema is the medical term for swelling. It is caused by excess fluid leaking from capillaries (tiny blood vessels) into the tissue.
- When this extra fluid builds up, the tissue swells.
- The swollen site may be red, painful, inflamed, and warm or hot to the touch.

Physiological Review of Fluid Compartment

- Fluid compartments in the human body are divided between the intracellular and extracellular spaces.
- The extracellular space constitutes about one-third of total body water, which is further divided into intravascular plasma volume (25%) and the extravascular interstitial space (75%).
- The fluid balance between these compartments is maintained by hydrostatic pressures and oncotic pressures.
- The other two factors that play an important role in fluid balance are vessel wall permeability and the lymphatic system.
- The lymphatic system collects fluid and filtered proteins from the interstitial space and returns that back to the vasculature.
- Any disturbance in this delicate homeostasis that results in net filtration out of the vascular space or impaired return of fluid by lymphatic's leads to the accumulation of fluid in the interstitial space that is called edema.

Causes of Edema

- Increased capillary hydrostatic pressure
- Regional venous hypertension (often unilateral), such as
- Deep vein thrombosis, compartment syndrome.
- Systemic venous hypertension (often bilateral) heart failure.
- Pericarditis, pulmonary hypertension, liver failure/cirrhosis.
- Increased plasma volume pregnancy, renal failure.
- Increased capillary permeability, burns, insect bites, cellulites, allergic reactions.
- Lymphatic obstruction, filariasis and malignancy involving lymph nodes leading to obstruction.
- **Others:** Myxedema in hypothyroidism.

Types of Edema

The following are the types of edema according to location and according to clinical findings:
- **According to location:**
  - *Localized edema:* The presence of excess fluid in the interstitial spaces. If the hydrostatic pressure is increased, particularly at the venular end of the capillary, the net movement of water will be disrupted. This is caused due to a thrombus, obstruction from pressure in the abdomen, for example, obesity, tumor, advanced pregnancy or immobility and lack of activity in the skeletal muscle

- *For instance:*
  - Pedal edema—affects lower legs, ankles, and feet. Possible causes: pregnancy, being older.
  - Peripheral edema/Lymphedema—affects the arms, legs, and feet. Possible causes: lymph nodes, kidneys or cancer treatment.
  - Pulmonary edema—affects lungs, makes it hard to breathe, especially when lying down. Causes: fluid in the lungs.
  - Cerebral edema—affects the brain. Causes: head trauma, blocked blood vessel, allergic reaction or tumor.
- *Generalized edema:* Edema that is widespread may be caused by sodium retention or decreased plasma proteins. Where sodium retention occurs, such as in Cushing's syndrome or advanced renal failure. When the kidneys are unable to secrete sufficient sodium, excess sodium moves into the interstitial interstitial space via diffusion Water will follow, causing, widespread edema.. This is referred as anasarca.
- ❖ **According to clinical findings:**
  - *Pitting edema* is described as an indentation that remains in the edematous area after pressure is applied. Its location, timing and extent are determined for treatment response. It is mainly assessed on the medial malleolus, the bony portion of the tibia and the dorsum of the foot.
  - *Non-pitting edema* is seen in lymphedema, myxedema, and lipedema.

Assessment of Edema

- ❖ **History collection:** While collecting the history of the patient the following points should be considered:
  - Timing of the edema.
  - Changes of edema with position.
  - Unilateral or bilateral edema.
  - Medication history.
  - Assessment of systemic diseases.
- ❖ **Physical examination:** In physical examination, pitting tenderness, skin changes, and temperature are evaluated.

Methods of Assessment of Peripheral Edema

- ❖ **Girth measurements** (with a tape measure), the circumferential method is one of the girth measurement techniques. For consistent measurements, each upper extremity or lower extremity is marked with a semi-permanent marker at a certain part with reference to the bony prominences.
- ❖ Pitting edema assessment is performed by pressing firmly with thumb for at least 2 seconds on each extremity.
  - Over the dorsum of the foot.
  - Behind the medial malleolus.
  - Lower calf above the medial malleolus.
  - Pit depth and the time needed for the skin to return to its original appearance (recovery time) are recorded.
- ❖ The grading of edema is determined by pit depth (measured visually) and recovery time from grade 0–4. The scale is used to rate the severity and the scores are as:

- *Grade 0:* No clinical edema.
- *Grade 1:* Slight pitting (2 mm depth) with no visible distortion that rebounds immediately.
- *Grade 2:* Somewhat deeper pit (4 mm) with no readily detectable distortion that rebounds in fewer than 15 seconds.
- *Grade 3:* Noticeably deep pit (6 mm) with the dependent extremity full and swollen that takes up to 30 seconds to rebound.
- *Grade 4:* Very deep pit (8 mm) with the dependent extremity grossly.

ELECTROLYTES REGULATION AND ELECTROLYTE IMBALANCES

Electrolytes

Introduction

- ❖ Electrolytes are those chemical substances whose molecules dissociate into ions when placed in water.
- ❖ These electrolytes are present both in extracellular fluid (ECF) and intracellular fluid (ICF), dissociate into electrically charged particles called ions, the positively charged ions are called cations, such as Na (sodium), K (potassium), Ca (calcium) and Mg (magnesium), H (hydrogen) and negatively charged ions are called anions such as bicarbonate (HCO_3^-), chloride (Cl) and phosphate (PO). The ionic charge is termed valence. Both cations and anions combine according to their valence, such as NaCl.
- ❖ Electrolytes in serum or fluid are expressed as mmol/L (millimoles per litre) or mEq/L (milliequivalent per liter).
- ❖ For example, serum potassium level is 3.5–5.5 mEq/L (mmol/L).

Functions of Electrolytes

- ❖ These regulate water and acid base balance.
- ❖ They maintain osmolarity of plasma and fluids.
- ❖ These help in neuromuscular activity, i.e., transmission of electrical impulses
- ❖ These help in muscle contractions.
- ❖ These help in clotting of blood.
- ❖ Calcium plays a role in clotting.
- ❖ These help in enzyme reaction.

Hyponatremia

Definition

- ❖ It is defined as a plasma sodium level less than 135 mEq/L. It is one of the common electrolyte disorders of adults.
- ❖ Normal serum Na level is 135–145 Eq/L

Causes

- ❖ Daily intake of sodium is 500 mg.
- ❖ The most common cause of hyponatremia is fluid overload seen in cardiac (CHF), renal (nephrotic syndrome) and liver (cirrhosis) diseases.
- ❖ The excess of fluid dilutes the sodium in blood, hence, called dilutional hyponatremia.

The common causes are:
- ❖ Poor dietary intake (dietary restriction).

- Loss of sodium in urine by diuresis, e.g., diuretics and in diabetes.
- GI tract loss of sodium due to gastroenteritis,
- Loss of sodium in patients with burns, sweating (heat stroke).
- Hypervolemia and edematous states (fluid overload) due to any cause as already discussed.
- Syndrome of inappropriate secretion of ADH (SIADH).

Clinical Manifestations
- The clinical manifestations of hyponatremia varies with the cause, type and rate of onset of sodium deficit.
- Acute onset of hyponatremia may be life-threatening.
- When plasma level of sodium is between 125–135 mEq/L, there may be no clinical manifestations.
- The clinical manifestations start when sodium level falls below 120 mEq/L.

The symptoms and signs are:
- GI tract manifestations, e.g., nausea, vomiting, abdominal cramps and diarrhea. The bowels sounds are increased.
- Neurological manifestations, e.g., headache, apprehension, confusion, hallucinations, seizures, coma and death.
- Cardiovascular manifestations, e.g., weak thready pulse, fall in BP, tachycardia.
- Respiratory manifestations, e.g., dyspnea, orthopnea, tachypnea, neurogenic hyperventilation or Cheyne-Stokes breathing.

Investigations
The diagnostic biochemical triad is:
- Plasma sodium levels below 135 mEq/L.
- Chloride level less than 98 mEq/L.
- Plasma osmolarity is low (<275 mOsm/kg).

Nursing Management
- Take a complete history of risk factors, and presenting manifestations.
- Collect complete information regarding diet and medications.
- The client and family members must be asked about behavior changes, headaches, dizziness, weakness and palpitations.
- Measure the client's body weight.
- Assess intake and output and vital signs every 4 hourly.
- Monitor plasma sodium levels and plasma osmolarity.
- **Restoration of sodium levels by:**
  - Fluids are restricted so as to allow sodium to regain balance. Fluids may be restricted to 1000–1500 mL if sodium level is <135 mEq/L.
  - Intake of balanced diet if patient is conscious, able to take and hyponatremia is mild.
  - Sodium replacement is needed if plasma levels falls below 125 mEq/L.
  - For sodium levels <125 mEq/L, IV saline therapy is needed.
  - Dietary supplementation of sodium is appropriate for clients who can take orally.
- Infuse IV normal saline or Ringer's lactate if sodium levels are below 120 mEq/L.
- A concentrated saline may be used if serum sodium is below 115 mEq/L. It should be continued till sodium level reaches 125 mEq/L.
- Rapid elevation of sodium concentrations to than 125 mEq/L is not desirable, as it may in hypernatremia and CNS damage.
- If the client is receiving tube-feeding, it is better to add extra salt through the tubing to achieve desired sodium results.
- Monitoring of the patient response is done by the level of consciousness, urine specific gravity, serum sodium and osmolarity.

Hypernatremia
Definition
It is defined as plasma sodium level mor than 145 mEq/L. It occurs in about 1% of hospitalized patients and carries a high mortality rate.

Causes
It results either from excessive water loss or sodium gain.

Causes of excess fluid loss: Osmotic diuretics, diuretics, burns, heat stroke cause more fluid less than sodium, hence, there will be hypernatremia. Increased sodium gain due to:
- Diabetes insipidus (free water loss)
- Administration of saline
- Hypertonic tube feedings
- Ingestion of excess salt from the table or food rich in salts.

Clinical Manifestations
The symptoms and signs are:
- GI symptoms, e.g., nausea, vomiting, weakness, anorexia, thirst.
- Neurological symptoms, e.g., restlessness, agitation, irritability, muscle weakness, disorientation, hallucinations, seizures, coma.
- Skin and mucous membrane, e.g., tongue dry and swollen, mucous membrane dry and sticky.
- Cardiovascular symptoms, such as tachycardia, high BP, arrhythmias.
- Pulmonary symptoms, such as cough, dyspnea, crackles can occur.

Investigations
- Serum sodium levels are greater than normal. Plasma osmolarity is greater than normal, i.e., 295 mOsm/kg.
- Plasma chloride level greater than normal.

Treatment
- For mild hypernatremia, treat the underlying cause followed by oral fluid replacement.
- Patient of severe hypernatremia with cardiovascular, pulmonary or neurological manifestations requires hospitalization and IV hypotonic infusion.
- To decrease total body sodium and replace fluid loss, either half saline (0.45% Nacl) or 5% dextrose in water (DW) is administered slowly with a goal of reducing plasma sodium levels at a rate of not more than 2 mEq/L/hr for the first 48 hours.

- Hypernatremia caused by sodium excess may be treated with a diuretic (furosemide). Hypernatremia due to diabetes insipidus is treated by nasal spray of desmopressin.

Nursing Management
- Assess the client for risk factors. Obtain a thorough diet and medication history, such as use of corticosteroids or over-the-counter medications containing sodium.
- Look for the clinical features and vital signs.
- Monitor intake and output chart and vital signs every 4 hourly
- Weigh the patient/client daily.
- Look at tongue and mucous membrane and skin to guide intervention.
- Identify the clients at high risk of hypernatremia.
- Maintain intake and output chart and chalk out fluid losses and gains every 4 hourly.
- Monitor changes in behavior, lethargy, restlessness and look for thirst and elevated body temperature.
- Monitor daily serum sodium levels and plasma osmolarity.
- If tube-feeding is being used, give sufficient water to keep the serum sodium and blood urea within normal range.
- Consult the physician in case of worsening hypernatremia or fluid overload.
- Care of mouth and mucous membrane by 2 hourly mouthwash.
- Soft tooth brush should be used to prevent mucosal injury.
- Moisten the client's lips every 1–2 hourly. Offer cool fluids, i.e., fruit juice.
- Teach the client how to keep the oral mucosa hydrated by keeping the fluids in the mouth for some time before ingestion.
- Prevent hypernatremia in debilitated clients by offering them fluids at regular intervals.
- If fluid intake remains insufficient, consult the physician regarding giving fluids by alternative route (parenteral or tube feeding).
- One must keep in mind that higher the osmolarity of feeding by tube, the greater is the need for water supplementation.

Hypokalemia

Definition
- Hypokalemia is defined as serum potassium level less than 3.5 mEq/L. It is a serious problem in sick hospitalized patients, especially on diuretics.
- Normal serum K level is 3.5–5.5 Eq/L

Causes
- The body does not conserve potassium efficiently, thus K^+ deficit commonly results from inadequate intake and excessive potassium excretion.
- Medications, e.g., diuretics, cathartics, steroids, aminoglycosides, amphotericin, digitalis, betablockers, etc., cause hypokalemia.

The common causes are:
- Reduced intake, e.g., inadequate dietary intake, starvation, clay ingestion, potassium free fluids.
- Shift of K into the cells, e.g., insulin therapy, metabolic alkalosis, hypothermia, hypokalemic periodic paralysis.
- Increased losses:
  - GI tract loss, e.g., vomiting, diarrhea, fistulae, ureterosigmoid anastomosis, laxative abuse.
  - Renal loss, e.g., diuretics, diuretic phase of acute tubular necrosis, renal tubular acidosis, diabetes, Cushing's syndrome, liquorice ingestion, hyperaldosteronism.
- Drug and medications, e.g., beta-agonists, steroids, aminoglycosides, amphotericin B, etc.

Clinical Features
- Normal daily intake of K^+ is 500–100 mEq. The clinical features may not be apparent with mild hypokalemia (K level between 3–3.5 mEq/L)
- **Early manifestations of hypokalemia** include anorexia, abdominal distention and constipation. Slow muscle contractions lead to weakness and leg muscle cramps, fatigue.
- **Moderate hypokalemia** leads to decreased conduction of nerve impulses resulting in fatigue, paresthesia, diminished reflexes and irritability. There may be polyuria and nocturia.
- **With severe hypokalemia,** ECG changes appear, i.e., ST segment depression, prolongation of QT, and prominent 'U' waves. Arrhythmias can occur. Progressive hypokalemia leads to confusion, depression, convulsions, areflexia and coma.

Investigations
- Serum K level <3.5 mEq/L.
- ECG may show prolonged QT, prominent U waves and arrhythmia.
- Acid base analysis may show alkalosis.

Treatment
- Identify the risk factors or cause of hypokalemia.
- Obtain detailed history focusing on dietary intake and use of diuretics and other medications, such as digitalis.
- Assess cardiac function and renal function every hourly for first few hours, then 4 hourly.
- Assess neuromuscular function (elicitation of deep tendon jerks) and bowel sounds every 4–8 hourly. If digitalis is the cause, then stop digitalis.

Restoration of Potassium Levels
- For mild to moderate hypokalemia treat the underlying cause or supplement potassium through potassium rich diet.
- Oral potassium is given in mild hypokalemia or potassium-wasting conditions.
- Severe hypokalemia is treated by I.V. potassium supplementation (e.g., KCl).
- A client with K level between 3–3.4 mEq/L needs 100–200 mEq of IV potassium to raise K level by 1 mEq/L.
- If plasma K level is <3 mEq/L, then 200–400 mEq of potassium may be given to raise K level by 1 mEq/L
- For severe potassium deficit, 10–20 mEq of potassium diluted in saline can be given hourly infusion.
- **Warning:** Larger veins should be used for infusion of higher concentration of K.

- Potassium must be diluted in saline not in dextrose.
- Potassium should not be given intramuscularly and never given as a bolus.
- Bolus IV push of K leads to severe hyperkalemia and cardiac arrest.
- Maintenance doses for clients not taking any source of K are 40–60 mEq/L in IV infusion.
- Larger doses are needed when there are co-existing potassium losses.
- If hypokalemia is refractory to usual measures then measure serum magnesium levels.
- Hypokalemia refractory to K supplementation is frequently associated with hypomagnesemia.

Nursing Management
- Assess the client for hypokalemia and find out the cause or risk factors
- Monitor the K levels every 4 hourly as a response to potassium supplementation.
- Maintain intake and output chart and urine output and monitor all the vital signs.
- Teach the client regarding intake of high potassium foods, such as fish, whole grain, nuts, vegetables (cabbage sprouts, brussels, carrots, mushrooms, potatoes, spinach, tomatoes) and fruits (apricots, bananas, guava, melons, oranges, prunes and strawberries).
- Take the K^+ as a preventive measure, when patient is at a risk to developing hypokalemia, for examples, receiving potassium losing diuretics and digitalis.

Hyperkalemia

Definition
- Serum potassium concentration more than 5.5 mEq/L is called hyperkalemia.
- **Pseudohyperkalemia or spurious hyperkalemia:** An artificially elevated K^+ concentration due to K movement out of cells immediately prior to or following venepuncture is called pseudohyperkalemia.

The causes are:
- Prolonged use of a tourniquet with or without repeated fist clenching.
- Hemolysis.
- Marked leukocytosis or thrombocytosis. The clot formation (clotted blood sample) results in release of K from the cells.

Causes
Hyperkalemia results due to the following causes:
- Retention of K^+ by the body because of decreased urine output (acute renal failure).
- Excessive release of potassium from the cells immediate after traumatic injury rhabdomyolysis, or burns or from cell lysis (Intravascular hemolysis, clot lysis) or acidosis (metabolic, diabetic ketoacidosis).
- Excessive infusion of IV potassium or high oral intake, especially in the presence of renal disease.
- Certain drugs, e.g., ACE inhibitor, ARBs (angiotensin receptor blockers retain K^+.)

Clinical Features
- **Mild to moderate hyperkalemia** (K^+ around 6 mEq/L) causes muscle weakness, paresthesias (numbness, tingling), intestinal colic, bradycardia and diarrhea.
- **Moderate to severe hyperkalemia** (K^+ levels above 7 mEq/L) leads to hypotension, convulsions, neuromuscular (Flaccid paralysis, ascending paralysis) and respiratory muscle paralysis and cardiac arrest.

Investigations
- Plasma level >5.5 mEq/L is diagnostic.
- ECG shows tall, tented T waves, AV blocks, QRS widening and sine-wave appearance of QRS (fusion of QRS with T waves).

Nursing Responsibility
- Blood samples for K^+ should be taken in a single prick without using tourniquet.
- Do not use force while aspirating the blood or while transferring the blood into test tubes.
- Under these conditions, K^+ comes out of cells into plasma raising the K^+ levels falsely (spurious hyperkalemia). Sample should be sent for processing and analysis immediately without any delay.

Treatment
- Treat the underlying cause, if found
- **Calcium gluconate:** Administration of calcium gluconate decreases membrane excitability thus antagonizes the effects of hyperkalemia on heart (arrhythmogenic action). It has an immediate onset of action. In the setting of hypotension or cardiac arrest, calcium chloride should be preferred because it releases calcium ions into circulation immediately.
- **Glucose with insulin:** Insulin causes K^+ to shift into cells and lowers the serum K^+ levels. For this purpose, insulin is administered with glucose (glucose neutralized drip) to prevent hypoglycemia. A commonly recommended combination is 10 IU of soluble insulin with 25 g of glucose (5% glucose).
- **Sodium bicarbonate:** Alkali therapy with IV can also shift the K^+ into the cells. This is the safest when administered as an isotonic solution. Alkali therapy is reserved for severe hyperkalemia associated with metabolic acidosis.
- Calcium gluconate and $NaHCO_3$ should not be mixed as they can precipitate from a solution.
- Nebulized B-adrenergic agonists (salbutamol) promote cellular uptake of K in patients with end stage renal disease (ESRD).
- Removal of the excess potassium the body. Excessive potassium burden can be removed by diuretics and hemodialysis.
- Cation exchange resin (sodium polystyrene sulphonate) given orally or by enema can reduce K^+ by exchange with Na^+.

Nursing Management
- Try to identify the risk factors for hyperkalemia by detailed history and physical examination.

- Review the laboratory reports in high-risk clients, i.e., cancer patients with/without chemotherapy.
- If K⁺ levels are between 5.5–6 mEq/L, dietary restriction of potassium is just sufficient.
- If K⁺ levels are higher or if the client is symptomatic, pharmacologic intervention is required.
- Check vital signs, bowel sounds, urine output, lung sounds before and after treatment of hyperkalemia every 4 hourly.
- ECG should be monitored continuously.
- Monitor K⁺ levels every 4 hourly.
- Teach the client the role of low potassium food items, i.e., vegetables (sweet potatoes, beans, fried potatoes), fruits (apple, blueberries, apple sauce, apple juice) and beverages (coffee, cola, beer, lemon soda).

Hypocalcemia

- Normal calcium level is 8.5–10.5 mg.
- About 50% of calcium is bound to albumin and 50% remains unbound and performs physiological actions.
- Changes in pH affect binding of calcium.
- Hypocalcemia is common in older persons.

Definition

- Hypocalcemia is defined as plasma calcium level less than 8.5 mg%. As calcium is bound to albumin, hence, its levels fluctuate with serum albumin levels. For accurate calculation of serum calcium level, following formula is adopted.
- **Correction formula:** Add 0.8 mg/dL to serum calcium level with every 1 g/dL fall in serum albumin level below 4 g/dL.

Causes

The common causes of hypocalcemia are:
- Parathyroidectomy or autoimmune destruction of parathyroids or hereditary defect
- Hypomagnesemia
- Chronic renal failure
- Vitamin D deficiency [(diet, diarrhea, lack of sun exposure for example in Muslim ipardah) ladies].
- Vitamin D antagonism by drugs, e.g., phenytoin
- Vitamin D resistant rickets
- Hyperphosphatemia due to tumor lysis, rhabdomyolysis, acute renal failure

Clinical Features

The symptoms and signs vary.
- **Mild hypocalcemia** may be asymptomatic called latent tetany which can be diagnosed by provocative tests.
- **Moderate hypocalcemia** produces neuromuscular excitability, such as tetany (carpopedal spasms, laryngeal muscle cramps, numbness seizures and fasciculations.
- **Severe hypocalcemia** can be life-threatening and may produce psychosis, convulsions, myopathy, heart failure, arrhythmias and prolonged QT intervals. Spontaneous fractures can occur due to depletion of calcium.

Provocative Tests for Latent Tetany

- **Trousseau's sign:** Raising BP above the systolic level by inflating the sphygmomanometer cuff produces typical carpopedal spasms within 3–5 minutes.
- **Chvostek's sign:** A tap at the facial nerve in front of ear at the angle of jaw produces facial twitching within 3 minutes.

Investigations

- Serum calcium levels are low <8.5 mg%.
- Serum ionized calcium level <2.36 mg/dL indicate hypocalcemia.
- ECG shows prolonged QT interval, arrhythmias.

Treatment

- **Asymptomatic hypocalcemia** is usually corrected with oral calcium gluconate, calcium lactate or calcium chloride. For increased absorption, the calcium supplement should be given with a glass of milk or with meals. The milk is source of vitamin D which improves calcium absorption.
- **Chronic mild hypocalcemia** can be treated by giving a diet rich in calcium, such as dairy products, cheese, milk, ice cream, other instant oat rhubarb, spinach. If hypocalcemia is due to parathyroid deficiency, then client must avoid high phosphate foods, such as milk products, beverages and excess protein.
- **Severe hypocalcemia** accompanied by tetany needs immediate I.V calcium gluconate or chloride slowly to avoid hypotension, arrhythmias and bradycardia. Calcium infusion can be given in 5% dextrose solution not in saline solution because later promotes calcium loss
- Maintenance doses of calcium and vitamin D can be used later or when emergency is over.
- Hypocalcemia due to hyperventilation can be overcome by rebreathing expired air in a paper bag or administering 5% CO_2 in oxygen.

Nursing Management

- Take a detailed history regarding illness, diet intake, medications to find out the cause.
- Check for Trousseau's and Chvostek's signs in high-risk clients.
- Assess the client's cardiovascular status by monitoring ECG and vital signs every 4 hourly. Monitor also for bleeding from the gums and petechiae, and ecchymosis in the skin.
- Examine urine for microscopic hematuria.
- Monitor plasma calcium levels for improvement or worsening.
- Monitor IV sites for infiltration or phlebitis when IV calcium is being infused.
- When possible, use fresh blood for transfusion.
- Avoid giving calcium and bicarbonate in the same IV solution, otherwise precipitates will form.
- Transfer or movements of the clients be restricted to avoid fractures.
- Teach the clients about food that are rich in calcium, such as milk, cheese, yogurt and green leafy vegetables and use them during maintenance therapy or self care.
- Encourage taking calcium supplements with milk during meals for better absorption of calcium.
- Take adequate precaution while taking the blood samples for calcium (instructions have already been discussed).
- Reinforce intake of well-balanced diet avoiding high protein diets or other non prescribed weight loss diets.
- Encourage weight bearing exercises to bone resorption.

Hypercalcemia

Definition

Hypercalcemia is defined as a plasma calcium level more than 10.5 mg/dL. It can occur at any age. It is a common electrolyte disorder which can produce life-threatening complications.

Causes

The causes of hypercalcemia are:
- Hyperparathyroidism due to any cause.
- Malignancy associated, e.g., malignancy of lung, breast, ovary, prostate, bone (multiple myeloma), bladder and blood (leukemias).
- Vitamin D excess, e.g., vitamin D intoxication, sarcoidosis.
- Increased bone resorption, e.g., thyrotoxicosis, thiazides, prolonged immobilization, Paget's disease.
- Associated with renal failure, e.g., secondary hyperparathyroidism, aluminum intoxication.

Clinical Features

The clinical features depend on the severity of hypercalcemia.
- **Mild hypercalcemia** (calcium above 11 mg/dL) is usually asymptomatic.
- **Moderate hypercalcemia** (serum calcium above 13 mg) produces nausea, vomiting, anorexia, polyuria, muscle weakness, fatigue, lethargy, dehydration and constipation. Calcification in the kidneys (renal stones) and other organs, i.e., skin, heart, lungs may also occur and renal insufficiency may develop.
- **Severe hypercalcemia** (serum calcium >15 mg%) produces confusion, depressed sensorium and eventually coma, cardiac arrhythmia due to shortening of QT intervals and cardiac arrest may occur.

Investigations

- Serum calcium and vitamin D (1-25 dihydroxycholecalciferol) levels are higher than normal.
- Serum phosphate and parathormone (PTH) levels are low to normal.

Treatment

- In mild cases, only hydration is often sufficient to reduce calcium levels.
- Immediate correction of moderate to severe hypercalcemia is essential.
- IV normal saline is given rapidly with furosemide (forced diuresis) to prevent fluid overload and to promote rapid urinary excretion of calcium.
- Anti-tumor antibiotics (mithramycin) may be given that inhibit the action of PTH on the bone in order to reduce decalcification and plasma calcium levels.
- Calcitonin decreases plasma calcium levels by inhibiting action of PTH on osteoclasts and increases calcium excretion in urine.
- Steroids decreases calcium levels by decreasing intestinal absorption of calcium by competing with vitamin D, hence useful in vitamin D intoxication, sarcoidosis and lymphomas
- Intravenous phosphate decreases plasma calcium levels is, however, used as a last resort because it may result in severe calcification of various tissues.
- Bisphosphonates (zoledronate, pamidronate) are the first line therapy for hypercalcemia secondary to cancer.
- Second-line therapy includes steroids, mithramycin, calcitonin and gallium nitrate.
- Dialysis removes the calcium rapidly and dramatically, is used to lower calcium in the presence of renal failure.

Nursing Management

- Assessment should be done regarding risk factors, medications by taking detailed history.
- Nurse should identify the high-risk clients and monitor serum calcium levels.
- Assess vital signs, apical pulse, ECG every 6–8 hourly depending on the severity of hypercalcemia.
- Look for bowel sounds, hydration and renal functional status (urine output) every 8 hourly.
- Encourage the client to take sufficient fluids orally to prevent dehydration.
- Discourage excessive consumption of milk products and high calcium diets.
- Encourage adequate bulk in the diet by taking dietary fibers (high fiber diets) to prevent constipation.
- Transfer and handle the client carefully.
- Be alert regarding the signs of digitalis toxicity (if digitalis is being used), cardiac arrhythmias can occur.
- Report any manifestation that indicates worsening of clinical status, such as an arrhythmia, disturbed sensorium, etc.
- Help prevent formation of calcium stones in clients with long-standing hypercalcemia or immobilization by adequate fluid intake and forced diuresis.
- Prevent urinary stasis by turning the immobilized patients, elevating the head of the bed or making the patient to sit up.

Hypomagnesemia

Definition

Hypomagnesemia is defined as a plasma magnesium level <1.8 mg/dL.

Causes

- Critically-ill patients, alcoholics, malnutrition
- Pregnancy and its related conditions
- Diabetes mellitus and infections
- Ischemic heart disease
- Hypomagnesemia also occurs due to loss of magnesium through GI tract, e.g., malabsorption, vomiting, diarrhea, GI suction, ileostomies, fistula, laxative abuse or radiation enteritis pancreatitis.
- Renal losses include the diuretic phase of acute renal failure, antibiotics, diuretics therapy, hyperphosphatemia.
- Prolonged LV or TPN therapy without magnesium substitution also increases the risk for hypomagnesemia.
- Cushing's syndrome, hyperaldosteronism, hyperparathyroidism and corticosteroid excess.
- Alkalosis.

Clinical Features

- **GI tract manifestations:** For example, nausea, anorexia, abdominal distention.

- **Neuromuscular manifestations:** For example, tetany, paresthesias, convulsions.
- **Cardiac manifestations:** These include prolongation of QT interval, premature ventricular contractions (PVC), atrial and ventricular fibrillation.
- Mental features, e.g., depression, confusion, psychosis.

Treatment
- Treatment of hypomagnesemia includes oral magnesium replacement in the form of magnesium—containing antacids in mild deficiency.
- Parenteral magnesium sulfate or chloride is used in critically-ill patients with acute magnesium deficiency.
- Increasing dietary intake of magnesium helps ensure balance and stability.

Nursing Management
- Monitor the vital signs and ECG every one hourly in critically-ill patients with hypomagnesemia.
- Assess the client's deep tendon reflexes.
- Initiate safety and seizure precautions for clients who are extremely confused or at risk for seizures.
- Monitor plasma magnesium, potassium and calcium levels.
- Avoid giving magnesium in saline solution.
- Magnesium infusion should be given slowly in seriously-ill patients as rapid infusion leads to hot and flushed feeling and phlebitis.
- Teach the clients and their family members about the necessity of food rich in magnesium to prevent magnesium deficiency or in treatment of mild deficiency.
- The high magnesium foods include cashews, chilli, halibut, and wheat germ.
- In alcoholism, magnesium should be given with thiamine to prevent neuropathy.

Hypermagnesemia

Definition
Hypermagnesemia is defined magnesium levels greater than 3 mg/dL.

Causes
- Excessive use of magnesium containing antacids or laxatives.
- Administration of potassium sparing diuretics, e.g., spironolactone.
- Excessive use of LV magnesium for controlling premature labor or pre-eclampsia or to treat intractable seizures or asthma or ventricular tachycardia.
- Severe dehydration and diabetic ketoacidosis.
- Renal failure.
- Hypoaldosteronism (Addison's disease, adrenalectomy).

Clinical Features
- The features are due to depressed neuromuscular activity. The symptoms and signs depend on the degree of hypermagnesemia.
- Mild hypermagnesemia leads to hypotension, ECG changes (prolonged PR and QT intervals).
- Severe hypermagnesemia leads to muscle weakness, lethargy, drowsiness, loss of deep tendon jerks, respiratory paralysis and loss of consciousness, cardiac signs tall, tented T waves, wide QRS, heart blocks and VPCS on ECG.

Treatment
It includes:
- Saline infusion with a diuretic increases excretion of magnesium, hence, lowers magnesium levels.
- IV calcium is used to antagonize the effects of hypermagnesemia.
- Albuterol also lowers magnesium levels, hence is useful.
- Respiratory failure is treated by assisted ventilation.
- Dialysis is useful for renal failure.

Nursing Management
- Assess vital signs, ECG, urine output, respiration and level of consciousness every 1–4 hourly.
- Monitor magnesium levels and elicit deep tendon jerks every 4 hourly.
- Keep the IV calcium in the emergency tray when magnesium is being given in critically-ill patients.
- Safety and seizure precautions must be observed.
- Teach the client to avoid constant use of magnesium containing antacids and laxatives.
- Encourage eating food with high fiber content and drink adequate fluids.

■ METABOLIC: ACIDOSIS AND ALKALOSIS

Metabolic Acidosis
- Metabolic acidosis is defined as, "The presence of a low serum bicarbonate concentration (normal range 22–26 mEq/L), although occasionally states can exist where the serum bicarbonate is normal with an elevated anion gap, e.g., patients with a lactic acidosis who have received a bicarbonate infusion or patients on hemodialysis".
- Metabolic acidosis is a serious electrolyte disorder characterized by an imbalance in the body's acid-base balance.

Types of Metabolic Acidosis
- **Diabetic acidosis:** It occurs in people who have diabetes, i.e., poorly controlled. If body do not get enough insulin and get dehydrated, ketones build up in the body. Lots of ketones in the body acidify the blood.
- **Hyperchloremic acidosis:** It results from a loss of sodium bicarbonate. This base helps to neutralize acids in blood. Severe diarrhea and vomiting can cause lower levels of bicarbonate.
- **Lactic acidosis:** It occurs when there is too much lactic acid in the body. The cells present in the body make this lactic acid when they do not have a lot of oxygen to use. Even prolonged exercise can lead to lactic acid buildup.
- **Renal tubular acidosis:** It occurs when the kidneys are unable to excrete acids into the urine. This causes the blood to become acidic. For example, kidney diseases as well as some immune system and genetic disorders can damage kidneys, so they leave too much acid in the blood.

Etiology
- It is rarely a primary disorder, usually develops during the course of another disorder.
- Lactic acidosis (acute)
- Diabetic ketoacidosis
- Acute and chronic renal failure
- Massive rhabdomyolysis
- Anaerobic carbohydrate metabolism
- **Intoxication:**
  - Organic acids, such as salicylates, ethanol, methanol, formaldehyde, ethylene glycol, paraldehyde and INH
  - Sulfate and metformin (Glucophage).
- Shock

Risk Factors
- Renal failure
- Starvation
- Prolonged diarrhea
- Lactic acidosis
- Aspirin or methanol poisoning.
- Pancreatic or biliary fistula.
- Normal saline I/V solution.

Pathophysiology
- Metabolic acidosis occurs, if there is an increase in extracellular hydrogen ion concentration that does not from net accumulation of carbon dioxide.
- Both the pH and serum bicarbonate decrease.

Clinical Manifestations
- Chest pain
- Palpitations
- Headache
- Fast heartbeat
- Lack of appetite
- Jaundice
- Sleepiness
- Abdominal pain
- Nausea/vomiting
- Muscle weakness
- Kussmaul's respirations (Deep and labored breathing pattern often associated with severe metabolic acidosis)
- Confusion
- Fatigue
- Breath that smells fruity, which is a sign of diabetic acidosis (ketoacidosis).
- Altered mental status, such as severe anxiety due to hypoxia.

Diagnostic Evaluation
If metabolic acidosis is suspected, patient needs to give a urine sample. Doctors will check the pH to see, it patient is properly eliminating acids and bases or not. Additional tests may be needed to determine the cause of metabolic acidosis.
- **Arterial blood gas:** It is essential for the diagnosis of metabolic acidosis. If the pH is low (<7.35) and the bicarbonate levels are decreased (<22 mEq/L) in compensated metabolic acidosis, metabolic academia is present and metabolic acidosis is presumed. Due to respiratory compensation (hyperventilation), carbon dioxide is decreased and conversely oxygen is increased.
- **ECG:** It is useful to anticipate cardiac complications.
- **Urinalysis:** It helps to reveal acidity (salicylate poisoning) or alkalinity (renal tubular acidosis type 1). In addition, it can show ketones in ketoacidosis urine pH >6) compensated.
- **Serum electrolytes:** Elevated serum potassium level and low magnesium level.
- Other tests, such as blood glucose and renal function tests.

Management
Medical Management
- A pH <7.1 is an emergency, due to the risk of cardiac arrhythmias and may warrant treatment with intravenous bicarbonate.
  - Bicarbonate is given at 50–100 mmol at a time under strict monitoring of the arterial blood gas readings.
  - This intervention however, has some serious complication in lactic acidosis and in case should be used with great care.
- If the acidosis is particularly severe and/or there may be intoxication, consultation with the nephrology team is considered useful, as dialysis may clear both the intoxication and the acidosis.

Nursing Management
- Monitor vital signs, peripheral pulses laboratory results and level of consciousness frequently.
- Auscultate bowel sounds, measure abdominal girth as indicated.
- Watch out for signs of decreasing level of consciousness
- Record intake and output accurately to monitor renal function.
- Monitor ECG for dysrhythmias and changes for hyperkalemia.
- Monitor heart and lung sounds, CVP and respiratory status.
- Assess edema particularly at the back, sacral, and periorbital area.
- Administer prescribed diuretics.
- Provide oral hygiene with sodium bicarbonate washes, lemon and glycerin swabs.
- Dialysis may be needed, if the patient is experiencing acidosis.
- Restriction of protein may be necessary to decrease production of acid waste products.
- Protect patient from injury resulting from confusion or disorientation.

Complications
- Arrhythmias
- Cardiac arrest
- Coma

Teaching Guidelines for Patient with Metabolic Acidosis
- Discuss about metabolic acidosis, its causes and treatment
- Explain how the prescribed therapy will decrease the acid in the blood.
- Explain that rapid deep breathing is the body's way of compensating for metabolic acidosis and it is a helpful process that will disappear when the extra acid is removed by the kidneys

- Explain the reduction of signs and symptoms indicates that therapy is working well.
- Explain how to prevent metabolic acidosis from recurring, if possible
- Teach how to detect early signs and symptoms of metabolic acidosis, in case it returns.

Metabolic Alkalosis

Metabolic alkalosis is a clinical disturbance characterized by a high pH [77.45 (decreased H' concentration)] and a high plasma bicarbonate concentration (726 mEq/L). It can be produced by a gain of bicarbonate or a loss of H.

Etiology
- Vomiting
- Overuse of antacids.
- Hyperadrenocorticism
- Fistulas
- Excessive intake of alkali, i.e., milk, baking soda, antacid, etc.
- Nasogastric tube drainage or lavage without adequate electrolyte replacement.
- Inherited diseases that can cause metabolic alkalosis are:
  - *Bartter syndrome:* An inherited salt-losing renal tubular disorder characterized by secondary hyperaldosteronism with hypokalemic and hypochloremic metabolic alkalosis and low to normal blood pressure.
  - *Gitelman syndrome:* It is also referred to as familial hypokalemia, hypomagnesemia, is characterized by hypokalemic metabolic alkalosis in combination with significant hypomagnesemia and low urinary calcium excretion.
  - *Liddle syndrome:* An autosomal dominant disorder characterized by early onset salt sensitive hypertension, hypokalemia, metabolic acidosis and suppression of plasma rennin activity and aldosterone secretion.
  - Glucocorticoid remediable aldosteronism
  - Apparent mineralocorticoid excess

Risk Factors
- Vomiting
- Gastric secretion
- Steroids
- Excess aldosterone
- Hypovolemia
- Iatrogenic base administration

Clinical Manifestations
- Confusion
- Nausea/Vomiting
- Diarrhea
- Cardiovascular abnormalities (atrial tachycardia)
- Dysrhythmia
- Compensatory hypoventilation
- Anxiety
- Seizures
- Muscle cramps.
- Tingling of fingers and toes.
- Tetany

Diagnostic Evaluation
- Medical history and physical examination.
- Arterial blood gases reveal pH greater than 7.45 and a serum bicarbonate concentration greater than 26 mEq/L. $PaCO_2$ is 45 mm Hg in compensatory hypoventilation.
- **Serum electrolyte:**
  - Serum phosphate <35 mEq/L
  - Chloride <95 mEq/L
- **Urine pH:** Low (1–3)
- Urinary chloride levels help to identify the cause of metabolic alkalosis, if patient's history provides inadequate information.
- Electrocardiogram may show low T wave, merging with a U wave and atrial or sinus tachycardia.

Management
Medical Management
- In patients with hypokalemia, potassium is administered as KCl to replace both K and Cl losses.
- Histamine 2 receptor antagonists, such as cimetidine (Tagamet), reduce the production of gastric HCl, thereby decreasing the metabolic alkalosis associated with gastric suction.
- Carbonic anhydrase inhibitors are useful in treating metabolic alkalosis in patients who cannot tolerate volume expansion.
- Sufficient chloride must be supplied for the kidney to absorb sodium with chloride (allowing the excretion of excess bicarbonate).

Nursing Management
- Maintain fluid and electrolyte balance.
- Monitor respiratory rate, depth, and effort.
- Monitor O_2 saturation level.
- Administer O_2, if required.
- Assess skin color for any cyanosis.
- Monitor mental status and level of consciousness.
- Provide Fowler's position to facilitate alveolar ventilation and gas exchange.
- Monitor the infusion rate to prevent damage and watch out for signs of phlebitis.
- Watch for signs of muscle weakness, tetany or decreased activity.
- Monitor vital signs frequently.
- Record I/O (Intake and output).

Complications
- Seizures
- Coma

Teaching Guidelines for Patient with Metabolic Alkalosis
- Describe about metabolic alkalosis and its treatment including specific cause in each patient's case
- Explain the need to improve metabolic alkalosis.
- Discuss how to prevent metabolic alkalosis from recurring if possible.
- Indicate that the patient should contact healthcare provider, if symptoms worsen.

RESPIRATORY: ACIDOSIS AND ALKALOSIS

Respiratory Acidosis

Respiratory acidosis is defined as "A condition that occurs when the lungs cannot remove all of the carbon dioxide (CO) the body produces"

It is characterized by:
- pH 7.35.
- $PaCO_2$ >45 mm Hg.

Carbon dioxide is produced constantly as the body's cells respire and this CO_2 will accumulate rapidly, if the lungs do not adequately expel it through alveolar ventilation.

Alveolar hypoventilation, thus, leads to an increased $PaCO_2$. The increase in $PaCO_2$ in turn decreases the $PaCO_2/HCO_3$ ratio and decreases pH.

Types of Respiratory Acidosis
- In acute respiratory acidosis, the $PaCO_2$ is elevated above the upper limit of the reference range (over 47 mm Hg) with an accompanying acidemia (pH <7.35).
- In chronic respiratory acidosis, the $PaCO_2$ is elevated the upper limit of the reference range, with a normal blood pH (7.35-7.45) or near normal pH secondary to renal compensation and an elevated serum bicarbonate (HCO, >30 mm Hg).

Etiology
- Asthma
- Chronic obstructive pulmonary disease (COPD)
- Severe obesity
- Obstructive sleep apnea
- Neuromuscular disorders, such as multiple sclerosis or muscular dystrophy.
- Pulmonary fibrosis
- Acute pulmonary edema
- Pneumonia
- Guillain-Barre syndrome (An inflammatory disorder of the peripheral nerves outside the brain and spinal cord).
- Atelectasis
- Chest wall trauma

Clinical Manifestations
- Headache
- Shortness of breath.
- Asterixis (an inability to maintain posture of part of the body).
- Tremors (shaking)
- Blurred vision
- Psychosis
- Seizures
- Warm and flushed skin.
- Confusion
- Coma
- Anxiety
- Sleepiness
- Fatigue
- Lethargy
- Dyspnea

Diagnostic Evaluation
- **Arterial blood gas:** It is used to measure oxygen and carbon dioxide levels in the blood.
- **Electrolyte testing:** It is a group of tests which helps to measure the levels of Na (sodium), K (potassium), Cl (chloride), and bicarbonate. One or more of the electrolytes will be increased or decreased in people with disorder of respiratory acidosis.
- **Chest X-ray:** It helps to reveal injuries or other problems likely to cause acidosis.
- **Pulmonary function test:** Performed to measure breathing and how well the lungs are functioning.
- Other tests include drug testing, a complete blood count (CBC), and a urinalysis (urine test).
- Assess level of consciousness.

Management

Medical Management
- Bronchodilator medicines and corticosteroids may be used to reverse some types of airway obstruction, such as those associated with asthma or COPD
- Oxygen therapy, if the blood oxygen level is low
- For severe cases, a breathing machine might be needed.
- Narcotic analgesics are inappropriate for patients who have respiratory acidosis because it may depress patient's respirations and worsen the acidosis.

Nursing Management
- Assess $PaCO_2$ level in the arterial blood gas.
- Monitor vital signs of the patient.
- Observe for the signs of respiratory distress, i.e., restlessness, anxiety, confusion and tachycardia.
- Assess mental status and orientation every hour.
- Monitor patient's anxiety level.
- Maintain a calm and quiet environment around the patient.
- Provide a position of comfort to allow ease of respiration
- Provide and monitor supplemental oxygen as needed.
- Maintain adequate hydration.
- Encourage the patient to take deep, slow breath or breath into a brown paper bag (inspire CO_2).
- Continuously monitor arterial blood gases.
- Remain alert for critical changes in patient's respiratory, CNS and cardiovascular functions.
- Instruct patient to avoid smoking as it leads to the development of many severe lung diseases that can cause respiratory acidosis.
- Provide reorientation and explain all activities.
- Encourage the anxious patient to verbalize his/her fear.

Complications
- Poor organ function
- Respiratory failure
- Shock

Teaching Guidelines for Patient with Respiratory Acidosis
- Describe the process that causes respiratory acidosis and explain that signs and symptoms result from too much carbon dioxide in the blood
- Explain the need to improve respiratory function
- Discuss how to prevent the underlying condition that caused respiratory acidosis from recurring, if possible

- Explain how to detect early signs and symptoms of the underlying condition and of respiratory acidosis in case they recur
- Indicate that the patient should contact health care provider, if symptoms worsen.

Respiratory Alkalosis

Respiratory alkalosis is defined as, "A medical condition in which increased respiration elevates the blood pH beyond the normal range (7.35–745) with concurrent reduction in arterial levels of carbon dioxide".

Types of Respiratory Alkalosis

- **Acute respiratory alkalosis:** It occurs within minutes and causes an acute decrease in the serum bicarbonate concentration. In acute respiratory alkalosis, the serum bicarbonate should fall by 2 mEq/L for every 10 mm Hg decline in the PCO.
- **Chronic respiratory alkalosis:** It occurs secondary to renal adaptations and takes 3–5 days as the kidneys reduce acid excretion and increase bicarbonate excretion, both of which increase the serum bicarbonate concentration. In chronic respiratory alkalosis, the serum HCO, concentration should fall by about 4–5 mEq/L for every 10 mm Hg reduction in the pCO_2.

Etiology

Hypoxemia or Tissue Hypoxia
- Lung disease
- Decreased atmospheric oxygen tension (e.g., high altitude)
- Severe anemia.
- Bacterial or viral pneumonia.
- Aspiration of food, foreign object, or vomitus.
- Laryngospasm
- Cyanotic heart disease
- Left shift deviation of oxyhemoglobin curve.
- Pulmonary edema

Central Nervous System
- Anxiety
- Psychosis
- Fever
- Cerebrovascular accidents
- Meningoencephalitis
- Tumor
- Trauma
- Voluntary hyperventilation

Pulmonary Causes
- Asthma
- Reduced lung volume (e.g., due to pneumothorax or pleural effusion)
- Pneumonia
- Pulmonary edema
- Pulmonary embolism
- Interstitial lung disease
- Chronic obstructive pulmonary disease on mechanical ventilation.

Iatrogenic Causes
Medications like progesterone, methylxanthines (e.g., theophylline), salicylates (also cause primary metabolic acidosis), catecholamines and nicotine as well as excessive minute ventilation provided by mechanical ventilation (especially in chronic obstructive pulmonary disease (COPD) or obstructive sleep apnea (OSA)/Obesity hypoventilation syndrome (OHS) patients who have chronic respiratory acidosis).

Medical Conditions Associated with Respiratory Alkalosis
- Pregnancy (due to progesterone)
- Hyperthyroidism
- Sepsis (due to cytokines)
- Chronic liver disease
- Heat exhaustion
- Congestive heart failure

Risk Factors
- Old age
- Mechanical ventilation
- Lung diseases failure
- Hepatic
- Infection
- Anxiety
- CNS infection
- Critically ill

Less Common Risk Factors
- Drugs, such as progesterone, methylxanthines, e.g., theophylline
- Poisoning

Clinical Manifestations

Central Nervous System
- Confusion
- Light headedness
- Generalized seizures
- Increased deep tendon reflexes
- Reduction in intracranial pressure.

Cardiovascular System
- Angina pectoris
- Cardiac arrhythmias
- Peripheral vasoconstriction
- Ischemic electrocardiographic changes
- Normal or decreased blood pressure.

Neuromuscular System
- Muscle cramps
- Carpopedal spasm
- Trousseau's sign
- Chvostek's sign
- Laryngeal spasm
- Circumoral numbness
- Numbness and paresthesia of the extremities.

Diagnostic Evaluation
- **Arterial blood gas:** This test helps to measure oxygen and carbon dioxide levels in the blood.

- **Pulmonary function tests:** Performed to measure breathing and how well the lungs are functioning.
- Other laboratory test and imaging studies that may be useful in respiratory alkalosis to find out the causes includes:
  - *Complete blood count:* Elevated WBC in sepsis.
  - *EKG and ECHO:* Performed for congestive heart failure.
  - *Thyroid function test:* It helps to rule out hyperthyroidism.
  - *Pulmonary function test:* It helps to rule out chest infections.
  - *VIQ scan:* Performed to rule out pulmonary embolism.
  - *Chest X-ray:* Performed to detect chest infection.
  - *CT scan:* Performed for pulmonary embolism.
  - *MRI brain:* It helps to rule out CNS cause of hyperventilation.

Management
Medical Management
To manage respiratory alkalosis, a healthcare provider needs to first find the underlying cause.
- For respiratory alkalosis caused by hyperventilation, into a paper bag allows patient to keep more carbon dioxide in his/her body, which improves the respiratory alkalosis.
- If the oxygen level is low, patient may receive oxygen.
- High altitude sickness is treated with acetazolamide 250 mg 12 hourly, dexamethasone 4 mg 6 hourly, oxygen therapy and descent to lower altitude in severe cases.
- For critically-ill patients on mechanical ventilation with respiratory alkalosis, tidal volume and respiratory rate needs to be decreased with adequate pain control.

Nursing Management
- Monitor vital signs, respiratory rate, depth, and ease and skin color.
- Monitor ABGs, primarily $PaCO_2$; a value less than 35 mm Hg indicates too little CO_2 (carbonic acid).
- Keep the patient warm and dry.
- Teach patient breathing techniques to slow down breathing, holding breath, rebreathing into a paper bag or rebreather mask.
- Be alert for signs of changes in neurologic, neuromuscular or cardiovascular functions.
- Institute safety measures for the patient with vertigo or the unconscious patient.
- If the respiratory alkalosis is related to a drug over-dose, the patient may require treatment for poisoning.
- Encourage the anxious patient to verbalize his/her fears.
- Discuss cause of condition (if known) and appropriate interventions and/or self-care activities.
- Instruct patient and family members to contact health care provider, if they notice the following
  - Loss of consciousness.
  - Rapidly worsening symptoms of respiratory alkalosis.
  - Seizures
  - Severe breathing difficulties.

Complications
- Cardiac arrhythmias
- Seizures

Teaching Guidelines for Patient with Respiratory Alkalosis
- Describe about respiratory alkalosis and its treatment, including its specific cause.
- Explain the need to improve respiratory alkalosis.
- Discuss how to reduce anxiety.
- Explain how to control breathing rate, if hyperventilation was anxiety related.
- Explain that the reduction of signs and symptoms indicates that therapy is working well.
- Indicate that the patient and family should contact healthcare provider, if symptoms worsen.

INTRAVENOUS INFUSION/INTRAVENOUS THERAPY

Definition
Intravenous infusion refers to the introduction of large amount of fluid into the body through a vein.

Purposes
- To restore the body fluid in case of bleeding and dehydration.
- To meet the basic requirements of the body, e.g., calories, water, minerals and vitamins.
- To overcome and prevent shock and collapse.
- To restore acid base balance.
- To monitor central venous pressure.

Indications
- Severe hemorrhage
- Vomiting
- Burns
- Septicemia
- Oral cancer
- Renal diseases
- Cardiac diseases
- Dehydration
- Fluid and electrolyte imbalance
- Shock
- Post-surgery
- Trauma
- Unconsciousness

Peripheral Venipuncture Sites

Criteria for Selection of Venipuncture Sites
- The condition of veins (collapsed or too small).
- The characteristics of tissues over the vein (edematous, injured, diseased, inflammed, etc.)
- Purpose and the duration of infusions.
- The type and the amount of IV fluids ordered.
- The diagnosis and the general condition of the patient
- The most convenient veins for venipuncture in the adult are the basilic and the median cubital vein in the antecubital fossa because these veins are large and superficial. However, for prolonged infusions, these veins cannot be used without limiting the movements at the elbow joints by the use of splints
- If the person is right handed, use of the left arm allows more independence and vice versa.

Sites of Venipuncture

The most commonly used veins in the order of their frequency of use are as follows **(Fig. 8.2)**:

Forearm: Basilic vein and cephalic vein.
- **Antecubital space:** Median cubital, basilic vein and cephalic vein.
- **Radial area:** Radial vein
- **Hands:** Metacarpal veins.
- **Foot:** Great saphenous and dorsal plexus.
- **Thigh:** Great saphenous and femoral veins.
- **Scalp veins:** Infants.

Types of IV Fluids

Isotonic: A solution that exerts the same osmotic pressure as that of plasma. It is used to expand intravascular compartment increasing circulating volume.
- 0.9% Normal saline
- Ringer lactate
- Blood components

Hypotonic: A solution that exerts the less osmotic pressure than that of plasma. It is used for patients who need extra hydration.
- 5% Dextrose
- 0.45% Saline
- 0.2% Saline

Hypertonic: A solution that exerts the more osmotic pressure than that of plasma. It is used for postoperative patients to maintain circulating volume and prevent edema.
- Dextrose 5% in normal saline
- 10% Dextrose
- 20% Dextrose

Plasma expanders: For example, dextran which is a long chain polysaccharide. These solutions are confined to the vascular compartment and preferentially expand this portion of the ECF.

Commonly used intravenous therapy solutions are described in **Table 8.3**.

Cannula Selection

Considerations

- Quality and size of vein and patient's clinical condition.
- Physician's order.
- Infusion viscosity.
- Diagnosis and/or expected procedures and duration of therapy.
- Volume, rate, irritability and viscosity of medication/solution to be administered.

Types of peripheral venous access devices:
- Plastic over the needle cannula (24–18 G, 3/4"–14" long) recommended for:
  - Short-term infusion therapy.
  - Restless patients.
  - Elderly patients with fragile veins.
  - Infants and children with small veins.
- Butterfly (winged metal needle 25–19 G, 2" to 1" long) recommended for:
  - Administering IV push medications when there is not a free flowing IV or an IV lock in place.
  - When there is an allergy to plastic.
- Scalp vein access (for infants less than 1 year old only). Used as alternative to over-the-needle cannula.

Calculation for Making IV Fluids

Definition

Intravenous (IV) fluid regulation refers to the manual or automatic pump control of the rate of flow of IV fluids as they are delivered to a patient through a vein.

Purposes

The purpose of intravenous fluid regulation is to control the amount of fluid that a patient is receiving, usually within a given hour of IV therapy.

Without fluid regulation, the IV would run in by gravity at a rapid rate and could cause fluid or drug overload.

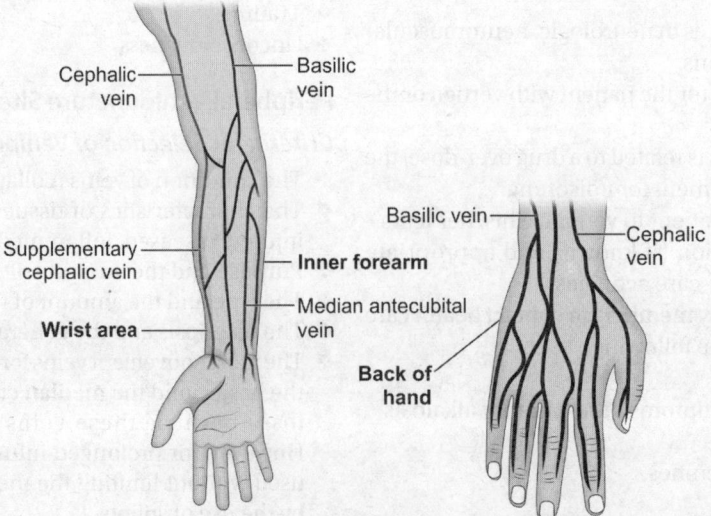

Fig. 8.2: Sites of venipuncture.

Chapter 8: Fluid, Electrolyte, and Acid-Base Balances

TABLE 8.3: Commonly used Intravenous therapy solutions.

Common intravenous therapy solutions	Benefits possible from administration intravenous therapy	Conditions requiring precautions
Carbohydrates in water (e.g., 3% dextrose in water)	• Prevents dehydrations. • Promotes sodium dieresis (particularly following excessive administration of electrolyte solution) • Prevents and treats ketosis. • Supplies water (for body needs) • Supplies calories (for energy)	• Water intoxication • Patients undergoing blood transfusion • Patients undergoing neurosurgical procedure
Carbohydrates in sodium chloride solution (e.g., 5% dextrose in half strength saline)	• Promotes diuresis • Corrects excessive fluid loss (due to perspirations) • Provides calories and sodium chloride • Prevents alkalosis	• Renal insufficiency • Edema from cardiac, hepatic, or renal disease.
Sodium chloride solutions. (e.g., 0.9% sodium chloride solution)	• Treats alkalosis • Treats adrenocortical insufficiency • Treats vomiting from pyloric stenosis • Corrects excessive fluid loss • Treats dehydration from reduced water intake, vomiting or diarrhea • Treats diabetic acidosis	• Hyponatremia • High sodium and plasma concentrations dehydration Edema
Ringer's solution (contains sodium, chloride, potassium and calcium)	• Treats mild alkalosis • Treats hypochloremia	• Addison's disease • Severe potassium or calcium deficiency
Lactated ringer's solution (contains sodium, potassium, calcium, chloride and lactate)	• Treats dehydration • Replaces daily extracellular electrolyte and water loss. • Restores normal fluid after extracellular fluid shift (from burns, infection etc.) • Moderates metabolic acidosis (from renal insufficiency, infant diarrhea, diabetic ketosis)	• Anoxia • Severe metabolic acidosis. • Severe metabolic alkalosis. • Hepatic disease
Multiple electrolyte solution (contains sodium, potassium magnesium, chloride, lactate phosphate)	Replaces gastric contents lost through gastric suctioning or vomiting.	• Severe renal disease • Diabetes insipidus • Severe hepatic disease
Plasma volume expanders (contain dextran, sodium, chloride)	Temporarily increases blood volume lost from trauma, hemorrhage, burns. surgery or anesthesia	Dextran allergy

Precautions

❖ There are varied types of IV administration sets and they deliver fluid at different amounts per drop.
❖ Nurses should always determine the type of drip chamber that they are using and calculate the IV flow per minute based upon the amount of fluid that the administration set delivers per drop.
❖ There are varied types of IV pumps and IV tubing used to deliver IV fluids.
❖ Nurses should be sure to use the correct tubing for the pump selected.
❖ The specific directions for the use of each individual pump should be followed.

Formula for Flow Rate Calculation

$$\text{Flow rate} = \frac{\text{Total volume infused in mL} \times \text{drops/mL}}{\text{Total volume infused in mL} \times \text{drops/mL}}$$

Example:
Total volume infused = 200 mL in 24 hours
Drops per mL = 15
Total time in minutes = 24 × 60 = 1440 minutes

$$\text{Flow rate} = \frac{2000 \times 15}{1440} = 20.8 \text{ drops}$$

Methods

Manual Regulation of IV Fluids

Manual regulation of IV fluids is performed by adjusting the roller adaptor on the IV tubing until it reaches the appropriate drip rate per minute. To manually regulate the IV rate, the nurse looks at her watch and times the number of drops that fall into the drip chamber over one full minute. If the rate is too slow, the adapter should be rolled to a looser position to speed the dripping of the IV. If the rate is too fast, the roller adapter should be tightened to decrease the dripping of the IV. Nurses should adjust the roller until the IV rate is set at the correct amount of drops per minute to deliver the IV fluids as ordered. The IV rate must be checked every hour or more often according to the policy of the medical setting to be certain that the rate remains accurate.

IV Fluid to be Delivered by an IV Pump

To regulate the IV fluid to be delivered by an IV pump, the tubing should be threaded into the machine correctly.

TABLE 8.4: Flow rates for intravenous infusions.

Flow rates for intravenous infusions	1000 mL/6 hr (drops/min)	1000 mL/10 hr (drops/min)	1000 mL/12 hr (drops/min)	1000 mL/24 hr (drops/min)
10	28	17	14	7
15	42	25	21	10
20	56	34	29	14
60	167	100	84	42

Nurses should dial in the hourly IV rate (cc to be delivered over an hour) and start the pump following the manufacturer's guidelines. I/V-rate and flow must be checked hourly when on a pump to be sure that the rate remains accurate and that the correct amount of fluid is delivered. Most pumps have a reading that shows how much fluid has been delivered over the past hour. The flow rates for intravenous infusions are tabulated in **Table 8.4**.

PERFORMING A VENIPUNCTURE

Definition

The purpose of puncturing a vein, with a needle, using aseptic technique.

Purposes

- To administer fluids intravenously
- To administer bolus medication of investigations or treatment
- To draw blood specimen
- To administer total parenteral nutrition
- To administer blood and blood products

Contraindications

- An arteriovenous fistula in the extremity
- Mastectomy on the same side of the arm/a surgically compromised extremity
- Presence of phlebitis, infiltration or sclerosis.

Articles Used

A clean tray containing:

- Sterile needle/angiocath/butterfly needle of appropriate size
- Sterile cotton swabs in a bowl with antiseptic/alcohol pads
- Tourniquet
- Tapes for fixing catheter/needle
- Syringe of required size for blood draws (optional)
- Specimen bottle (optional)
- Syringe loaded with medicine (optional)
- Infusion made ready for administration
- Towel/mackintosh for protecting linen
- Gloves
- IV pole
- Kidney tray/paper bag.

Procedures

- Check physician's order and nursing care plan.
- Identify plan.
- Explain procedure to patient that there will be a slight discomfort initially. If required, demonstrate procedure on a doll for children.
- Make sure that clothing can be removed over IV tubing if needed. Provide client with a gown if necessary.
- Wash hands.
- Select venipuncture site. Unless contraindicated select the nondominant arm of the client. Look for veins that are relatively straight. Consider catheter length so that the wrist/elbow will be away from the catheter tip.
- **Dilate the vein:**
  - Place extremity in a dependant position (lower than heart).
  - Apply a tourniquet firmly about 15–20 cm (6–8 inches) above the vein puncture site, explain that tourniquet will feel tight. The tourniquet must be tight enough to obstruct venous flow but not tight enough to obstruct arterial supply.
  - If the vein is not sufficiently dilated, massage/stroke the vein distal to the site in the direction of venous flow towards the heart.
  - Encourage the client to clench and unclench the fist.
  - Lightly tap the vein.
  - If all the steps fail, remove the tourniquet and apply heat to the entire extremity for 10–15 minutes.
- Don clean gloves.
- **Clean venipuncture site:**
  - Clean with antiseptic swab from center outward in circular motion for several inches.
  - Permit solution to dry on the skin.
- **Insert the needle/catheter:**
  - Use nondominant hand to pull the skin below the entry site.
  - Hold catheter/needle at a 15–30° angle with level up, insert the catheter through the skin and into vein. A sudden lack of resistance is felt as needle enters the vein.
  - Once blood is seen in the lumen or when a lack of resistance is felt, reduce the angle of catheter approximately 0.5–2 cm.
  - Remove needle from inside the angiocath completely and attach syringe with medication
  - Syringe for blood draws/IV infusion tube as required.
- **Tape the catheter using 3 strips of adhesive tapes:**
  1. Place one strip with sticky side up under the catheter hub. Fold over each side so that sticky sides are against the skin.
  2. Place second strip sticky side down over catheter hub.
  3. Place 3rd strip sticky side down over hub/infusion tubing.

- ❖ **Dress and label the venipuncture site as per agency policy:**
  - Place a sterile gauze piece with povidone iodine over the venipuncture site. Apply pad over the site. Apply occlusive dressing over site.
  - Label the dressing with date, time of insertion, size of needle used, catheter used and initials.
- ❖ Remove gloves and wash hands.
- ❖ Discard all soiled equipment appropriately.
- ❖ Document all relevant data and report any observation.

COMPLICATIONS OF IV FLUID THERAPY

Local Complications

Phlebitis

Phlebitis is the inflammation of the vein's inner lining, the tunica intima. Clinical indications are localized redness, pain, heat, and swelling, which can track up the vein leading to a palpable venous cord.

- ❖ **Mechanical causes:** Inflammation of the vein's inner lining can be caused by the cannula rubbing and irritating the vein. It is recommended to use the smallest gauge possible to deliver the medication or required fluids.
- ❖ **Chemical causes:** Inflammation of the vein's inner lining can be caused by medications with a high alkaline, acidic, or hypertonic solutions. To avoid chemical phlebitis, follow the Parenteral Drug Therapy Manual (PDTM) guidelines for administering IV medications for the appropriate amount of solution and rate of infusion.
- ❖ **Treatment:**
  - Immediately remove cannula. May elevate arm or apply a warm compress.
  - Document findings in chart.
  - Initiate a new peripheral IV, if necessary.

Infiltration

Infiltration occurs when a non-vesicant solution (IV solution) is inadvertently administered into surrounding tissue. Signs and symptoms include pain, swelling, redness, skin surrounding insertion site is cool to touch, change in quality or flow of IV, tight skin around IV site, IV fluid leaking from IV site, and frequent alarms on the IV pump.

- ❖ **Treatment:**
  - Stop infusion and remove cannula.
  - Follow agency policy related to infiltration.
  - Always secure peripheral catheter with tape or IV stabilization device to avoid accidental dislodgement.
  - Avoid areas of flexion and always assess IV site prior to giving IV fluids or IV medications.

Extravasation

Extravasation occurs when vesicant solution (medication) is administered and inadvertently leaks into surrounding tissue, causing damage to surrounding tissue. Characterized by the same signs and symptoms as infiltration but also includes burning, stinging, redness, blistering, or necrosis of the tissue.

- ❖ **Treatment:**
  - Stop infusion and remove cannula.
  - Follow agency policy for extravasation for specific medications. For example, toxic medications have a specific treatment plan.

Hemorrhage

Hemorrhage is defined as bleeding from the puncture site.
Treatment: Apply gauze to the site until the bleeding stops, then apply a sterile transparent dressing.

Local Infection at IV Site

Local infection is indicated by purulent drainage from site, usually two to three days after an IV site is started.
Treatment: Remove cannula and clean site using sterile technique. Monitor for signs and symptoms of systemic infection.

Systemic Complications

- ❖ **Pulmonary edema:** Pulmonary edema, also known as fluid overload or circulatory overload, is a condition caused by excess fluid accumulation in the lungs, due to excessive fluid in the circulatory system. It is characterized by decreased oxygen saturation, increased respiratory rate, fine or coarse crackles at lung bases, restlessness, breathlessness, dyspnea, and coughing up pinky frothy sputum. Pulmonary edema requires prompt medical attention and treatment. If pulmonary edema is suspected, raise the head of the bed, apply oxygen, take vital signs, complete a cardiovascular assessment, and notify the physician.
- ❖ **Air embolism:** Air embolism refers to the presence of air in the vascular system and occurs when air is introduced into the venous system and travels to the right ventricle and/or pulmonary circulation. An air embolism is reported to occur more frequently during catheter removal than during insertion, and the administration of up to 10 mL of air has been proven to have serious and fatal effects. Small air bubbles are tolerated by most patients.
  - *Signs and symptoms of an air embolism:*
    - Sudden shortness of breath
    - Continued coughing
    - Breathlessness
    - Shoulder or neck pain
    - Agitation
    - Feeling of impending doom
    - Lightheadedness
    - Hypotension
    - Wheezing
    - Increased heart rate
    - Altered mental status
    - Jugular venous distension.
  - *Treatment:*
    - Occlude source of air entry.
    - Place patient in a Trendelenburg position on the left side (if not contraindicated)
    - Apply oxygen at 100%
    - Obtain vital signs
    - Notify physician promptly.

- **Prevention:** To avoid air embolisms, ensure drip chamber is one-third to one-half filled, ensure all IV connections are tight, ensure clamps are used when IV system is not in use, and remove all air from IV tubing by priming prior to attaching to patient.
- **Catheter embolism:** A catheter embolism occurs when a small part of the cannula breaks off and flows into the vascular system. When removing a peripheral IV cannula, inspect tip to ensure end is intact.
- **Catheter-related bloodstream infection:** Catheter-related bloodstream infection (CR-BSI) is caused by microorganisms that are introduced into the blood through the puncture site, the hub, or contaminated IV tubing or IV solution, leading to bacteremia or sepsis. A CR-BSI is a nosocomial preventable infection and an adverse event.
  - *Signs and symptoms:* CR-BSI is confirmed in a patient with a vascular device (or a patient who had such a device in the last 48 hours before the infection) and no apparent source for the infection other than the vascular access device with one positive blood culture.
  - *Treatment:* IV antibiotic therapy
  - *Prevention:* To avoid CR-BSI, perform hand hygiene prior to care and maintenance of an IV system, and use strict aseptic technique for care and maintenance of all IV therapy procedures.

Other Complications

- **Circulatory overload:** The intravascular compartment contains more fluid than the normal. Circulatory overload results in cardiac failure and pulmonary edema.
- **Hematoma formation:** The walls of blood vessels may be damaged due to careless introduction of the needle into the body.
- **Pyrogenic reaction:** It is characterized by temperature elevation, chills, headache, nausea, vomiting and circulatory collapse in severe cases.
- **Serum hepatitis:** Infectious hepatitis have been attributed to improperly disinfected syringes and needles.
- **Allergic reaction:** This may due to certain drugs administered along with the IV fluids.

MEASURING INTAKE AND OUTPUT (FLUID INTAKE)

Definition

It is defined as the measuring and recording of fluid intake and output (I and O) during a 24 hour period which provides important data about a patient's fluid and electrolyte balance.

Normal Intake and Output

- **Daily intake:** An adult human at rest takes approximately 2,500 mL of fluid daily.
- **Levels of intake:** Approximate levels of intake include fluids 1,200 mL. foods 1,000 mL, and metabolic products 300 mL.
- **Daily output:** Daily output should approximately equal in intake.
- **Normal output:** Normal output occurs as urine, breathing, perspiration, feces, and in minimal amounts of vaginal secretions.

Significance

- Determining intake and output is an important component in assessing daily fluid balance.
- Intake and output (I&O) indicate the fluid balance for a patient.
- The goal is to have equal input and output.
- Too much input can lead to fluid overload.
- Too much output can cause dehydration.
- A change in urine volume is an indicator of fluid alterations or kidney diseases.
- It is important to know the exact amount of fluid intake and urinary output because it may be an aid in diagnosis and in assessing the treatment of the patient.
- It is the responsibility of the nurse to record each and every intake and output of the patient
- The entire fluid intake even the parenteral means should be measured and recorded.

Intake and Output

- **Intake includes:** Water, tea/coffee, intravenous fluids, nasogastric feeds, water used to flush NGT after feeds, juices, ice creams, soups, gelatin and syrups if taken in considerable amounts frequently
- **Output includes:** Urine, watery diarrhea stools, drainage, vomitus, bleeding, excessive perspiration (approximately), aspirated stomach contents
  - The urinals with measuring up or for the catheterized patient the urine bag with graduations can be used to measure the urine output
  - The patient and his family members need to be taught about the importance of intake and output charts.

Intake and Output should be Maintained for the following Patients

- Postoperative patients
- Unstable, deteriorated patients
- Patients with fever (febrile)
- Patients on fluid restriction
- Patients receiving intravenous fluids, diuretics
- Patients with chronic illnesses, cardiopulmonary, renal diseases, diabetes.

Purposes

- To assess patient's general health
- To monitor specific disease conditions
- To assess the fluid and electrolyte balance.

Articles

- Intake and output from a bedside
- Intake and output graphic record in chart
- Bedpan or urinal or bedside commode
- Graduated drinking cup/tumbler
- Graduated container for output

- Clean gloves
- Sign at bedside that patient is on intake and output measurement.

Procedures

- Identify the patient.
- Explain the methods of maintaining, Intake and output. All fluids taken orally must be recorded on the patient's intake and output from (intake and output flow sheet).
- Wash hands every time prior to giving oral fluids.
- Measure all oral fluids in accordance with institutional policy
  - *Example:*
    - Water glassful = 200 mL
    - Cupful = 20 mL
  - *Paper cup*
    - Large = 200 mL
    - Small = 120 mL
    - Soup bowl full = 180 mL
    - Water pitcher full = 1000 mL
  - Measure all fluids in the graduated cup/tumbler before giving to patient.
- Record time and amount of fluid intake in the designated space on bedside chart. Include all semisolid and liquid food rich in fluids (oral, IV, tube feedings and IV fluids).
- Transfer eight hours total fluids intake from bedside intake and output chart of 24 hour, intake and output record in patient's chart.
- Record all fluid intakes in the appropriate column of the 24 hour record.
- Complete 24 hour intake record by adding as eight hour totals.
- For measuring output intake, urinary output and other drainage from patient.
- **Urinary output:** After each voiding measure the urine, using a measuring container and record it with the time of voiding on the intake and output form.
  - For patients with retention catheter empty the drainage bag into a measuring container at the end of the shift or at prescribed times if output is measured more often. Note and record it.
  - For infants and incontinent patients the output may be measured by first weighing diapers or incontinent pads that are dry and then subtracting this weight from the weight of soiled items.
- The amount and type of fluid (urine, drainage from NG tube, drainage tube) are recorded in the intake and output form.
- Transfer 8 hour output total to 24 hours intake and output record on the patient's chart.
- Complete 24 hours output record by totalling all 8 hours total.

Special Considerations

- Proper aseptic technique should be taken while handling patient's body fluid output viz. blood, urine, etc.
- Remember that fluids taken to swallow pills must be recorded as intake.
- Do not have visitors or family members empty bedpan, urinal or catheter bags.

ADMINISTERING BLOOD AND BLOOD COMPONENTS

Definition

- Blood transfusion consist of administration of compatible donor's whole blood or any of its components to correct/treat any clinical condition.
- Blood transfusion therapy refers to the process of administering whole blood or blood components to a patient through an intravenous (IV) needle or catheter placed in a patient's vein. Blood and blood products may be autologous (comprised of the patient's own blood), homologous (blood donated from another person) or synthetic (blood products developed in a laboratory).

Purposes

- To restore circulating blood volume
- To correct platelet and coagulation factor deficiencies
- To correct anemia.

Types of Blood Products for Transfusion

Whole Blood

- **A whole blood contains:**
  - Up to 510 mL total volume (volume may vary in accordance with policies).
    - 450 mL donor blood.
    - 63 mL anticoagulant preservative solution.
  - Hemoglobin approximately 12 g/mL.
  - Hematocrit 35–45%.
  - No labile coagulation factors (V and VIII).
  - No functional platelets.
- **Unit of issue:** 1 donation, also referred to as a "unit" or "pack".
- **Infection risk:** Not sterilized, so capable of transmitting any agent present in cells or plasma which has not been detected by routine screening for transfusion transmissible infections, including HIV-1 and HIV-2, hepatitis B and C, other hepatitis viruses, syphilis, malaria and Chaga's disease.
- **Storage:** Between +2°C and +6°C in approved blood bank refrigerator, fitted with a temperature chart and alarm.
  - During storage at +2°C and +6°C, changes in composition occur resulting from red cell metabolism.
  - Transfusion should be started within 30 minutes of removal from refrigerator
- **Indications:**
  - Patients needing red cell transfusions where red cell concentrates or suspensions are not available.
  - Exchange transfusion.
  - Red cell replacement in acute blood loss with hypovolemia.
- **Contraindications:**
  - Risk of volume overload in patients with:
  - Chronic anemia.
  - Incipient cardiac failure.

❖ **Administration:**
- Must be ABO and RhD compatible with the recipient.
- Never add medication to a unit of blood.
- Complete transfusion within 4 hours of commencement.

Red Cell Concentrate (Packed Red Cells, Plasma-reduced Blood)

❖ **Contains:**
- 150–200 mL red cells from which most of the plasma has been removed.
- Hemoglobin approximately 20 g/100 mL (not less than 45 g per unit).
- Hematocrit 55–75%.

❖ **Unit of issue:** 1 donation
❖ **Infection risk:** Same as whole blood.
❖ **Storage:** Same as whole blood.
❖ **Indications:**
- Replacement of red cells in anemic patients.
- Use with crystalloid replacement fluids or colloid solution in acute blood loss.

❖ **Administration:**
- Same as whole blood.
- To improve transfusion flow, normal saline (50–100 mL) may be added using a Y pattern infusion set.

Red Cell Suspension

❖ **Contains:**
- 150–200 mL red cells with minimal residual plasma to which 100 mL normal saline, adenine, glucose mannitol solution (SAC-M) or an equivalent red cell nutrient solution has been added.
- Hemoglobin approximately 15 g/100 mL (not less than 45 g per unit).
- Hematocrit 50–70%
- *Unit of issue:* 1 donation

❖ **Infection risk:** Same as whole blood.
❖ **Storage:** Same as whole blood.
❖ **Indications:** Same as red cell concentrate.
❖ **Contraindications:** Not advised for exchange transfusion of neonates. The additive solution may be replaced with plasma, 45% albumin or an isotonic crystalloid solution, such as normal saline.

❖ **Administration:**
- Same as whole blood.
- Better flow rates are achieved than with red cell concentrate or whole blood.

Leukocyte Depleted Red Cell

❖ **Contains:**
- A red cell suspension or concentrate containing $<5 \times 10^6$ white cells per pack, prepared by filtration through a leukocyte depleting filter.
- Hemoglobin concentration and hematocrit depend on whether the product is whole blood, red cell concentrate or red cell suspension.
- Leukocyte depletion significantly reduces the risk of transmission of cytomegalovirus (CMV).

❖ **Unit of issue:** 1 unit (350 mL)

❖ **Infection risk:** Same as whole blood for all other transfusion transmissible infections.
❖ **Storage:** Depends on production method—consult blood bank
❖ **Indications:**
- Minimizes white cell immunization in patients receiving repeated transfusions but, to achieve this, all blood components given to the patient must be leukocyte depleted.
- Reduces risk of CMV transmission in special situations.
- Patients who have experienced two or more previous febrile reactions to red cell transfusion.

❖ **Contraindications:** Will not prevent graft-vs-host disease—for this purpose, blood components should be irradiated where facilities are available (radiation dose = 25 – 30Gy).

❖ **Administration:**
- Same as whole blood.
- A leukocyte filter may also be used at the time of transfusion if leukocyte depleted red cells or whole blood are not available.
- Complete transfusion within 4 hours of commencement

Fresh Frozen Plasma

❖ **Contains:**
- Pack containing the plasma separated from one whole blood donation within 6 hours of collection and then rapidly frozen to -25°C or colder.
- Contains normal plasma levels of stable clotting factors, albumin and immunoglobulin.
- Factor VIII level at least 70% of normal fresh plasma level.

❖ **Unit of issue:**
- Usual volume pack is 200–300 mL.
- Smaller volume packs may be available for children.

❖ **Infection risk:**
- If untreated, same as whole blood.
- Very low risk if treated with methylene blue/ultraviolet light inactivation.

❖ **Storage:**
- At -25°C or colder for upto 1 year.
- Before use, should be thawed in the blood bank in water which is between 30-37°C. Higher temperatures will destroy clotting factors and proteins.
- Once thawed, should be stored in a refrigerator at +2°C to +6°C

❖ **Indications:**
- Replacement of multiple coagulation factor deficiencies.
- Liver disease.
- Warfarin (anticoagulant) overdose.
- Depletion of coagulation factors in patients receiving large volume transfusions.
- Disseminated intravascular coagulation (DIC). Thrombotic thrombocytopenic purpura (TTP).

❖ **Precautions:**
- Acute allergic reactions are not uncommon, especially with rapid infusions.
- Severe life-threatening anaphylactic reactions occasionally occur.

- Hypovolemia alone is not an indication for use.
- Dosage Initial dose of 15 mL/kg

❖ **Administration:**
- Must normally be ABO compatible to avoid risk of hemolysis in recipient.
- No compatibility testing required.
- Infuse using a standard blood administration set as soon as possible after thawing.
- Labile coagulation factors rapidly degrade; use within 6 hours of thawing

Platelets (Table 8.5)

❖ **Single donor unit in a volume of 50–60 mL of plasma should contain:**
- At least 55×10^9 platelets.
- $<1.2 \times 10^9$ red cells.
- $<0.12 \times 10^9$ leukocytes.

❖ **Unit of issue:** May be supplied as either:
- *Single donor unit:* Platelets prepared from one donation.
- *Pooled unit:* Platelets prepared from 4–6 donor units "pooled" into one pack to contain an adult dose of at least 240×10^9 platelets.

❖ **Infection risk:**
- Same as whole blood, but a normal adult dose involves between 4 and 6 donor exposures.
- Bacterial contamination affects about 1% of pooled units.

❖ **Storage:**
- Up to 72 hours at 20–24°C (with agitation) unless collected in specialized platelet packs validated for longer storage periods; do not store at 2–6°C
- Longer storage increases the risk of bacterial proliferation and septicemia in the recipient.

❖ **Indications:**
- *Treatment of bleeding due to:* Thrombocytopenia.
- Platelet function defects.
- Prevention of bleeding due to thrombocytopenia, such as in bone marrow failure.

❖ **Contraindications:**
- Not generally indicated for prophylaxis of bleeding in surgical patients, unless known to have significant pre-operative platelet deficiency.
- *Not indicated in:*
  - Thrombocytopenia associated with septicemia, until treatment has commenced or in cases of hypersplenism.
  - Untreated disseminated intravascular coagulation (DIC).
  - Idiopathic autoimmune thrombocytopenic purpura (ITP).
  - Thrombotic thrombocytopenic purpura (TTP).

❖ **Dosage:**
- 1 unit of platelet concentrate/10 kg body weight in a 60 or 70 kg adult, 4–6 single donor units containing at least 240×10^9 platelets should raise the platelet count by $20 - 40 \times 10^9/L$
- Increment will be less, if there is:
  - Splenomegaly.
  - Disseminated intravascular coagulation.
  - Septicemia.

❖ **Administration:**
- After pooling, platelet concentrates should be infused as soon as possible, generally within 4 hours, because of the risk of bacterial proliferation.
- Must not be refrigerated before infusion as this reduces platelet function.

TABLE 8.5: Platelet products.

Parameters	Platelet concentration (PC)	Apheresis platelets (SDAP)
Description	Platelet concentrates are prepared from either 350 mL or 450 mL whole blood. They are also random donor platelets (RDP)	Platelet concentrate derived from blood donor using an apheresis machine and disposable lot. It also called single donor apheresis platelets (SDAP)
Volume	50–90 mL	200–300 mL
Platelet contents	3.5–4.5 $10^{''}$/unit	$3–7 \times 10^{''}$/unit (6–8 times the content in RDP).
Dosage	1 unit of platelet concentrate/10 kg body weight: In a 60 or 70 kg adult, 4–6 single donor units.	One pack of platelet concentrate collected from a single donor by apheresis is usually equivalent to one therapeutic dose.
Storage and shelf life	3–5 days at 20°C to 24°C (with agitation).	5 days at 20–24°C (with agitation).
Do not store at 2°C to 5°C in refrigerators as it makes them non-functional		
Indications	• Thrombocytopenia. • Platelet function detects. • Prevention of bleeding due to thrombocytopenia, such as in bone marrow failure.	• Same as for RDPs. • Patients experiencing frequent febrile. • Reactions with platelet concentrate.
Administration	• Transfuse using standard blood transfusion set with 170 mm filter. • Initiate transfusion slowly for first 15 minutes unless massive blood loss.	Same as random do not platelets, but ABO compatibility is more important.

Caution: Platelets are prone to develop bacterial contamination, transfusion should be started immediately after receiving the units in the ward and should be completed over a period of about 30 minutes.

- 4-6 units of platelet concentrates (which may be supplied pooled) should be infused through a fresh standard blood administration set.
- Special platelet infusion sets are not required.
- Should be infused over a period of about 30 minutes.
- Do not give platelet concentrates prepared from RhD positive donors to an RhD negative female with child bearing potential.
- Give platelet concentrates that are ABO compatible, whenever possible.

Indications of Blood Transfusion

- External bleeding
- **Internal bleeding:**
  - *Non-traumatic:*
    - Peptic ulcer
    - Varices
    - Ectopic pregnancy
    - Antepartum hemorrhage
    - Ruptured uterus
  - *Traumatic:*
    - Chest
    - Spleen
    - Pelvis
    - Femur
- Red cell destruction: For example, malaria, sepsis and HIV
- Disseminated intravascular coagulation.
- Anemia.
- Thrombocytopenia.
- Hemophilia.
- Congenital clotting deficiencies.
- Pre-eclamptic toxemia.
- Renal failure.
- Cardiorespiratory disease.
- Chronic lung disease.
- Acute infection.
- Diabetes.
- Treatment with beta blockers.

Articles

- Blood transfusion set
- Normal saline
- Blood/blood components 9 sterile in appropriate container
- Cannula No. 18/19 (adult)
- Alcohol/iodine swabs (disinfectant)
- Sterile gauze
- Tourniquet
- Adhesive tape
- Scissors
- Roller bandage and splint (optional)
- Infusion stand
- Disposal bag/kidney tray
- Disposable gloves
- Pressure bag (optional in case of severe bleeding)
- Specimen container.

Procedure

- Check physician's orders, patient's condition, and history of transfusion/transfusion reaction, reason for present transfusion, etc.
- Identify patient.
- Check availability of blood with the blood bank.
- Explain the procedure to the patient, need for
- transfusion, blood product to be given, approximate length of time, desired outcome, etc. Emphasize the need for patient to report unusual symptoms immediately. Obtain informed consent from patient.
- Obtain blood from blood bank in accordance with agency policy. If transfusion cannot begin immediately, return product to blood bank. Blood out of refrigerator for more than 30 minutes, above 10°C cannot be reused. Never store blood in unauthorized area-like ward refrigerator. Blood must be stored in refrigerated unit at carefully controlled temperature (4°C).
- Encourage patient to empty bowel and bladder and assist to a comfortable position. Collect urine specimen.
- Ensure privacy.
- Wash and dry hands.
- Check vital signs and record.
- Don disposable gloves.
- Insert IV cannula (18G/19G) if not already present in a large peripheral vein and initiate infusion of normal saline solution using blood transfusion set.
- **Inspect the blood product (By 2 nurses) for:**
  - Identification number
  - Blood group and type
  - Expiry date
  - Compatibility
  - Patient's name
  - Abnormal color, clots, excess air, etc.
- Warm blood if needed using special blood warmer or immerse partially in tepid water.
- If blood product is found to be correct. Stop the saline solution by closing roller clamp. Remove insertion spike from saline container and insert spike into blood container.
- Start infusion of blood product slowly, at the rate of 25–30 mL per hour for the first 15 minutes. Stay with patient for first 15 minutes. Check vital signs every 15 minutes for first 30 minutes, or as per agency policy.
- Increase infusion rate if no adverse reactions are noticed. The flow rate should be within safe limits.
- Assess the condition of patient every 30 minutes and if any adverse effect is observed stop transfusion and start saline. Send urine sample, blood sample and remaining blood product in container with transfusion set, back to the blood bank.
- Complete transfusion and administer saline (as per physician's order) if no adverse reaction is observed.
- Dispose blood product container and set in appropriate receptacle.
- Wash hands.

- ❖ **Record the following product and volume transfused number and blood group:**
  - Time of administration. Started and completed.
- ❖ Name and signature of nursing staff carrying out procedure and patient's condition, if agency policy requires remove label from blood bag and paste in on patient's record
- ❖ Assist patient to comfortable position.

Special Considerations

- ❖ Do not administer medication through the same line, where blood product is transfused. Start another IV line if medications are to be infused, because of possible incompatibility and bacterial contamination. Blood transfusion should be completed over a period of 4 hours from the time of initiation.
- ❖ Cover the blood bag with a towel when it hangs on the IV pole.
- ❖ Gently rotate the blood bag periodically to prevent clumping of cells.
- ❖ When re-warming the blood by immersing in tap water, do not immerse the blood fully into the water as it may cause hemolysis.

Complications of Blood Transfusion

Acute Reactions

Because many reactions exhibit similar clinical manifestations, every symptom should be considered potentially serious and the transfusion discontinued until the cause is determined. When a reaction is suspected, blood bags with tubing from all products transfused within 4 hours should be returned to the blood bank for re-evaluation

- ❖ **Allergic reactions:**
  - *Clinical manifestations:*
    - Flushing
    - Itching, rash
    - Urticaria, hives
    - Asthmatic wheezing
    - Laryngeal edema.
    - Anaphylaxis
  - *Management:*
    - Stop transfusion immediately. Keep vein open with normal saline.
    - Give antihistamine as directed (diphenhydramine).
    - Observe for anaphylaxis and prepare epinephrine, if respiratory distress is severe.
    - If hives are the only clinical manifestation, the transfusion can sometimes continue at a slower rate.
- ❖ **Hemolytic reactions:**
  - *Clinical Manifestations:*
    - Chills, fever.
    - Low back pain.
    - Feeling of head fullness, flushing.
    - Oppressive feeling.
    - Tachycardia, tachypnea.
    - Hypotension, vascular collapse.
    - Hemoglobinuria, hemoglobinemia.
    - Bleeding.
    - Acute renal failure.
    - Death.
  - *Management:*
    - Stop transfusion immediately. Keep vein open with 0.9% saline.
    - Notify physician and blood bank.
    - Treat shock, if present.
    - Draw testing samples, collect urine sample.
    - Maintain BP with IV colloid solutions. Give diuretics as prescribed to maintain urine flow, glomerular filtration and renal blood flow.
    - Insert indwelling catheter to monitor hourly urine output. Patient may require dialysis, if renal failure occurs.
- ❖ **Non-hemolytic febrile reactions:**
  - *Clinical manifestations:*
    - Sudden chill and fever
    - Headache
    - Flushing
    - Anxiety
  - *Management:*
    - Stop transfusion immediately and keep vein open with normal saline. Notify physician and blood bank.
    - Send blood sample and blood bags to blood bank.
    - Collect urine sample for testing.
    - Check temperature 1/2 hour after chill and as indicated thereafter.
    - Give antipyretics as prescribed. Treat symptomatically.
- ❖ **Circulatory overload:**
  - *Clinical manifestations:*
    - Rise in venous pressure.
    - Distended neck veins
    - Dyspnea
    - Cough
    - Crackles at base of lungs
  - *Management:*
    - Stop transfusion and keep vein open with normal saline. Notify physician
    - Place patient upright with feet in dependent position.
    - Administer prescribed diuretics, oxygen, morphine and aminophylline.
- ❖ **Septic reactions:**
  - *Clinical manifestations:*
    - Rapid onset of chills
    - High fever
    - Vomiting, diarrhea
    - Marked hypotension
  - *Management:*
    - Stop transfusion immediately and keep vein open with normal saline. Notify physician and blood bank.
    - Obtain cultures of patient's blood and return blood bags with administration set to blood bank for culture.
    - Treat septicemia as directed: Antibiotics, IV fluids vasopressors and steroids

Delayed Reactions

Transfusion complications can occur days to months post-transfusion. Symptoms exhibited within this time frame should be investigated thoroughly to rule out a delayed transfusion reaction. Examples of delayed reaction include:

❖ **Delayed hemolytic reaction:**
  • *Clinical manifestations:*
    ▪ Fever
    ▪ Mild jaundice
    ▪ Decreased hematocrit
  • *Management:* Generally, no acute treatment is required, but hemolysis may be severe enough to cause shock and renal failure. If this occurs, manage as outlined under acute hemolytic reactions.

❖ **Iron overload (hemosiderosis):**
  • *Clinical manifestations:*
    ▪ Diabetes
    ▪ Decreased thyroid function
    ▪ Arrhythmias
    ▪ Congestive heart failure and other symptoms related to major organ failure.
  • *Management:* Treat symptomatically. Deferoxamine (Desferal); an iron chelator that removes accumulated iron through the kidneys, may be administered IV, IM or subcutaneously.

❖ Graft versus host disease.
❖ **Infectious diseases:**
  • Hepatitis B
  • AIDS
❖ Thrombophlebitis.

❖ Pulmonary embolism.
❖ Microbial contamination.

Blood Transfusion and Nursing Management
Refer **Table 8.6**.

RESTRICTING FLUID INTAKE

❖ Fluid restriction means that patient need to limit the amount of liquid per day. Fluid restriction is needed if body is holding water, i.e., fluid retention. Fluid retention can cause health problems, such as tissue and blood vessel damage, long-term swelling and stress on the heart. So, following nursing interventions are used:
❖ Explain the need for fluid restriction to patient. Involving patients in the therapeutic regimen enhance the cooperation from the patient.
❖ Plan out the amount of liquid prescribed during the day for the patient.
❖ Using a small cup for providing fluid to patient.
❖ Maintain good oral care by brushing teeth after meals, rinsing with alcohol free mouthwash, chewing sugarless gum or sucking on hard candy you may be able to decrease dry mouth and urges to drink.
❖ Avoid foods with high levels of sodium (salt) these types of foods will increase thirst.
❖ Provide gum or hard candy as by consuming these mouth feel less dry.
❖ Frozen liquids may help with thirst, and can help to provide liquids more slowly, for example, ice chips. count these also in patient's daily consumption of fluid intake

TABLE 8.6: Nursing observation and management during blood transfusion.

Reaction	Signs and symptoms	Nursing management
Allergic reaction	• Hives • Itching • Anaphylaxis	• Stop transfusion immediately and keep vein patent with normal saline. • Notify physician fast. • Administer antihistamine parenterally as necessary.
Febrile reaction: fever, developing during infusion	• Fever and chills • Headache • Malaise	• Stop transfusion immediately and keep vein patent with normal saline. • Notify physician. • Treat symptoms.
Hemolytic transfusion reaction: Incompatibility of blood product.	• Immediate onset • Facial flushing • Fever, chills • Headache • Low-back pain Shock	• Stop transfusion immediately and keep vein patent with normal saline. • Notify physician stat. • Obtain blood samples from site. Obtain first voided urine. • Treat shock if present. • Send remaining blood in bag, tubing and filter to lab. Draw blood sample for serologic testing and send urine specimen to lab
Circulatory overload	• Dyspnea • Dry cough • Pulmonary edema	• Slow/stop infusion. • Monitor vital signs. Notify physician. • Place patient in upright position with feet dependent.
Bacterial reaction: Bacteria present in blood	• Fever • Hypertension • Dry, flushed skin. • Abdominal pain.	• Stop transfusion immediately. • Obtain culture of patient's blood and return blood bag to lab. • Monitor vital signs. • Notify physician. • Administer antibiotics stat.

- Recording fluid intake will help make sure that patient are not taking in more fluids than expected.

■ ENHANCING FLUID INTAKE

- Explain the patient the need for increase water intake as understanding of patient will increase the effort for taking adequate fluid, educate the patient to drink at least 8-10 cups (2-2½ liters) of fluid daily throughout the day.
- Educate the patient to drink most of fluids between meals so you will not be replacing food with fluid.
- Drink a water-based beverage (water, juice or milk) with every meal and snack
- Avoid drink caffeinated beverages (coffee, tea and sodas), alternate decaffeinated beverage intake throughout the day as caffeinated beverages and alcohol are diuretics. Diuretics increase the excretion of water from the body rather than hydrating
- Add variety by using calorie-fee, fruit-flavored waters.
- Adding citrus to water such as a slice of lime to water improves the taste and increase the fluid consumption.
- **Keep a "water intake record:** Educate the patient to tracking and recording of water intake helps to motivate to maintain fluid intake.

Administration of Medications

MEDICATION

- *"Medication is medicine that is used to treat and cure illness."*
- *"A medication is a substance administered for the diagnosis, cure, treatment, or relief of a symptom or for prevention of disease."*
- A dosage form that contains one or more active and/or inactive ingredients.
- Medications come in many dosage forms, including tablets, capsules, liquids, creams, and patches.
- They can also be given in different ways, such as by mouth, by infusion into a vein, or by drops that are put into the ear or eye.
- The form with the active ingredient is used to prevent, diagnose, treat, or relieve symptoms of a disease or abnormal condition.
- A medication that does not contain an active ingredient and is used in research studies is called a placebo. Also called drug product.

ADMINISTRATION OF MEDICATION

Introduction

- Administration of medicine is one of the great responsibilities of a nurse.
- Nurse should see that all medicines are administered in such a way as to obtain best results.
- For this, she should have a knowledge of the drugs that is administered by her to patient.

Definition

- **Medication administration** means *"the physical act of giving medication to a client by the prescribed route."*
- **Medication administration** means *"an act in which a single dose of a prescribed medication or biological is given by application, injection, inhalation, ingestion, or any other means to a resident by an authorized person in accordance with all laws and regulations governing the administration of medications and biologicals."*
- **Medication administration** means *"the provision or application of a medication to the body of a patient by a medical practitioner or a nurse or as otherwise provided by law."*
- **Medication administration** means *"the delivery of medication, by an individual delegated to and supervised by a licensed nurse, to a client whose use of that medication must be monitored and evaluated applying specialized knowledge, skills, and abilities possessed by a licensed nurse."*
- **Medication administration** means *"an act in which a drug or biological is given to a resident by an individual who is authorized in accordance with state laws and regulations governing such acts, and may include a licensed healthcare practitioner, licensed nurse, or medication assistant."*

General Principles

- The nature of the drug, i.e., the name, classification, types of preparations, effects, dosage, absorption and excretion, routes of administration, time of administration and indications.
- Essential parts of a medication order.
- Abbreviations and symptoms are used in writing a medication order.
- Weights and measures are used.
- Preparation of solutions and calculation of fractional doses.
- Storing of medicines.
- Factors of safety in the administration of medicines.
- Rules for the administration of medicines.
- Ethical and legal aspects.
- Nurse's role in the administration of oral medicines.

DRUGS NOMENCLATURE

Drugs may be known by several names:

Chemical Name

- Chemical name is the name by which a drug is known to the chemists; usually, it indicates the ingredients of the drug.
- It identifies the molecular structure.
- It describes in chemist's terms, the placement of atoms or atomic groupings.
- For example, the chemical name of the anti-inflammatory agent ibuprofen is 2-4 (isobutyl phenyl) propionic acid.

Generic Name

- Generic name or non-proprietary name is the name assigned by the manufacturer who first developed the

drug and is assigned by the United States Adopted Names Council.
- Subsequent manufacturers of the drug use the same generic name. Often the generic name is derived from the chemical name.
- Each drug has only one generic name, which is simpler than the chemical name, from which it is derived.
- Examples of drugs known by their generic name include morphine sulphate, ibuprofen, etc.

Official Name

- Official name is the name by which the drug is identified in the official publications.
- For example, BP (British Pharmacopoeia), USP (United State Pharmacopoeia), NF (National Formulary), publications officially approved by FDA.
- Official name is the name assigned by the Food and Drug Administration (FDA) after approval of a drug and is often the same as the generic name.

Trade Name

- Trade name or brand name or proprietary name is the registered name assigned by the manufacturer and is copyrighted.
- Brand names are nouns with the first letter capitalized and marked with a circled R.
- One drug may be manufactured by several companies and so may be known by several different trade names.
- For example, Paracetamol (chemical name) have different trade names, such as Crocin, Calpol, Ifimol, Metacin, etc.

EFFECTS OF DRUGS ON THE BODY

Therapeutic Effects

- It is the effect which is desired or the reason a drug is prescribed.
- Therapeutic effects are the medication's desired and intentional effects.
- These effects vary with the nature of medications, the length of time the client has been receiving it and the client's physical condition.
- Interaction with other drugs also can affect a drug's therapeutic action.

The drugs are administered for the following purposes:
- **To promote health:** Drugs are given to the individual to increase the resistance against diseases, e.g., vitamins.
- **To prevent diseases:** For example, vaccines and antitoxins.
- **To diagnose disease:** For example, barium used in the X-ray studies.
- **To alleviate diseases:** Certain drugs are given for the palliative effect or for the temporary relief of distressing symptoms but does not remove the cause or cure the disease, e.g., analgesics.
- **To treat or cure a disease:**
  - By restoring normal functions, e.g., digoxin.
  - By supplying a substance that is deficient in the body, e.g., insulin.
  - By destroying the causative organisms, e.g., Quinine in malaria.
  - By counteracting with a toxic substance circulating in the body, e.g., antidotes.
  - By stimulating the functions of an organ or a system, e.g., stimulants.
  - By depressing the functions of an organ or a system, e.g., sedatives.

Local and Systemic Effects

- Local effects of a drug are expected when they are applied topically to the skin or mucus membrane.
- A drug used for systemic effect must be absorbed into the blood stream to produce the desired effect in the various systems and parts of the body.

Adverse Effects

- Adverse effect is any effect other than the therapeutic effect.
- Some adverse effects are minor, whereas some other may cause very serious health problems.
- Adverse effects may be more in a very seriously-ill client or a client who receives more medications.

Side Effects

- Side effects are the minor adverse effects. Side effects can be harmful or harmless.
- These are the effects other than the principal action desired.

Allergic Reactions

- A client can react to a drug as a foreign body and thus develop symptoms of allergic reaction.
- Allergic reaction can be either severe or mild.
- A severe allergic reaction usually occurs immediately after the administration of the drug, it is called anaphylactic reaction.
- A mild reaction has a variety of symptoms from skin rashes to diarrhea.
- **Anaphylaxis:** This is an immediate and severe reaction marked by a decreased blood pressure, local edema, prickling feeling in the throat, edema of the face and hands, cyanosis, chocking cough, dyspnoea and wheezing due to accumulated fluids and edema in the respiratory tissues. This is an emergency. Unless acted quickly, death may follow within few minutes. Sera and penicillin, etc., should be administered only after a sensitivity test has been done to prevent such reactions.
- **Skin rashes (Urticaria):** Edematous pinkish elevations with itching may occur due to reaction of a drug. Rash is usually generalized over the body.
- **Pruritis:** Itching of the skin with/without a rash.
- **Angioedema:** Edema due to increased permeability of the blood capillaries.
- **Rhinitis:** Excessive watery discharge from the nose.
- **Lacrimal tearing:** Excessive tears from the eyes.
- **Nausea and vomiting:** Due to stimulation of these centres in the brain.

- ❖ **Nausea and vomiting:** Due to stimulation of these centers in the brain.
- ❖ **Diarrhea:** Irritation of the mucosa of the intestines.
- ❖ Shortness of breath and wheezing due to laryngeal Edema.
- ❖ **Atropine-like side effects:**
  - Certain drugs cause dryness of the mouth and nose, flushing and dryness of the skin, tachycardia, urinary retention and blurring of vision.
  - The client may need to be reassured that the effects will disappear when the drug is withdrawn.
  - Clients, after taking drugs, producing these side effects should not operate dangerous machinery.
- ❖ **Liver damage:** This is characterized by jaundice especially in the sclera of the eyes, hemorrhages under the skin, dark urine and pruritis. Since many drugs are detoxicated by the liver and may become harmful if liver damages are present for any reason.

Effects on the Urinary System

- ❖ Certain drugs may cause renal damage which is characterized by anuria, oliguria, hematuria, crystalluria, albuminuria, etc.
- ❖ Accurate recording and intelligent observation of the intake and output is indicated.
- ❖ Frequent urine analysis and chemistry studies can prevent such occurrences.
- ❖ Clients should be asked to take plenty of fluids to prevent stone formations.

Effects on the Cardiovascular System

- ❖ **Arrhythmias:** Any change in the rate, rhythm, volume or character of the pulse. Counting pulse for one full minute will reveal such irregularities,
- ❖ **Hypotension:** It is characterized by decrease in the blood pressure, dizziness, syncope and shock. Checking BP before and after the administration of the drug is indicated. The client should be warned about postural hypotension.
- ❖ **Hypertension:** This is characterized by elevated blood pressure, epistaxis, emotional irritability, headache, visual disturbances and dizziness.

Blood Dyscrasias

- ❖ **Aplastic anemia:** Characterized by pallor, weakness, dyspnoea, anorexia, fever, headache, bleeding from mucus membrane, etc. Bone marrow functions may be affected.
- ❖ **Thrombocytopenia:** It is characterized by purpura, petechia, melaena epistaxis, hematuria and other symptoms of internal bleeding.
- ❖ **Granulocytosis, leukopenia:** It is characterized by chills, fever, sore throat, cough, malaise and lesions in the mouth.
- ❖ Education of the public is essential to refrain from taking drugs without physician's orders and supervision, prolonged and unnecessary use of drugs, etc.

Effects on the Nervous System

- ❖ **Abnormal involuntary movements:** Tremor, chorea, dystonia, alterations in the muscle tone, difficulty in preserving equilibrium in erect and sitting position.
- ❖ **Stimulations of the central nervous system:** These are characterized by anxiety, nervousness, insomnia, headache, double vision, etc. Stimulation of the nervous system may precipitate convulsions if the client has the history of epilepsy.
- ❖ **Depression of the central nervous system:** It is characterized by dizziness, vertigo, drowsiness, fatigue and ataxia. Restriction of ambulation and use of bed rails may be necessary. The persons taking such medications should not drive a car or operate machinery.

Effects on the Gastrointestinal System

- ❖ **Irritation of the gastric mucosa:** This is characterized by nausea, vomiting, anorexia. This can be prevented some extent by not giving the drug in an empty stomach. Give the drug with or the meals or it should be given along with one glass of milk or an antacid. These drugs are contraindicated if the client has a history of peptic ulcer.
- ❖ **Small bowel ulceration:** It is characterized by abdominal pain, melena, distension and diarrhea, constipation.

Hypersensitivity Reaction

This develops in a client who is sensitive to a medication's therapeutic effects or secondary effects.

Toxicity

- ❖ High levels of the drug in the blood stream produce toxic effects.
- ❖ Often the toxic effects of the drug occur due to the cumulative effect of the drug or due to the excess intake of the drug than what is needed for the therapeutic effects.
- ❖ Cumulative effect occurs when a person is unable to metabolize the previous dose of the drug.
- ❖ Some of the toxic effects are fatal for the client.
- ❖ Toxicity can affect and permanently damage organ function.
- ❖ Common drug toxicities include, nephrotoxicity (kidney), neurotoxicity (brain), hepatotoxicity (liver), immunotoxicity (immune system), ototoxicity (hearing), cardiotoxicity (heart).

Interactions

Medication interaction occurs when a medication's effects are altered by the concurrent presence of other medications or food.

The interaction can result in the following:

Synergism

- ❖ Synergistic effect occurs when a combination of medications is given.
- ❖ In synergistic effect, the combined effect of two or more drugs is different from the effect of each drug when taken alone.
- ❖ The combined effect may be less than what would be expected or greater than the effect of each drug.
- ❖ Synergism may be a desired therapeutic effect or an undesirable complication, e.g., alcohol and barbiturates

are potentially lethal; Phenytoin (Dilatin) has an inhibitory effect upon digitalis.

Antagonism
- It results in decreased drug effectiveness.
- Sometimes food influences a drug.

Drug incompatibility
Drug incompatibility is a condition in which a drug precipitates from solutions if mixed with other medications.

Toxic Effects
Drug toxicity occurs when a person has accumulated too much of a prescription drug in their bloodstream, leading to negative effects. This can happen if the dose taken exceeds the prescribed amount, or if prescribed dosage is too high. The toxic effects of a drug are dose-dependent and can affect an entire system as in the CNS or a specific organ such as the liver.

Tolerance
It occurs when a client develops decreased response to a drug, requiring increased dosage to achieve the therapeutic effects.

Drug Intolerance
Drug tolerance refers to the inability of person to tolerate a drug and is unpredictable. Tolerance is a person's decreased response to a drug, which occurs when drug is used repeatedly and the body adapts to the continued presence of the drug. When drug intolerance is develop, the person requires high dose of the drug to maintain the therapeutic effect of the drug. Repeated administration of certain drugs can result in a decrease in their pharmacological effect. Hence, higher doses of such drugs are needed to produce a given response, e.g., ephedrine, organic nitrates, opioids, etc.

Types of Tolerance
- **Natural tolerance:** Blacks are tolerant mydriatics (racial tolerance).
- **Acquired tolerance:** It develops on repeated exposure to a drug, e.g., on repeated use of morphine, tolerance develops to its euphoriant and analgesic effects.

Idiosyncratic Effects
Drug idiosyncrasy refers to untoward reactions to drugs that occur in a small fraction of patients and have no obvious relationship to dose or duration of therapy. Idiosyncratic drug reactions, also known as type B reactions, are drug reactions that occur rarely and unpredictably amongst the population and may be individual to a patient.

Teratogenic Effects
Appearance of fetal anomalies and/or developmental defects due to exposure to a teratogenic agent during fetal development when administered during pregnancy. Drugs that can cause birth defects are said to be teratogenic drugs.

Cumulative Effect
A cumulative effect is the increasing response to repeated doses of a drug that occurs when the rate of administration exceeds the rate of metabolism or excretion. As a result, the amount of the drug builds up in the client's body unless the dosage is adjusted. Toxic symptoms may occur.

FORMS OF MEDICATIONS

Solid Form
- **Caplet:** Shaped like a capsule coated for easy swallowing
- **Capsule:** Powdered, liquid or oily drug enclosed in a gelatine shell.
- **Pills:** Tablets containing one or more drugs shaped into ovoid or oblong form.
- **Tablet:** Powdered dosage compressed into hard disc
- **Lozenges:** Flat, round form containing drug flavouring sugar and mucilage. It dissolves in mouth.
- **Suppository:** Solid dosage form mixed with gelatine for insertion in the body cavity, melts at body temperature, releasing the drug for absorption.

Liquid Form
- **Injections:** Liquid drugs in the ampoule or vial for IM, IV, SC, ID use.
- **Drops:** Liquid drugs for instillation in eyes, ears, nose.
- **Elixir:** Clear fluid containing water or alcohol, usually has sweetener for easy swallowing
- **Syrup:** Drug dissolved in concentrated sugar solution.
- **Suspension:** Finely divided drug particles in a liquid medium.
- **Lotion:** Drug in liquid suspension used externally onto the skin.
- **Tincture:** Water or alcohol drug solution.
- **Emulsion:** Mixture of two liquids uniformly dispersed throughout each other.

Semi-Solid Form
- **Ointment:** Preparation made for external use usually containing gone or more drugs.
- **Paste:** Thick and stiff preparation absorbed through skin more slowly than ointment.
- **Cream:** A non-greasy semi-solid preparation used onto the skin.

DRUG PREPARATIONS

- Medications are available in the market in different types of preparations.
- The preparations may determine the method of administration.
- When a medication is ordered, it is important that the nurse must use the correct preparations.

The following is the list of pharmaceutical preparations of drugs:
- **Aqueous solution:** One or more drugs soluble in water
- **Aqueous suspension:** One or more drugs finely divided in a liquid, such as water.
- **Capsule:** Powdered drugs or liquids within a gelatine cover.
- **Extract:** Concentrated preparation of a drug from raw material generally used to preserve a drug for use in a medication.

- **Elixir:** Solution containing alcohol, sugar and water. May or may not have active medicines.
- **Emulsion:** An emulsion is a mixture of two or more liquids that are normally immiscible, e.g., dispersion of fat globules in water or water globules in fat.
- **Fluid extract:** Alcoholic liquid extracts of drugs made by percolation so that I mL of the fluid extract contains 1 g of the drug. This is the most concentrated forms of all fluid preparations, only vegetable drugs are used.
- **Lotion:** Drugs in liquid suspension intended for external use.
- **Liniments:** Mixture of drugs with oil, soap, water or alcohol and intended for external use.
- **Lozenges:** A combination of drugs having some sugar or soothening material which relieves the tickling sensation at the back of the throat and stops a cough.
- **Mucilages:** Aqueous preparations containing viscous substances, such as gums and starches.
- **Ointment:** Semi-solid preparations of a drug or drug in petrolatum (Vaseline).
- **Pill:** Single dose units made by mixing the powdered drug with a liquid, such as syrup and rolling the mixture into round or oval shape. It is replaced today by tablets and capsules.
- **Powder:** A finely ground drug or drugs. Some are used internally and some are used externally.
- **Paste:** Preparations like an ointment for external use, frequently thick and stiff, penetrates the skin less than ointments.
- **Plaster:** Solid preparation is used as a counter-irritant or as an adhesive used externally.
- **Poultice:** Soft moist preparations that supply moist heat to the body used externally.
- **Solutions:** Liquid preparations containing one or more substances completely dissolved in a solvent
- **Suppository:** A drug or several drugs mixed with a firm base, such as glycerinated gelatine and shaped for insertion into the body cavities. The base dissolved slowly at body temperature releasing the drug
- **Spirits:** A concentrated alcoholic solutions of a volatile substance. Also known as essences.
- **Syrup:** An aqueous solution of sugar is often used to disguise unpleasant tasting drugs and soothe irritated membrane (demulcent effect).
- **Spansule:** A drug made up in a capsule in such a way that there is slow release of its contents.
- **Tincture:** Alcoholic or hydro-alcoholic solution prepared from drugs derived from plants or animals' material
- **Tablet:** Single dose units are made by compressing powdered drugs into small hard discs. Some are readily broken along a scored line; some are enteric coated to prevent irritation to gastric mucosa or to prevent the effect of the gastric secretions upon the drug.
- **Waters:** Saturated solutions of volatile oils.

PURPOSES OF MEDICATIONS

- To diagnose the disease
- To cure an illness or condition
- To support and correct disturbed physiologic function
- To relieve pain and symptoms
- To prevent the disease
- To promote health status
- To depress or to stimulate the activity of some organ or system of organs
- To supply a missing or deficient material such as a vitamin or a hormone
- To restore and maintain normal body function

PHARMACODYNAMICS AND PHARMACOKINETICS

- Pharmacology is the scientific field that studies how the body reacts to medicines and how medicines affect the body.
- Pharmacokinetics and pharmacodynamics are two broad divisions within pharmacology
- Pharmacokinetics is "what the body does to the drug", whereas pharmacodynamics is "what drug does to the body."
- Pharmacokinetics and pharmacodynamics are the key to the development and approval of every drug.

Pharmacodynamics

- The term pharmacodynamics is comes from the Greek words "pharmakon," meaning "drug" and "dynamikos," meaning "power."
- Pharmacodynamics is defined as the body's biological response to drugs.
- The term pharmacodynamics refers to the relationship between drug concentrations at the site of action (receptor) and pharmacologic response.
- Pharmacodynamics includes the biochemical and physiologic effects that result from the interaction of the drug with the receptor.
- The most common mechanism is by the interaction of the drug with tissue receptors located either in cell membranes or in the intracellular fluid.
- A receptor is the drug's specific target, usually a protein located on the surface of a cell membrane or within the cell.
- As the drug binds to the receptor, it enhances or inhibits the normal cellular function.
- Drug receptors interact only with drugs of specific chemical structure, and the receptors are classified according to the type of pharmacodynamic response induced.
- Drugs may be considered a full agonist, partial agonist, or antagonist, depending upon the type of drug interaction with the receptor and the resulting pharmacodynamic response.
- When a drug produces the same type of response as the physiological or endogenous substance, it is referred to as an agonist.
- A drug that inhibits cell function by occupying receptor sites is called an antagonist.

Pharmacokinetics

- The term pharmacokinetics is derived from the ancient Greek words "pharmakon" and "kinetikos", meaning "drug" and "putting in motion" respectively.

Chapter 9: Administration of Medications

- Pharmacokinetics is the study of the absorption, distribution, metabolism, and excretion of drugs to determine the relationship between the dose of a drug and the drug's concentration in biological fluids.
- Pharmacodynamics, described as what a drug does to the body, involves receptor binding, post-receptor effects, and chemical interactions.
- Drug pharmacokinetics determines the onset, duration, and intensity of a drug's effect. Pharmacokinetics of a drug depends on patient-related factors as well as on the drug's chemical properties.

■ DRUG ACTION

- Drug action refers to a drug's ability to combine with a cellular drug receptor. Depending on the location of different cellular receptors affected by a given drug, a drug can have a local effect," systemic effect, or both local and systemic effects **(Fig. 9.1)**.
- During administration, the nurse must pay close attention to the desired effect and therapeutic patient response, as well as the safe dose range for any medication.
- Drug actions are dependent on four properties: absorption, distribution, metabolism, excretion.

Absorption

- Absorption is the process in which a pharmaceutical substance enters the blood circulation in the body.
- The rate and extent of drug absorption depend on multiple factors, such as route of administration, the formulation and chemical properties of a drug and drug-food interactions.
- The administration of a drug influences bioavailability, the fraction of the active form of a drug that enters the bloodstream and successfully reaches its target site.
- When a drug is given intravenously, absorption is not required, and bioavailability is 100% because the active form of the medicine is delivered immediately to the systemic circulation.
- Orally administered medications have incomplete absorption and result in less drug delivery to the site of action. For example, many orally administered drugs are metabolized within the gut wall or the liver before reaching the systemic circulation. This is referred to as first-pass metabolism, which reduces drug absorption.

Distribution

- Distribution is the process in which a pharmaceutical substance is dispersed through the fluids and tissues in the body.
- Most often, the bloodstream is the vehicle for carrying medicines throughout the body.
- During this step, side effects can occur when a drug has an effect at a site other than its target.
- Many factors could influence this, such as blood flow, lipophilicity, molecular size, and how the drug interacts with the components of blood, like plasma proteins.
- To be distributed to the tissue, the drug must cross the cell membrane.
- Some membranes act as a barrier for distribution of medications.
- Drugs with certain characteristics, like high lipophilicity, small size, and molecular weight will be better able to cross the blood brain barrier.
- Other factors that can influence distribution include protein and fat molecules in the blood that can put drug molecules out of commission by latching onto them.

Metabolism

- Metabolism, also known as biotransformation or detoxification, is the process in which a pharmaceutical substance is transformed into other substances, called metabolites, in the body.

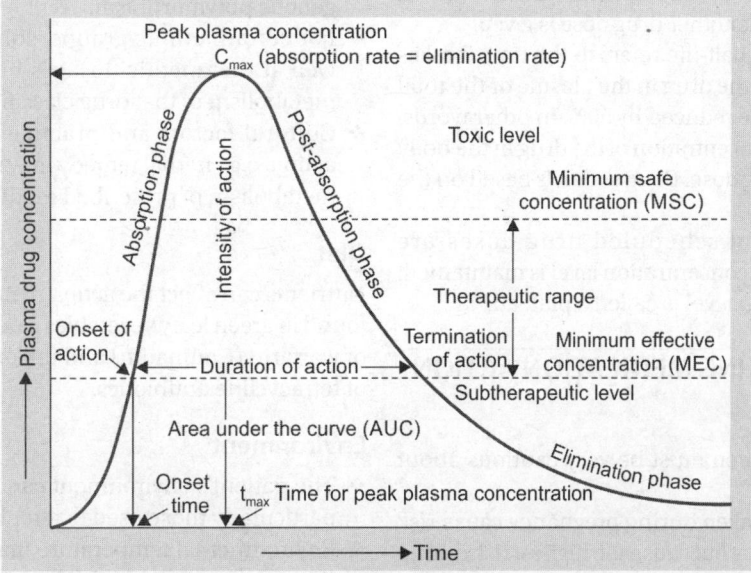

Fig. 9.1: Graphical representation of plasma drug concentration with time.

- After a medicine has been distributed throughout the body and has done its job, the drug is broken down, or metabolized.
- Most drugs are metabolized in the liver.
- The presence of enzymes in the liver that detoxify the drugs determine the rate of metabolism.
- Drug interactions can lead to decreased drug metabolism by enzyme inhibition or increased drug metabolism by enzyme induction.
- The pharmacokinetic parameters for metabolism include: metabolic clearance, drug metabolism rate/drug concentration in plasma.

Excretion

- Excretion is the process in which a pharmaceutical substance is removed from the body.
- Drug excretion refers to the movement of a drug or its metabolites from the tissues back into circulation and from the circulation into the organs of excretion.
- Excretion of drugs or chemicals from the body can occur through the lungs, intestines, kidney and bile.
- However, renal excretion is a major pathway for the elimination of most water-soluble drugs or metabolites.
- Changes in renal function may have a profound effect on the clearance and apparent half-life of the parent compound or its active metabolite(s).
- In the kidneys, drugs may be cleared by passive filtration in the glomerulus or secretion in the tubules, complicated by reabsorption in some compounds.

Key terms related to drug actions are as follows:
- **Onset of action:** The onset of medication refers to when the medication is administered and the body initially responds to the drug. Onset is affected by route of administration and pharmacokinetic factors
- **Peak plasma level:** The peak plasma level refers to the maximum concentration of drug in the body, and the patient shows evidence of greatest therapeutic effect. Once the peak plasma" level is achieved, the blood concentration level will decrease steadily unless another drug dose is given.
- **Drug half-life:** A drug's half-life refers to the time it takes for the concentration of the drug in the plasma or the total amount in the body to be reduced by 50%. In other words, after one half-life, the concentration of the drug in the body will be half of the starting dose. Drug action is based on the half-life of a drug.
- **Plateau:** If a series of scheduled drug doses are administered, the blood concentration level is maintained; maintenance of a certain level is called a plateau.

FACTORS INFLUENCING MEDICATION ACTION

Developmental Factors

- During pregnancy, women must be very cautious about taking medication.
- Some drugs which are taken during pregnancy cause risk throughout the pregnancy but cause the highest risk during first trimester, due to the formation of vital organs and function of the foetus during this time.
- Most drugs are contraindicated during pregnancy because of many adverse effects on foetus.
- Infants usually require small dosages because of their body size and immaturity of their organs, especially the liver and kidneys.
- In adolescence or adult hood, allergic reactions may occur to drugs formerly tolerated.
- Older adults have different responses to medication due to physiologic changes that accompany aging.
- These changes include decreased liver and kidney functions, which can result in accumulation of drug in the body. In older adult, gastric mobility, gastric acid production and blood flow is decreased, which can cause impairment in drug absorption.

Gender

- There are two main reasons that men and women respond to medications differently: Difference in fat and water distribution and differences in hormones.
- Although women have weight less than men, they have proportionally more adipose tissue, men have more body fluid than women.
- Some medications are more soluble in fat, whereas others are more soluble in water.
- So, the men absorb some medication more rapidly than women and due to hormonal changes, have more effects of drugs actions in women.

Cultural, Ethnic and Genetic Factors

- A client's response to a drug is influenced by age, gender, and body size and body composition.
- This variation in response is called drug polymorphism.
- Genetically, the genes that controls liver metabolism vary and some clients may have slow metabolism, whereas others have rapid metabolism, so the metabolism effects the absorption of drug.
- So, the race may affect a drug response. This is called genetic polymorphism.
- For certain ethnic groups, some medication may work well at therapeutic dosages but can be toxic for others metabolism of that drug classification.
- Cultural factors and practices can also affect a drug's action, e.g., herbal remedy may speed up or slow down the metabolism of prescribed medications.

Diet

Nutrients can affect the action of medications, e.g., vitamin K found in green leafy vegetables can decrease the effectiveness of warfarin (Coumadin) and milk interferes with absorption of tetracycline antibiotics.

Environment

- The patient's environment can affect the action of drugs, particularly those used to alter behaviour and mood.
- Environmental temperature may also affect drug activity. When temperature is high, the peripheral blood vessels dilate, thus intensifying the action of vasodilators.

- In contrast, cold environment causes vasoconstriction which inhibits the action of vasodilators but enhance action of vasoconstrictors.
- A client who takes a sedative or analgesic in a busy, noisy environment may not benefit as fully as if the environment were quiet and peaceful.

Psychological Factors

A client's expectations about what a drug can do can affect the response to medication. For example, a client who believes that codeine is ineffective as an analgesic may experience no relief from pain after it is given.

Illness and Disease

- Illness and disease can also affect the action of drugs. For example, Aspirin can reduce the body temperature of a client with fever but has no effect on the body temperature of a client without fever.
- Drug action is altered in clients with circulatory, liver/kidney dysfunction.

Time of Administration

- The time of administration of oral medication affects the relative speed with which they act.
- Orally administered medications are absorbed more quickly if the stomach is empty.
- Thus, oral medications taken two hours before meals act faster than those taken after meals.
- However, some medications, e.g., iron preparations, irritate the gastrointestinal tract and need to be given after a meal, when they will be better tolerated.
- A client's sleep-wake rhythm may affect the action of a drug.
- Circadian variations in urine output and blood circulation, may affect client's response to a drug.

Dose

Very small dose of drug will not be effective while overdose may cause harmful effects. Some drug produces its beneficial effect only in proper therapeutic doses.

The Route of Administration

Drug by mouth has less effect. In injection from whole of drug goes to blood.

Techniques of Administration

For optional effect of drug, it should be given by proper route by proper technique in correct dose.

MEDICATION ORDERS AND PRESCRIPTIONS

- Prescriptions and medication orders are the primary means by which prescribers communicate with pharmacists regarding the desired treatment regimen for a patient.
- Medication orders typically contain similar information that would be included on a prescription
- A medication order is written by a doctor for a medication that will be administered.
- Medication orders are require before a nurse may administer medications.
- A medication order, drug order or physician's order is a request for a drug product for inpatients in institutional settings.
- It must include specific information before the medication order can be carried out.
- A medication order may be written, typed or it may be given verbally or by telephone to a licensed nurse.
- A prescription is a lawful order of a practitioner for a drug or device for a specific patient. It means a written request for preparation and administration of any medication for an outpatient.
- Prescriptions are used in the outpatient, or ambulatory, setting, whereas medication orders are used in the inpatient or institutional health system setting.
- Prescriptions and inpatient orders are legal orders that can be used for medications, devices, laboratory tests, procedures, and the like.

Components of Medication Order

- All orders must be written clearly and legibly.
- The nurse must ensure these components are included in the prescription before administering the medication.

When a medication order is written, it must contain the following 7 important parts or it is considered invalid or incomplete:

- **Patient's name:**
  - The medication order should always include the patient's full name.
  - The nurse should also be aware of the patient's middle name or initial if they have one.
  - This can help the nurse to avoid any confusion with another patient that has the same last name.
  - Nurse must be careful when administering medications when there is more than one person with the same last name on unit.
- **Date and time of the medication:**
  - The date and time the order is written should always be included in the medication order.
  - The date and time of the order include the month, day, year, and the time the order was written.
  - This will help in determining the start and stop of the medication order.
  - The date and time are also important for medications given over a specific time period and needs to be discontinued on a specific day.
  - When the medication order is dated and time the nurse will know which dose will be the last dose.
  - The date and time will help prevent medication errors.
  - It also helps prevent missed doses.
- **Name of the medication:**
  - The name of the medication to be administered must be written in the medication order.
  - To avoid confusion with another medication, the name of the medication should be written clearly and spelled correctly.

- The name of the medication may be written as the brand name or the generic name.
- It is important for a nurse to be familiar with the brand name and the generic name of a medication.

❖ **Dose of the medication:**
  - The dosage is the strength of the medication.
  - The medication order should include the medication dose, and its dosage form.
  - The dosage of a medication is normally stated using the metric system.
  - The metric system is the most widely used system.
  - It is also considered to be the safest system for the measurement of medication dosage.
  - There are certain abbreviations used to indicate medication amounts.
  - However, it is considered safe practice to avoid other abbreviations and include the full words in prescriptions to avoid errors.

❖ **Route the medication:**
  - The route of medication administration is included in the medication order.
  - Specifying the route is important because some medications can be given via more than one route.
  - Some medications may be safe for administration to a patient via one route and not safe for a different patient via the same route.
  - Common routes of administration and standard abbreviations include the following: oral (PO), sublingual (SL), rectal (PR), intramuscular (IM), intravenous (IV) and transdermal (TD)

❖ **Frequency of the medication:**
  - The frequency a medication is to be administered is included in the medication order.
  - Frequency prescriptions is indicated by how many times a day the medication is to be administered.
  - Most time the frequency is written using medication dosage abbreviations.
  - There are several common abbreviations for frequency such as OD mean once daily, BD means twice daily, TID means three times QID means four times daily and PRN which means as needed.

❖ **Signature of person writing the order:**
  - The medication order must include the signature of the person who prescribed the medication.
  - The signature whether handwritten or computer generated makes this order a legal part of the patient's chart.
  - Verbal orders from a prescriber are not recommended.
  - If permitted verbal orders, the nurse repeat back the order to the prescriber for confirmation.

Types of Medication Orders

❖ Medications are prescribed differently, depending on their purpose.
❖ There are several types of medication orders.
❖ They are based on when the medication must be given and the urgency of the dose.

Medications can be Prescribed in Following Types of Orders

Routine Order
❖ A routine order is a prescription that is followed until another order cancels it.
❖ Detailed order for a medication given on a routine or regularly scheduled basis such as every morning at 10 AM.

Standing Order
❖ This is one that should be carried out for a specified number of days or until another order cancels it.
❖ This allows the nurses to administer certain medication without a physician order.
❖ These orders usually contain the number of treatments to be given and how long the treatments should last.

Stat Order
❖ A Stat order is used in emergency situation when the medication must be administered immediately.
❖ These orders are for a single dose of medication.
❖ The nurse should assess and document the patient's response to all stat medications.

One Time Order or Single Order
❖ A one-time order is a prescription for a medication to be administered only once at a specific time.
❖ Medications used to treat an acute symptom may be given as a single one-time order.
❖ And medications used for diagnostic procedures are given as a single one-time dose.

PRN Orders
❖ PRN means as needed or necessary. A PRN order is a prescription for medication to be administered when necessary or as needed by the patient.
❖ This type of order is commonly written for analgesics, antiemetic and laxatives.
❖ PRN orders usually have instructions and guidelines for when, what dose, and how often the medication should be administered.

■ SYSTEMS OF MEASUREMENT

❖ The system of medication measurements involves various calculations and conversions of the formulation, ingredients and components of a medication dosage.
❖ The system of medication measurements are the metric, apothecary and household system.
❖ Nurse should be proficient in the use of these systems of medications measurements to administer medications safely.
❖ It is important for a nurse to have knowledge of the systems of medication measurements to calculate drug dose and prepare medications for administration safely.
❖ Incorrect measurements, conversions or calculations will affect the dose of the mediation.
❖ Mistakes in calculating medication dose often led to foetal errors.
❖ These mistakes in measuring and calculating medications could cause harm to the patient.

Systems of Drugs Measurement

Calculation of medication dosages requires knowledge of the three systems of measurement. All three systems are used currently. They are:
1. Metric system
2. Apothecary system
3. Household measurements

Metric System

- The metric system was introduced in Europe in the late 18th century and is widely used throughout the world.
- The metric system, developed in 1799 in France, is the chosen system for measurements in the majority of European countries.
- The metric system is based on the decimal system, which is organized in units of tens.
- The basic unit can be multiplied or divided to form secondary units or subdivisions.
- Calculation of multiplies are done by moving the decimal to the right and divisions are done by moving the decimal to the left.
- The basic units used in metric system include the liter (L)—volume of fluid, the gram (gm) eight of the solid and the meter (M)—measure of length.
- The subdivision of metric basic unit are designated with prefix as follows—deci 1/10 or 0.1 of the unit, centi 1/100 or 0.01 of unit and milli 1/1000 or 0.001 of unit.
- In clinical practice, the subdivision milligram (mg), kilograms (kg) are solely used for measurement of weight.
- This allows conversions to be made by moving the decimal point to the right or left.
- The decimal point moves to the right when the nurse multiply and to the left when the nurse divide.
- However, gram and litre are the only measurements from the metric system that are used in medication administration.
- The metric system measures length, volume and weight. The meter is a unit of distance, the gram (abbreviated g or gm) is a unit of weight, and the later (abbreviated L) is a unit of volume.
- Meters, letters and grams are the basic units of measures.
- All have larger and smaller units of measures.
- In clinical practice, the subdivision milligram (mg), kilograms (kg) are solely used for measurement of weight.
- For example, grams express weight.
- Most of us familiar with kilograms to measures body weight.
- A kilogram is larger than gram. 1 kilogram = 1,000 grams.
- We may also use the prefix kilo for meters and liters.
- Therefore, a kilometers = 1000 meters and a kiloliters = 1000 liter.

Metric System Units of Weight and Equivalents one kilogram (kg)

- 1 gram (g)
- 1 milligram (mg)
- 1 microgram (µg)

$$1 \text{ kg} = 1000 \text{ g}$$
$$1 \text{ g} = 1000 \text{ mg}$$
$$1 \text{ mg} = 1000 \text{ µg}$$

Metric System Units of Volume and Equivalents

- 1 later (L)
- 1 milliliter (mL)
- 1 cubic centimetre (cc)

$$1 \text{ L} = 1000 \text{ mL}$$
$$1 \text{ mL} = 1 \text{ cc}$$

Apothecaries' System

- The apothecary's system is older of three system of measurement, although this system is slowly being replaced by metric system.
- In apothecaries' system the basic unit of weight is the grain (gr), followed in ascending order with the scruple, the dram, the ounce, and the pound, although the scruple and dram are seldom used for measurement.
- The basic unit of volume is the minim (m), followed by fluidum, the fluid ounce, the pint, the quart, and the gallon.
- The apothecaries' system, older than the metric system, was brought to the United States from England during the colonial period.
- The apothecary system is a system of measuring and weighing drugs and solutions in which fractions are used to identify parts of the unit of measure.
- The basic units of measurement in the apothecary system include weights and liquid volume.
- The basic unit of volume is the minim (m), followed by fluidum, the fluid ounce, the pint, the quart, and the gallon. The word minim means "the least."

Apothecary System Units of Weight and Equivalents

- 1 pound (lb)
- 1 ounce (oz)
- 1 dram (dr)
- 1 grain (gr)

$$1 \text{ lb} = 16 \text{ oz}$$
$$1 \text{ oz} = 8 \text{ dr}$$
$$1 \text{ dr} = 60 \text{ gr}$$

Apothecary System Units of Volume and Equivalents

- 1 gallon (gal)
- 1 quart (qt)
- 1 pint (pt)
- 1 fluid ounce (fl oz)
- 1 fluid dram (fl dr)
- 1 minim (M)

$$1 \text{ gal} = 4 \text{ qt}$$
$$1 \text{ qt} = 2 \text{ pt}$$
$$1 \text{ pt} = 16 \text{ fl oz}$$
$$1 \text{ fl oz} = 8 \text{ fl dr}$$
$$1 \text{ fl dr} = 60 \text{ M}$$
$$1 \text{ fl oz} = 1 \text{ oz}$$
$$1 \text{ fl dr} = 1 \text{ dr}$$

Household System

- The household system of measurement is similar to the apothecary system of liquid measures and is the least accurate of the three systems.
- The use of household measurements is considered inaccurate because of the varying sizes of cups, glasses, and eating utensils, and this system generally has been replaced with the metric system.

- Measures used for the household system include drops (gtts), teaspoons (tsp), tablespoon (tbsp), cups, pints and quarts.
- Household units are often used to inform patients of the size of a liquid dose.
- It is once again necessary for the nurse to have an understanding of the household measurement system to be able to use and teach it to clients and families.
- Pints and quarts are also household measure, but are defined as apothecaries's measurement.
- This system of measurement is least accurate of three systems.

Household Measurement System and Equivalents
- 1 cup
- 1 tablespoon (tbsp or T)
- 1 teaspoon (tsp or t)
- 1 drop (gtt)

$$1 \text{ cup} = 8 \text{ ounces (oz)}$$
$$2 \text{ Tbsp} = 1 \text{ oz}$$
$$3 \text{ tsp} = 1 \text{ tbsp}$$
$$1 \text{ tsp} = 60 \text{ gtt}$$

MEDICATION DOSE CALCULATION

Drug Dosage Calculations

Drug dosage calculations are required when the amount of medication ordered (or desired) is different from what is available on hand for the nurse to administer.
Formula:

Tablet

$$\text{Required amount } (x) = \frac{\text{Ordered dose (D)}}{\text{Stock dose (A)}}$$

Example: A client is ordered 150 mg soluble aspirin. 'Disprin' tablets containing 300 mg aspirin are available. How many tablets will you give?

$$\text{Required amount } (x) = \frac{150}{300}$$
$$\text{Required amount } (x) = 0.5 \text{ mg}$$

Solution/Liquid

$$\text{Required amount } (x) = \frac{\text{Ordered dose (D)}}{\text{Stock dose (A)}} \times \text{Quantity (Q)}$$

Example: You are required to give 6 mg morphine. In your stock ampoule, there is 15 mg per 1 mL. How much of the ampoule will you need?

$$\text{Required amount } (x) = \frac{6}{15} \times \frac{1 \text{ mL}}{1}$$
$$\text{Required amount } (x) = 0.4 \text{ mL}$$

Dosage Calculations Based on Body Weight

Dosage calculations based on body weight are required when the dosage ordered and administered is dependent on the weight of the patient. For example, many pediatric drugs are ordered and given per weight (usually in kg).

Step 1

Weight (kg) × Dosage ordered (per kg) = Required dosage (X)

Calculation of Intravenous Drip Rates

In these types of calculations, for a given volume, time period, and drop factor (gtts/mL), the required IV flow rate in drops per minute (gtts/min) is calculated.

Note: Since a fraction of a drop is not possible to give to a patient, it is usual to round the answers to the nearest whole number.

$$\text{Drop per min} = \frac{\text{Total volume}}{\text{Total time (min)}} \times \text{Drop factor}$$

Note: Drop factor for macro drip = 20 drops/mL; micro drip = 60 drops/mL.

Example: A client is ordered an intravenous infusion of 1000 mL normal saline to run over 24 hours, using a macro drip. Calculate the drip rate. (Drip rate 20)

$$\text{Drop per min} = \frac{1000}{26 \times 60} \times 20$$

$$\text{Drop per min} = 13.8 = 14$$

Preparation of Solutions and Calculations

- These are three methods of expressing and calculating the strength of solutions and dosage of medicines.
- Ratio method or proportion method, e.g., 1:20 carbolic lotion means in every part of the solution, 1 part is carbolic acid and nineteen parts are water.
- Percentage method, e.g., 5% carbolic lotion means out of every 100 parts, 5 parts are carbolic acid and 95 parts are water.
- The amount of solute in a particular number of relevant means—a particular amount of drug in a particular amount of solution, e.g., Quinine Sulphate Solution label may be 5 grains (grs) Quinine Sulphate OM 4 mL of solutions [one drachme (dr)]
- Numerical Ratio—proportions

Example: Prepare 500 mL of 2 % boric lotion 2% means 2 gm in 100 mL

$$2 : 100 :: x : 500$$
$$100x = 500 \times 2$$
$$x = 1000$$
$$x = 100$$
$$x = 10$$

Example:
- Prepare 5% solution of 600 mL of Dettol.
- How much sodium chloride is required to prepared 500 mL of normal saline?
- Percentage method.
- How much glucose powder is require to prepare 600 mL of 20 % glucose solution?
- (20 % means 20 parts of glucose and 80 parts of water

$$\text{To prepare 600 mL} = \frac{20 \times 600}{100} = 120$$

- Take 120 gram of glucose and add 480 mL of water).

Calculate the Pediatric Dosage

Most of the drugs are available in the adult dose. The nurse needs to know how to prepare the pediatric dosage.

Young's rule: For children over 1 year up to 12 years.

$$\frac{\text{Age in years}}{\text{Age in years} + 12} \times \text{Adult dose} = \text{Child's dose}$$

Clark's rule: According to the weight of the child, therefore, it can be used for children of all ages.

$$\frac{\text{Weight of child (pounds)}}{150} \times \text{Adult dose} = \text{Child's dose}$$

Fried's rule: For children under 1 year of age.

$$\frac{\text{Age in months}}{150} \times \text{Adult dose} = \text{Child's dose}$$

GENERAL PRINCIPLES FOR ADMINISTRATION OF MEDICATIONS

While Preparing the Medicines

- Read the physician's orders before preparing the drug.
- No medicine should be prepared without the doctor's written orders.
- Verbal orders are carried out only in emergency.
- Check the medicine card against the physician's orders
- Be sure that the medicine is copied correctly on the medicine card and the nurse's record.
- Concentrate on the preparation of medicines.
- Avoid conversations during the preparation of medicines.
- Calculate the fractions of dosage accurately. If there is doubt, consult the physician or at least seniors.
- Give the medication only from a clearly labeled container.
- **Read the label of the container and compare it with the medicine card thrice:**
  - Before the medicine container is taken from the shelf.
  - Before pouring the drug.
  - Before replacing the container in the shelf.
- Always use a calibrated measure in order to measure the accurate dose.
- Make sure that the medicine glasses are dean and dry before the medicine is taken.
- Shake the fluid medication before pouring it into the ounce glass.
- Wipe the mouth of the bottle, close it tightly and replace the bottle in the proper place after use.
- Pour the from the bottle on the side opposite to the label.
- Hold the ounce glass at eye level and place the thumb on the mark on the ounce glass to which the medicine is to be poured. Read the lower meniscus of the fluid level in the medicine glass.
- When taking tablets and capsules do not touch them with hand.
- Drop the tablets or capsules from the container to its lid and then into the medicine cup to be taken to the bedside.
- Once the medication is poured out of a bottle, it should not be poured back into the same bottle to prevent contamination of the whole medicine.
- Do not use the medicine that differs in color, taste, odor and consistency.
- Prepare the drug just before the time of administration of medicine. Never leave the drug in the medicine tray without proper identification.

Regarding the Administration

- Observe the ten rights
- Observe for the symptoms of over dosage of the drugs before it is administered, e.g., a bradycardia observed in the clients getting digoxin tablets.
- Identify the client correctly—by the bed number, room number, calling the name of the client, asking the client to repeat his name, asking others who know the client.
- Give the drugs one by one.
- Stay with the client until he has taken the medication completely.
- Observe for any contraindications in oral administration of medicine, such as nausea, vomiting, unconsciousness, etc., whether the drug can safely be administered through the oral route.
- Always give the medicine you have prepared yourself.
- Remove the unpleasant taste of medicines from the mouth by the use of orange syrups, lemon juice or by mouthwash.
- Do not allow the medicine glass to touch the mouth of the client when the medicine is administered to the client.
- Always provide a drink of fresh water to the client after giving an oral medicine.
- Report an error in medication immediately to the charge nurse and the physician.
- Do not leave the medicine with the client.
- Prepare a fresh dose of medicine, if the medication is to be given later.
- The drugs that stimulate appetite should be given before food.
- The drugs that are irritant to the gastric mucosa should be given only after meals. he drugs given for the local effect in the stomach, (e.g., an antacid) should be given after meals to prevent quick absorption of the drug
- Never give water after administering the cough syrups, as it leaves a soothing effect on the throat and prevent coughing sensation.
- If the client has a nasogastric tube for feeding purposes, the nurse can powder the medications and dissolve it in a solution and feed the client. The capsules can be opened to mix the powder with the other medications.
- Enteric coated tablets should never be chewed or broken or crushed for ease of administration, because it has irritating effect on the mucosa of the stomach. Some drugs are destroyed by the action of the gastric juice.
- The lozenges are to be sucked and not chewed until they are completely dissolved in the mouth.

Regarding the Recording of Drugs

- Record each dose of medicine soon after it is administered.
- Use standard abbreviations in recording the medications.
- Record only those medicines which you have administered.
- Record the date, time, name of the drug administered the dose of the medicine and the strength.
- Never record a medication, before it is given to the client.

- Record the effect observed the local and systemic effects, the side effects, the symptoms of toxicity, etc.
- Record the medications that are vomited by the client, refused by the client and those drugs that are not administered to the client and the reason for not giving the medication.

Ethical and Legal Aspects

- Under the law, nurses are responsible for their own actions regardless of a written order. It is expected that the nurse should know the minimum and the maximum dose of every medicine that she administers. If a nurse gives an injection of Pethidine 500 mg to a client instead of 50 mg, the nurse is responsible for the harm that has taken place to the client. She cannot justify her deed in spite of a written order for the same dosage.
- The nurse should know the law about the use of narcotics. The narcotics should be kept under the safe custody of nurses and an account should be maintained for the administration of these drugs. The following information should be recorded when the narcotics are administered the name of the client, name of the drug, dosage, date and time of administration, signature of the person who prepared and gave the narcotic and the name of the physician who ordered the drug.
- Narcotics should be stocked only by the persons/institutions who possess licence to do so. (Narcotics are controlled because of the problems of drug addiction).
- The nurse's responsibility includes prevention of medication errors by observing the "Ten rights" of giving medications.
- Charting the administration of medication or its omission is the legal responsibility of the person who gives the medication. Since observation and reporting untoward effects or errors is a nursing responsibility, the nurse must observe and record her observations in the client's permanent record.
- The nurse should know what is and what is not acceptable practice in her own institution, e.g., leaving medications at the bedside of the client is strictly prohibited in certain institutions; in others, certain medications may be left with the clients.
- Another legal responsibility of the nurse is when she is involved in the experimental drug program. She has the legal obligation to be fully informed about any investigational medications which she will be administering to a client. In addition, prior to administering any experimental drug, the nurse must witness that the client has received a complete explanation about the benefits, side effects, toxic effects of the medications.

10 RIGHTS OF MEDICATION ADMINISTRATION

The Ten Rights" ensures safety in giving drugs:

1. Right Client

- Read the physician's orders to make sure for whom the medicine is ordered.
- Read the client's name on the client's chart and on the medicine card.
- Call the client by name and ask him to repeat his name. Be very careful if the client is deaf or otherwise does not understand your language.

2. Right Drug

- Read the physician's orders to study the correct name of the drug. If the order is not clear consult the physician or at least seniors.
- To make sure the drug is copied correctly on the medicine card, on the nurse's record, etc.
- Be careful of drugs whose names sound alike.
- **Select the right drugs from the cupboard:** Read the label of the medicine container and the name of the medicine in the medicine card thrice.
- Before taking the drug from the shelf.
- Before measuring it.
- When returning the container to the shelf and before removing the hand from the container.
- Look for the color, odor and consistency of the drug. Unusual characteristics of the drugs should be questioned.
- Administer medicine only from a clearly labeled container.
- Avoid conversation or anything that distracts the mind.
- Be familiar with the trade names. If there is doubt, consult the physician or at least seniors or medicine books.
- Avoid accepting verbal orders. Verbal orders should be accepted only in emergencies. But it should be written on the chart as early as possible.
- Always identify the client before giving medication.
- Make sure that the drug has not been discontinued by the physician.

3. Right Dose

- Read the physician's orders to know the correct dose.
- Consider the age and weight of the client. This may help to find an error in the physician's orders.
- Know the minimum and maximum dose of the medicine administered. Calculate the fraction of dosage correctly.
- Measure accurately. Always use a calibrated measure in order to measure accurate doses. Use ounce glasses instead of teaspoons to measure ounces.
- Have the medicine card or written order in hand before you prepare the drug.
- Avoid conversation or anything that distracts the mind.
- Consider how many tablets or capsules are required for the dose.
- Know the abbreviations and symbols used.
- Make sure that the medicine glasses are dry before pouring or measuring the medications.
- Hold the ounce glass at the eye level and place the thumb at the mark up to which the medicine is to be poured. Read the lower meniscus of the fluid level when measuring the fluid medications.
- Help the client to take all the medicine that is ordered for him.
- The medicine should be carried to the client without spilling it out of the container.

4. Right Time
- Read the physician's orders.
- Know the hospital routines for the intervals.
- Give at stated intervals for blood levels.
- Know the abbreviations for the time, e.g., BD, TDS, etc.
- Give the medicine near the time ordered—15 minutes before or after the designated time.
- Give the medicine as ordered in relation to the food intake, e.g., before food or after food.
- Give the medicines according to the action expected, e.g., sleeping pills are given at bedtime; the diuretics are given in the morning hours, so that the client will not be disturbed in the night.

5. Right Method
- Read the physician's orders to determine the route of administration.
- Dilute the medicine if indicated.
- Know the method of giving drugs, e.g., orally, parenterally, rectally, etc.
- Know the abbreviations used to designate the route of administration, e.g., IV, IM, PO, etc.
- Identify the client correctly.
- Stay with the client until he/she has taken the medication.
- Never leave any medicine with the client.
- An error in the medication should be reported immediately.

6. Right Patient Education
- Check if the patient understands what the medication is for.
- Make them aware that they should contact a healthcare professional if they experience side-effects or reactions.

7. Right Documentation
- Ensure you have signed for the medication after it has been administered.
- Ensure the medication is prescribed correctly with a start and end date if appropriate.

8. Right to Refuse
- Ensure you have the patient consent to administer medications.
- Be aware that patients do have a right to refuse medication if they have the capacity to do so.

9. Right Assessment
- Check if your patient actually needs the medication.
- Check for contraindications.
- Baseline observations if required.

10. Right Evaluation
- Ensure the medication is working the way it should.
- Ensure medications are reviewed regularly.
- Ongoing observations if required.

■ ERRORS IN MEDICATION ADMINISTRATION

Medication error can be defined as any error or mishappening during prescribing, dispensing, transcribing or administering a drug. A medication error is any preventable event that may cause or lead to inappropriate medication use.

Sources of Medication Error
- Misidentification of patient.
- Unclear labelling of drugs.
- Verification errors.
- Use of inadequate knowledge.
- Time and performance pressure.
- Inaccurate recording and transcribing error.

Classification of Medication Error
Medication errors may be classified according to where they occur in the medication process:
- Prescribing error
- Transcribing error
- Dispensing error
- Administering or monitoring error

Prescribing Error
These include the errors or mishappening during prescription of a drug.

Contributing Factors for Prescribing Error
- Lack of knowledge of the prescribed drug
- Illegible hand writing
- Inaccurate medication history taking
- Confusion with the drug name.
- Inappropriate use of decimal.
- Use of irrelevant abbreviations.
- Use of verbal orders.
- Work environment/pressure
- Room communication within the team.
- Organizational factors, such as inadequate training

Measures to Reduce Prescribing Errors
- Electronic prescribing may help to reduce the risk of prescribing errors resulting from illegible hand writing
- Organization should organize training sessions at regular intervals and awareness of errors should be created.
- Avoid verbal orders.
- Use of standard abbreviation should be encouraged
- Work environment should be calm, quiet and stress free.
- Always use leading zeros for decimal points. For example, Digoxin 0.5 mg

Transcribing Error
- Transcribing is defined as the encoding process/generation of electronic prescription sheet to reduce the incidence of error
- This part of work is performed by computer operators or medicine transcriptionist.
- Due to poor/inadequate knowledge about clinical pharmacology, they often can produce typing error in the electronic prescription sheet.
- So, it is the responsibility of staff nurse and duty doctor to keep a check on them and supervise their sheets before indenting to pharmacy.

Dispensing Error

- It is defined as the error from the receipt of the prescription in the pharmacy to the supply of a dispended medicine to the patient.
- This occurs primarily with drugs that have a similar name or appearance.
- For example, Lasix (frusemide) and Losec (omeprazole).

Measures to Reduce Dispensing Error

- Ensuring a safe medication dispensing procedure.
- Separating drugs with a similar name or appearance, i.e., LASA drugs (look alike and sound alike).
- Adequate training of the staff regarding storage of LASA drugs and high-risk medications.
- Introducing safe systematic procedures for dispensing medicines in the pharmacy.
- Maintain the workload of the person dispensing the medication.
- Keep the dispensing area free from any kind of interruptions.
- Avoid sepsis and moisture contamination.

Administration Errors

It is defined as any error between the drug prescribed by the prescriber and the drug received by the patient.

Causes of Administration Error

- Lack of perceived risk
- Lack of available technology.
- Lack of knowledge of the preparation or administration procedures.
- Wrong calculation.
- Lack of knowledge of the route of administration prescribed.
- Wrong patient.
- Environmental factors such as noise and poor light.
- Workload.

Approaches to Reduce Administration Error

- Check correct identification of the patient.
- Ensure correct dosage calculation before administering
- Ensure medicine is been administered at right time to the right patient.
- Minimize interruptions during medication administration.

Steps to be taken to Prevent Medication Error

- Follow the ten rights of medication administration,
- Be sure to read labels at least 3 times—before, during and after administration of the drug.
- Check the expiry date of the drug before administration.
- Prepare the medicine in a well-lighted room.
- Double check all the dosage calculations before administration.
- Do not make assumptions of illegible hand writing.
- Do not accept incomplete orders or telephonic/verbal orders.
- Avoid the use of irrelevant abbreviations.
- Double check patient who has allergies and about all new drugs as they are added in treatment plan.
- Document all the medications as soon as they are given.
- Attend in-service training programs for drug administration and calculations.
- Evaluate the patient for medication error.
- Routinely refer to drug interaction charts.
- Beware about ambiguous orders or drug names, consult the physician in case of any doubt.
- Do not allow any activity to interrupt you during medication administration.

STORAGE AND MAINTENANCE OF DRUGS

General Guidelines

- To stock the medicines, each ward should be provided with a medicine cabinet.
- It should be large enough to accommodate all drugs to be stocked in the ward.
- As far as possible, the medicine cabinet should be kept in a separate room adjacent to the nurse's room.
- A washing sink with running water should be provided in that room for hand washing facilities.
- Adequate lighting should be provided within the cabinet to read the labels clearly.
- There should be separate compartments for different categories of drugs for mixtures, tablets, powders, etc.
- Drugs used for external use should be kept separate from the drugs used for internal use.
- The containers should be arranged alphabetically, so that it is easy to find them.
- Poisonous drugs should be kept in a separate cupboard which must have separate lock and key.
- A senior nurse should be responsible for the poisonous medicines in the cupboard.
- A register should be maintained to keep the account of the poisonous drugs.
- A daily inventory should be taken to prevent theft of narcotics.
- All the poisonous drugs should be marked "poison" in red ink.
- No drug should be stored without labels, even for a day.
- All the containers should have labels written neatly and legibly.
- The labels should contain the name of the drug, the ingredients, the strength, the dose, etc.
- All medicine containers should be kept closed always. The containers keeping the capsules, alcoholic preparations, volatile drugs, etc., should have airtight caps.
- The tablets and pills tend to disintegrate if exposed to air.
- The drugs that are unusual in color, odor and consistency should be returned to the pharmacy and replaced with fresh ones.
- Check the expiry date of every drug and make use of it before its expiry date is over or send it to the dispensary and get it replaced.
- The drugs which are destroyed in the room temperature such as vaccines, sera, antibiotics, etc., should be kept in the refrigerators.
- Emergency drugs should be kept in a place where they are readily obtainable for emergency use.

- When indenting for drugs, indent only the required quantity—the request for new supply of medicines should be signed by the ward sister. All medicines should be checked and signed as they are received from the dispensary.
- The medicine cabinet should always be kept neat and clean and all equipment should be kept clean and dry after their use.
- The medicine cabinet should always be kept locked and the key should be kept where only doctors and nurses have access to it.
- The oily medicines should be kept in a separate tray or on a piece of waterproof paper to prevent soiling the shelf. Special oil cups or spoons are used which are helpful in keeping the oily odors away from medicine glasses.

Storage System of Medication

Once the pharmacy delivers the drugs to a nursing unit, the nurse is responsible for their safe storage. The nurse should always refer to the pharmacists for correct instruction on storage of medicines to ensure treatment can optimized.

Certain guidelines for safe medication storage are as follows:

Cabinet

- Store all medications according to the classification in a locked, secure cabinet or container.
- Place the locked cabinet in bright and ventilated place to check and identify easily, but should be free of direct shine and keep it clean, tidy and dry.
- Do not mix different medicines in the same container.
- Oral medication should be kept separately from medicines for external use.
- Ward nurse in-charge carries asset of keys for the cabinet.
- Key should be available only to authorized personnel who are assigned medication-related responsibilities.
- Checks the quantities and the qualities of the medications regularly.
- Replenish the stock medication following the policies of institution and discard the medication with problems.

Placement of Medications

- Store and place medications separately according to manufacturers, according to pharmacological action and alphabetically.
- The drugs should be arranged in such a way that they are easily traceable as and when required.
- Store look-alike and sound-alike drugs separately.
- Do not remove the original medicines label with information, such as name of the medication, strength, dosage, method of administration, method of storage and expiry date.

Label the Container of Medications

- Store drugs in conditions required per labeling or other official guidelines.
- Different medications should be labeled with different colorful strips.
- Blue strip labels oral medications, red strip labels external medications, and black strip labels virulent toxicants.
- Keep each medication in its original labeled container, and keep the labels and specifications legible.
- If the labels are soiled or illegible, discontinue using the medications.
- In addition, label drug name, concentration and dosage.
- Adequate lighting should be provided within the cabinet to read the labels clearly.

Check the Medications Carefully

- Check the expiry date and nature of medications carefully.
- Discontinue using the medications if they become deposited and cloudy, smell abnormal, change color, get deliquescence or mildew.
- Medications must not be administered, and products and equipment must not be used beyond their expiry dates.

Storage Conditions

- The quality of medicines may be affected due to improper storage.
- As a result, the treatment might be ineffective.
- Store the drugs products as per drug product storage condition to avoid contamination or deterioration, prevent or reduce pilferage, theft or losses and maintain integrity of packaging and so guarantee quality and potency of drugs during shelf life.
- Stability of medications depends on both environmental factors, such as temperature, air, light and humidity and drug-related factors such as the active ingredient itself, the dosage form (tablet, solution, etc.) and the manufacturing process.
- It is therefore necessary to respect storage instructions given by manufacturers.

Temperature

- The medications which are destroyed in the room temperature should be kept in the refrigerators such as vaccines, sera, antibiotics, etc.
- Maintain temperature between 15–25°C for non-refrigerated medications.
- Where refrigeration is necessary maintain temperature between 2–8°C.
- **The cold chain must be strictly respected during transport:**
  - *2–8°C:* Keep in the middle of refrigerator (insulin, eye drop, antibiotic suspension)
  - *8–15°C:* Keep in cool dry place in the house (soft gel capsule)
  - *15–30°C:* Room temperature, away from sunlight (tablet and capsule)

Air and Humidity

- Drugs to be stored under condition that prevent contamination as far as possible, deterioration.
- Protected from moisture means that the product is to be stored in air tight container.
- Relative humidity should not be above 65%.
- Air is a factor of deterioration due to its content of oxygen and humidity.
- All containers should remain closed.

- In airtight and opaque containers, drugs are protected against air and light.
- Medications which tend to volatilize. deliquesce, or effloresce should be kept in airtight bottles, e.g., ethanol, iodine, sugar-coated tablets.
- Medications that will be oxidized if exposed to air and be denatured if exposed to light should be kept in airtight colored bottles.

Light

- The medication must not get exposed to direct sunlight.
- Protected from light the drug is to be stored either in a container made of material that absorbs actinic light sufficiently to protect the contents from change induced by such light.
- Drugs should be protected from light, particularly solutions.
- Parenteral forms should be preserved in their packaging. Colored glass may give illusory protection against light.
- Cover the container with shade paper box if necessary and store it in the shady and cool area, e.g., vitamin C.
- Biologic products and antibiotics that will be destroyed and decomposed if exposed heat should be kept in the dry, and shady and cool area.

Nursing Responsibility

Nurses are the persons who are delivering services round the clock and they have the main responsibility for the storage and maintenance of the drugs.

- The medicines should be stored in the medicine cabinet. Each ward should be provided with this medicine cabinet. The medicine cabinet should be large enough to accommodate all the drugs. The drugs should be arranged alphabetically, so that it can be found easily.
- All drugs are to be kept and stored in the containers in which they are received. The separate boxes or the compartments should be there for different categories of drugs. No drug is to be transferred from one container to another. Never keep and mix different medicines in the same container.
- All the stored drugs should be stored with labels. The labels should contain the name of the drug, the ingredients, the strength and dose, etc.
- All medicines supplied to the patient in a labelled container should include the name of the patient, date and place of issue, full directions for use and the words "keep out of reach and sight of children".
- All patients should receive advice on how to take their medication, common side effects and any special dosage instructions.
- All drugs are to be stored in a secure and orderly manner without crowding.
- Drugs are to be accessible only to licensed nursing and pharmacy personnel.
- The medicine cabinet should be kept in a separate room, near to the nurse's room. The hand washing facilities should be available in that room.
- Poisonous drugs should be kept in the separate area which must have separate lock and key and should be marked 'Poison' with the red ink.
- The head nurse should be responsible for the poisonous drugs. All the poisonous drugs should be entered in a register and that should be checked regularly.
- The containers of the drugs should have air tight caps.
- The drugs should be regularly checked and replaced/returned to pharmacy that is unusual in color, odor and consistency.
- Never keep medication in a place that expose to direct sunlight, place with high temperature and moist areas such as near the windows, on the refrigerator or in the bathroom.
- Drugs are to be stored at proper temperatures.
- Drugs requiring storage at room temperatures are to be stored at a temperature of not less than 15°C or more than 8°C.
- Drugs stored in a multipurpose refrigerator are to be kept in a closed, separate container labeled drugs.
- One refrigerator should be available for the vaccines, sera, antibiotics, etc., because these drugs can be destroyed at the room temperature.
- Lunches and other foods not used in passing medication may not be kept in the medication refrigerator in the medicine room under any circumstances.
- Emergency drugs should be kept in a place where they are readily available for emergency use. This prevents delays in accessing medications.
- Drugs are not to be kept on hand after the expiration date which appears on the label.
- Outdated, contaminated, or deteriorated drugs and those in containers which are cracked, soiled or without secure closures are to be immediately withdrawn from stock.

TERMINOLOGIES

- **Analgesics:** Drugs used for relieving pain, e.g., Aspirin.
- **Anesthetics:** Drugs which cause loss of sensation or insensibility to paid, e.g., Ether.
- **Antacids:** Drugs which neutralize the acidity of the stomach, e.g., magnesium trisilicate.
- **Anti-helminthic or vermifuge:** Kill worms (or weaken them so that they can be easily purged out, e.g., Piperazine.
- **Antibiotics:** Are Antibacterial substance of biologic origin, e.g., penicillin.
- **Antidote:** Are the substances used to counteract the effects of poison, e.g., dilute alkali for acid poisoning.
- **Antihistamines:** Are useful in the case of allergic reactions and they also cause sleepiness, e.g., phenergan.
- **Aperients:** Drugs which stimulate peristalsis and cause evacuation of the bowel. Laxatives have a mild action, e.g., liquid paraffin. Purgative have a more power action, e.g., castor oil.
- **Antipyretics:** Are drugs which reduce fever, e.g., metacin
- **Anti-inflammatory:** Those that help to reduce inflammation, e.g., brufen.
- **Antidiarrheals:** Agents used to treat diarrhea.
- **Anticoagulants:** Substances which inhibit or decrease the blood clotting process either by inhibiting the formation of the clotting substances in the liver or by interfering with the peripheral action of these substances, e.g., heparin.

- **Anti-infection:** Act either to inhibit, kill or retard the growth of microorganisms.
- **Antiasthmatics:** Drugs which provide symptomatic relief of asthmatic attacks by relaxing the smooth muscle or the bronchioles, e.g., deriphyllin.
- **Antitussives:** Drugs which inhibit the cough reflex.
- **Androgens:** Hormones secreted by testis and adrenal cortex. They are steroids/produce secondary male.
- **Antiseptics:** Substances that inhibit growth of bacteria.
- **Antiemetics:** Drug that stop vomiting, e.g., stemetil
- **Astringent:** A drug that causes the contraction of tissue and arrest discharges.
- **Antifungal (Antimycotic):** Drugs which prevent the growth of fungi or the destruction of fungi.
- **Antispasmodic:** An agent that relieves the spasmodic pains or spasm of the muscle.
- **Antitubercular:** Specific drugs used in the treatment of tuberculosis.
- **Antirheumatic:** To treat rheumatism.
- **Bronchodilator:** Medicines which relax muscles of the bronchioles by reducing smooth muscle spasm or mucosal edema.
- **Caustics:** Substances that are destructive to living tissues.
- **Coagulants:** Those drugs that help in the clotting of blood either by the increased formation of liver precursors by the clotting factor present in the drug administered.
- **Corticosteroids:** Hormonal drugs extracted from adrenal cortex material and draw fluids from the tissues of the body, e.g., hydrocortisone.
- **Cardiac tonic:** Drug which strengthens the cardiac muscle and improves cardiac output, e.g., digoxin.
- **Carminatives:** Relieves flatulence (gas in the stomach or intestine) e.g., ginger.
- **Cardiac stimulant:** Drugs that stimulate the heart, make the heart to function strongly – used in shock and collapse, e.g., adrenalin.
- **Diuretics:** Drugs which increase the urine output, e.g., Lasix.
- **Diaphoretics:** Drugs which increase the action of sweat glands and induce perspiration.
- **Detergent:** A cleaning agent.
- **Demulcent:** Substance that softens, soothes and protects mucous membranes.
- **Decongestant:** Drugs which produce shrinkage of the engorged mucosa and relieves.
- **Emetics:** Substance that produces vomiting, e.g., strong salt solution.
- **Expectorants:** Are cough helpers. They loosen bronchial secretions and help to bring them out, e.g., benadryl.
- **Beta cholics or oxytocin:** Drugs which stimulate, e.g., Pitocin.
- **Fungicides:** Destroy fungal infection, such as ringworm.
- **Germicides:** Drugs that kill the germs, e.g., chlorine.
- **Hypnotics:** Drugs which produce, sleep but may not lessen the pain, e.g., barbiturates.
- **Hematinics:** Agent which tends to increase the hemoglobin.
- **Hypotensive:** Substance capable of decreasing the blood pressure, e.g., aldomet
- **Hemostatics:** An agent to check.
- **Hypoglycemics:** Drugs that lower the blood sugar level.
- **Keratolytics:** Drugs which softens horny layer of the skin.
- **Laxatives (Aperients):** Drugs having mild action on the bowel and produce stools that are formed and normal in character usually given at night, e.g., liquid paraffin.
- **Mydriatics:** Drugs that dilate the pupil of the eye.
- **Myotic:** Drugs which contract the pupil of the eye.
- **Muscle relaxants:** Agents used for diminution of tension or functional activity of muscles.
- **Narcotics:** Drugs which relieve pain and produce sleep, e.g., morphine.
- **Sedatives:** Are drugs which produce sleep, e.g., codeine phosphate.
- **Scabicides:** Topical anti-infective used in the treatment of scabies, e.g., benzyl benzoate.
- **Tranquilizers:** Drugs which reduce anxiety and nervous tension, e.g., largactil valium.
- **Tonics:** Medicines taken to strengthen the body and make up nutritional deficiency, e.g., iron and vitamin preparation.
- **Oral contraceptives:** Oral drugs that prevent conception.
- **Vesicant:** A blistering agent.
- **Vasodilators:** Drugs which dilate the blood vessels, e.g., sorbitrate.
- **Vasoconstrictor:** Drugs that cause constriction of the blood vessels.

ABBREVIATIONS

Used in Prescribing Medications (Table 9.1)

TABLE 9.1: Abbreviations used in prescribing medications.

Abbreviation	Derivations	Meaning
ac	Ante cibum	Before meals
pc	Post cibum	After meals
am	Ante meridian	Morning
pm	Post meridian	Afternoon
Alt die	Alternies diebus	Alternate days
Alt not	Alternies notes	Alternate night
Alt hor	Alternies horis	Alternate hours
Met N	Maine et nate	Morning and night
om	Omni mane	Each Morning
od	Omni die	Daily
on	Omni night	Each night
hs	Hora Somni	At sleeping time
hn	Hac note	To night
h	Hora	Hour
q	Quaque	Every
cm	Gas Mane	Tomorrow morning
hd	Arora decubitus	At bed time

Contd...

Abbreviation	Derivations	Meaning
prn	Propsenate	When required
qh	Quaqua hora	Every hour
bid	Bis in die	Twice a day
Q2h., Q3h, Q4h		Every two, three and four days
qid or 4 d	Quarter in die	Four times in a day
stat	Statin	At once
tds	Ter in die	Three times a day

Preparation of Drug (Table 9.2)

TABLE 9.2: Abbreviations used in drug preparation.

Abbreviation	Derivations	Meaning
aq	Aqua	Water
aq dest	Aqua destillatu	Distilled water
comp.	Compositum	Compound
dil	Dilutio	Dilute
et.	Et.	And
fl.	Fludium	Fluid
inf.	Indusum	Inform
Lin.	Linementum	Liniment
empl.	Emplastrum	Plaster
Liq.	Liquor	Liquid
let.	Lotion	Lotion
mist.	Mistura	Mixture
ol	Oleum	Oil
pil	Pilula	Pill
puli	Puliva	Powder
sp.	Spirutys	Spirit
syr.	Syrups	Syrup
Tinet or Tr.	Tincturu	Tincture
ung.	Unguentum	Ointment

Dosage and Application (Table 9.3)

TABLE 9.3: Abbreviations used for drug dosage and applications.

Abbreviation	Derivations	Meaning
aa	ana	of each
add	adde	add to
add part del	Adde Parts dolents	to the painful part
ad lib.	ad Libitun	as much as desired
gal.	gallon	gallon
C	centigrade	centigrade
-c	cum	with
cc		cubic centimeter
gm	gram	gram, grams
gr.	granum,	grana grain

Contd...

Contd...

Abbreviation	Derivations	Meaning
gtt.	gutta	a drop, drops
garg	gargarisma	a gargle
kg	kilogram	One thousand grams
L	liter	liter
LB	Libra	Pund
m	Minimus	Minim
ml.	Milliliter	1 cc
no.	numero	number
(.)	octarius	a pint
part vio.	partitis vicibus	in divided doses
qs	quantum suffiut	as much as is sufficient
Rx	receipe	take thou
-s	sine	without
sos	si opus sit	if necessary
ss	semis	one half
tsp	teaspoon	teaspoon full
z	drachma	dram
oz	unica	ounce

Miscellaneous (Table 9.4)

TABLE 9.4: Miscellaneous abbreviations.

Abbreviation	Meaning
Hypo	Hypodermic
IM	Intramuscularly
Per	Through or by means of
PV	Per vagina
SC or SQ	Subcutaneously
IV	Intravenously
Pr	Per rectum
i.e.,	that is

DEVELOPMENTAL CONSIDERATIONS IN MEDICATION ADMINISTRATION

Developmental Age (1 Month to 1 Year)

- Poor head control requires support to minimize choking
- Hands should be monitored to prevent interference.
- Drug agents require precise measurement
- Physical comfort during administration.
- Initial response to medication is to spit or drool.
- Allow parent to give medication with nurse watching.

Developmental Age (1–2 years)

- Allow child to choose a position to take the medication
- Follow routine of home
- Taste of medication may be disguised
- Use single commands
- Allow child to familiarize self with dosing device
- Giving medications at this age may be a real challenge

- Give simple choices: a cup or a spoon, but you need to do it now.
- Do not over negotiate.

Pre-School (3–6 years)
- Tablets and capsules should be crushed—most children this age are unable to swallow pills.
- Allow child to make decisions about how to take

ROUTES OF DRUG ADMINISTRATION

There are number of different routes of administration of drugs into the body. The routes prescribed for administering a medication depend on the drug properties, desired effect and on the patient's physical and mental condition.

Drugs could be administered by following routes:
- Local route or topical route
- Oral route or enteral route
- Parenteral route

Local Route or Topical Route

Types:
- Local dermal application
- Insertion
- Insufflations
- Instillation
- In this route, drug acts at the site of application and might enter the systemic circulation.
- To have local effects, drugs are applied on skin and mucous membranes

These be done by variety of ways:
- By directly applying a liquid or ointment, e.g., eye drops, gargling or swabbing the throat.
- By inserting into body cavity, e.g., placing suppository in rectum or vagina.
- By inserting fluid into body cavity, e.g., ear drops, nasal drops or bladder and rectal instillation.
- By irrigating a body cavity, e.g., flushing ear, vagina, bladder or rectum with drug-based fluid.
- By spraying, e.g., instillation into nose and throat.

Advantages
- Provide local and systemic effect.
- Painless with limited side effects.
- Indicated when oral route is contraindicated.
- Inhalation provides easy access to respiratory tract.

Disadvantages
- Skin applications leave oily or paste like substance on skin.
- Mucous membranes are highly sensitive to some drugs.
- Insertion of rectal and vaginal drugs causes embarrassment.
- Contraindicated, if had ruptured ear drum, rectal surgery, etc.
- Some inhalation drugs cause serious systemic effects

Oral Route or Enteral Route
- This is the easiest and commonly used route.
- Drugs are given orally usually swallowed with water.
- These have slower but prolonged effect than parenteral route.
- Common dose formed for oral administration are tablets, capsules, liquids, solutions, suspensions, syrups and elixirs.

Advantages
- Convenient and comfortable for patient.
- Economical and easy to administer.
- Produce local or systemic effects.
- Rarely cause anxiety for patient.

Disadvantages
Oral drugs can irritate lining of gastrointestinal tract, discolored teeth and cause unpleasant taste.

Oral route cannot be prescribed in some cases like:
- Unconscious or confused patient
- Alterations in gastrointestinal function, (e.g., nausea, vomiting), reduced motility (after general anesthesia).
- Patient has gastric suction or surgery of gastrointestinal tract.

Parenteral Route
- The term "Parenteral" comes from Greek words Para means 'outside, enteron means the intestine.
- This route of administration bypasses the alimentary canal.
- Parenteral drug administration means, "Any non-oral means of administration" but is generally interpreted as relating to injecting, directly into the body, bypassing the skin and mucous membranes.
- Administration of drug through any route other than oral route is called as parenteral route.

Some common parenteral routes of drug administration are:
- Injection
- Transmucosal
- Transdermal
- Inhalations

A route of administration is the path by which drug, fluid or other substance is brought into contact with the body.

Advantages
- Means of administration when oral route is contraindicated.
- Rapid absorption than oral or topical route.
- Do not irritate the gastrointestinal tract.

Disadvantages
- Risk of introducing infection or tissue damage.
- Anxiety due to repeated needlesticks.
- Sometimes, IM and IV routes are dangerous due to rapid absorption.
- Self-medication is not possible.

Injection

Injections can be given by various routes:
- **Intradermal (ID):** The drug is injected into the dermis: layer of skin below the epidermis.
- **Subcutaneous (SC):** The drug is injected into the subcutaneous tissue of skin below the dermis.

- **Intramuscular (IM):** The drug is injected into the muscle
- **Intravenous (IV):** The drug is injected into a vein
- **Intrathecal:** Drugs are administered through a catheter into sub-arachnoid space or into one of the ventricles of the brain.
- **Epidural:** Drugs are injected in the epidural space via a catheter
- **Intraosseous:** The drug is administered directly into the bone marrow.
- **Intraperitoneal:** The drugs are injected into the peritoneal cavity.
- **Intrapleural:** The drugs are injected into the pleural space
- **Intraarterial:** The drug is administered directly into the artery.
- **Intracardiac:** The drug is administered directly into the cardiac tissue.
- **Intraarticular:** The drug is injected into the joint.
- **Intramedullary:** Drugs are injected into bone marrow.

Transmucosal

Transmucosal is the, "Absorption of drugs across the mucous membrane".

Transmucosal administration includes the following:
- **Nasal route:** Nasal administration of drugs include numerous compounds, peptides and protein drugs. Drugs are cleared rapidly from nasal cavity after intranasal administration resulting in systemic drug absorption.
- **Sublingual route:** In sublingual route, drug is placed under the tongue. Rapidly absorbed by sublingual mucosa.

Advantages
- Economical
- Quick termination
- Less pain
- Quick drug absorption

Disadvantages
- Unpalatable in bitter drugs
- Irritation of oral mucosa
- Few drugs are absorbed

Rectal: Rectal administration uses the rectum as a route of administration for medication and other fluids, which are absorbed by the rectum's blood vessels and flow into body's circulatory system which distributes the drug to the body's organs in bodily systems.

Transdermal

The drugs delivery through the skin (for systemic effect) is commonly known as Transdermal Drug Delivery (TDD).

Methods for transdermal drug delivery are as follows:
- **Adhesives (patches):** Transdermal adhesives (patches) are dosage forms designed to deliver a therapeutically effective amount of drug from outside the skin through its layers into the bloodstream
- **Inunction:** Drug is rubbed into skin and get absorbed to produce systemic effects.
- **Iontophoresis:** Iontophoresis is a process of transdermal drug delivery by use of a voltage gradient on the skin.

Molecules are transported across the stratum corneum by electrophoresis and electro-osmosis and the electric field can increase the permeability of skin. This phenomenon, directly and indirectly, constitute active transport of matter due to an applied electric current.
- Therapeutically, Electromotive Drug Administration (EMDA) delivers a medicine or other chemical through a skin.
- In other words, it is an injection without a needle, and may be described as non-invasive method of drug administration.
- It is different from dermal patches, which do not rely on an electric field.
- It drives a charged substance, usually a medication or bioactive agent, transdermally by repulsive electromotive force through the skin. For example, salicylate fluoride iontophoresis in dental hypersensitivity.
- **Implantation:** Implantation means some solid drugs are planting or putting into body tissue for systemic effect.
- **Jet injection:** Jet injector is a type of medical injecting syringe that uses a high-pressure narrow jet of the injection liquid instead of hypodermic needle to penetrate the epidermis.

Inhalations
- During general anesthesia, volatile liquids and gases are given through inhalation route to sedate the patient. Inhaled fumes moved to the lungs which further leads to local or systemic effect.
- Inhaled drugs have local as well as systemic effect.

ORAL MEDICATION

Oral medications are defined as the administration of medication by mouth and ensuring that patient swallows the medicine.

Purposes
- To prevent the disease
- To cure the disease
- To promote the health
- To give palliative treatment
- To give as a symptomatic treatment.

Nurse's Responsibility in Administration of Oral Medication
- Check the diagnosis and age of the patient
- Check the purpose of medication
- Check the identification of the patient, the name and bed number
- Check the physician's orders for the correct name of the drug, dosage and method of administration
- Check the nurse record for the time at which the last dose was given
- Check for any contraindications present in the patient for an oral intake of the medicines, such as nausea, vomiting, unconsciousness, etc.
- Check the character of the drug—whether it can be taken safely by the oral method

- Check the form of the drug available and the correct method of administration
- Check the level of consciousness of the patient and ability to follow instructions
- Check the abilities and limitations in swallowing the medications.

Equipment

A trolley containing:
- A bowel of clean water
- Ounce glass, medicine glass, dropper, teaspoon to measure the medicine
- Drinking water in a feeding cup
- Mortar and pestle to crush and powder the tablets if necessary
- Duster/towel to widen the outside of the bottle after pouring the medicine ordered
- Kidney tray and paper bag to discard the waste
- Medicine cards to write the medication order from patient's order sheet

Preparation of the Patient

- Explain the procedure to the patient. Tell the advantages and needs of medication
- If patient is allowed to sit assist him to sit
- Never give medication in flat position as there is a danger of aspiration of drug and fluid when swallowed
- Give a mouthwash, if necessary
- If medication is ill tasting, prepare a drink to mask the taste of the medication
- Protect the bed clothes and garments with a towel placed under the chin across the chest.

Procedures

- Keep the patient comfortable in bed
- Arrange the articles at the bedside
- Identify patient by name and check the name board at bedside
- Check the nurse's record to find out when drug was last administered
- Check for special instructions and check vital signs if needed
- Select medicine from patient's locker and check medication label thrice
- Encourage patient to sit-up and make sure medicines are swallowed
- First give little water to moisten the mouth and then give medicine one at a time
- Stay with the patient until the medicine has been swallowed; give him a drink of water after it.

Aftercare of the Patient and Articles

- Remove the towel and wipe the face with it
- Position the patient for good body alignment
- Take all articles to the utility room. Wash and dry all articles and replace them in their proper place
- Wash hands
- Record medications given in medication sheet and also nurses record
- Record any reaction observed after the administration of the drug
- Report any reaction to the ward sister and doctor in charge.

Contraindications

- Continuous vomiting
- Gastric or intestinal suction
- Unconscious patient
- Patient who are unable to swallow
- Patient on nil per oral.

Advantages

- This method is safe and convenient
- It is effective method
- There is no pain while administering the drug
- Allergic reactions are very less.

Disadvantages

- Sometimes the patient may not swallow the medicine
- The drug may only be partially observed
- It may irritate the gastric mucosa and can cause vomiting or diarrhea and the effect is lost.

SUBLINGUAL AND BUCCAL MEDICATION ADMINISTRATION

Definition

- Sublingual and buccal medications are drugs administered by placing them in the mouth, either under the tongue (sublingual) or between the gum and the cheek (buccal).
- The medications dissolve rapidly and gets absorbed through the mucous membranes of the mouth, where they enter directly into the bloodstream.
- The medications are compounded in the form of small, quick-dissolving tablets, sprays, lozenges or liquid suspensions.

Sublingual Administration

- A drug that is placed under the tongue, where it dissolves.
- When the medication in capsule form is ordered sublingually, the fluid must be aspirated from the capsule rip and placed under the tongue.
- A medication given by the sublingual route should not be swallowed as desired effects will not be achieved.

Buccal Administration

- A medication is held in the mouth against the mucous membranes of the cheek until the drug dissolves.
- The medication should not be chewed, swallowed or placed under the tongue, (e.g., sustained release nitroglycerine, antiemetic, tranquilizer, sedatives).
- Patient should be taught to alternate the cheeks with each subsequent dose to avoid mucosal irritation

Purpose

The most common sublingual medication is the nitroglycerine tablet. Its rapid action to relax the blood vessels reduces the workload on the heart and relieves the pain of angina pectoris. Other buccal and sublingual medications, however, serve a variety of purposes, such as narcotic pain relief, migraine pain relief, blood pressure control and mental decline due to dementia (i.e., ergoloid mesylates). This form of medication is extremely effective, because it bypasses the digestive system and is absorbed into the bloodstream in minutes.

Advantages

- Administration usually does not cause stress.
- Can be administered for local effect
- Drug is rapidly absorbed into bloodstream,
- Safe, does not break skin barrier.
- Usually less expensive.
- Most convenient.

Disadvantages

- Inappropriate for the patient with nausea and vomiting.
- Drugs may have unpleasant taste and odor.
- If swallowed, drug may be inactivated by gastric juice.
- Drug must remain under the tongue until dissolved and absorbed.

Steps of Procedure

- Check the medication orders and assess the patient's ability to take medication (examine the mucous membrane of patient's mouth for irritation or sores).
- Check the written medication orders and confirm the identity of patient.
- Wash hands.
- Collect equipment and check dosage and amount of medication.
- Explain the procedure to patient. Nothing should be eaten, drank, swallowed or chewed until the tablet dissolved.
- To administer sublingual tablets, the patient open his or her mouth and raise the tongue. The tablet should then be placed under the tongue
- Administration of buccal tablets is similar to that of sublingual tablets. First, the patient should open his or her mouth. The tablet should be placed between the gum and the wall of the cheek.
- With the mouth closed, the tablet should be held in this position for 5–10 minutes or until it has dissolved.
- When administering a liquid suspension, the bottle should be shaken before the appropriate dose is poured. Liquid suspensions may be given in a medicine cup into the patient's mouth using a medicine syringe with no needle. The patient should be directed to hold and swish the liquid in the mouth for the amount of time designated by the physician's order. Some liquid suspensions are then swallowed and some expectorated into a sink or basin.
- When administering sprays, the container also needs to be shaken and the top taken off before the medication is given.
- The patient should be reminded not to breathe while the nurse is spraying the medicine. If the spray is ordered sublingual, the spray should be held about one inch (2.5 cm) away from the site and directed toward the tongue
- If the spray is ordered buccal, the tongue should be held out of the way, the cheek held outward and the spray directed into the gum area between the cheek and the teeth.
- Observe the patient for medication action.
- Discard the disposables.
- Wash hands and document medication administered on medication record.

Special Considerations

- Sublingual medications should not be administered, if the gums or mucous membranes have open sores or areas of irritation. Rather, the physician should be notified and medication should be held.
- The patient should be placed in a sitting position to prevent accidental aspiration of the medication.
- Buccal or sublingual medication should not be used when a patient is uncooperative or unconscious.
- The patient should not eat, drink, chew or swallow until the medication has been absorbed; swallowing the medication must be prevented, as it will decrease the drug's effectiveness.
- The patient should not smoke while taking sublingual or buccal medication, because smoking causes vasoconstriction of the blood vessels. This will decrease the absorption of the medication.

ADMINISTRATION OF PARENTERAL MEDICATIONS

Types of Parenteral Therapies

- Parenteral administration refers to giving medication by injection into or under the skin.
- **Injections may be (Figs. 9.2 and 9.3):**
  - Intradermal—into the dermis layer of the skin
  - Subcutaneous—under the skin into the adipose tissue
  - Intramuscular—into muscle tissue
  - Intravenous—into the blood through a vein
  - Intrathecal—into the spinal canal
  - Intracardial—into the heart
  - Intraarticular—into a joint.

ROUTES OF PARENTERAL THERAPIES

Injections

- Injections are parenteral therapy. It means giving of therapeutic agents including food outside the alimentary tract.
- An injection is the forcing of a fluid into a cavity, a blood vessel or body tissue through a hollow tube or needle.

Purposes

- To get a rapid and systemic effect of the drug.
- To provide the needed effect even when the patient is unconscious.

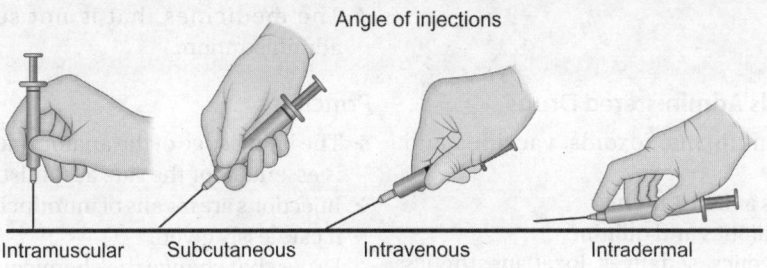

Fig. 9.2: Angle of injections.

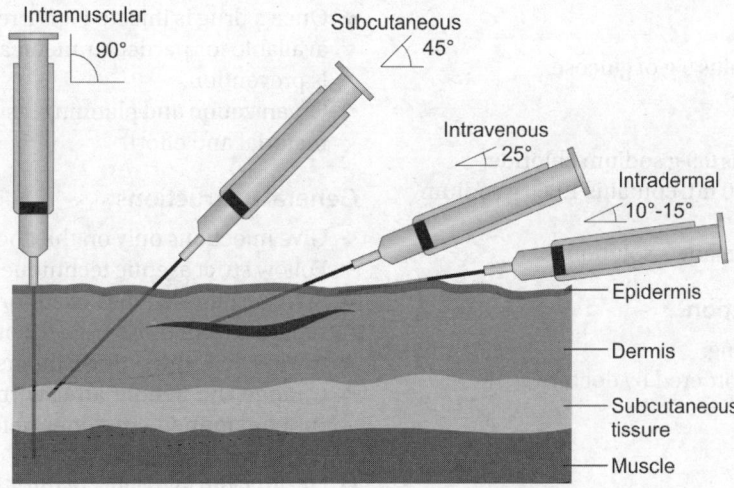

Fig. 9.3: Angle and route of injection administration.

- Assures that the total dosage will be administered and
- the same will be absorbed for the systemic action of the drug.
- Provides the only means of administration for medications that cannot be given orally.
- To obtain a local effect at the sight of the injection.
- To restore blood volume by replacing the fluid, e.g., in shock conditions.
- To give nourishment when it cannot be taken by mouth.

Types of Injections

- **Intradermal:** Drug introduced into the dermis.
- **Subcutaneous:** Drug introduced into the subcutaneous tissue.
- **Intramuscular:** Injected into the muscles.
- **Intravenous:** Introduced into the vein.
- **Intraspinal:** Introduced into the spinal cavity.
- **Intraosseous:** Introduced into the peritoneal cavity.
- **Venesection:** Opening a vein and introducing a tube or wide bore needle and introducing medicines and fluids or taking out blood.
- **Infusions:** When a large quantity of medicines is fluids are to be introduced into the body.
- **Transfusions:** It is the introduction of whole blood or plasma into a vein or artery.

Factors that Favors Absorption

- **Blood supply to the area:** Fluids injected into the blood stream will act quicker than any other methods used.
- **The composition of the fluid injected:** Solubility and diffusibility of the fluid.
- **Application of heat:** Heat dilates the blood vessels; therefore, the heat applied over the site of injection increases the rate of absorption.
- **Massage:** It stimulates the local blood supply and increases the rate of absorption.
- **Circulation time of the blood:** Adsorption of medicines and fluids injected to the body will diminished in a person who has venous congestion (edema).
- **Physical condition:** The local disease condition of the skin and underlying tissues, such as skin lesions, inflammations, etc., delays the absorption of the drug.
- **Addition of the substances:** That tends to breakdown the natural resistance of the tissues can increase the rate of absorption.

Complications of Injections

- Allergic reactions certain drugs, e.g., penicillin
- Infections (abscess formation)
- Pyrogenic reactions (producing fever)
- Tissue trauma
- Psychic trauma
- Pain
- Accidental intravascular injections
- Foot drop and persistent paralysis of the limb
- Air embolism
- Over dose and under dose of the medication
- Errors in the administration of the medication

- Infectious hepatitis
- Circulatory overload.

Types of Drug and Fluids Administered Drugs

- **Preventive action:** Antitoxins, toxoids, vaccines and antibiotics
- **Diagnostic acids:** Dyes and histamines
- **Remedial action:** Antibiotics and quinine
- **Palliative action:** Narcotics, sedatives, local anesthetics and general anesthetics
- **Substitution:** Hormones, fluids, minerals and vitamins.

Fluids

- **D5W:** Each 100 mL contains 5 g of glucose.
- **D10W, D25W, D50W.**
- **DNS:** Dextrose 5% saline.
- **NS:** Each 100 mL contains 0.9 g sodium chloride.
- **Sodium lactate:** Each 100 mL contains 1.866 g sodium
- **Ringer lactate.**
- **Ringer's solution or Hartmann's solution.**

Selection of Site for Injection

It depends upon the following:
- Route of administration ordered by doctor
- Quantity of the drugs
- Condition of the patient
- Muscular development
- Knowledge of anatomical position of the nerves
- Rotation of the site is necessary to avoid tissue trauma.

Technical Skill Needed

- Arrange the required equipment for the procedure.
- Nurse must be very skilful while giving the injection according to the route ordered
- Select correct sit for injection
- Prepare the medication dose accurately.

Criteria for Selection of Syringes and Needles

- **Intradermal:** Tuberculin syringe or 1 mL calibrated in 0.01 mL units. 26- or 27-gauge diameter and 3/8–5/8 length size of needle used.
- **Subcutaneous:** Insulin syringe or 1 mL calibrated in 40- or 80-unit's syringe. 25 gauge and ½ to 5/8 inches syringe is used.
- **Intramuscular:** 2.5 mL syringe is used it calibrated in 0.2 mL. 21, 22, 23 gauge 1–2 inches in length needles are used.
- **Intravenous:** The size depends upon the amount of fluids to be injected, 18–20 gauge 1–2 inches needles use.

INTRAMUSCULAR INJECTION

Intramuscular injection is defines as introduction of medicine into the muscle in form of solution.

Purposes

- To obtain a quick effect of medicine than is obtained by oral administration and subcutaneous administration.
- Assures that the total dosage will be administered and the same will be absorbed for the systemic action of the drug.
- The medicines that is not suitable for intravenous administration.

Principles

- The knowledge of the anatomy and physiology of the body is essential for the safe administration of the injection.
- Injections are means of introducing infection into the body, if carelessly given.
- Drugs that change the chemical composition of the blood will endanger the life of the patient, if not used cautiously.
- Any unfamiliar situation produces anxiety.
- Once a drug is injected it is irretrievable. Antidote may be available for particular medications but the best antidote is prevention.
- Organization and planning results in the economy of time, material and effort.

General Instructions

- Give injections only on the doctor's written orders.
- Follow strict aseptic techniques.
- Syringes and needles used for injections should be kept separate from those used for other purpose.
- Always have the syringe and needles in good order.
- Change the needle after withdrawing the drug from a rubber stopped container before giving injection to the patient.
- Observe the five rights of the administration of medicines.
- Never use a drug whose expiry date is over.
- Always have a patient relaxed and placed in a comfortable position.
- Never allow the patient to walk soon after the injection.
- Always give a test dose in case of penicillin and all types of sera.
- Expel the air from the syringe before the injection.
- Select the appropriate sit for giving injections.
- Rotate the site for patients getting insulin to prevent lip dystrophy.
- **Use correct technique of injection:** The needle inserted gently and quickly, and the drug injected slowly.
- After inserting the needle, always withdraw the piston to make sure that it is not in a blood vessel in case of intramuscular and subcutaneous injections.
- Solution for injection should be clear, sterile, nearly neutral in reaction.
- Massage the area at the site of injection except in case of intradermal injections.
- Injection should be charted immediately.

Site of Intramuscular Injections

Dorsal gluteal site: Find out the greater trochanter of the femur and the posterior superior iliac spine drawn an imaginary line between these two bony prominences. Site will be upper and outer quadrant.

Ventrogluteal site: Place the tip of the index finger on the anterior superior iliac spine of the patient the middle finger just below the iliac crest (**Fig. 9.4**).

Vastus lateralis site: The site is at the outer aspect of the thigh. It is the area between mid-anterior thigh and mid-lateral thigh

Chapter 9: Administration of Medications

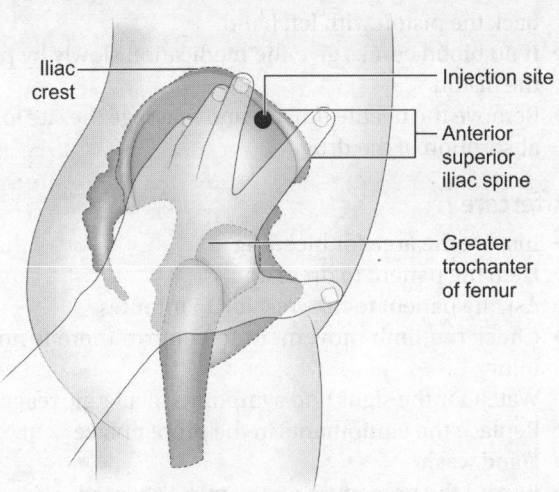

Fig. 9.4: Ventrogluteal site.

one hands span from elbow and great trochanter to one hand span above knee **(Figs. 9.5A and B)**.

Mid-deltoid site: Locate the lower edge of the acromion process and form a rectangle. The deltoid area is used to inject very small quantities of non-irritating drugs **(Fig. 9.6)**.

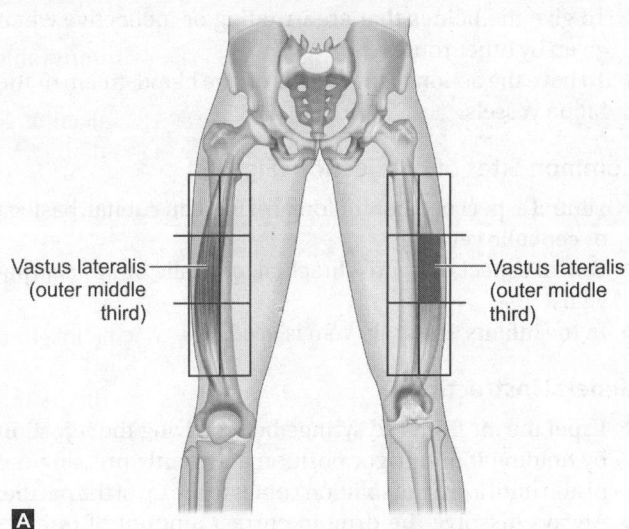

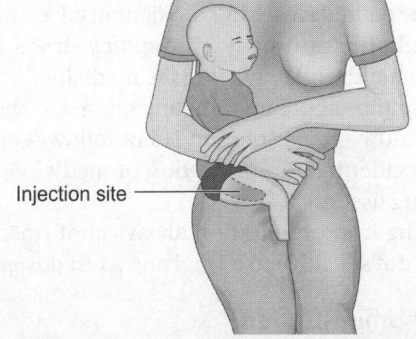

Figs. 9.5A and B: (A) Vastus lateralis site, (B) Marking the vastus lateralis site on baby.

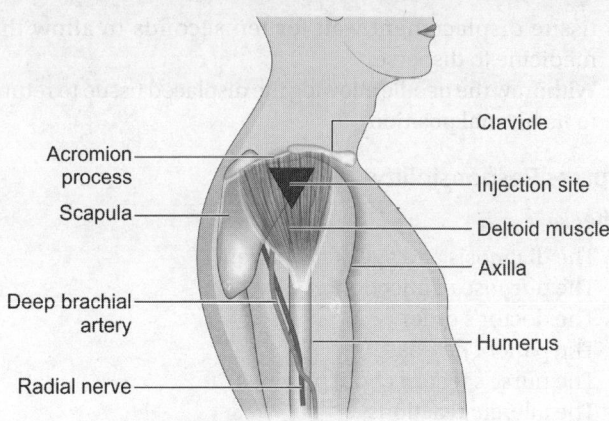

Fig. 9.6: Mid-deltoid site.

Methods of IM Injection Administration
Air lock method (Fig. 9.7)
- Expel the air from the syringe leaving 0.2 mL, stretch the skin lightly with the index finger.
- Insert the full needle quickly into the muscle.
- Withdraw the piston to confirm that the need is not in the blood vessel.
- Push the piston gently to give the medicine very slowly.

Z–Tract Method (Fig. 9.8)
- Expel the air from the syringe, displace the skin laterally using the side of your left hand, insert the needle as pirate the placement, inject the medicine very slowly, marinating

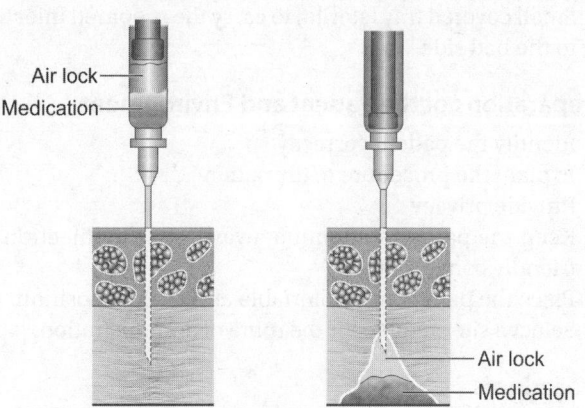

Fig. 9.7: Air lock method injection administration.

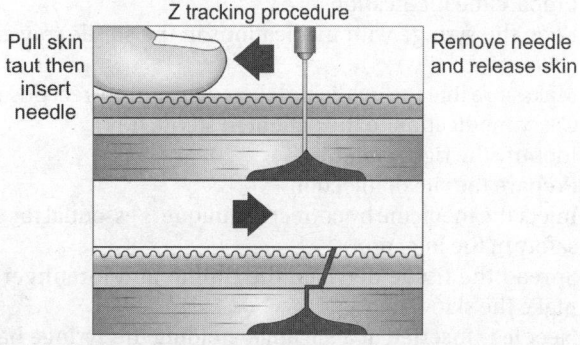

Fig. 9.8: Z-track method.

tissue displacement wait for ten seconds to allow the medicine to disperse.
- Withdraw the needle allowing the displaced tissue to return to its normal position.

Nurses Responsibility

Check
- The diagnosis and age of the patient
- The purpose of injection
- The doctor's order
- The patient details
- The nurse's record about previous
- The allergic reactions
- The necessity for giving test dose
- The levels of consciousness and the ability to follow instructions
- The site of injection
- The patient's previous experiences.

Equipment
A tray containing:
- Syringe and needles of various size (sterile)
- Transfer forceps in a jar containing antiseptic solution
- Sterile cotton swabs and gauze pieces in sterile container
- Methylated spirit in container
- Bowl with water
- Kidney tray and paper bag
- Drug order sheet
- Water for injection
- File to cut upon the ampoules
- Small covered tray (sterile) to carry the prepared injection to the bed side

Preparations of the Patient and Environment
- Identify the patient correctly
- Explain the procedure to the patient
- Provide privacy
- Keep the patient's attention away from the injection by friendly conversation
- Place the patient in comfortable and relaxed position
- Select a site suitable for the route of administration.

Procedures
- Select the medication
- Hand wash
- Prepare the medication
- Keep the syringe with medications in the sterile tray and cover it
- Make sure that the medicine taken right and correct dosage
- Carry medication to the patient in sterile tray
- Identify the right patient
- Prepare the site of injection
- Inject the medicine by correct technique is essential for the safety of the injection
- Spread the tissue between the thumb and forefinger to make the skin taut
- Needle is inserted at a 90° angle holding the syringe back the piston with the left hand
- Using a steady push on the needle and aspirate by pulling back the piston with left hand
- If no blood comes give the medication slowly by pushing the piston
- Remove the needle quickly and massage the site for quick absorption of the drug.

Aftercare
- Inspect the area for bleeding
- Help the patient to dress up
- Ask the patient to take rest for 15 minutes
- Check the limb movement to confirm there is no nerve injury
- Watch for the signs and symptoms of allergic reaction
- Replace the equipments in the proper place
- Hand wash
- Record the procedure on the nurse's record.

■ INTRAVENOUS INJECTION

Intravenous injection is the introduction of a small quantity of drug into the vein by venous puncture.

Introduction of drug directly into the bloodstream is called intravenous injection.

Purposes
- To have a fast action of the medicine as in emergency.
- To give medicines that are irritating or ineffective when given by other routes.
- To have the action of medicines on the bloodstream or the blood vessels.

Common Sites of IV Injection (Fig. 9.9)
- Ventral aspect of elbow or forearm median cubital, basilica or cephalic veins.
- Dorsal aspect of hand—brachial, cephalic or metacarpal veins.
- In the infants, the scalp vein is used.

General Instructions
- Expel the air from the syringe before giving the injection by holding it in upright position and gently pressing the piston until a drop of solution comes to the tip of the needle.
- Always dissolve the drug in correct amount of fluid to minimize the risk of adverse effect of the medicine.
- Observe the patient closely for the signs of adverse reaction of the medicine and have emergency drugs and the antidote in hand while injecting the medicine.
- Do not give the medicine if the injection site shows any edema or intravenous solution is not following properly to avoid accidental administration of medicine into the surrounding tissues.
- When giving iron preparation always confirms that the patients is not sensitive to it by giving a test dose.

Types of IV Administration
- Adding the medicine in intravenous solution bottle (intravenous infusion).

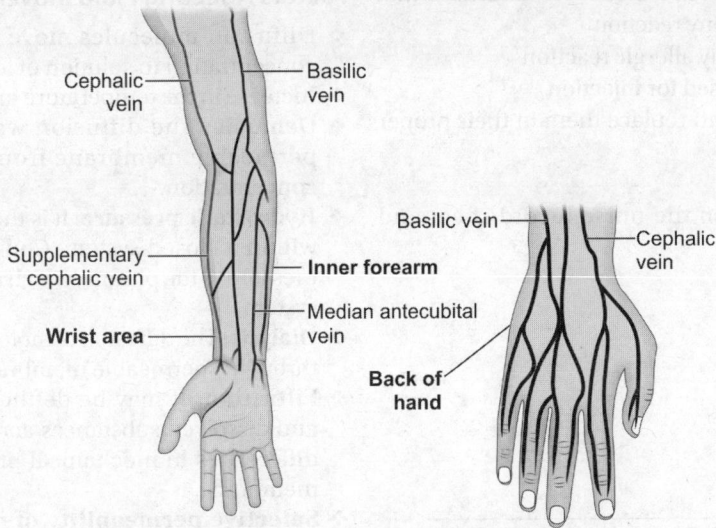

Fig. 9.9: Common sites of IV injection.

- Existing intravenous line for continuous infusion.
- **Bolus:** Direct intravenous push for immediate or fast action.

Selection of Syringe and Needle
- The size of syringe used for intravenous infusion depends upon the amount of fluids to be injected.
- Size of the needle used are 18–21 gauge or 1–2 inches.

Preliminary Assessment
Check
- The diagnosis and age of the patient
- The purpose of injection
- The doctor's order for the type, dosage, time and route of administration
- The patient's name and bed number
- The nurse's record to find out the time at which the last dose was given.
- The symptoms of overdose or allergic reaction
- The necessity for giving test dose
- The form of the medicine available and correct method of administration
- The level of consciousness of the patient
- The site and previous experience of the patient.

Equipment
A Tray Containing
- Syringe and needles of various sizes according to the need in a covered tray (sterile)
- Transfer forceps in a jar containing antiseptic solution.
- Sterile cotton swabs and gauze pieces in sterile containers
- Methylated spirit in a container
- Bowl with water
- Tourniquet
- Water for injection
- Drug order sheet
- File to cut open the ampules
- Small covered tray (sterile).

Preparations of the Patient and Environment
- Identify the patient correctly
- Explain the procedure to the patient
- Provide privacy
- Place the patient in comfortable and relaxed position suitable of intravenous injection
- Select a site suitable for the route of administration, quantity of medication to be given and characteristics of medication.

Procedures
- Read the doctor's order and select the medication
- Wash hands
- Select appropriate syringe and needle and check whether they are in good working order
- Recheck the order, medicine card with the label of the medicine, expiry date, etc.
- Mix well and take out the required amount of solution in the syringe
- Carry medicine to the patient.

Methods of Administering IV Injection
- Apply a tourniquet on the upper arm
- Ask the patient to clean the hand
- Pull the skin taut and place the needle in line with vein at a 15–45° angle
- Insert the needle, a bit below the point where the needle will pierce the vein
- When the back flow of blood occurs into the syringe release the tourniquet and injects the medicine very slowly
- Pressure apply with swab at the puncture site after the needle is withdrawn to prevent bleeding.

Aftercare
- Observe the area for bleeding if bleeding occurs apply pressure but do not massage
- Give comfortable position to the patient

- Ask the patient to take rest at least 15–30 minutes so that you can observe him for any reaction
- Observe the patient for any allergic reaction
- Replace the equipment used for injection
- Clean all other articles and replace them in their proper place
- Wash hands
- Record the procedure on the nurse record sheet and medication sheet.

Complications
- Allergic reactions
- Pain
- Injection abscess
- Injury to nerves
- Air embolism.

INTRAVENOUS INFUSIONS

An introduction of a large amount of fluid into body via veins is called as intravenous infusion.

Intravenous infusion is puncturing vein with sterile cannula/needle into a vein to supply the body with fluids electrolyte, nutrients and medication.

Purposes
- To supply fluids and electrolytes
- To restore fluid volume due to dehydration, hemorrhage, vomiting, diarrhea, etc.
- To meet patient's basic requirements, e.g., calories, vitamins, etc.
- To maintain hemostatics balance
- To treat in emergency conditions some medications are given intravenously
- To prevent and treat shock and collapse.

Indications
- To save the patients in life-threatening situations, e.g., extensive burns
- To introduce a drug into the circulation for diagnostic purpose, e.g., IVP (intravenous pyelogram)
- To supply fluids and nutrients to the patients who are unable to digest or absorb a diet administered mouth or through the nasal tube
- To dilute toxins in case of toxaemia or septicaemia
- When blood or blood products are to be given, e.g., anemia, hemorrhage.

Solutions Used
- Isotonic solutions—sodium chloride 0.9% commonly used
- Hypotonic solution or buffer substances sodium/potassium, calcium chlorides and lactic acid
- Nutrient solutions dextrose 5, 10, 25, 50%
- Alkalinizing and acidifying solutions
- Blood volume expanders—plasma substitutes and contain large molecular substances, e.g., dextran, lomodex, hemocele, etc.

Factors Affecting Fluid Movement
- Diffusion molecules move from a solution of higher concentration to solution of lower concentration.
- Increase in the temperature increases the rate of diffusion.
- **Osmosis:** The diffusion water molecules through a permeable membrane from an area of lesser solute concentration.
- **Hydrostatic pressure:** It is the pressure exerted by a fluid within a closed system. Counter balancing the osmotic pressure of the plasma, which attract fluid into the vascular system.
- **Dialysis:** The diffusion of molecules of soluble constituents through a permeable membrane is known as dialysis.
- **Filtration:** It may be defined as the passage of fluids and dissolved substances across membranes because of differences in mechanical pressure on two sides of the membrane.
- **Selective permeability of membranes:** In body, the capillary and the cell membranes are described as selective permeable.

Factors that Favors Absorption
- **Warmth:** Application of heat over the site of injection or the use of warm solution.
- **Massaging:** Massaging the part gently increases the local supply and increase absorption.
- Diffusibility and solubility of the drug.

VENIPUNCTURE SITE

The selection of site depends upon following facts:
- The condition of veins
- The characteristics of tissues over the vein
- Purpose and durations of infusions
- The type and amount of IV fluids ordered
- The diagnosis and general condition of the patient.

The Commonly Used Veins
- Basilica and cephalic veins (forearm)
- Median cubital, cephalic and basilica veins (Antecubital fossa)
- Radial vein (radial area)
- Dorsal metacarpal veins (the hand)
- Veins in the foot
- Femoral and saphenous veins (thigh)
- Veins in the scalp (for infants).

Complications of IV Infusion
- **Circulatory overload:** The intravascular compartment contains more fluid than the normal. Circulatory overload results in cardiac failure and pulmonary edema.
- **Infiltration:** It is the escape of fluid into the subcutaneous tissues due to dislodgement of needle.
- **Hematoma formation:** The walls of blood vessels may be damaged due to careless introduction of the needle into the body.
- **Thrombophlebitis:** It is caused by mechanical trauma to the vein or the chemical irritation of some substances introduced into the veins such as potassium chloride.

- **Pyrogenic reaction:** It is characterized by temperature elevation, chills, headache, nausea, vomiting and circulatory collapse in severe cases.
- **Air embolism:** The vascular collapse occurs due to occlusion of the vessel by embolism. The signs of pulmonary embolism are dyspnea, cyanosis, low blood pressure, shock and collapse, tachycardia and unconsciousness.
- **Infection at the needle site:** Contamination occurs during insertion or left exposed for a long period.
- **Serum hepatitis:** Infectious hepatitis have been attributed to improperly disinfected syringes and needles.
- **Allergic reaction:** This may due to certain drugs administered along with the IV fluids.

Fluid Rate Calculation

$$\text{Flow rate} = \frac{\text{Total volume infused in mL} \times \text{drops mL}}{\text{Total time of the infusion in minutes}}$$

General Instructions

- Follow strict aseptic technique thought the procedure.
- Administer IV fluids only with a clearly written prescription.
- Maintain the specified rate of flow to prevent circulatory overload.
- Constant and continuous observation for any unfavorable symptoms.
- Observe the rights during administration.
- Check the expiry date before opening the bottles.
- If fluids are discolored, cloudy in appearance that should not be used for infusion.
- Do not use any site that is tender, red, edematous and inflamed.
- Never allow the bottle to get empty completely to prevent the entry of air into the tissues.
- Keep the patient warm and comfortable with blankets if necessary.
- Immobilize the joints with splints when the needle is placed near a joint.
- Frequent observation of the vital signs throughout the procedure will help to detect many complications.
- Allow the patient to void before the IV infusion is started.

Observation Needed Throughout the Procedure

- Flow rate and potency of IV tubing
- Dislodgement of needle
- Signs of circulatory overload
- Urinary output
- Needle site
- Fluid level in the bottle
- Vital signs at frequent intervals.

Preliminary Assessment

Check

- Patients name, age, bed no and diagnosis
- Purpose of infusion
- Doctor's order
- Level of consciousness
- General conditions
- Abilities and limitations
- Need for additional restraints
- Articles available
- Previous experience.

Equipment

A Tray Containing

- Sterile IV solution
- Sterile IV infusion set
- Sterile needle of choice (butterfly or cannula)
- Sterile syringe (2 or 5 mL)
- Sterile transfer forceps in a jar
- Sterile cotton swabs and gauze pieces
- Surgical spirit
- Kidney tray and paper bag
- Bowl with water
- Tourniquet
- Adhesive tape and scissors
- Specimen bottles
- Mackintosh and towel
- IV pole
- Restrainer (splint with roller bandages).

Preparations of the Patient and Environment

- Explain the procedure
- Sent the visitors outside
- Provide privacy
- Allow the patient to empty the bladder
- Check the vital signs
- Adjust the height of the bed
- Arrange the articles at the bedside
- Place the patient in comfortable and relaxed position
- Provide adequate light in the room.

Procedures

- Hand wash
- Prepare the IV solution; insert the drip set, and the air went into the bottle openings
- Hang the bottle on the IV pole about 18–24 inches high
- Over the clamp and flush the IV fluid through the tubing and needle into the kidney tray until all air is removed.
- Prepare few strips of adhesive tapes and keep ready for use.
- Apply tourniquet firmly 6–8 inches proximal to the venipuncture site.
- Encourage the patient to clench and unclench rapidly.
- Lightly tap the vein with your fingertips.
- Clean the area with surgical spirit.
- Insert the needle into the vein by holding the needle at a 30° angle with the hovel up.
- Pierce the skin lateral to the vein.
- When back flow of blood occurs into the needle and tubing, insert the needle further up into the vein about 3/4 or 1 inch.
- Release the tourniquet and open the clamp to allow the fluid to run in.
- Secure the scalp vein needle by H method or by crises cross method.
- Secure the scalp vein tubing and IV tubing.

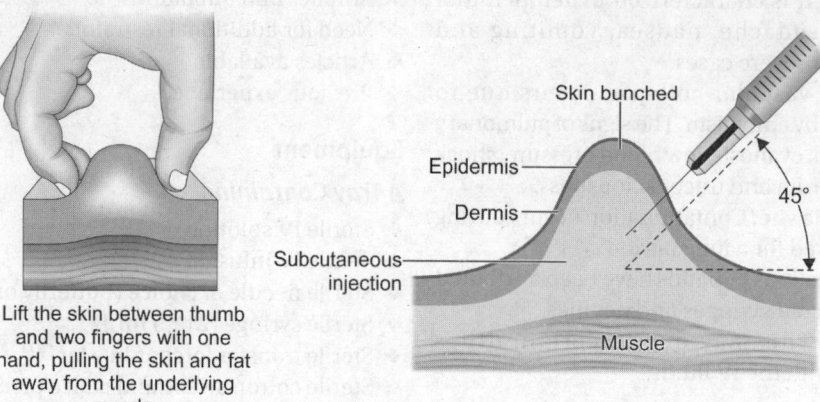

Fig. 9.10: Subcutaneous injection administration.

■ SUBCUTANEOUS INJECTION

Definition
A subcutaneous injection is administered as a bolus into the subcutis, the layer of skin directly below the dermis and epidermis, collectively referred to as the cutis.

Subcutaneous injection involves placing medication into the loose connective tissue under the dermis.

Subcutaneous injection means the introduction of medicine into the subcutaneous tissues beneath the upper layers of the skin.

Purposes
- To administer the medication that is ineffective in the gastrointestinal tract by the action of the digestive juice
- To administer smaller doses
- For slow drug absorption
- To obtain a prompt action of a medicine that is obtained by oral administration.

General Instructions
- A 90° angle is normally used with a 5/8-inch needle is used with a 5/8-inch needle for obese patients
- A 45° angle is used with a needle 3/4 inch long or longer for an average patient are in a thin patient
- The techniques of giving injection for hypodermic injections will be same as in IM injection
- Use only non-irritating medications
- Use only small quantity of medication
- Deposit the medication in a fold formed by picking up a layer of skin and fat
- Be sure to insert the needle beyond the thickness of the skin (The medication is to be deposited in the subcutaneous tissue) **(Fig. 9.10)**.

Equipment
- One mL calibrated in 40 or 80 units, e.g., insulin syringe.
- Hypodermic needles (24–25 gauge, 1/2 – 5/8 inches length).
- Sterile cotton scubas
- Methylated spirit in container
- Kidney tray with paper bag
- Drug ordered sheet
- Small covered tray (sterile) to carry the prepared injections to the bedside.

Criteria for Selection of Site
- The skin and underlying tissues are free of abnormalities
- Not over bony prominences
- Free of large blood vessels and nerves.

Common Sites Subcutaneous Injection (Fig. 9.11)
- Outer aspect of the upper arm
- Posterior chest wall below the scapula
- Anterior abdominal wall from below breast to iliac crests
- Anterior and lateral aspect of the thigh.

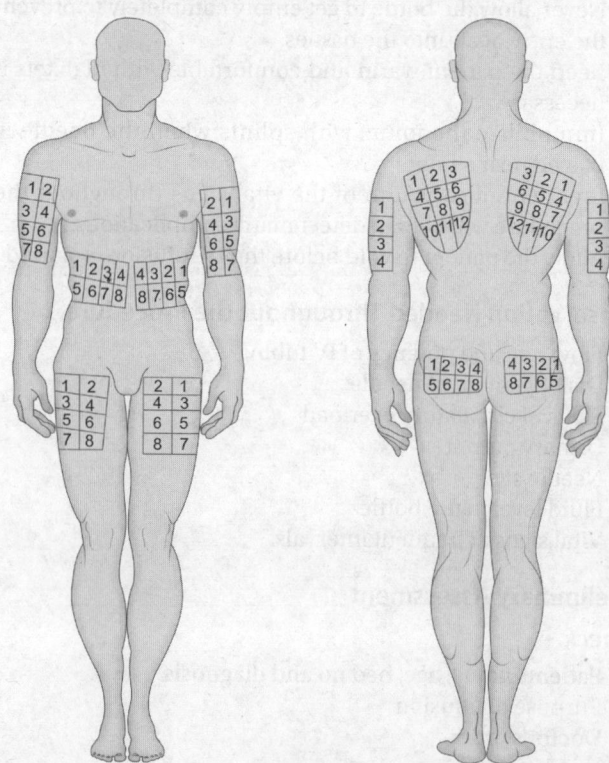

Fig. 9.11: Common sites of subcutaneous injection.

Procedure (Table 9.5)

TABLE 9.5: Steps of procedure for subcutaneous injection administration.

Nursing action	Rationale
Assemble equipment and check physician's order.	Avoids medication error from occurring.
Identify patient carefully	Ensures that right procedure is done on right patient
Explain procedure to patient, the drug that is to be administered, site, and how he has to cooperate.	Encourages cooperation and allays anxiety.
During procedure: Wash hands	Reduces spread of microorganisms.
Withdraw medication from an ampoule/vial as prescribed.	
Assemble all equipment including loaded medication in syringe near the patient's bedside.	
Pull curtains.	Provides privacy.
Help patient assume position depending on site selected: • Outer aspect of upper arm-arm relaxed and at the sides of the body. • Anterior thigh-sitting or lying down with muscles relaxed. • Abdomen-patient in semi recumbent position.	Ensures free access to injection site.
Assess the area. Check for lumps, nodules, tenderness, hardness, swelling, scarring, itching, burning sensation and localized inflammation in the area.	Good visualization helps in establishing the correct location of site and avoids damage to tissues. Nodules and lumps indicate that there is inadequate absorption at previous injection site.
Don gloves.	Reduces spread of microorganisms
Clean the area around injection site with an alcohol swab Use firm circular motion, while moving outward (5 cm diameter) Allow the site to dry. Keep alcohol swab in the tray for reuse. (When withdrawing needle.)	Friction helps to clean the skin.
Remove needle cap with non-dominant hand, pulling straight off	Lessens risk of an accidental needle prick.
Grasp and pinch the area surrounding the injection site or spread skin at site.	Provides for easy and less painful entry into subcutaneous tissue.
Hold the syringe in dominant hand between thumb and forefinger. Inject needle quickly at an angle of 45–90°, depending on amount of tissue, turgor of tissue, and length of needle. For thin people, an angle of 45 is preferred. When using an insulin syringe with a 26G needle, an angle of 90° can be used in normal and obese people	Subcutaneous tissue is abundant in well nourished, well hydrated people and sparse in emaciated, dehydrated or very thin people.

Contd...

Contd...

Nursing action	Rationale
After insertion, release the tissue and immediately move your non-dominant hand to steady lower end of syringe. Slide your dominant hand to top of the barrel.	Injecting solution into compressed tissue results in pressure against nerve fibres and creates discomfort. The non-dominant hand secures the needle and allows for smooth aspiration.
Aspirate if recommended, by pulling back gently on the plunger to determine whether needle is in a blood vessel. If blood appears, withdraw needle and discard. Prepare medication again. Do not aspirate for heparin/insulin.	Discomfort and serious reactions may occur if a drug intended for subcutaneous administration enters into the bloodstream. Heparin is an anticoagulant and can cause bruising on aspiration. Insulin needle is very small and hence aspiration will not give relevant information regarding placement of needle.
Inject medication slowly if no blood appears	Rapid injection of the medication creates pressure in the tissues and results in discomfort.
Withdraw needle quickly at the same angle as it was inserted, while applying counter traction around the injection site with non-dominant hand.	Slow withdrawal of the needle pulls tissue and causes discomfort. Applying counter traction around the injection site helps in preventing pulling of tissues when needle is withdrawn. Removing needle at the same angle minimizes trauma to tissues and discomfort to the patient.
Massage the area gently with alcohol swab Do not massage a heparin/insulin injection site.	Massaging helps to distribute the medication and hastens its absorption. Massaging a heparin site can lead to bruising.
Do not recap needle. Discard syringe and needle in appropriate receptacle.	Proper disposal prevents accidental needlestick injury.
After procedure: Assist patient to a comfortable position.	
Wash hands after removing gloves.	
Document medication administration with date, time, dosage, route, site and nurse's signature.	
Evaluate response of the patient to medication	

Aftercare

❖ Inspect the area but do not massage
❖ Help the patient to dress up
❖ Watch for signs and symptoms of any allergic reaction
❖ Replace the equipment used for injection
❖ Clean all other articles and replace them in their proper place
❖ Wash hands
❖ Record the procedure on the nurse's record and drug sheet

INTRADERMAL INJECTION

Intradermal Located between the epidermis and the hypodermis.

Sensitivity: A sensitivity analysis is a test that determines the "sensitivity" of bacteria to an antibiotic. It also determines the ability of the drug to kill the bacteria.

Bleb wheat: A suddenly formed elevation of the skin surface or a blister (often hemispherical) filled with serous fluid.

Definition

- Intradermal injection is a shallow or superficial injection of a substance into the dermis which is located between the hypodermis and epidermis.
- An intradermal injection is the introduction of a hypodermic needle into the dermis.
- Intradermal medicine when introduced into the dermis (under the epidermis).

Purposes

- To obtain a local effect at the site of injection of local anesthesia such as xylocaine and novocaine.
- Diagnostic purpose as in sick test, tuberculin test, etc.
- To test for allergic reaction to a drug, e.g., penicillin serum, etc.
- Vaccination

Selection of Syringe and Needle

- Size of syringe used for intradermal injections are 1 mL calibrated in 0.01 mL units (tuberculin syringe).
- Size of needle used for intradermal injections are 26–27-gauge diameter and 3/8–5/8-inch length.

Equipment

A Tray Containing

- Syringe and needles of various sizes according to the need in a covered tray (sterile)
- Sterile cotton swabs and gauze piece in sterile containers
- Methylated spirit in a container
- Kidney tray and paper bag
- Drug order sheet
- Small covered tray (sterile) to carry the prepared injections (syringes and needles with medication) to the bedside.

Preparation of the Patient and Equipment

- Identify the patient correctly
- Explain the procedure to the patient
- Provide privacy
- Place the patient in comfortable and relaxed position suitable for the type of injection.
- Select a site suitable for the route of administration, quantity of medication to given to the characteristics of medication.

Methods of Administration

- This method is used for skin tests to detect allergies
- Hold the skin tight by grasping it water the forearm
- With the bevel of the needle facing up insert the needle at an angel of 10–15° to the skin
- The needle enters between the two layers of the skin.
- The bevel should be practically visible through the skin
- Inject the medication slowly to produce wheel on the skin to 0.1 mL of medication injected intradermal
- Take out the needle quickly do not clean or massage the area.

General Instructions

- As skin contains sensory nerve ending only a small amount of solution can be injected into the skin as it is painful
- The skin should be healthy, free of any skin infection such as edema or irritation, the cloths should not irritate the skin.
- Separate syringe and needles should be used for giving injections.

Observation of the Site after Intradermal Injection

Tuberculin Test

- If tuberculin test is done, ask the patient to report after 48 hours.
- Reddened raised area at the site of injection shows a positive reaction.
- If the area is not discolored or raised, it is a negative reaction.

Penicillin Test

- If the test dose is given for penicillin observes the area for reactionary changes after 20 minutes to 1 hour.
- The area will be reddened the wheel will be increases in case of reactionary changes.
- If the patient is sensitive to penicillin, he may develop the signs and symptoms of anaphylactic shock within few minutes after the injection.

Mantoux Test

A test for immunity to tuberculosis using intradermal injection of tuberculin, it is also abbreviated as PPD test for purified protein derivative

Procedure (Table 9.6)

TABLE 9.6: Steps of procedure for intradermal injection administration.

Nursing action	Rationale
Check physicians order for medication administration and identify patient	Eliminates medication error
Explain procedure to patient, the purpose, the site of injection and how he has to cooperate	Explanation encourages cooperation and reduces apprehension
Wash hands	Reduces spread of microorganisms
Prepare medication from ampoule/vial.	
Wash hands and don gloves	Reduces spread of microorganisms
Assemble equipment at the bedside.	

Contd...

Contd...

Nursing action	Rationale
Position patient and locate site for intradermal injection (inner aspect of forearm, upper chest or upper back beneath scapulae).	Forearm is the most convenient and easily located and hence the commonly used site
Cleanse the site with alcohol swab in circular motion moving outward. Allow skin to dry. Keep cotton in the clean tray for reuse when taking out the needle.	Avoids introduction of pathogens into the tissues
Remove needle cap with the non-dominant hand by pulling it straight off	Reduces chances of contamination of needle
Use non-dominant hand to spread skin taut over injection site.	Taut skin provides an easy entrance into skin
Place needle almost flat against patient's skin and insert the needle into the skin so that the point of the needle can be seen through the skin. Insert needle only about 1/8 inch.	Needle position facilitates insertion into intradermal tissue
Slowly inject the drug (0.01–0.1 mL). Watch for a bleb/blister to develop. If not present, withdraw needle slightly and inject medication.	Appearance of a bleb/wheal indicates that needle is in intradermal tissue
Withdraw needle quickly in the same angle as it was inserted.	Reduces tissue damage and discomfort of patient
Do not massage the area.	Massaging the area will lead to spread of medication to subcutaneous tissue and false results may occur
Do not recap the needle after injection. Drop the needle after cutting, into the needle cutter. Drop the needle after cutting, into the needle cutter. Drop the syringe (piston and barrel) into the receptacle with bleach or red color bin as per agency policy.	Reduces risk of accidental puncture with needles
Assist patient to comfortable position.	
Remove gloves and wash hands	Reduces spread of microorganisms
Record medication administration-the medication administered, amount, dose, site and patient's response.	Reduces chances of medication errors
Draw a circle using blue/black pen around injection site. Write date and time of administration of medication and medication name on a piece of adhesive tape and stick near to the site. Check reaction within specified time period.	Helps in identifying exact site for checking reaction to medication

Aftercare

- Inspect the area but do no massage
- Help the patient to dress up
- Watch for the signs and symptoms of any allergic reaction
- Replace the equipment used for injection
- Clean all other articles and replace them in their proper place
- Wash hands
- Record the procedure on the nurse's record and drug sheet.

Special Considerations

- Ensure that the injection was given using the correct techniques which is evidenced by the appearance of tip of needle directly beneath the skin surface; resistance during injecting the medicine and formation of white wheal of 5–10 mm in diameter at the point of the contact of needle and skin.
- In case of test for patient allergy to dust, pollen, or similar substance, the reaction will take place after few minutes only
- In case of Mantoux test evaluation of whether the patient has been exposed tuberculosis, is done after 48–72 hours.

■ EQUIPMENTS

Syringe

Syringes are cylindrical barrels with plunger and tip for attaching needle it acts as a medium for storing and measuring required medications for administration.

Types of Syringes

- There are several types of syringes.
- **The most common are:**
  - The standard hypodermic syringe
  - The tuberculin syringes
  - The insulin syringe.
- Some syringes are made of glass and resterilised after each use.
- Plastic syringes are available in sterile, individual packets and are meant for disposal after one use.

Parts of Syringes (Fig. 9.12)

- Syringes have two parts:
  1. A Barrel
  2. A Plunger That Fits Insides
- The plunger has a wide, flat surface at the top called the flange, Only the flange portion of the plunger may be touched when preparing and giving an injection.

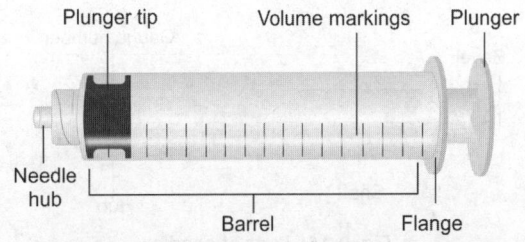

Fig. 9.12: Parts of syringe.

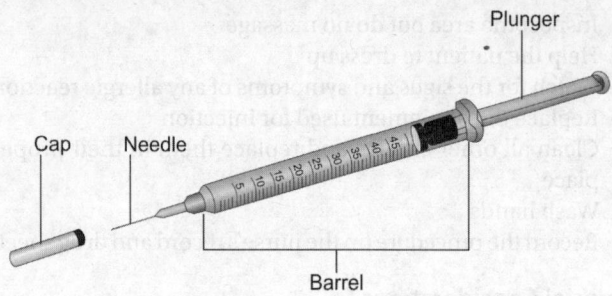

Fig. 9.13: Parts of tuberculin syringe.

- The barrel may be touched anywhere on the outside except the tip.
- The outside of the barrel contains markings in milliliters.
- The most commonly used sizes of hypodermic syringes for giving injections are the 2 mL and 5 mL size.
- 10 mL and 20 mL sizes are used in special cases.
- Tuberculin syringes have a small, slender barrel holding 1 mL (**Fig. 9.13**).
- It has markings to make it easy to give very small amounts of medication.
- An insulin syringe is the same size and shape of a tuberculin syringe, but with marking in units especially for insulin.

Needle

It a hollow solid tube which delivers/introduces the medication into the body.

Parts of Needles (Fig. 9.14)

- Have a hub, that fits on the tip of a syringe, and a long slender shaft.
- The shaft has a flat surface diagonally across the end called the bevel.
- The tip of the bevel is very sharp for piercing the skin. It should not be painful when inserted.
- There is an opening through the inside of the shaft through which medication goes into the tissues. It is called the lumen of the needle.
- Only the hub of the needle may be touched when preparing to give and injection.

Size of Needles (Table 9.7)

- The size of needles is according to the diameter of the lumen. Common sizes of needles are from 18–26 gauge, with the largest number being for the smallest size lumen.
- The gauge of the needle is selected according to the viscosity of the medication to be given. Some thick, oily preparations may require a 20- or 18-gauge needle.

TABLE 9.7: Size and specifications of needle.

Specification	ID (mm)	OD (mm)	Color	Size	Qty
14G	1.55	2.1	Olive	1/2"	12Pcs
15G	1.36	1.8	Amber	1/2"	12Pcs
18G	0.84	1.27	Green	1/2"	12Pcs
20G	0.6	0.92	Pink	1/2"	12Pcs
21G	0.51	0.82	Purple	1/2"	12Pcs
22G	0.41	0.72	Blue	1/2"	12Pcs
23G	0.34	0.64	Orange	1/2"	12Pcs
25G	0.26	0.52	Red	1/2"	12Pcs
27G	0.21	0.42	Clear	1/2"	12Pcs
30G	0.16	0.31	Lavender	1/2"	12Pcs

- Water-based preparations are given easily with a 22- or 25-gauge needle.
- The length of needles varies from 0.6–5 cm for most injections.
- The length of the needles selected is according to the site of the injection and the size of the patient.
- A very short needle (0.6 cm) is best for an intradermal injection.
- An intramuscular injection for an adult will require 3.5–5 cm needle, but for a baby, a 2.5 cm needle is sufficient.

IV Cannula

Cannula is a tube that can be inserted in body mainly to administer of remove fluid. IV cannula comes with trocar to puncture skin and vein in order to get into the intended vein (**Fig. 9.15**).

Indications of IV Cannula

- To administer long-term IV therapy; fluids, injections.
- Before surgery large bore cannula is inserted.
- For blood and blood product transfusion.
- For blood collection, when donating blood.

Gauge Size Color Code

Injection port caps are color coded for instant identification of cannula gauge size (**Table 9.8**).

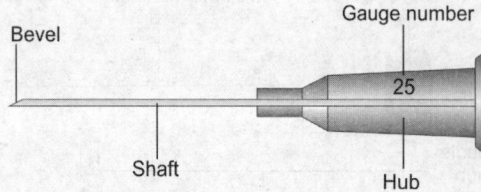

Fig. 9.14: Parts of needle.

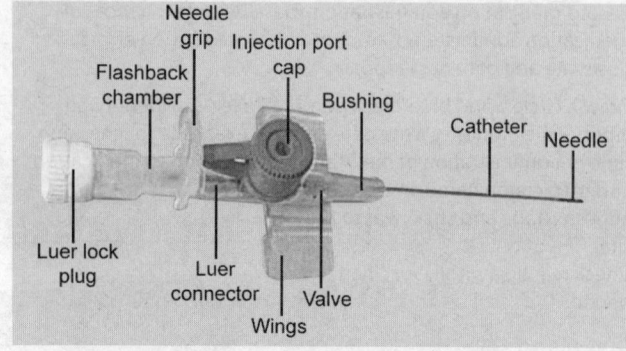

Fig. 9.15: Parts of intravenous cannula.

TALE 9.8: Color coding and gauge of cannulas.

Gauge	Color code	Ext. Dia. (mm)	Length (mm)	Flow rate (mL/min)
14G	Orange	2.1	45	240
16G	Gray	1.8	45	180
18G	Green	1.3	35/45	90
20G	Pink	1.1	32	60
22G	Blue	0.9	25	36
24G	Yellow	0.7	19	20
26G	Violet	0.6	19	13

Special Considerations

The size of cannula effects four factors:
1. Needle gauge
2. External diameter of cannula, i.e., its catheter
3. Length of catheter
4. Flow rate, i.e., mL/min

Securing of IV Cannula

- Dressing to peripheral intravenous (PIV) sites are the first line of defense against infections and must be kept secure clean and dry
- The type of secure dressing for the PIV cannula depends upon the child's age, condition of the skin, site of the IV, child's activity and/or mobility.
- Consider placing a small piece of cotton wool ball or gauze underneath the hub of the cannula to reduce pressure.
- Cover the cannula site with sterile transparent or semi-permeable occlusive dressing (e.g., Tegaderm, IV 3000) placed aseptically over the catheter.
- If desired, place sterile tape over the hub and wings of the device before placing the transparent dressing.
- IV board/splints are recommended to secure PIV cannula placed in or adjacent to areas of flexion. This will adequately immobilize the joint and minimize the risk of venous damage resulting from flexion:
  - When using splints, ensure these are positioned and strapped with the limb and digits in a neutral position to prevent restricting blood or nerve supply and pressure sores.
  - Inspect the splint at least daily and change, if soiled by blood or fluid leakage.
- Cover with gauze or non-compression tubular bandage:
  - When using non compression tubular bandage (e.g., Tubifast), ensure there is a clear window where the cannula enters the skin so the site can be viewed.
  - It is secure.
  - The site is visible.
  - The child can't injure himself/herself on the connections.
  - The child can't remove or dislodge the cannula.
  - That tapes are not too tight
- Change the dressing only if it becomes insecure or if there is blood or fluid leakage.

Changing Cannulas

Re-cannulation should be avoided where possible, as this will cause the child and family further distress. There is no limit to the length of time that a cannula may remain in situ and with appropriate care, several days may be possible. Cannulas only need to be replaced when there is accidental dislodgment, occlusion, phlebitis and infection.

Removal of IVs

The possible reasons for removal of cannula includes:
- Infiltration,
- Extravasations
- No longer be required
- No longer be functioning effectively
- It may be causing the child excessive discomfort,
- Signs of phlebitis or infection.

Steps

- Perform hand hygiene, wearing non-sterile gloves, carefully remove the dressing, holding the cannula in place at all times.
- Hold a piece of sterile gauze or cotton wool over the exit site but do not apply pressure.
- Slowly withdraw the cannula, maintaining a neutral angle with the child's skin.
- Cover site with cotton wool and tape or band-aid.
- Advise the child and family that the cotton wool and tape or band-aid should remain in situ for 24 hours.
- Document date and reason of removal.

Prevention of Infections

- Good hand hygiene before Peripheral Intravenous (PIV) catheter insertion and maintenance, combined with proper aseptic technique during catheter manipulation provides protection against infection.
- Prior to accessing PIV cannula, clean with an approved antiseptic wipe.
- All children with a capped PIV access device in situ should have the site inspected at commencement of shift and least every six hours for signs of infusion phlebitis.
- Where children are receiving continuous IV fluids/medication, site should be inspected hourly and documented on the fluid balance chart for the duration

Documentation

Any complications:
- Record the date and time of the infusion when extravasation was noted, the type and size of catheter, the drug administered, the estimated amount of extravasated solution and the administration technique used.
- Record the patient's signs and symptoms, treatment and response to treatment. Include the time you notified the patient's primary care provider and the primary care provider's name.

INFUSION SET

- Intravenous fluids are administered through thin, flexible plastic tubing called an intravenous infusion set.
- Intravenous infusion sets are used for the controlled infusion of medications, typically over long periods of time.
- IV sets are used to connect the medication to the needle inserted into the patient. IV extension sets are also used to extend IV lines without risk of contamination.

Principle of Intravenous Set

- The intravenous infusion set operates on the action of gravity. When the IV bottle/bag is fixed at a higher position in comparison to that of the patient level, the gravitational force pulls down the fluid. Thus, the fluid flows into the veins of the patients.
- The rate of flow of fluids is controlled with the help of the roller clamp. Generally, when the clamp is moved upward, the tube will open. Similarly, by rolling the clamp downward, the internal diameter of the tubing can be narrowed. Thus, by rolling the clamp to a suitable position, the rate of flow of fluid can be controlled.

Parts of Intravenous Set (Fig. 9.16)

- **Spike:** Spike allows the flow of fluid from the reservoir bag/bottle to the drip chamber. It is a hollow device and has a dual-channel with a sharp tapering cannula, located at the proximal end of the IV set, ensuring a safe seal between the IV line and the fluid container. Spike should be able to pierce the bottle stopper of the infusion bag or bottle, and it should not produce debris.
- **Solution filter:** The filter is used to filter out the particles in the liquid and protect the patient from the infection caused by the particles. The filtration rate of latex particles by the filter should not be less than 90%.
- **Drip chamber:** The drip chamber is located just below the IV bag. Inside the drip chamber, we can see the fluid, drip down into the IV tube. The drip chamber must always be half full. If the drip chamber is too full, we will not be able

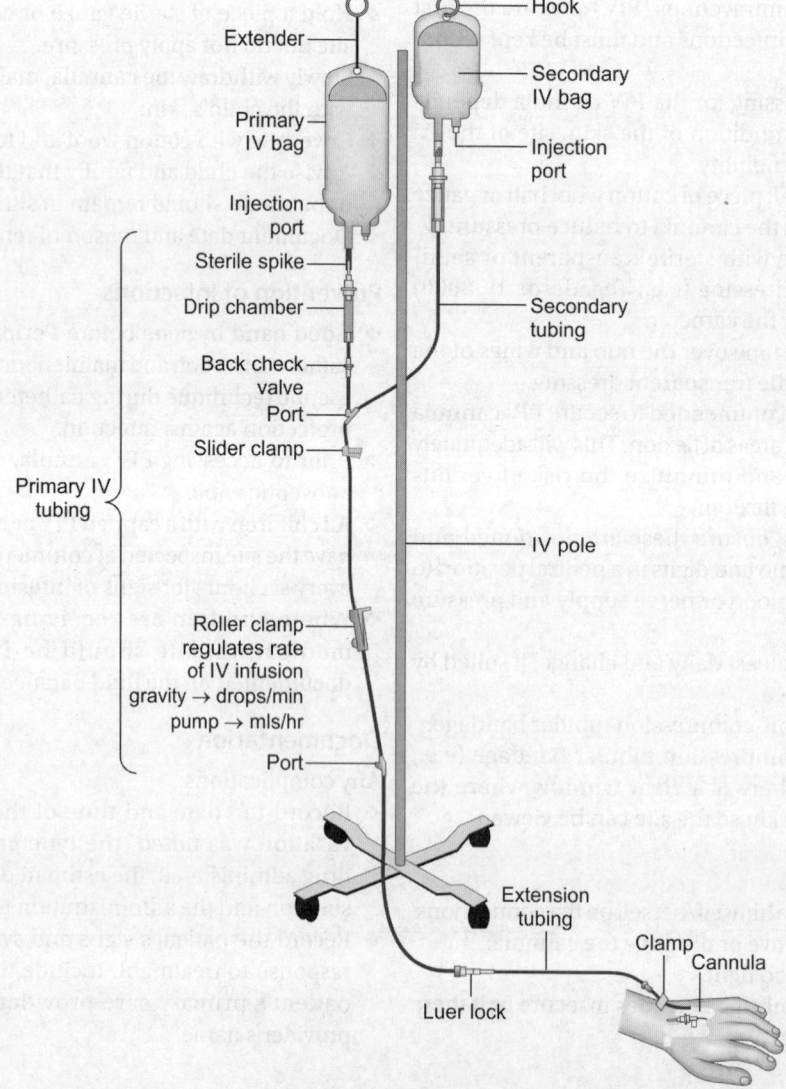

Fig. 9.16: Parts of intravenous set.

to see the drops to count them. By counting the number of drops per minute, the rate of flow can be measured.
- ❖ **Roller clamp (regulator):** It is a small wheel between the drip-counting chamber and the IV connector. The roller clamp use to control the rate at which the IV fluid infuses. It also allows the fluid to stop whenever required.
- ❖ **Tubing:** Allows the fluid to travel from the reservoir bag to the patient. The tube is transparent so that when the air bubbles pass through the infusion, the interface between water and air can be easily and clearly distinguished with normal vision.
- ❖ **Cap:** Cap prevents microbes and foreign particulate matter from entering the infusion. One of the safety practice recommendations includes covering IV tubing's exposed end with a sterile cap between uses in intermittent infusions.
- ❖ **Luer connector:** This connects to the IV cannula. The Luer taper is a standardized system for making leak-free connections.

Piggyback Infusion

It is a small IV bag or bottle (25–250 mL) connected to short tubing lines these lines to the upper Y port of a primary infusion line. The piggyback tubing is a micro drip or macro drip system. This set is called piggyback because the small bag is set higher than the primary infusion bag. In the piggy back set up, the main line does not infuse when the piggybacked medication is infusing. The port of the primary IV line contains a back check valve that automatically stops the flow of primary infusion when the piggyback infusion starts. After that the piggyback solution infuses and the solution within the tube falls below the level of primary infusion drip chamber, the back check valve opens and the flow of primary infusion starts again.

Tandem

It is a setup of a small IV bag or bottle, i.e., 25 mL to 100 mL, connected to the short tubing line to the lower Y port of a primary infusion line. The tandem set is placed at the same height as the primary infusion bag. In the tandem, the main line infuse simultaneously, the nurse monitors the tandem sets closely. But if the tandem set is not clamped immediately, the IV solution from the primary line will back up into the tandem line.

Volume Controlled Administration

These are small sets containers, i.e., 50–150 mL that attach just below the primary infusion bag. The set is attached and filled in a manner similar to that used with a regular IV infusion. The primary filling of the set depends upon the type of filter used within the set.

Mini Infusion Pump

It is a battery-operated pump and allows the medication to be given in a small amount of fluid within the controlled infusion times using standard syringes.

Intravenous Tubing Calibration

The size of a drop in an IV setup depends upon the width of the IV tubing thinner tubing produces smaller drops and wider tubing produces larger ones. IV tubing is pretty standard, and so there are two major categories of IV tubing:
1. **Macro drip:** Macro drip tubing is wider and so produces larger drops. The macro drip tube is suitable for normal applications and is most commonly used for routine IV administration, such as infusion of IV fluids without any medication. Macro drip tubing comes in 3 sizes: 10 gtt/mL, 15 gtt/mL, and 20 gtt/mL.
2. **Micro drip:** Micro drip tubing is narrower and so produces smaller drops. It is used for children and infants, or to infuse sensitive medications where precision in the flow rate is essential. Micro drip tubing comes in only one size: 60 gtt/mL. This implies that 60 drops of liquid make a total volume of 1 mL.

■ TYPES OF VIALS AND AMPOULES

Parenteral medications are available in prepacked sterile solutions in ampoule or vial containers.

Parenteral medications for intramuscular or intravenous use are most frequently supplied in ampoules and vials.

Ampoule
- ❖ Ampoule is a small vial that is sealed after filling and used chiefly as a container for a hypodermic injection solution.
- ❖ Ampules are small glass containers containing liquid medication ranging from 1 mL to 10 mL sizes that hold a single dose of medication.
- ❖ Ampoules are usually made of glass.
- ❖ The neck of an ampoule is sealed using an open flame in order to prevent contamination.
- ❖ This leads to an airtight obstruction for prevention of air, moisture and water from contaminating the liquid inside the ampoule.
- ❖ **Each ampoule is provided with two parts:** The upper portion (stem) and lower portion (base) in between these two contractions is present (from where) it can be cut and opened with filer.
- ❖ These glass ampoules are designed as single dose containers because once an ampoule has been opened, there is no way to pressure the medication for future use.

Mechanisms for Breaking Ampoule
- ❖ Mechanisms for breaking ampoule have been developed in an attempt to decrease percutaneous injuries and contamination of contents.
- ❖ They have a scored neck to indicate where to break the ampoule.

There are two types of breaking systems, such as rupture disk (VIBRAC) and OPC (One-Point Cut Ampoules) with optimized opening forces.

VIBRAC (Fig. 9.17)
- ❖ It is the most common system. This mechanism can be found in 85% of ampoules.

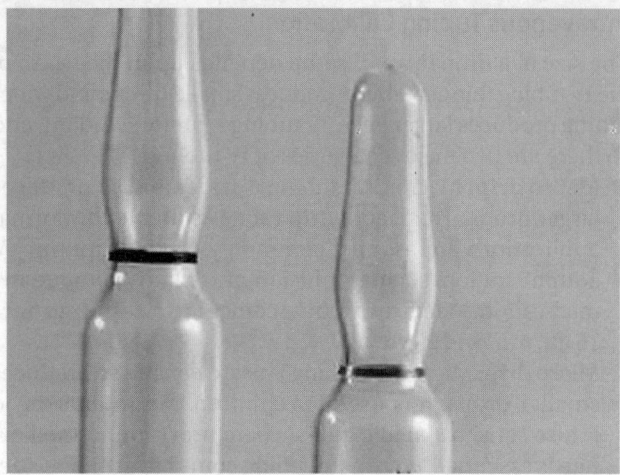

Fig. 9.17: Rupture disk (VIBRAC) in ampules.

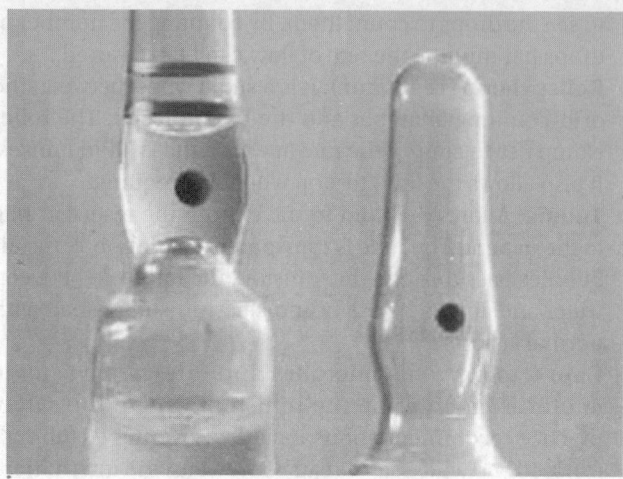

Fig. 9.18: OPC in ampules.

- It implies applying a ring of paint after the cure/tempera process of ampoule manufacture.
- It partially penetrates in the glass, causing fragility of the area of application.
- This fragility is located at the strangulation point of the ampoule (between the head and body of the ampoule).

OPC (Fig. 9.18)

- In this system, a small incision is made in the strangulation area of the ampoule.
- A small point of paint is placed few millimeters above the incision.
- This point orients the correct opening position.
- Because there is risk of being cut by glass when opening a glass ampoule, the nurse should use an ampoule breaker or wrap an alcohol swab package around the neck of the ampule for protection **(Fig. 9.19)**.

Vials

- A vial is a small multi-dose container, cylindrical, usually made of glass or plastic and may or may not be sealed.
- It may be shaped like a tube or bottle and have a flat bottom so that it can be rested on a flat surface.

- Vial, in the form of container possesses a screw on cap or a rubber plug.
- Vials are typically used to store medicines or laboratory samples.
- The vials are single or multiple dosage dispensing container.
- The solution in the vials are protected with a soft metal cap which can be removed before the medication is taken from the vial.
- The rubber seal, which is the route of entrance into the vial, remains intact to protect the sterility of succeeding doses, providing principles of aseptic technique are used in withdrawing each dose.

Vial Materials

Vials are available in different material, such as glass, plastic and silicone.

Glass Vials (Fig. 9.20)

- Glass is the ideal material to store delicate medicines and injectable products.
- Glass keeps medicines and formulas safe from environmental factors like light and moisture and allows a long shelf life.

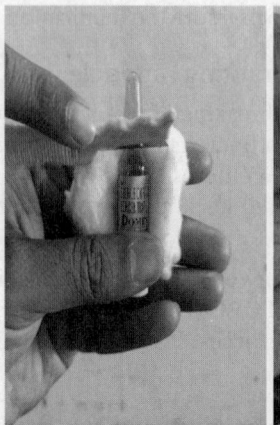 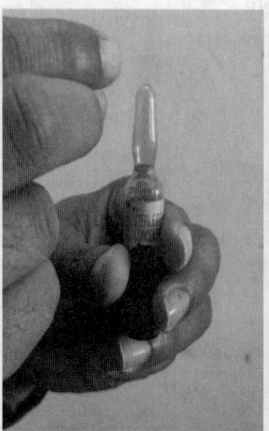 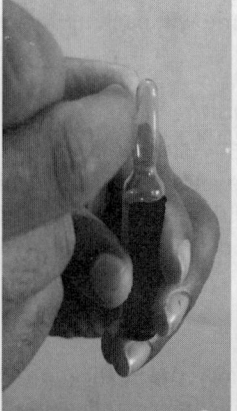 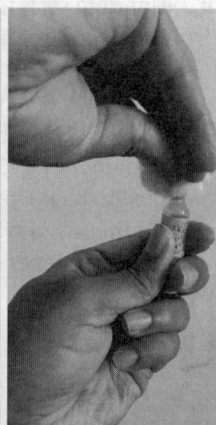

Fig. 9.19: Process of breaking the ampule.

Chapter 9: Administration of Medications

fluids from sticking to the internal surface of the vial and increases transparency
* Siliconization can be used to treat amber, borosilicate or soda-lime glass vials and bottles.

Vial Inserts
* Vial inserts enable maximum sample retrieval and make it easier to remove the contents of a vial.
* Inserts offer a solution when there is a limited sample amount.

Inserts are typically available in borosilicate glass or polypropylene, and they come in various shapes. Common insert styles include:

Conical (Fig. 9.22)
Conical inserts feature a tapered bottom and may come with shock-absorbing springs.

Flat (Fig. 9.23)
* Flat inserts have a flat bottom and cylindrical shape.
* They have the greatest capacity and might be the most economical choice.

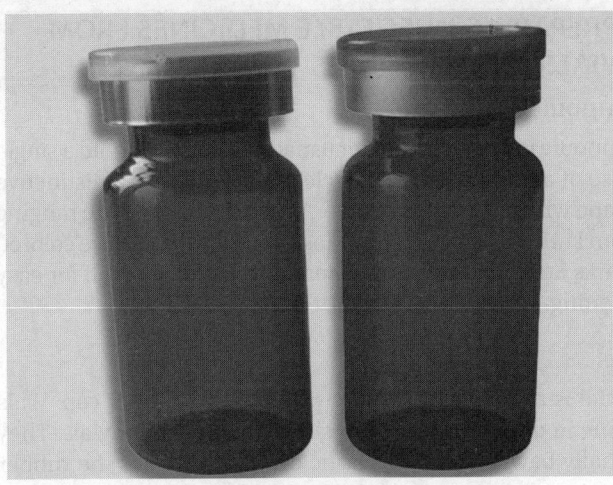

Fig. 9.20: Glass vials.

* Vials may be made of soda-lime glass, the most common and least expensive type of glass, or borosilicate glass.
* There are many benefits of glass vials; clarity, inertness, heat resistance, nonporous surface and recyclable material.

Plastic Vials (Fig. 9.21)
* Plastic vials are typically made of polypropylene or polyethylene.
* Polypropylene is a rigid material that may be translucent or pigmented.
* It is valued for its flexibility and excellent resistance to impact.
* Both of these plastics are used in a vast range of applications, including and pharmaceutical uses.
* Benefits of plastic vials include—chemical resistance, high melting point, durable, light weight and affordable.

Silicone Vials
* Some glass vials undergo a process called siliconization.
* Siliconization involves applying a silicone solution to the surface of the glass to create a protective layer.
* The benefits of silicone vials include: minimal interaction between the sample and the vial, prevents high viscosity

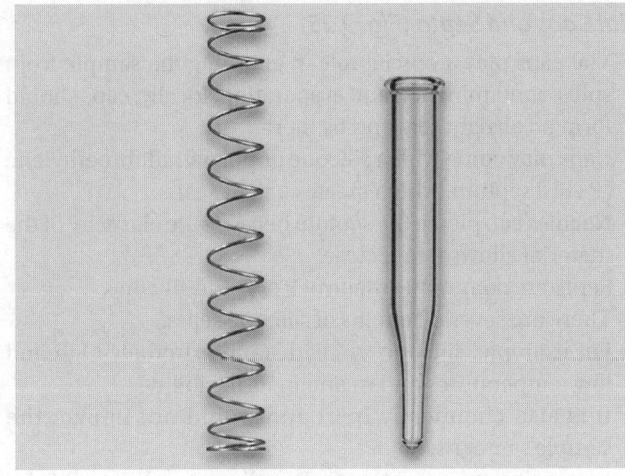

Fig. 9.22: Conical vial inserts with spring.

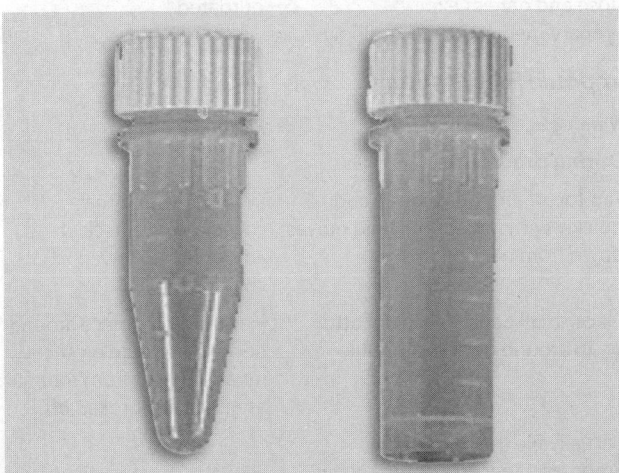

Fig. 9.21: Plastic vials.

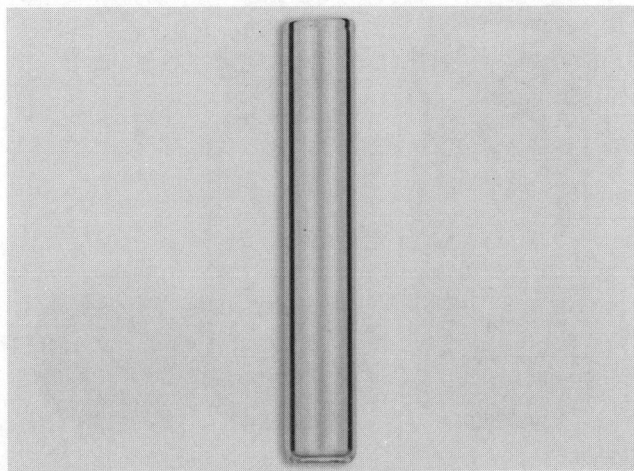

Fig. 9.23: Flat vial insert.

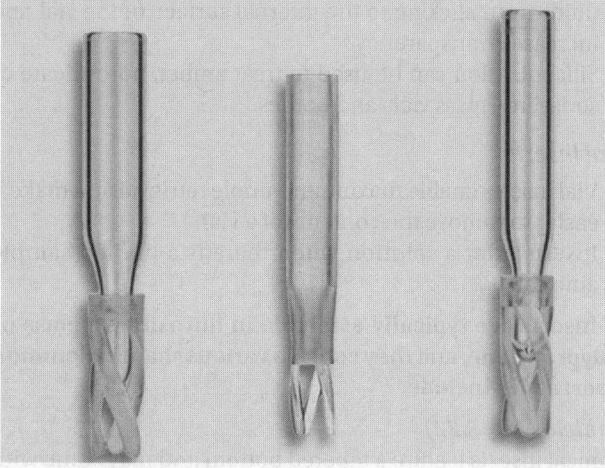

Fig. 9.24: Mandrel vial insert.

Mandrel (Fig. 9.24)
- Mandrel inserts have precise tips to reduce the insert's residual volume.
- It might use when require maximum recovery of a sample.

Vial Caps and Septa (Fig. 9.25)
- Vial caps play a crucial role in guarding the sample from spills, contamination and evaporation. Ideally, caps should form an airtight seal and be inert.
- Caps may come with a silicone or polytetrafluoroethylene (PTFE) septum, which creates a tight seal.
- Needles can pierce the septum because the elasticity of the material allows it to reclose.
- Septa are commonly made of PTFE and silicone.
- There are several benefits of silicone septa.
- For example, silicone can withstand extremely high and low temperatures and maintain its flexibility.
- It is also chemically inert and would not impact the sample's integrity.
- Lastly, silicone is resistant to UV radiation and is suitable for various sterilization methods, including steam autoclaving.

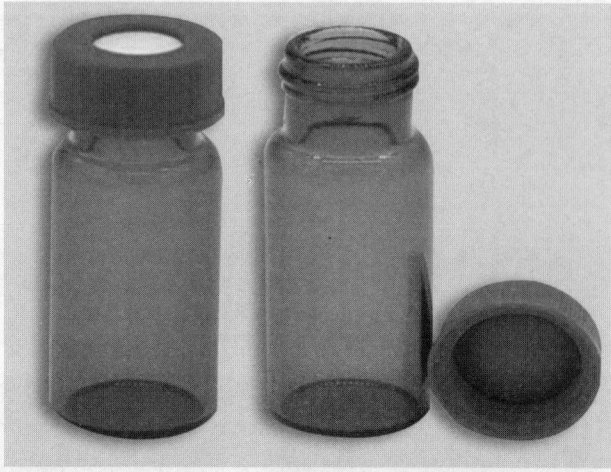

Fig. 9.25: Vial caps and septa.

PREPARING INJECTABLE MEDICINES FROM VIALS AND AMPOULES

Ampoule
Ampoule is a glass container usually designed to hold a single dose of a drug. It is made of clear glass and has a distinctive shape with a constrictive neck Ampoules vary in size ranging from I mL to 10 mL or more. Most ampoule necks have colored marks around it indicates where they are pre scored for easy opening.

Vial
A vial is a small glass bottle with a sealed rubber cap. Vials come in different sizes from single to multi-dose vials. They usually have a metal or plastic cap that protects the rubber seal.

Articles
- Medication in an ampoule or vial.
- Syringe, needle.
- Small gauze piece.
- File.
- Medication chart/medication card.
- Kidney tray.
- Alcohol swabs.

Procedure
Refer **Tables 9.9 and 9.10**.

TABLE 9.9: Steps of procedure for preparing injectables medications from vials and ampoules.

Nursing action	Rationale
During procedure	
Check patient's name and medication order, including medication name, dose and route of administration	Ensures correct administration of medication
Perform hand washing and assemble equipment	Reduces transmission of microorganisms
Check medication order and check label for the name of medication, dose and date of expiry Prepare medication accordingly	Medication potency may increase or decrease when outdated

Ampoule Preparation

Nursing action	Rationale
During procedure	
Tap top of ampoule lightly and quickly with finger until fluid moves down from neck of ampoule	Drains any fluid that collects above neck of ampoule into lower chamber
Place small gauze piece or cotton swab around neck of ampoule	Placing gauze piece around neck of ampoule protects nurse's fingers from trauma as glass tip is broken off
Partially file the neck of the ampoule, if necessary, for a clean break	

Contd...

Contd...

Nursing action	Rationale
Snap neck of ampoule quickly and firmly away from hands	Protects nurse's fingers and face from shattering glass
Place the ampoule on a flat surface Insert needle into centre of ampoule opening. Do not allow needle tip or shaft to touch rim of ampoule	Broken rim of ampoule is considered contaminated
Aspirate medication into syringe by gently pulling back on plunger	Withdrawal of plunger creates negative pressure within syringe barrel, which pulls fluid into syringe
Keep needle tip under surface of liquid. Tilt ampoule to bring all fluid within reach of the needle	Prevents aspiration of air bubbles
If air bubbles are aspirated, do not expel air into ampoule	Air pressure may force fluid out of ampoule and medication will be lost
Expel excess air bubbles: Remove needle from ampoule. Hold syringe with needle pointing up Tap side of syringe to cause bubbles to rise toward needle. Draw back slightly on plunger and then push plunger upward to eject air. Do not eject fluid	Withdrawing plunger too far will remove it from barrel. Holding syringe vertically allows fluid to settle in bottom of barrel. Pulling back on plunger allows fluid within needle to enter barrel so fluid is not expelled
If syringe contains excess fluid, use kidney tray for disposal. Hold syringe vertically with needle tip up and slanted slightly toward kidney tray Slowly eject excess fluid into kidney tray. Recheck fluid level in syringe by holding it vertically at eye level	Medication is safely dispersed into kidney tray. Position of needle allows medication to be expelled without flowing down needle shaft. Rechecking fluid level ensures proper dose
Cover needle with its safety sheath or cap. Replace the needle with another needle for injection	Prevents contamination of needle. The outer surface of the needle may be coated with medication which may cause tissue irritation, if used for injection

Preparation from Vial

Nursing action	Rationale
Prepare the medication vial for withdrawing drug. Mix the solution, if necessary, by rotating the vial between the palms of the hands, not by shaking	Some vials contain aqueous suspensions, which settle when they stand in some instances, shaking is contraindicated because it may cause the mixture to foam
Remove cap covering top of unused vial to expose sterile rubber seal in a multi-dose vial which has been used before, cap is already removed. Firmly and briskly wipe surface of rubber seal in a circular motion with alcohol swab and allow it to dry	Seals must be swabbed with alcohol before preparing medication Allowing alcohol to dry prevents needle from being coated with alcohol and mixing with medication

Contd...

Contd...

Nursing action	Rationale
Pick up syringe and remove needle cap Pull back on plunger to draw amount of air into syringe equivalent to volume of medication to be aspirated from vial	Air must be injected into vial to prevent build-up of negative pressure in vial when aspirating medication
With vial on flat surface, insert tip of needle with beveled tip entering first through centre of rubber seal. Apply pressure to tip of needle during insertion	Center of seal is thinner and easier to penetrate. Injecting bevelled tip first and using firm pressure prevents cutting of rubber seal which could enter vial or needle
Inject air into the vial keeping the bevel of the needle above the surface of the medication	The air will allow the medication to be drawn out easily because negative pressure will not be created inside the vial. Avoids creating bubbles in the medication
Invert vial while keeping firm hold on syringe and plunger. Hold vial between thumb and middle fingers of non-dominant hand. Grasp end of syringe barrel and plunger with thumb and forefinger of dominant hand to counteract pressure in vial	Inverting vial allows fluid to settle in lower half of container. Position of hands prevents forceful movement of plunger and permits easy manipulation of syringe
Keep tip of needle below fluid level	Prevents aspiration of air
Allow air pressure from the vial to fill syringe gradually with medication. If necessary, pull back slightly on plunger to obtain correct amount of solution	Positive pressure within vial forces fluid into syringe
When desired volume has been obtained, position needle into vial's air space, tap sides of syringe barrel carefully to dislodge any air bubbles	
Remove needle from vial by pulling back on barrel of syringe taking care not to pull the plunger	Accidentally pulling plunger rather than barrel causes plunger to separate from barrel, resulting in loss of medication
Hold syringe at eye level at 90° angle to ensure correct volume and absence of air bubbles. Remove any air bubbles if present Draw back slightly on plunger, then push plunger upward to eject air. Do not eject fluid Recheck volume of medication	Holding syringe vertically allows fluid to settle in bottom of barrel. Pulling back on plunger allows fluid within needle to enter barrel so fluid is not expelled. Air at top of barrel and within needle is then expelled
Change needle to appropriate gauge and length according to route of medication.	Inserting needle through a rubber stopper may dull bevelled tip. New needles are sharper and will not track medication through tissues
For multi-dose vial, make label that includes date of mixing. concentration of medication per millilitres, and nurse's initials.	Ensures that future doses will be prepared correctly.

Vial Containing a Powder (Reconstituting Medications)

TABLE 9.10: Steps of procedure for vial containing a powder (reconstituting medications).

Nursing action	Rationale
Remove cap covering vial of powdered medication and cap covering vial/ampoule of proper diluent. Firmly swab both seals with alcohol swab and allow it to dry	Maintains sterility and allows alcohol to dry
Withdraw an equivalent amount of air from the vial before adding the solvent unless otherwise indicated in the directions by the manufacturers	Reduces pressure inside the vial when injecting the diluent
Draw up diluent into syringe from vial or ampoule	Prepares diluent for injection into vial containing powdered medication
Insert tip of needle through centre of rubber seal of vial containing powdered medication. Inject diluent into vial. Remove needle	Diluent begins to dissolve and reconstitutes medication
Mix medication thoroughly by rolling in palms. Do not shake	Ensures proper dispersal of medication throughout the solution Shaking produces bubbles
Reconstituted medication in vial is ready to be drawn into new syringe. Read label carefully to determine dose after reconstitution	Once diluent has been added, concentration of medication determines dose to be given
Clean work area and perform hand washing	Controls transmission of infection

CARE OF EQUIPMENT: DECONTAMINATION AND DISPOSAL OF SYRINGES, NEEDLES, INFUSION SETS

Sharp Collection

- Sharps should be collected in puncture-resistant sharps containers with 1% sodium hypochlorite solution.
- Before discarding the needles, the tip of needle should be burned or destroyed with the help of needle tip burner or destroyer.
- Disposable sharps containers are made of cardboard or plastic, reusable sharps containers are made of plastic or metal.
- Low-cost options include clearly marked reuse of plastic bottles or metal cans.

Handling Sharps Containers

- Check all sides for any holes or protruding needles before lifting the container
- Place the needles carefully in a puncture-resistant container.
- Sharps containers should only be filled up full.
- Do not recap needles or bend the needle.
- Always destroy sharps
- Never pass used sharps from one person to another.
- Locate needle destroyer near point of generation to facilitate disposal of sharp waste.

Collection of Syringes and IV Infusion

- The syringes are collected separately into thick plastic bag with sign of biohazard.
- IV infusions sets are cut with scissors and collected in red bin.

Waste Treatment

- Syringes are disinfected either by chemical disinfection, autoclaving, or microwaving.
- Disinfected syringes can be shredded and re-melted.
- Encapsulation—concrete vault filled 3/4th with sharps and the remaining space filled with cement or Sharps placed in drums, sealed in cement, and then buried in landfills.

Sharps Handling Recommendations: Sharps Waste Management

- Devices for needle destruction are called as needle melters
- Needle is melted and often the plastic hub of the syringe is cut.
- These could be electrical or battery-operated.
- Syringes still need to be disinfected.
- **Needle cutters:** Needle is cut manually and collected in a container.
- Some needle containers may contain a chemical disinfectant.

PREVENTION OF NEEDLESTICK INJURIES

- Needlestick injuries (NSIs) are defined as percutaneous injuries with sharp objects contaminated with blood or other body fluids.
- Needlestick injuries are one of the most serious occupational accidents among nurses due to the possible severe consequences, such as the transmission of infectious diseases and inducing of mental impairment.
- Needlestick injuries are a hazard for people who work with syringes and other needle equipment
- These injuries can occur at any time when people use, disassemble, or dispose of needles.
- When not disposed of properly, needles can hide in linen or garbage and injure other workers who encounter them unexpectedly.
- Needlestick injuries are caused by sharps, such as hypodermic needles, blood collection needles, IV cannulas or needles used to connect parts of IV delivery system.

Activities with Potential for Needlestick Injuries

Home healthcare workers can be at risk for needlestick or sharps injuries when they:

- Handle needles that must be taken apart or manipulated after use.

- Dispose of needles attached to tubing.
- Manipulate the needle in the client.
- Recap a needle.
- Use needles or glass equipment to transfer body fluid between containers.
- Fail to dispose of used needles in puncture-resistant sharps containers.
- Lack proper workstations for procedures using sharps.
- Work quickly.
- Bump into a needle, a sharp, or another worker while either person is holding a sharp article

Prevention

- Avoid recapping or bending needles that might be contaminated.
- Recapping needles has led to the transmission of infection.
- If possible, always use devices with safety features (safety shield) and engage the needle's safety system.
- If absolutely necessary, use the scoop method of recapping.
- Dispose of the needle immediately after injection. Immediately dispose of used needles in a sharp's disposal container (puncture-proof and leak-proof) to avoid unsafe disposal of a sharp.
- Healthcare workers should cover open skin areas or lesions on hands and arms with a dry dressing at all times.
- Hand hygiene is still essential, so consultation is necessary if the dressing interferes with this procedure.
- Reduce or eliminate all hazards related to needles. Avoid using needles, if possible.
- Use a needle only when performing an SC, ID, or IM injection.
- Use of new, single-use disposable injection equipment for injections is highly recommended.
- Sterilizable injection should only be considered if single-use equipment is not available
- Needle-free systems should be used to access intravascular devices.
- The device must be easy to use and require little change of technique on the part of the health professional
- Avoid the use of needles where safe and effective alternatives are available.
- Evaluate devices with safety features that reduce the risk of needlestick injury.
- Report all needlestick and sharps-related injuries promptly to ensure that you receive appropriate follow up care.
- Remember that latex gloves do not protect you against needlestick injuries.
- Do not bend or snap used needles.
- Never re-cap a used needle.
- Provide training on injury prevention strategies, adequate information and discussion on blood-borne disease and their modes of transmission and the use of PPE.
- Wear gloves when cleaning equipment prior to sterilization or disinfection, when handling chemical disinfectant and when cleaning up spillages.

Needlestick Injury Management

If anyone experience a needlestick or sharps injury or are exposed to the blood or other body fluid of a patient during the course of work, immediately follow these steps:
- Wash needlesticks and cuts with soap and water.
- Flush splashes to the nose, mouth, or skin with water.
- Irrigate eyes with clean water, saline, or sterile irrigants
- Report the incident to supervisor.
- Reporting any injury from an accidental needlestick not only helps get the right kind of care, it helps shape guidelines for future needle handling so other people stay safe, too.
- Immediately seek medical treatment at the nearest ER or treatment facility.
- **Get immunization shots:** Some vaccine shots, like those for hepatitis B, diphtheria, and tetanus, help your body's immune system kick in and protect from those infections.
- **Post-exposure prophylaxis:** Antiretroviral drugs don't kill viruses. But a short course of these HIV medications, taken within 72 hours of exposure to the virus, may keep it from taking hold in body.

The Needlestick Safety and Prevention Act

- As part of the Needlestick Safety and Prevention Act passed into law in November 2000, new provisions of the blood borne pathogens standard took effect July 17, 2001.
- The revised provision specifies the types of engineering controls, such as safer medical devices, in the health care setting and adds new requirements for employers. Employers must:
  - Review their exposure control plans annually to reflect changes in technology that will help eliminate or reduce exposure to blood borne pathogens.
  - Involve non-managerial workers in evaluating and selecting, safety engineered devices.
  - Maintain a sharps injury log that ensures employee privacy and contains, at a minimum, the type and brand of device involved in the incident, if known; the location of the incident; and a description of the incident.

Safe Injection Practices as per Universal Safety Precaution

- Proper hand hygiene.
- Use personal protective equipment.
- Avoid the use of needles where safe and effective alternatives are available.
- Avoid recapping needles.
- Plan for safe handling and disposal before beginning of any procedure using needles.
- Dispose of used needles promptly in appropriate puncture proof sharps disposal containers.
- Use devices with safety features.
- Report all NSI/sharps-related injuries and blood exposure promptly to ensure that you receive appropriate follow up care.
- Tell the hospital about hazards from needles that you observe in your work environment.

- Participate in blood-borne pathogen training.
- Follow recommended infection prevention practices, including hepatitis B vaccination.
- Regard all waste soiled with blood/body substances as contaminated and dispose off according to relevant standards.

TOPICAL ADMINISTRATION

- In topical administration, the medications are applied directly to the body surfaces, including the skin and mucous membranes of the eyes, ears, nose, vagina, and rectum.
- Topical medication are usually available as creams, ointments, gels, lotions sprays, powders, aerosols, liniments, and drops.
- The topical medication generally provides a local effect but can also cause systemic effects.
- The rate and degree of the drug's absorption at determined by the vascularity of the area.
- Topical drugs are usually given to provide continuous absorption to produce different effects to relieve pruritus (aching), to protect the skin, to prevent or treat an infection, to provide local anesthesia, or to create a systemic effect.
- Medications that can be administered via a topical route include antibiotics, narcotics, hormones, and even chemotherapeutics.

Types of Topical Medications

Ointments
Ointments are mixtures of various fats that can be easily spread. They are made of fat, oil or wax or a combination of these. These semi-solid mixtures tend to be greasy and sticky. but they are incredibly effective in skin defence because they produce a barrier against environmental influences.

Pastes
Pastes are special ointments that contain fat as well as a large amount of powder additives. Pastes are ointment-like type of form where drugs and other solid substances (e.g., zinc oxide) are mixed together with an adhesive fatty base (e.g., petroleum jelly). Pastes are semi-solid preparations intended for topical application affected areas of the skin. Usually they are thick (contain 25% of solids by weight) and do not melt at normal temperature. Remain on the area for longer duration than ointments and are therefore generally more effective.

Lotions
Lotions are liquid forms, which are applied to the skin to protect, cool, cleanse, act as emollient and even provide antipruritic treatment. Most formulations contain oil and water with an emulsifier, like alcohol, to make the active medical ingredients soluble.

Creams
Creams are topical mixtures that contain water and oil. Oil in water creams spread easily, and are not as greasy, while water in oil creams are slightly greasier with a lower melting point, meaning they absorb more rapidly and can better penetrate the outer layer of the skin. Creams always contain emulsifiers that add viscosity. They may also, in some cases, contain preservatives.

Gels
Gels are a special type of water-based cream. Gels are usually relatively transparent, being made from cellulose ethers mixed into a mixture of water and alcohol. They turn into a liquid almost the instant they come into contact with skin, leaving a faint film of medication on the surface after the bulk of the formula evaporates. Most gels contain alcohol or similar ingredients that evaporate faster than water, this makes them a bit drying, but also improves convenience by leaving no greasy or sticky coating after application.

Powders
Powders are sprinkled on the skin and stick there. Powders are essentially the same drugs found in pills and capsules, they are just crushed into a powder form and/or mixed into a carrier, like corn starch. Medicated talcum powder, for example, is a common treatment for athlete's foot.

Tinctures
Tinctures are topical medications in liquid form. They are made by dissolving or diluting dried extracts, often of plant material. Alcohol is commonly used as a solvent. One well-known example is tincture of iodine, which is used for disinfecting wounds.

Transdermal Patches (Fig. 9.26)
Transdermal patches have an adhesive base. Patch is applied to the certain areas of the body, such as the upper arm, stomach, thigh, or lower back for particular period of time that allow the skin to absorb small amounts of medication over the course of several hours or days.

Purposes
- Used to nourish the skin and protect it from harm
- To deliver directly onto the area that are inflamed, irritated or infected
- Used for local treatment
- Used to treat pain or other problems in specific parts of the body

Advantages of Topical Administration
- Alternative to oral administration
- Useful for local delivery of medication

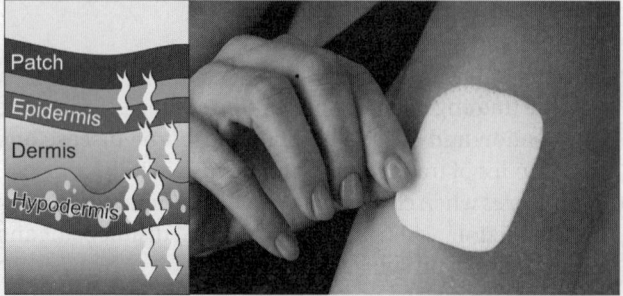

Fig. 9.26: Transdermal patch.

- Target affected area for rapid treatment and relief
- Used for most dermatologic and ophthalmologic preparations
- Avoidance of first pass metabolism
- Easy to apply and convenient to use
- Fewer risk of gastrointestinal difficulties
- Easy termination of medications when needed
- Suitable for self-medication.

Disadvantages of Topical Administration

- Possibility of local skin irritation at the site of application
- Some drugs are not absorbed easily through the skin
- Possibility of an allergic reaction
- Application site must be monitored for reactions
- Effectiveness may be impacted by temperature, humidity, and other environmental factors
- Contact dermatitis due to some drug and/or excipients may occur
- Can be used only for those drugs which require low plasma concentration for action.

APPLICATION TO SKIN AND MUCOUS MEMBRANE

- Medications are given topically through the skin and absorbed because of the skin's relatively rich blood supply.
- Because skin thickness and blood flow to the skin vary with age, the potential for toxic effects of the drug must be considered
- Children have a larger body surface area and thinner layer of cutaneous and subcutaneous tissue than adults, so there is an increased risk for systemic absorption and effects through topical application.
- Drugs applied to the skin must overcome the phospholipid barrier created by the squamous epithelium of the skin surface.
- The speed of absorption of the drug depends on the size of the epithelium and on the transfer through the stratum corneum.
- Dermatological medications (applied to the skin) can also be applied to the nose, ears and rectum.
- Resorption of the drug through the mucosa is similar to absorption through the skin, with the difference that the mucosal epithelium does not contain a calloused layer. Therefore, the permeability of a drug through the mucosa is considerably higher.

Purpose

Dermatological medications are administered for the purpose of moisturizing and softening the skin, relieving itching, increasing or decreasing skin secretion, creating a protective coating on the skin, creating local vasoconstriction or vasodilatation, etc.

Application

They are applied to the skin in the form of ointments, pastes, creams, foams, solutions, gels, transdermal therapeutic plasters, etc.

Equipment

- Prescribed medication
- Nonsterile gloves
- Washcloth
- Basin of warm water
- Gauze (if needed)
- **Appropriate applicator:** Wooden spatula, cotton swab, tongue depressor, or other
- Sterile dressing (if needed)

Preparation of the Patient

- Inform the patient of the type of medicament applied, the reason of its use and the application procedure. Inform the patient about the effects of the administered drug
- Assess the skin integrity before administration of topical medication. Observe for cleanliness and clean off dirt and excess lotions as needed.
- Assess the condition of the skin, noting areas of healing, excoriation, edema, rashes, or increased redness.
- Instruct the patient not to scratch the areas where the drug was applied.
- Assess for drug allergy and inform the patient of the need to report any side-effects (e.g., burning, redness, severe itching, etc.)
- Inform the patient of the need to avoid sunlight during treatment, e.g., in tar preparation treatment.
- Provide appropriate privacy during the procedure.

Procedure

- **Verify the order with the medical record, including:**
  - Calculation of appropriate dose
  - *Check for allergy to drug:* If present, do not administer drug and notify the doctor.
- Obtain the ordered topical medication and read the label to verify with the order.
- Check for expiration date; if expired, do not administer.
- Use topical medication at room temperature unless specified.
- Perform hand hygiene and Don gloves to reduce transmission of microorganisms. Using gloves protects health care provider from contact with medication.
- Cleanse the skin, as ordered or per reference manual recommendations, before application of the medication.
- **Use a basin of warm water and a washcloth only:** If an open wound is present, use gauze instead of a washcloth. Dry skin well after washing.
- Apply topical medication to the site. Use the correct amount as ordered and administration technique for the type of topical medication. An excessive amount of medication may result in irritation of the skin and adverse systemic effects.
- Instruct the patient that initial application may feel cold. Apply medication using long even strokes that follow the direction of the hair. Do not rub vigorously.
- Wrap the hand of the patient in gauze if topical medicines are applied to skin on the hands to prevent the patient

from accidentally rubbing the medicine into their eyes or mouth If ordered, cover the affected site with the prescribed dressing. A covering prevents the medication from being rubbed off, protecting clothing and site
- Remove the gloves and perform hand hygiene to prevent transmission of microorganisms. All changes in the skin are recorded during the course of treatment. Any changes are immediately reported to a doctor.

After Care
- Assess the patient's response after applying the dermatological medication
- Help the patient to get dressed
- Assess the patient's response after the expected time of drug onset
- All used aids are disposed of in the designated waste bins.
- Instruments are placed into the prepared disinfectant solution.
- Ensure safe disposal of disposable and biological materials.
- Record the procedure

■ DIRECT APPLICATION OF LIQUIDS

Gargle
- Washing out of throat with a stream of solution.
- Gargling is the act of bubbling liquid in the mouth.
- It is also the washing of one's mouth and throat with a liquid, such as mouthwash, that is kept in motion by breathing through it with a gurgling sound.
- Gargle helps clear out bacteria from parts of mouth that cannot reach during brushing or flossing.
- It can also help prevent upper respiratory infections.

Salt Water Gargle
- Salt water gargles help reduce the inflammation and pain of sore throats and mouth ulcers.
- It helps stop bacteria growth, prevents upper respiratory infections and dislodges food particles.
- Make this home remedy by combining ½ teaspoon of salt to 1 cup of warm water.

Purposes
- To soften and remove discharges
- To relieve pain and swelling
- To apply heat.

Advantages
- Help with sore throats, colds, and mouth ulcers.
- Reduce throat inflammation and clearing nasal passageways.
- Help relieve throat pain and irritation by reducing inflammation.
- Prevent the growth of harmful bacteria in mouth
- Prevent upper respiratory tract infections
- Less abrasive or irritating to the mucosal lining of the throat
- One of the best ways to disinfect oral wounds, especially after having dental surgery, because it works as an antiseptic and it inhibits bacterial growth.

Solutions Used
- Normal Saline
- Potassium permanganate—1:5000–1:6000
- Sodium bicarbonate.

Procedures
- Prepare a solution in drinking glass at the temperature tolerated by the patient and go to the bedside.
- Instruct the patient to hold solution as far back in throat as possible.
- Gargle a few seconds and put into kidney tray.
- Repeat until whole glass is used.

Swabbing the Throat (Painting of Throat)
- Swabbing or painting the throat is the application of medication through spraying and painting to the throat.
- **The medicines are applied for the following reasons:**
  - To relieve pain, inflammation and congestion,
  - To treat infection
  - To anesthetize the part.

Purposes
- To relieve pain, swelling and congestion
- To anesthetize the part.

Articles
In a tray containing:
- Tongue depressor
- Applicators
- Kidney tray
- Head mirror
- Towel
- Mask
- Medication

Procedures
- Explain the procedure to the patient
- Take all equipment to the bedside
- Ask patient to sit on a chair comfortably
- Wear mask if required
- Adjust light
- Take the medication on the applicator.
- Instruct the patient to open the mouth
- Depress tongue with the tongue depressor and paint tonsil, pillar or pharynx.
- Avoid painting any other part of the mouth or throat, except the necessary area.
- Touch gently and quickly
- Remove mask and wash hand thoroughly
- Record the procedure on the chart.

■ INSERTION OF DRUG INTO BODY CAVITY

Rectal Suppositories
- Suppositories are cone-shaped or bullet-shaped medication which are gelatine or glycerine based solid at room temperature and melts at body temperature **(Fig. 9.27)**.
- These are used to create local or systemic effects in the body.

Chapter 9: Administration of Medications

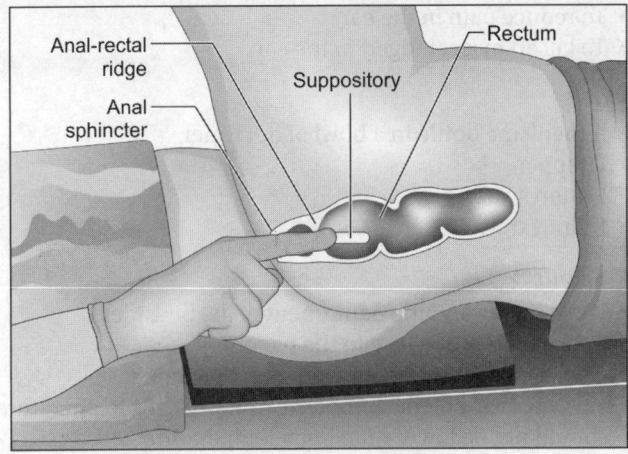

Fig. 9.27: Insertion of rectal suppository.

Purpose
To create localized effects and treat infections or inflammation.

Equipment
- Medication (rectal suppository)
- Lubricant jelly
- Gauze pieces
- Gloves
- Kidney tray

Advantages
- Avoid first pass metabolism
- Suitable for formulations with unpleasant taste
- Beneficial for patients suffering from severe nausea and vomiting. Can be administered to unconscious patients
- Allows achieving rapid systemic effects by giving a drug
- The absorption rate of the drug is not influenced by food or gastric emptying.
- Preferred route when drugs are administered to relieve constipation or hemorrhoids.

Disadvantages
- Inconvenient and embracing
- Absorption is slow and irregular
- Defecation may interrupt the absorption process
- Chances of rectal mucosal irritation
- Placement too high into rectum may lead to first pass metabolism
- It is possible the degradation of certain drugs by microorganisms in the rectum

Procedure
Refer **Table 9.11**.

Vaginal Medication/Suppositories
These are cone shaped medicated tablets that are inserted in the vagina for producing systemic or local effects.

Advantages
- Allows for the administration of lower doses. Avoid first pass metabolism

TABLE 9.11: Steps of procedure for rectal suppository insertion.

Nursing action	Rationale
Review medication orders and confirm the identification of the patient. Gather equipment	To reduce error during medication administration
Drape the patient exposing only the anal area	To provide privacy to patient and avoid unnecessary exposure
Provide side-lying/sim's position with upper leg flexed upward	Facilitate proper insertion of suppository
Wash hands and Don gloves	To prevent cross infection and maintain sterility during procedure
Lubricate both the index finger (of dominant hand) with suppository	Reduce friction and facilitate easy insertion
Educate the patient to take deep breath and relax anal sphincter	Cause difficulty while inserting suppository
Retract patient's buttocks and gently insert suppository with gloved index finger	Facilitate proper absorption and therapeutic action
After insertion of suppository, wipe off patient's anal area	Provide patient's comfort and prevent soiling
Ask the patient to remain in supine position	To prevent expulsion of suppository
Provide bed pan or assist patient to reach toilet	If laxative actions are caused by suppository
Remove gloves, dispose off articles in proper receptacle. Wash hands. Document the procedure. Provide comfortable position to the patient	To prevent cross infection

- Self-administration of drugs
- Does not cause nausea and vomiting due to gastric irritation in case of oral therapy.
- Beneficial for patients suffering from severe vomiting
- Can be administered to unconscious patients. Drug absorbed systemically, because due to the presence of dense network of blood vessels in vaginal wall

Disadvantages
- Inconvenient and embracing
- Chances of vaginal mucosal irritation
- Unwanted ejection of the rings used to administer the drug
- Potential local infections. Only a few drugs are administered
- Influence with sexual intercourse

Equipment
A medication tray containing:
- Vaginal suppository/vaginal cream
- Lubricant
- Gauze pieces
- Gloves
- Perineal pad

Procedure
Suppository (Table 9.12).

TABLE 9.12: Steps of procedure for vaginal suppository insertion.

Nursing action	Rationale
1. Review the medication order and confirm the identity of patient	To reduce error during medication administration
2. Gather all the equipment and explain the procedure to the patients	It reduces patient's anxiety
3. Give dorsal recumbent position and drape the patient exposing only genital area	Facilitates proper insertion of suppository to prevent unnecessary exposure
4. Wash hands and don gloves	It reduces transmission of microorganisms
5. Lubricate both the suppository and index finger of gloved hand (of dominant hand)	Reduce friction and facilitate easy insertion
6. Retract labial fold (with non-dominant gloved hand) and insert the suppository	Facilitate proper absorption
7. Clean the orifice and labia with gauze piece	To prevent sorting and provides comfort

Vaginal Cream (Table 9.13)

TABLE 9.13: Steps of procedure for vaginal cream application.

Nursing action	Rationale
1. Fill the applicator and insert into vagina	For proper insertion
2. Instruct the patient to lie in supine position for 10–15 minutes	To prevent expulsion of suppository
3. Offer perineal pad to the patient	To prevent soiling of bed sheet
4. Remove gloves and dispose off articles	
5. Wash hands. Document the procedure	
6. Provide comfortable position to the patient	

INSTILLATIONS—EAR, EYE, NASAL, BLADDER AND RECTAL

Instillation of Ear Drops
Definition
"Instillation of ear drops into the auditory canal for local effects."
- Sterile solutions are used for instillation as the administration of non-sterile solutions causes infections.
- The internal ear is sensitive to extreme temperatures, it may cause vertigo or nausea in the patient.

Purposes
- To soften the ear wax
- To reduce infection
- To reduce pain in the ear
- To kill an insect lodged in the ear.

Articles
- A medicine bottle in a bowl of hot water
- Dropper
- Cotton swabs
- Kidney tray.

Procedures
- Wash hands and the equipment of the bedside
- Explain the procedure to the patient
- Give dorsal recumbent position to the patient.
- Take medicine in the dropper, test on wrist, the temperature should not be lower than body temperature
- Straighten the auditory canal by pulling the pinna upward and backward in case of adults. Downward and backward in case of children
- Instill medication drop by drop on the side wall of the canal to allow the air to escape from the auditory canal
- Ask patient to remain in this position for few minutes
- Plug the ear with a cotton swab
- Record the medication on the chart.

Instillation of Eye Drops
Definition
"Eye drop instillation is the dispensation of a sterile ophthalmic medication into a patient's eye."

Purposes
- To dilate pupils and paralyze the ciliary muscles
- To contract the pupil
- To apply medication to the eye for local effects
- To relieve inflammation and infection of the eyes
- To produce local anesthesia prior to operation.

Articles
- Eyedrops according to the physician's order.
- Sterile eyedropper
- Sterile eye swabs in a sterile container
- Kidney tray or paper bag.

Procedures
- Wash hands and collect the required articles and keep it to the bedside locker
- Put on mask
- Explain the procedure to the patient and relatives
- Ask patient to tilt head slightly backward and a little to the side of the affected eye. Separate the lids gently, drawing lower lid and ask the patient to look up
- Take drops in the dropper. Hold the dropper from 1–3 cm, above the eye
- Instill the ordered number of drops in the centre of the lower lid
- Release lid. Ask the patient to close the eyelids and move the eyeballs from side so that medication will spread all over the conjunctival sac
- Wipe off the excess medications
- Record the medication on the temperature chart.

Complications
- Irritation in some patients that might result in eye redness of burning
- **Stronger medications can cause more extreme allergic symptoms, such as:**
  - Dizziness
  - Disorientation.
- **Some cycloplegic drops can cause such severe reactions as:**
  - Delirium
  - A rapid pulse
  - Difficulty in swallowing

Application of the Eye Ointment
Purpose
To relieve inflammation of the conjunctiva, lids and the cornea.

Articles
- Eye ointment tube
- Eye swabs

Procedures
- Explain the procedure to the patient
- Wash hands thoroughly and take articles to the bedside locker of the patient
- Clean the lids with eye swabs
- Pull down lower lid with left hand thumb and ask patient to look up
- Press ointment from the tube laying it gently on the mucous membrane of the lower lid. (Apply the ointment from inner aspect to the lateral aspect)
- Ask the patient to close the eye and move the eyeball around so that eyeball will be covered with the ointment.
- Record treatment on the temperature chart.

Instillation of Nasal Drops
Purposes
- To relieve inflammation, pain, swelling and congestion
- To arrest hemorrhage
- To give local anesthesia
- To diagnose nasal conditions.

General Instructions
- It is a clean procedure.
- Avoid touching the tip of nose with dropper since it may contaminate
- Avoid touching the inner surface of the nose with dropper since it may cause the patient to sneeze
- Position the patient as necessary to provide medicine flow to the affected area
- Do not use oily solution as nasal drops since it interferes with the normal ciliary's action.
- Do not use decongestant excessively or frequently as they become ineffective and may actually worsen the patient's nasal congestion
- Instruct the patient remain in the same position for some time following instillation to allow the medicine to act on mucous membrane of anterior nares and then drain into the posterior nares.

Articles
- Medicine dropper
- Medication as ordered.
- Cotton swabs
- Kidney tray

Procedures
- Wash hands and collect the articles and take it to the bedside.
- Explain the procedure to the patient
- Give comfortable position to the patient
- Take medication in the dropper and instill not more than 3 drops into each nostril
- Keep patient in the same position for 5 minutes and avoid blowing the nose
- Give handkerchief or cotton swabs to wipe
- Give sputum mug to spit any medication that have reached the mouth and throat.

Aftercare
- Place the patient in comfortable position
- Replace the articles
- Hand wash
- Record the procedure in the nurse's record.

Instillation of Bladder
- Bladder instillation is also known as bladder baths or bladder washes.
- Bladder instillation is the treatment used for painful conditions, e.g., interstitial cystitis, a chronic disorder of bladder which may be inflammation of bladder wall.
- In this procedure the bladder is filled with solution which the patient holds for some time (few seconds to 15 minutes).
- Then the bladder is drained with catheter.
- The drugs mainly used for bladder instillation are:
  - Dimethyl sulfoxide
  - Heparin
  - Sodium hyaluronate

Purposes
- To reduce inflammation and infection in urinary bladder
- To relieve pain, discomfort and irritation.

Articles
- Double lumen Foley's catheter in place in the patient
- A small tray containing:
  - Sterile syringe (asepto syringe or 50 mL syringe) in a sterile bowl containing medicine as ordered
  - Antiseptic swabs in a sterile bowl
  - Sterile gloves
  - Clean container.

Procedures
- Put on clean gloves, and clean the opening of free end of catheter

- Fill the syringe with medicine solution and attach to the catheter. Instill slowly into the bladder. Plug the catheter
- Allow the medicine to remain in bladder for the prescribed time. Remove plug from catheter to drain the bladder and collect the drainage in the clean container
- Place the patient in comfortable position
- Remove, clean, boil, dry and replace the supplies
- Wash your hands.
- **Recording:**
  - Date
  - time medicine dose (amount)
  - Duration for the medication remained in the bladder
  - Patient's reaction

Rectal Instillation

- In rectal administration, rectum is used as a route drug administration for medications, semisolid preparations and liquids.
- This route is used as an alternative for the patients with digestive tract mobility problems such as dysphagia or bowel obstruction.

Forms of Rectal Administration

Rectal semisolids: Rectal cream, gels and ointments- these are used topically to the perianal area for insertion within the anal canal. They largely are used in the treatment of local conditions such as anorectal pruritus, inflammation and pain associated with hemorrhoids.

Rectal liquids:
- Rectal suspensions, emulsions and solutions. Solutions, suspensions or retention enemas represent rectal dosage forms with very limited application, largely due to inconvenience of use and poor patient compliance.
- These formulations are utilized to administer contrast media and imaging agents for cancer GI visualization.
- **This dosage forms are mainly used as enemas:**
  - *Retention enema:* For systemic or local effect.
  - *Evacuation enema:* For cleansing of bowel.

Rectal aerosols:
- **Rectal aerosols or foams:** Rectal aerosols foams products are also accompanied by applicators to facilitate administration.
- The applicator is attached to the container and filled with a measured dose of product.
- Metered dose aerosols are available. In this, inserter is inserted into the anus and the plunger is pushed to deliver the drug product.

Advantages

Useful for:
- Pediatric geriatric or unconscious patient.
- The drugs causing severe nausea and vomiting in oral administration can be used.
- When oral intake is restricted.

Disadvantages

- Inconvenient for patients.
- The absorption of drugs is frequently irregular and difficult to predict.

Procedure

Refer **Table 9.14**.

TABLE 9.14: Steps of procedure for rectal instillation.

Nursing action	Rationale
Review medication orders and confirm the identification of the patient. Gather equipment	To reduce error during medication administration
Drape the patient exposing only the anal area	To provide privacy to patient and avoid unnecessary exposure
Provide side-lying/sim's position with upper leg flexed upward	Facilitate proper insertion of suppository
Wash hands and don gloves	To prevent cross infection and maintain sterility during procedure
Lubricate both the index finger (of dominant hand) with suppository	Reduce friction and facilitate easy insertion
Educate the patient to take deep breath and relax anal sphincter	Cause difficulty while inserting suppository
Retract patient's buttocks and gently insert suppository with gloved index finger	Facilitate proper absorption and therapeutic action
After insertion of suppository, wipe off patient's anal area	Provide patient's comfort and prevent soiling
Ask the patient to remain in supine position	To prevent expulsion of suppository
Provide bed pan or assist patient to reach toilet	If laxative actions are caused by suppository
Remove gloves, dispose off articles in proper receptacle	To prevent cross infection
Wash hands	
Provide comfortable position to the patient	
Document the procedure	

IRRIGATIONS—EYE, EAR, NASAL, RECTAL AND BLADDER

Eye Irrigation

Eye irrigation is the washing of the conjunctival sac by a stream of liquid.

Purposes

- To cleanse the eye of foreign matter, chemical or discharge
- To reduces inflammation and congestion
- To prepare for ophthalmic surgery
- To reduce infection
- To apply medications
- To apply heat or cold to the eye.

Articles

- Sterile undine with irrigation solution
- Sterile solution in a jug
- In a covered sterile tray eye swab, eye pads, eye bandage
- Sterile wet swabs in container

- Kidney tray and paper bag
- Mackintosh and draw sheet
- Eye ointment or eye drops.

Solutions Used
- **Plain water:** To clean the eye
- **Normal saline:** To clean the eye
- **Boric acid 2%:** As an antiseptic
- **Silver Nitrate 1%:** As an antiseptic
- **Acriflavin 1%:** As an antiseptic
- **Mercurochrome 1%:** As an antiseptic.

Temperature of the Solution
It should be about 98–100°F. in order not to injure the conjunctiva.

General Instructions
- Main aseptic technique throughout the procedure to prevent introduction of infection into the eye.
- Use all sterile articles and solutions for eye irrigation.
- Wash your hands thoroughly before and after the procedure.
- Irrigate least infected eye first and then another eye or use separate equipment and solution for each eye to prevent cross infection.
- Clean the eyelids to remove any particles of dust or secretions adhering to the lashes.
- Separate the eyelids very gently using the thumb and four fingers of the left hand, so that fluid will reach all parts of the conjunctiva. While separating the eyelids, the pressure should be on the cheek and eyebrows and not on the eyeball.
- Never touch eye with an undine.
- Keep the pressure as low as possible in order to secure a steady flow of solution to avoid the injury to the eye.
- Test the temperature of the solution at the inner surface of the wrist to avoid injury to the eye.
- The flow of the fluid should be from inner canthus to the outer canthus. It will prevent the infection into the nasolacrimal duct.
- Medications should be instilled immediately after the eye irrigation.

Procedures
- Explain the procedure to the patient to win his confidence and get the cooperation.
- Keep the patient in a supine position. His head should be slightly turned to the side to be irrigated.
- Use Mackintosh and draw sheet to protect bed linen.
- Wash hands to prevent cross infection.
- Take equipment to the bedside.
- Place kidney tray to catch flow of solution. Patient may help hold tightly to cheek, if able.
- Clean the eyelids and eyelashes from the inner to outer corner of the eye by using wet swabs.
- Irrigate the eye using the solution which is at body temperature.
- Ask the patient to close the eyes and allow a small amount of fluid to run over the lid.
- Separate the lids gently by using thumb and fore-finger and irrigate eye. Have patient to look up.
- Holding undine quite close to the eye about 10 cm above eye. Continue irrigation until the eye is clear of discharge.
- Ask the patient to look up while irrigating the part of the lower lid and to look down while the inner part of the upper lid is irrigated.
- Repeat the procedure on the other side if required, using separate equipments and solution.

Aftercare
- Dry lids with dry cotton swabs
- Dry cheeks if needed after irrigation
- Observe the eyes for effect of the irrigation
- No pus should remain after the irrigation, if it is irrigation for inflammatory conditions
- Instill the eyedrops or ointment according to order. Apply dressing if it is ordered
- Make the patient comfortable
- Remove articles from bedside
- Clean it, dry and replace to their usual places.
- Wash hands

Recording, Reporting
- Record the procedure on the temperature chart and on the nurse's record with date and time and sign.
- Record the solution used, temperature of the solution, condition of the eye before and after the irrigation, medications instilled, etc.
- Record any abnormality to the ward sister and physician.

Ear Irrigation
Ear irrigation is the washing of the external auditory canal with a continuous return flow.

Purposes
- To clean
- To remove foreign body or wax
- To relieve inflammation, congestion and pain
- To apply heat.

Articles
- Sterile ear syringe in a bowl
- Solution in a pint major
- Swabs, swab stick and ear forceps in a container
- Ear medications according to order
- Mackintosh and draw sheet
- Kidney tray and paper bag
- Head mirror.

Solutions Used
- Sodium bicarbonate—1%
- Normal saline—0.9%
- Boric acid—2–4%
- Hydrogen peroxide—2%
- Plain water.

Temperature of the Solution
It should be about 90–100°F.

General Instructions

- Explain the procedure to the patient to win his confidence and get the cooperation.
- Prepare the solution at 105°F. So that it will be close to the body temperature at the time of irrigation and will not stimulate the semicircular canals and cause giddiness, vomiting, etc.
- Hold the pinna of the ear upward and backward in case of adults, and in children pull it downwards and backward to straighten the external auditory canal.
- Obtain written order from doctor for irrigation.
- While irrigating the ear, direct the stream of solution against the wall of the external auditory canal and never against tympanic membrane to prevent injury to the ear drum because it will cause deafness.
- Watch the patient for vertigo, if this occurs stop the procedure immediately.

Procedures

- Explain the procedure to the patient.
- Examine the ear for any perforation of the ear drum.
- Wash hands and take articles to the bedside.
- Protect patient and bed with Mackintosh and towel.
- Give dorsal recumbent position to patient with head near edge of the bed, slightly to affected side. Ask patient to hold kidney tray under ear to collect return flow.
- Cleanse pinna of the ear and external auditory canal with the cotton applicators.
- Test the temperature of the solution on the inner aspect of the wrist.
- Irrigate the ear using ear syringe. In adults, hold ear upward and backward, take firm but gentle hold of the cartilaginous portion of the auricle.
- Place the tip of the syringe at the opening of the canal, but do not block the ear canal.
- Direct slow even stream into the ear using low pressure.
- When thoroughly cleansed, stop the procedure.

Aftercare

- Turn the patient on the affected side, for the drainage from the ear.
- Plug the ear with cotton swabs to collect the drainage.
- Dry the skin around the ear, and instill the medications according to order.
- Remove Mackintosh and towel, collect all articles and make the patient comfortable.
- Clean the articles with soap and water, dry and keep ready for next use.
- Ask for any giddiness or discomfort to the patient.
- Wash hands.

Recording, Reporting

- Record the procedure on the temperature chart and on the nurse's record with date and time and sign.
- Record the type of solution used, effect to treatment.
- Record any untoward reaction to the patient and report it or doctor and ward sister.

Nasal Irrigation

Nasal irrigation is not done now-a-days.

Vaginal Irrigation

It means washing out the vagina with a liquid at low pressure.

Purposes

- To clean the vaginal canal
- To relieve congestion, inflammation, and pain in vaginal tissues
- To treat vaginal infection
- To prepare the patient for vaginal surgery
- To stop bleeding.

Articles

- **A tray containing:**
  - Irrigation can with tubing, clamp and douche nozzle
  - Jug with irrigating solution
  - Lubricant and medicine
  - Sterile gloves-one pair
  - Sponge holding forceps and vaginal speculum
  - Wet swabs in a bowl containing Dettol 2%
  - Dry swabs in a bowl and cotton applicators
  - Protective sheet and towel
  - Bath sheet, dress and linen as required
  - Kidney tray and paper bag.
- Bedpan.

Procedures

- Explain the procedure to the patient enlist her cooperation.
- Take supplies to the bedside.
- Ask the patient to void.
- Arrange the screen and the irrigation stand near the patient.
- Arrange to provide adequate light.
- Replace the top clothes with bath sheet and fanfold top clothes to the foot end of bed.
- Remove the bottom dress or raise it above the waist level, drape the patient as for any gynaecological examination and expose only the perineum.
- Place bedpan under the patient and position, her in the modified dorsal recumbent position. Hips are kept higher than the shoulders by placing a pillow under the back.
- Wash your hands.
- Pour solution into the can, unclamp the tubing to allow little solution to run through the tubing to expel the air from tubing and re-clamp.
- Hang the can on the irrigation stand and adjust the height not more than 12 inches/30 cm from the level of the patient's hips.
- Put on sterile gloves.
- Clean the patient's perineum with Dettol swabs using sponge holding forceps. Start cleaning from the outer edges of labia in smooth downward strokes. Use each swab once discard.
- Connect douche nozzle to the tubing and lubricate the nozzle with water-soluble lubricant.
- Allow some solution to flow over the vulva and regulate the flow of the solution with the help of screw clamp.

- Separate the patient's labia with thumb and forefinger of your left hand and gently insert the nozzle into the vagina about 2 inches/5 cm angling it upward and then downward toward the patient's back.
- Unclamp the tubing and allow the solution to flow into the vagina in a steady stream.
- Gently rotate the nozzle during irrigation.
- Continue to irrigate until the desired effect is achieved.
- Clamp the tubing, gently remove the douche nozzle, disconnect it and place in the kidney tray.
- Help the patient to sitting position on the bedpan for a few minutes to completely drain the solution from the vagina.
- Remove bedpan, turn the patient to one side and dry the perineum and buttocks.
- If medication is ordered, insert the vaginal speculum to visualize the cervix, apply medicine with the help of cotton applicator and apply a perineal pad to prevent medicine stains on the patient's dress.
- Remove gloves.
- Remove protective sheet and towel.
- Change patient's dress and linen as necessary. Remake the bed and make the patient comfortable.
- Remove supplies, discard those which need so. Empty the bedpan and clean as usual, rinse douche nozzle in cold water first, then in warm soapy solution rinse again, boil or disinfect. Clean other supplies dry and replace.
- Wash hands thoroughly.

Recording

Record in the nurse's notes:
- Date and time of the procedure
- Amount and type of vaginal discharge present, if any
- Type and amount of solution used and character of return flow
- Patient's reaction to procedure.

Guidelines

- Doctor's order is required for the procedure.
- Never give douche during menstruation, pregnancy and puerperium to prevent spread of infection to uterus.
- Follow clean technique but wear sterile gloves. Use sterile technique when indicated.
- Observe through hand washing before and after the procedure to prevent cross infection.
- Remove and destroy the patients pads carefully.
- Douche nozzle has holes on the side to minimize the risk of solution passing through the cervical to the uterus.
- Examine douche nozzle for any cracks to prevent injury to vaginal wall.
- When irrigating, rotate the douche nozzle to ensure through flushing of vaginal canal but never rotate, if the patient is with recent vaginal surgery or cervical cancer.
- Have the solution at 100–105°F/38–40.5°C for most of the irrigations and higher in case of congestion, inflammation and bleeding unless otherwise specified.
- Do not elevate the irrigating can more than twelve inches above the patients' buttocks to regulate the pressure of solution flowing and vice versa (sitting position) when solution is out-flowing.
- Check the patient's perineum for lesions as lesions such as excoriation are painful when comes in contact with the solution. So, consult the doctor before proceeding.
- **Following solution are used for vaginal irrigation:**
  - Distilled water
  - Normal saline
  - Sodium bicarbonate 2%
  - Savlon 1:1000
  - Dettol 2%
  - Acetic acid 1%
  - Potassium permanganate 1:4000
  - Boric acid 2%
  - Acriflavine 1:4000.

Bladder Irrigation

It is dealt in unit 5 (elimination need)

Rectal Irrigation

Rectal irrigation is the treatment of washing out of the rectum with large quantities of solution in order to clean the bowel.

Purposes

- To empty the bowel of feces, gas, excess mucus, barium.
- To dilute and remove any toxic agent.
- To apply medications.
- To prepare the colon for diagnostic aids and surgery.

Articles Required

- Irrigation kit (irrigation bag with clamp and tubing)
- Water soluble lubricant
- IV pole (or another suspending hook)
- Soap and water
- Waste receptacle
- Wash cloth and towel
- Prescribed irrigating solution, usually 500–1000 cc warm (100–105°F) tap water
- Glass connection
- Disposable gloves/apron
- Rubber sheet
- Towel

Procedure

- Explain the procedure to the patient.
- Bring all the articles near the bedside.
- Ensure privacy for the procedure.
- Wash and dry hands thoroughly.
- Apply disposable gloves.
- Place the patient on the left side with knees bent, the upper leg higher than the lower.
- Place the rubber sheet and towel under the buttocks.
- Expose the required area.
- Keep the bucket on a low stool to receive the outflow of fluid.
- Fill the irrigation bag with the prescribed solution and hang it on the IV pole or hook.
- The bottom of the bag should be placed 18–20 inches above the bed.
- Open the clamp on the irrigation tubing and allow the solution to fill the tubing. Re-clamp.

- Lubricate the catheter with Vaseline.
- Ask the patient to be easy and take deep breath by mouth.
- Insert the rubber catheter 7–10 cm into the rectum, open the stop-cock and allow the fluid to flow slowly.
- Remove the connection and allow the return flow in the bucket.
- Reconnect and repeat the steps.
- Continue the procedure until all the fluid ordered has been given or until the return flow is clear.

Contraindications
- Loose sphincter
- Painful and bleeding hemorrhoids
- Anal fistula
- Anal narrowing
- Intestinal polyps
- Rectal infections
- Rectal tumours
- Painful skin lesions around the rectum

Throat Irrigation
It is the process of flushing the throat with an irrigating

Purposes
- To clean the mouth and pharynx.
- To relieve congestion.
- To relieve dryness.
- To relieve pain.
- To combat infection.
- To provide antiseptic effect

Equipment
- A tray containing
- Irrigating solution
- Sterile cotton swabs
- Gauze pieces
- Small towel
- A mackintosh and towel
- A kidney tray
- 2 Paper bag
- Hot and cold water
- IV stand
- Salt or boric powder or soda bicarbonate.

Procedure
- Check physician's order to obtain specific instruction.
- Identify the patient to prevent the regarding irrigation.
- Explain procedure to the patient.
- Position the patient with his or her head bent slightly forward and tilted to one side.
- Cover his or her shoulder and neck with a mackintosh and towel.
- The patient should be given kidney tray.
- The normal saline or water irrigation solution should be heated.
- Then the temperature of the solution should be checked before the irrigation is started.
- Hang the irrigation not more than 12 inch above the patient's mouth.
- Introduce the irrigating tip from the sides reaching behind the tongue avoiding the uvula. Rotate the tip to direct the flow of fluid in all directions.
- When the irrigation is complete, stop the procedure.
- The irrigation apparatus should be removed and the patient assisted with drying off.
- The mouth should be wiped with cotton swabs.
- Irrigation fluid should be discarded.
- Disposable equipment should be placed in a trash bag that can be sealed and discarded.
- Wash hands once the procedure is completed.
- Record the time of irrigation, kind and amount of solution used, nature of return flow, effect of treatment.

SPRAYING: NOSE AND THROAT

Nasal Spray
- Nasal sprays are medicines that you spray into your nose to reduce inflammation.
- They are sprayed directly into the nostrils (nasal passage).
- Nasal sprays are commonly used to treat asthma, allergies of the nose and persistent rhinitis (inflammation of the nose).
- Nasal sprays are available as either over the counter or as prescriptions.
- Also, they come in two types of containers. pressurized canisters and pump bottles.

Steps for Using a Pressurized Canister
- Gently blow your nose to clear it of mucus before using the medicine.
- Make sure canister fits snugly in its holder. Shake canister several times just before using it.
- Keep your head upright. Breathe out slowly.
- Hold nasal spray canister in one hand. Insert the canister tip into nose, aiming the tip toward the back of head.
- Use a finger to close the nostril on the side not receiving the medicine.
- Press the spray to release the dose and breathe in gently and steadily through nose.
- Do not sniff hard.
- Repeat these steps for the other nostril. If you are using more than one spray in each nostril, follow all these steps again.
- Try not to sneeze or blow your nose just after using the spray.

Steps for Using a Pump Bottle
- Gently blow your nose to clear it of mucus before using the medicine.
- Remove the cap. Shake the bottle. Do this by squirting it a few times into the air until a fine mist comes out.
- Tilt your head forward slightly. Breathe out slowly.
- Hold the pump bottle with your thumb at the bottom and index and middle fingers on top.
- Insert the canister tip in nose, aiming the tip toward the back of head.
- Use a finger on other hand to close nostril on the side not receiving the medicine.

- Squeeze the pump as you begin to breathe in slowly through nose.
- Repeat these steps for the other nostril. If you are using more than one spray in each nostril, follow all these steps again.
- Try not to sneeze or blow your nose just after using the spray.

Throat Spray

- Throat spray is the spraying the medication directly into the throat to relieve the irritation, pain of a sore throat, not to treat the cause of it.
- Apply to the affected area (one spray)
- Allow to remain in place for at least 15 seconds, then spit out
- Use every 2 hours or as directed by a doctor or dentist
- **Stop using the spray if:**
  - Sore mouth symptoms do not improve in 7 days
  - Irritation, pain or redness persists or worsens
  - Swelling, rash or fever develops

■ INHALATIONS

Inhalation is the act of drawing in air, vapor or gas into the lungs. Drugs are inhaled either for a local effect (e.g., steam inhalations to relieve congestion in the respiratory tract) or for a general effect, e.g., inhalation of oxygen and an aesthetics. Inhalations are given either dry or moist.

■ DRY INHALATIONS

It is the inhalation of gases, fumes from volatile drugs or burning drugs. Examples of dry inhalation are:
- **Inhalation of general aesthetics:** Ether, chloroform, nitrous oxide, etc., are given by using a mask.
- **Oxygen and carbon dioxide inhalations:** These are administered by using a mask, tent or catheter.
- **Inhalation of volatile drugs:**
  - Amyl nitrite contained in an ampoule is broken and emptied into a gauze piece or handkerchief and is held under the nose of the patient and the patient inhales the fumes. This is used to relieve the pain in angina pectoris.
  - Volatile drugs such as menthol, aromatic spirits of ammonia eucalyptus, etc., are administered in the same way. When aromatic spirits are administered, care should be taken that the drug neither touch the skin nor its fumes irritate the conjunctiva of the eyes. Therefore, it be held away from the nose and eyes.
- **Inhalation of stramonium and belladonna:** These are burned and the patient breathes the fumes.
- **Aerosol spray:** An aerosol is a fine suspension of liquid or a powder that deliver medications topically into the respiratory tract. Atomizers and nebulizers are used for spraying medication into the respiratory passages.

Refer to Nebulization therapy in unit 7 for more information.

■ MOIST INHALATIONS

Breathing warm and moist air produced by a vaporizer is called steam/moist inhalation. The value of steam inhalation lies chiefly in the moisture and heat, although the medicines used are also helpful as they are acting as respiratory antiseptics.

Purpose of Steam Inhalation

- To relieve the inflammation and congestion of the mucous membranes of the respiratory tract and paranasal sinuses, thus to produce symptomatic relief in acute cold and sinusitis.
- To soften thick, tenacious mucus and help its expulsion from the respiratory tract, thus to relieve cough in bronchitis, and in postoperative cases, etc.
- To provide heat and moisture and to prevent the dryness of the mucous membranes of the lung and upper respiratory passages following operations such as tracheostomy.
- To aid in the absorption of oxygen.
- To relieve spastic conditions of the larynx and bronchi.
- To provide antiseptic action on the respiratory tract, e.g., by using menthol, Tr. Benzoin, eucalyptus, etc.

Drugs Used

- Tr. Benzoin 5 mL per 500 mL of boiling water
- Eucalyptus 2 mL per 500 mL of boiling water
- Methyl salicylate few drops per 500 mL of boiling water
- Menthol few crystals per 500 mL of boiling water
- Camphor few crystals per 500 mL of boiling water.

Methods for Giving Steam Inhalation

- By jug method
- By steam tent
- By electric steam inhaler.

Jug Method

- In this method, a Nelson's inhaler is used.
- The boiling water is filled in the jug and the patient breathes the vapor.
- At home situations, where a Nelson's inhaler is not available the patients can be advised to improvise a jug.
- A tea kettle or a mug is filled with boiling water and the inhalant.
- A 'cone' is made with a cardboard paper and is fitted over the kettle or the mug.
- Through a small hole made on the top of the cone the patient breathes in the steam. (Remember if Tr. Benzoin is used in the kettle, it forms stains in the kettle).

Steam Tent

- When a high concentration of steam is required, a steam tent may be used.
- There are different ways of making a tent.
- A quick and easy method is to place a screen on either side on the patient's bed and stretch blankets or sheets across them, fixing them with safety pins, and forming a canopy.
- Woollen blankets are preferred to sheet because they absorb moisture and will not drip over the patient.
- For a child, the blankets can be stretched across the top of the cot.
- The steam can then be directed into the tent from the spout of a kettle.

- Care must be taken that the stove and the kettle are placed far away from the screen and the bed clothes to prevent the danger of catching fire.
- Never point the spout towards the face of the patient.
- A child should never be near enough to the steam generating apparatus to get his hands into the steam jet.
- The steam may be given for 20–30 minutes at a time and it may be repeated every four hours or it may be given continuously, in special cases. Tr. Benzoin and water are added necessarily.
- Continuous observation is essential to avoid scalding of the patient.

Electric Steam Inhaler

- Small electric vaporizers can be used to give steam inhalation.
- It consists of a small jar with a heating element extending into the jar.
- The jar is filled with water.
- On the top of the jar is a removable perforated cup to which is attached a small metal spout.
- Cotton saturated with medication is placed inside the cup and the metal spout is fitted over the cup.
- As the water boils, the medicated steam is directed through the spout which is inhaled by the patient.

General Instructions

- Always remember the danger involved of scalding the patient either with the steam or with the water coming out of the inhaler. This is particularly important when the patient is very young, very old, acutely ill or in a state of confusion. In these cases, the spout of the inhaler must be placed in such a way that the patient cannot touch it or put his face too nearby.
- When jug or kettle is used, fill it only 2/3rds with boiling water to prevent scalding of the patient. If the inhaler is filled to the brim, there is possibility of drawing water into the mouth and scalding the patient. The water should remain just below the spout. If the spout is filled with the water, it will not act as an air inlet. The patient will not get warmed air.
- Always remember the danger of fire. If a stove is used with a kettle to generate steam continuously, as in the case of steam tent, the blankets used may fall on the stove and catch fire.
- Have the water in the jug method at a moderate temperature. The temperature is maintained between 120–160°F (54.4–76.7°C). If the water is cold, it will not generate steam. If the water is too hot, it may cause scalding of the patient.
- Keep the patient warm and prevent draught before, during and after the inhalation. During the treatment, the blood vessels of the skin and mucous membranes are dilated and the patient is easily chilled when exposed to draught. This predisposes him to a more severe and prolonged attack of inflammation and congestion. Therefore, the patient should not go into a cold atmosphere for several hours after the treatment. The windows and doors are closed and the fan is put off during the treatment to prevent draught.
- Ask the patient to empty the bladder to ensure that the patient will remain on the bed for several hours after inhalation.
- When volatile drugs are used, e.g., menthol, warn the patient to keep his eyes closed to prevent the drug irritating the conjunctiva.
- Watch the patient closely throughout the procedure for any adverse effects. Provide a calling device near the patient to call the nurse in case of necessity.
- When giving inhalation by jug method, keep the spout away from the patient. This is a precaution to prevent scalding of the patient, should the patient tilts the jug during inhalation.
- Place a sputum cup in the reach of the patient to spit the sputum that is coughed up during the inhalation.
- Explain the procedure to the patient before the preparation of the inhalation, so that no time is lost to start the inhalation once the inhaler with boiling water is taken to the bedside. If the time is lost for explanations the temperature of the water will be reduced.

Preparation of the Patient and the Environment

- Explain the procedure to the patient to win his confidence and cooperation. Explain the sequence of the procedure and tell him how he can take the inhalation.
- Make the patient to understand that he has to remain in the bed one to two hours more after the inhalation.
- Ask the patient to go to the toilet and empty the bladder and bowels, if necessary. For a bedridden patient, offer bedpan or urinal, so that he will not be disturbed during the procedure. Emptying the bladder and bowels ensures that the patient will remain on the bed for several hours after the inhalation.
- Place the patient in Fowler's position with a cardiac table in front. If the movements are restricted, place him in a side lying position, or place him in any; position which is comfortable to him (e.g., sitting with a pillow on the lap).
- Close the doors and windows and put off the fan to prevent draught.
- Place the sputum cup in a convenient place within the easy reach of the patient.
- Provide a face towel to the patient to wipe the sweating from the face during the inhalation.

Articles

See **Table 9.15**.

Preliminary Assessment

- Check the patient's name, bed number and other identifications.
- Check the diagnosis and the general condition of the patient.
- Check the physician's orders to see the specific precautions for the patient's movement and positioning.
- Assess the patient's ability for self-care, his ability to move and to maintain the desired position.
- Assess the level of consciousness and the ability to follow instructions.
- Check the articles available in the patient's unit.

Chapter 9: Administration of Medications

TABLE 9.15: Articles required for stem inhalation.

Articles	Purpose
A tray containing:	
Nelson's inhaler with a mouth-piece tightly fit to the neck of the inhaler	To use as vaporizer
Bowl or basin large enough to hold the inhaler	To place the inhaler safely
A flannel piece or a towel	To wrap around the inhaler is prevent the heat loss
Face towel	To wipe the face of the patient
Bath blanket or bath towel	To put over the patient's head and the jug to prevent the loss of steam
Tr. Benzoin or any other inhalant ordered	Used as a respiratory antiseptic
Teaspoon or a minim glass	To measure the inhalant
Kettle with boiling water	
Gauze piece in a container	To wrap around the mouthpieces
Cotton swabs in a container	To plug the spout
Kidney tray and paper bag	To receive the wastes

Procedure

Refer **Table 9.16**.

Aftercare of Patient and the Articles

* Continue the treatment for 15–20 minutes, or as long as the patient gets the vapours.
* Remove the inhaler from the patient after the stated time. Wipe off the perspiration form the face.
* Remove the back rest and the cardiac table. Adjust the position of the patient in bed. Make him comfortable. Tidy up the bed.
* Instruct him to remain in bed for 1–2 hours to prevent draught.
* Take the articles to the utility room.
* Empty the inhaler, clean it inside with spirit to remove Tr. benzoin.
* Then wash it with warm soapy water. Rinse with clean water.
* Remove the gauze covering the mouth piece and clean the mouth piece thoroughly.
* Boil it to prevent cross
* infection. All the other articles are cleaned with warm soapy water and then with clean water.
* Dry and replace them in their proper places.
* Wash hands.
* Record the procedure on the nurse's record with date and time. Record the patient's response to the procedure.
* Return to the patient to assess his comfort and to observe any untoward reactions in him. Offer hot drinks if needed.

For Oxygen administration refer Unit 7

TABLE 9.16: Steps of procedure for steam inhalation.

Nursing action	Rationale
Explain the procedure to patient and ensure that patient has emptied his bowel and bladder	Helps in promoting relaxing. Patients will have to remain in bed for 1 hour
Warm the inhaler by pouring a little hot water into the inhaler and emptying it after one minute	Reduces loss of heat from inhaler during procedure
Pour the required amount of inhalant into the inhaler and fill into to a level below the spout with boiling water. The water should remain just below the spout	If the inhaler is filled up to the level of spout there is possibility of drawing water into the mouth when inhaling and cause scalds. If the spout is filled with water, it will not act as an air inlet
Place sterile mouthpiece and close the inhaler tightly. See that the mouthpiece is in the opposite direction to the spout	This keeps the spout away from the patient when inhalations are taken in
Cover the mouth piece with a gauze piece and plug the spout with a cotton ball	Covering the mouthpiece with a gauze piece will prevent burns of the lips. Cotton ball in the spout will prevent escape of steam Covering the mouthpiece with a gauze piece will prevent escape of steam
Place a towel around the inhaler and position it in the bowl	Insulates the inhaler and prevents heat loss
Take it to the patient without losing time	
Switch off fan/AC and close window and door	
Position the patient in high fowlers or sitting position	
Place the apparatus conveniently in front of the patient on cardiac table with spout opposite to the patient. Remove the cotton plug and discard it into the kidney tray	Keeping the spout opposite to the patient reduces the changes of burns. Removing the cotton plug helps to open spout, so that it can act as an inlet for air
Instruct the patient to place lips on the mouthpiece and take deep breath. After removing the lips from the mouthpiece, breathe out air through nose	Directing the steam out through the nostril relieves the congestion of the mucous membranes of the nostril
Continue the treatment for 15–20 minutes as long as patient gets the vapors. Observe the patient during procedure	Helps in effectiveness of the procedure
Remove inhaler from the patient after the stated time wipe off perspiration from the patient's face	Enhances comfort of patient
Give chest physiotherapy and encourage to bring out sputum by coughing	To facilitate removal of mucus and sputum
Instruct the patient to remain in the bed for 1–2 hours	Reduces chances of dizziness and effects of sudden temperature variation

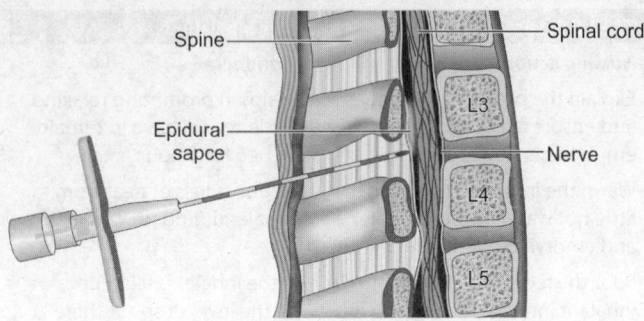

Fig. 9.28: Epidural route.

EPIDURAL ROUTE

- ❖ Epidural administration is a medical route of administration in which a drug such as epidural analgesia and epidural anesthesia or contrast agent is injected into the epidural space around the spinal cord **(Fig. 9.28)**.
- ❖ A thin, tube-like catheter is inserted through the lower back into the area just outside the membrane covering the spinal cord (called the epidural space).
- ❖ An epidural is a nerve blocker.
- ❖ A doctor can give an epidural for a variety of reasons, including for pain relief during labour, back pain, such as sciatica, and chronic leg and arm pain associated with an irritated spinal nerve root.

Benefits

- ❖ Temporary or prolonged pain relief (analgesia) for labor and childbirth.
- ❖ Provide anesthesia for certain surgeries as an alternative to general anesthesia.
- ❖ Temporary or prolonged reduction of inflammation in the region of the spine causing pain.
- ❖ Improved ability to perform daily activities without the restrictions previously caused by pain.
- ❖ May reduce the need for invasive procedures.

Risks

- ❖ Temporary increase in pain.
- ❖ Headache is also extremely rare, but possible.
- ❖ Reaction to the medications, such as hot flashes or rash.
- ❖ Infection at the injection site.
- ❖ Bleeding if a blood vessel is inadvertently damaged.
- ❖ Injury to the nerves at the injection site.
- ❖ Temporary paralysis of the nerves leading to the bladder and bowel, causing temporary bladder or bowel dysfunction.

INTRATHECAL ADMINISTRATION

- ❖ Intrathecal drug administration is the administration of medication into the cerebrospinal fluid by injection into the subarachnoid space of the spinal cord to bypass the blood-brain barrier **(Fig. 9.29)**.
- ❖ The blood brain barrier and the blood-cerebrospinal fluid barrier often slow the entrance of drug into the CNS.

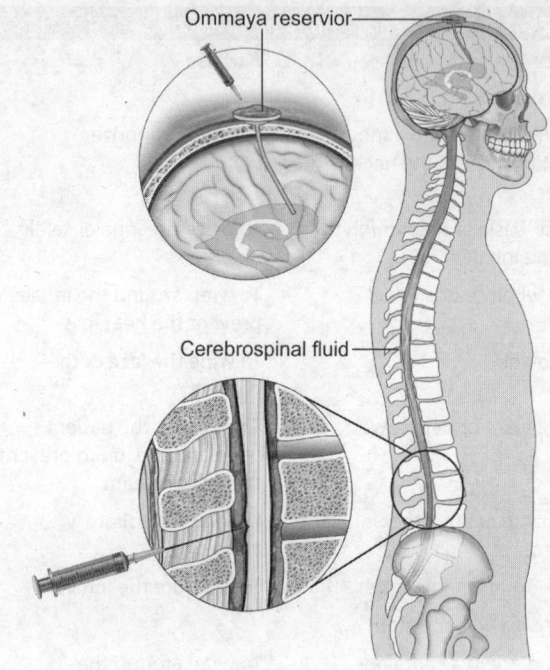

Fig. 9.29: Intrathecal administration.

- ❖ Intrathecal route of drug administration is well established in anesthesia and pain management.
- ❖ It provides a route for drug transport deep into the brain via CSF.
- ❖ The drug will be accessible to the meninges and cerebrospinal axis.
- ❖ The injection made in the lumbar area or in the cisterna magna.
- ❖ An intrathecal injection can reduce the amount of other medicines needed to control pain.
- ❖ This route is also used to introduce drugs that fight certain infections, particularly post-neurosurgical.
- ❖ This route is used for diagnostic procedures (myelography) and treatment of meningoencephalitis.
- ❖ Local anesthetics are sometimes administered intrathecally to produce region or spinal anesthesia.

Advantages

- ❖ Direct administration of drugs into the subarachnoid space
- ❖ High availability of the drug in the CSF as the blood brain barrier and blood—CSF barrier is bypassed.
- ❖ Drug acts directly on the central nervous system (CNS)
- ❖ Provides the advantage of using comparably low daily dosages to achieve the desired analgesic effect.

Disadvantages

- ❖ Strict aseptic precautions are needed
- ❖ Expertise needed
- ❖ An invasive technique that requires surgical implantation of a drug delivery system
- ❖ Contraindicated in some patients based on their medical comorbidities.

Indications

Diagnostic
- **Absolute:**
  - Meningitis
  - Subarachnoid hemorrhage
- **Relative:**
  - Neurosyphilis
  - Unexplained coma
  - Guillain-Barre syndrome
  - Multiple sclerosis
- **Radiological:**
  - Myelography
  - Pneumoencephalography (PEG)

Therapeutic
- **To introduce drugs:**
  - Methotrexate 0.25 mg/kg biweekly in leukaemia
  - Gentamicin 10–20 mg in gram-negative meningitis.
  - Crystalline penicillin 10,000–20,000 units in pyogenic meningitis.
- To reduce raised intracranial tension in hypertensive encephalopathy.
- To administer spinal anesthesia.

Contraindications
- Raised intracranial tension (as shown by papilledema) because of the risk of herniation of brain through foramen magnum, and damaging the vital medullary centres causing death.
- Marked spinal deformity
- Local infections
- Suspected cord compression.

Procedures
- **Position:** The patient is placed on his side at the edge of the bed with the knee drawn up and the head flexed. It can also be done with the sitting and bending forward.
- **Site:** In the 3rd lumbar space. This space lies in the plane which joins the highest points on the iliac crest. The skin over the back from the lower thoracic vertebrae to the coccyx is sterilized with Cetavlon, ether, iodine and spirit. The part is draped.
- **Local anesthesia:** The skin to be punctured is infiltrated with 5 mL of 2% lignocaine. Infiltration is done up to ligamentum flava.
- **Puncture:**
  - A lumbar puncture needle with a stylet is introduced after 2–3 minutes into the anesthetized space, with the cutting edge of the bevel in the direction parallel to the fibres of the ligamentum flava.
  - The needle is introduced (slightly upwards and forwards at 5° to avoid injury to the disk) through the resistance of supraspinous ligament. The interspinous ligament is then easily negotiated.
  - At about 4–7 cm the firmer resistance of ligamentum flavum popping sensation as the dura is breached.
  - The stylet is then withdrawn and the fluid is collected slowly in 4–5 bulbs for biochemical, cytological and serological tests.
- **Seal:** The needle is withdrawn and the puncture mark is sealed with a tincture benzoin seal.
- **Post-procedure orders:**
  - Plenty of fluids are to be taken by mouth
  - Head low position with half to one block to prevent headache
  - Salicylates if headache.

INTRAOSSEOUS ROUTE

- This involves direct administration of drugs into the marrow of a bone.
- The needle is injected through the bone's hard cortex and into the soft marrow interior which allows immediate access to the vascular system **(Fig. 9.30)**.
- Intraosseous route is an alternative method to providing venous administration of drugs and fluids.
- In most cases, the antero-medial aspect of the upper tibia is used as it lies just under the skin and can easily be palpated and located.
- The anterior aspect of the femur, the superior iliac crest and the head of the humerus are other sites that can be used.
- The intraosseous infusions use the medullary cavity to the bone as a route of infusion when no other site is accessible due to severe shock and the patient requires immediate parenteral therapy.
- Drugs injected intraosseously are as rapidly absorbed as intravenously. Most emergency drugs, such as saline, blood, plasma, 5% or 10% dextrose, sodium bicarbonate, dopamine and various antibiotics can be given by this route during an emergent situation.
- This route may also be utilized for taking blood culture and gasometry samples in such critically-sick patient.

Advantages
- Venous access when no other sites can be found
- Useful if difficult, delayed, or impossible IV access
- Used in burns or other injuries preventing alternate access

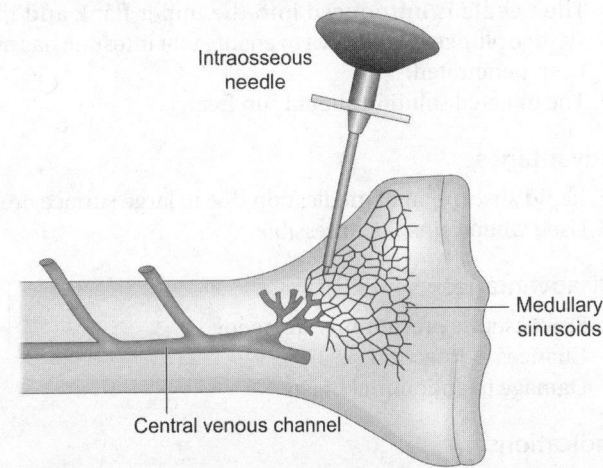

Fig. 9.30: Intraosseous route.

Disadvantages
* Need for special equipment and skill
* Requires pressure bag to provide reasonable flow of fluids
* Strict aseptic precautions are needed

Sites
* Intraosseous infusion using a bone marrow needle may be given in the midline on the flat surface of the tibia about 2–3 cm below the tibial tuberosity.
* Lower one-third of the femur may also be used as an alternative site.

Method
* Under all aseptic conditions the bone marrow needle is introduced into the marrow and the stylet is removed.
* The needle is directed away from the knee and pushed a few millimetres further into the marrow.
* If the needle feels firmly inserted in the bone, attach a syringe of saline and attempt aspiration. In case the needle is in place the marrow is aspirated and saline can be infused easily from the syringe.
* Attach the infusion set to the needle and tape it in place.

Complications
* Local cellulitis
* Osteomyelitis and sepsis
* Leakage around the needle.

Remember
Intraosseous route is used only in case of dire emergencies till some vascular access is achieved.

INTRAPERITONEAL ROUTE
* Intraperitoneal administration is the injection of a substance into the peritoneum (**Fig. 9.31**).
* The injection is given in the peritoneal space leading to a high absorption rate credited to the available large surface area.
* This route may cause infections in the peritoneal cavity and is painful and risky.
* The needle is introduced into the upper flank and the syringe plunger withdrawn to ensure that intestine has not been penetrated.
* The injected solution should run freely.

Advantages
* Rapid absorption of medication due to large surface area
* Used when veins not accessible.

Disadvantages
* Strict aseptic precautions are needed
* Chances of infection
* Damage to abdominal organ

Indications
* Marked abdominal discomfort and cardiorespiratory embarrassment.

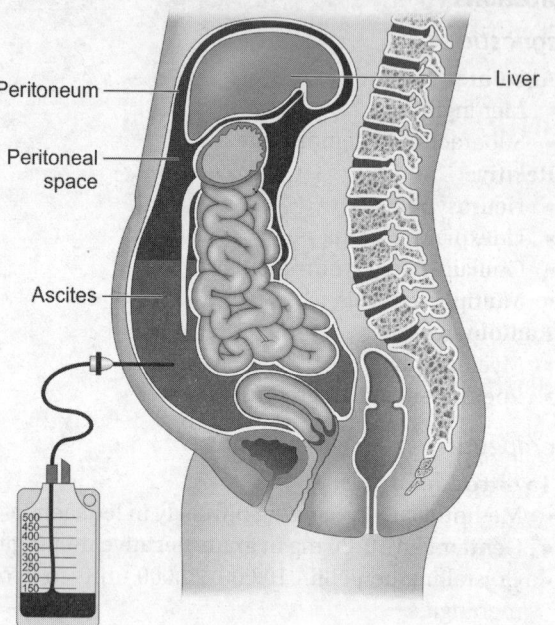

Fig. 9.31: Intraperitoneal route.

* Ascites refractory to medical line of treatment
* For diagnosis the nature of the ascitic fluid
* Ascites with anorexia, dyspepsia, hematemesis or oliguria.

Contraindications
Severe jaundice with impending hepatic coma.

Prerequisite
The patient must be asked to evacuate the bladder.

Procedures
* **Preanesthetic medication:** Injection atropine 0.6 mg and injection phenobarbitone 50 mg must be given intramuscularly half an hour before the procedure.
* **Position:** Supine or semi-reclined with a backrest.
* **Site:** In the flank midway between the anterior superior iliac crest and umbilicus.
* **Local anesthesia:** Skin, subcutaneous tissue and parietal pleura are infiltrated with 2% lignocaine.
* **Puncture:**
  * A large bore needle about 3½ inches in length is introduced and the ascites fluid is drained slowly through the rubber tubing connected to the needle.
  * An abdominal binder may be placed and tightened as required.
* **Seal:** After the biopsy, the punctured skin is sealed with a tincture benzoin seal.
* **Post-procedure orders:** TPR, BP to be recorded half hourly and the patient should not be given feeds for the next 4 hours. If there is pain, analgesics may be given.

Complications
* **Fainting:** If the fluid is removed to rapidly
* Acute liver cell failure and precipitation of hepatic coma

- **Infection:** Peritonitis
- **Perforation of a viscus**
- **Depletion of proteins.**

INTRAPLEURAL ROUTE

An intrapleural drug is injected through the chest wall into the pleural space or instilled through a chest tube placed intrapleurally for drainage. Doctors use intrapleural administration to promote analgesia, treat spontaneous pneumothorax, resolve pleural effusions, and administer chemotherapy **(Fig. 9.32)**.

Indications

- Large pleural effusion up to the clavicles
- Bilateral pleural effusion
- Cardiorespiratory embarrassment
- When pleural effusion is suspected to the infected (persistence of fever and constitutional symptoms) or hemorrhage
- Acute pulmonary edema.
- Persistent pleural effusion in spite of antituberculosis.

Contraindications: None

Procedures

- **Preanesthetic medication:** Injection atropine 0.6 mg and injection phenobarbitone 50 mg must be given intramuscularly half an hour before the procedure.
- **Position:** Patient sits-up against a backrest or leans forward resting the arm on the tip of a bed-table.
- **Site:** Seventh or eighth intercostals space in the midaxillary or scapular line. The part is prepared with Cetavlon, ether, iodine and spirit.
- **Local anesthetic:** Skin subcutaneous tissue and parietal pleura are infiltrated with 2% lignocaine.

- **Puncture:**
  - The aspiration needle is introduced at right angles to the skin, midway between the two ribs, and advanced till parietal pleura is punctured which is indicated by a 'give in'.
  - The needle is now attached to a 50 mL syringe with a two way stop cork and about 800–1000 mL of fluid is removed at a time.
  - Aspiration must be stopped if the patient coughs or complains of tightness in the chest.
- **Seal:** After the biopsy, the punctured skin is sealed with a tincture benzoin seal.
- **Post-procedure orders:** TPR, BP to be recorded half hourly and the patient should not be given feeds for the next 4 hours. If there is pain, analgesics may be given.

Complications

- Pleural shock due to vagal inhibition
- Air embolism
- Pulmonary edema
- Circulatory collapse due to a high negative intra-pleural pressure, which may occur if there is pulmonary fibrosis as this prevents expansion of lung
- Injury to the intercostal vessels
- Pneumothorax
- Hemoptysis
- Infection

INTRA-ARTERIAL ROUTE

- Intra-arterial route involves direct administration of medication into an artery.
- This route is used when localized effect of a drug in a particular tissue or organ is desired.
- Intra-artery route is especially used when high drug concentration in specific tissue is required

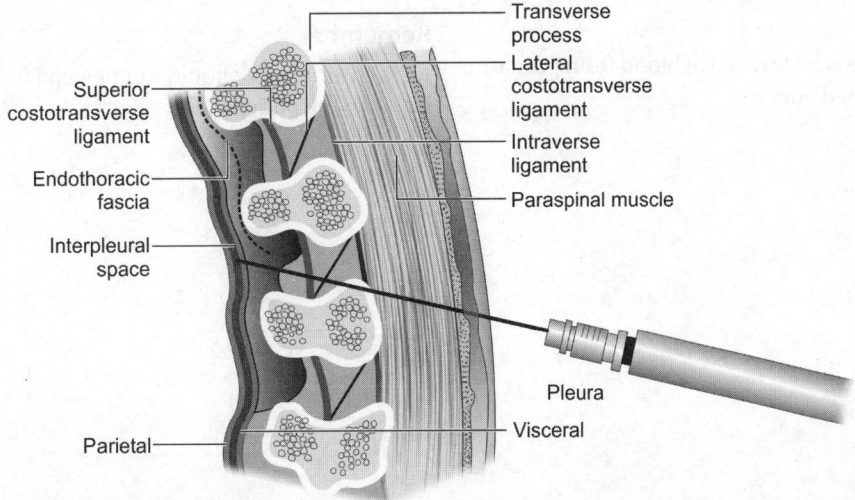

Fig. 9.32: Intrapleural route.

- Diagnostic purpose and for chemotherapy.
- The sites of injection commonly used are radial artery, brachial artery, and femoral artery.

Advantages
- The first pass and cleansing effects are by-passed
- Bioavailability is 100%
- It is of great clinical value in administering anticancer drugs

Disadvantages
- Intra-arterial injection requires great and expertise
- If the drug is of adverse effect there might be great danger.

Sites for Arterial Puncture
- Radial and brachial arteries are commonly used.
- The posterior tibial and temporal arteries may also be used in small infants.
- The radial artery is palpated on the lateral aspect of forearm and the wrist.
- The site is cleaned with iodine and spirit and the operator should also sterilize tips of his index and second finger similarly.
- A small 24G or 25G needle is attached to 2 mL syringe flushed with heparin.
- After feeling for the radial artery pulsations.
- The needle is aggressively advanced at a 45° to 60° angle piercing both walls of the artery.
- Negative pressure is applied with syringe and re-entry into the arterial lumen is signalled by appearance of blood in the needle hub.
- Arterial blood can usually be recognized by its bright red color and by easy filling of the syringe without requiring any negative pressure.
- Once the specimen is collected the needle is remove rapidly and site is pressed with a sterile cotton ball for 5–10 minutes.

Important
Please ensure that there is no leakage of blood from puncture site before leaving the bedside.

Method of Intra-arterial Cannulation
- The ulnar artery is identified and checked for collateral flow before radial artery cannulation.
- The artery is punctures with an arterial catheter at an angle of 30–45° as described above.
- The stylet is removed and there is no blood back until pulsatile blood flow from it signalling re-entry into the arterial lumen.
- The catheter is then advanced further into the artery.
- The arterial line may be kept patent with intermittent heparin solution irrigation.

Intra-arterial Cannulation Steps
- After puncturing the skin, insert the cannula into the artery by transfixing method of illustrated here.
- When the needle has punctured the posterior wall of the artery it should be partially withdrawn, held by the grip. While holding the wing of the cannula to keep it stationary.
- Bring the cannula back until blood rectum indicates that the cannula tip is in the lumen of artery.
- Advance the cannula into the artery at the same time drawing the needle back. Once the needle has been completely withdrawn. The red thumb switch can be pushed forwards to close off the cannula.
- If required, connect up a 3-way stopcock. After checking successful cannulation by aspirating blood, flush the system with saline.
- Fix the cannula securely in position with sterile tap. The cannula is now ready for use.

Risks of Intra-arterial Puncture
- Arterial thrombosis
- Arterial embolism
- Skin ischemia proximal to catheter site
- Arterio-spasm
- Hematoma and persistent bleeding
- Gangrene of the digits.

Remember
Intra-arterial line should not be used for giving any drugs or fluids to the patients.

CHAPTER 10

Sensory Needs

■ INTRODUCTION

- An individual's senses are essential for growth, development and survival.
- Human being uses sensory organs to learn about the environment in which he lives.
- Stimulation of the sensory organs also promotes development of these organs and contributes to the overall well being of the individual.
- Sensory stimuli give meaning to events in the environment.
- Any alteration in people's sensory functions can affect their ability to function within the environment.
- To interact with our environment we rely on information coming in from our senses.
- This includes the five senses that most of us are familiar with—sight (visual), hearing (auditory), smell (olfactory), touch (tactile), and taste (gustatory).
- The body also has a kinesthetic sense that enables a person to be aware of the position and movement of body parts without seeing them.
- The senses form the perceptual base of our world.
- When the sensory function is altered, an individual's ability to function within the environment is drastically changed.
- Hospital is a place of unfamiliar sights, smells, and sounds, and minimal contact with family and friends.
- If patients are unable to receive meaningful stimuli and feel depersonalized, serious sensory alterations may develop.
- Nurses play an important role to identify patients with existing sensory alterations and recognize those most at risk of developing sensory problems.
- A person's senses are vital to the survival, growth and development and the experience of environmental stimuli
- Many patients who have sensory impairment are at risk for injury and decreased well-being.
- Moreover, the stress of illness or trauma and the need for diagnosis and treatment may quickly result is sensory deprivation or overload, with serious disturbances in visual, perceptual, cognitive or emotional functioning.
- Nurses are in position to use knowledge of sensory functioning to support positive outcomes for patients.

■ COMPONENTS OF SENSORY EXPERIENCE

Introduction
- The nervous system continuously receives information from sensory nerve organs and relays the information through appropriate neurological channels and integrates the information into a meaningful response.
- Three components of sensory experience includes Reception, perception and reaction

Reception
- It begins with stimulation of a nerve cell for sight, smell, taste, sound, etc.
- In the case of special senses, the receptors are located in specialized organs such as the taste buds of the tongue or the retina of the eye.
- The nerve impulse is created; it travels along the pathways to the spinal cord or directly to the brain.
- Reception begins with stimulation of a nerve cell called a receptor, such as touch, taste, smell, vision or sound.
- When a nerve impulse is created it travels along pathways to the spinal cord or directly to the brain.
- Sensory nerve pathways usually cross over to send stimuli to the opposite side of the brain.

Perception
- The perception or awareness of unique sensations depends on the receiving regions of the cerebral cortex, where specialized neurons interpret the quality and nature of sensory stimuli.
- When a person receives the information, perception takes place.
- Perception includes the integration and interpretation of stimuli based on individual experiences.
- Any factors lowering consciousness impair sensory perception.
- The actual perception or awareness of sensations depends on the receiving region of the cerebral cortex, where specialized cells analyze the quality and nature of sensory stimuli.

- When a person becomes conscious of the stimuli and receives the information, perception takes place.
- Perception includes integration and interpretation of the stimuli based on the person's experiences.
- A person's level of consciousness influences how well stimuli are perceived and interpreted.
- Any factors lowering consciousness influences impair sensory perception.
- If sensation is incomplete, e.g., blurred vision the person may react inappropriately to the sensory stimuli.

Reaction

- It is not possible to react to all stimuli entering the nervous system.
- A person usually reacts to the most meaningful stimuli at a time.
- After continued reception of the same stimulus, a person stops responding, and the sensory experience goes unnoticed.
- For example, a person reading a favorite book is not aware of background music.
- A person usually react to a stimuli that are most meaningful and significant at the time
- After continued reception of the same stimuli, however a person stops responding and the sensory experience goes unnoticed.
- This adaptability phenomenon occurs with most sensory stimuli except for those of pain.
- A balance between sensory stimuli entering the brain and those actually reaching a person's conscious awareness maintains a person's wellbeing.

■ AROUSAL MECHANISM

Introduction

- Arousal is the physiological and psychological state of being awaken or of sense organs stimulated to a point of perception.
- It involves activation of the ascending reticular activating system (ARAS) in the brain, which mediates wakefulness, the autonomic nervous system, and the endocrine system, leading to increased heart rate and blood pressure and a condition of sensory alertness, desire, mobility, and readiness to respond.
- Arousal is mediated by several neural systems.
- Wakefulness is regulated by the ARAS, which is composed of projections from five major neurotransmitter systems that originate in the brainstem and form connections extending throughout the cortex; activity within the ARAS is regulated by neurons that release the neurotransmitters acetylcholine, norepinephrine, dopamine, histamine, and serotonin.
- Activation of these neurons produces an increase in cortical activity and subsequently alertness.
- Arousal is important in regulating consciousness, attention, alertness, and information processing. It is crucial for motivating certain behaviors, such as mobility, the pursuit of nutrition, the fight-or-flight response, and sexual activity.

It holds significance within emotion and has been included in theories, such as the James-Lange theory of emotion.

Reticular Activating System (RAS)

- Reticular activating system of cells is the formation of the medulla oblongata that receive collaterals from the ascending sensory pathways and project to higher centers; they control the overall degree of central nervous system activity, including wakefulness, attentiveness and sleep.
- The reticular activating system (RAS) is involved in most central nervous system activity, including control of wakefulness, sleep and part of our ability to direct attention towards specific areas of our conscious minds.
- The RAS is a primitive network of interlacing nerve cells and fibers that receives input from multiple sensory pathways.
- It extends from the spinal cord to the lower brainstem, upward through the mesencephalon and thalamus and then is distributed throughout the cerebral cortex.
- RAS fibers affect the autonomic and motor system.
- They integrate the regulation of cardiovascular, respiratory and motor response to external stimuli.
- The RAS diffusely distributes incoming sensory stimulation throughout the CNS, regulating and preparing the system to respond to a loud noise.
- Once regulated, the CNS begins to search for more data and coordinates information to locate and deal with the cause of the noise.
- Without a functioning RAS, the noise might remain as isolated and unrelated stimulation within various CNS structures.

Reticular Formation

- The brainstem also contains networks of neurons, known collectively as the reticular formation, that project up into the cerebral cortex and basal ganglia and affect general arousal.
- The reticular formation is also involved in inducing and terminating the different stages of sleep.

Ascending Reticular Activating System

- The ascending reticular activating system is a postulated group of neural connections that receives sensory input and projects to the cerebral cortex through the midbrain and thalamus from the reticular formation. Two structures must remain intact for a person to be conscious:
- Ascending reticular activating system located in the brainstem; extends from mid-pons to the hypothalamus; responsible for arousal.
- Cerebral cortex responsible for cognitive abilities.

■ FACTORS AFFECTING THE SENSORY FUNCTION

Many factors influence the capacity to receive or perceive. These are as follows:

Age

- Infants are unable to discriminate sensory stimuli because their because their nerve pathways are immature

- Normal changes associated with ageing include reduced visual fields, increased glare sensitivity, impaired night vision, reduced accommodation and depth perception and reduced color discrimination.
- Older adults face tactile changes, including decreased sensitivity to pain, pressure and temperature.
- Infants and children are at high risk for visual and hearing impairment due to genetic, prenatal, and postnatal conditions.
- Visual changes during adulthood include presbyopia and astigmatism and may require glass for reading.
- Normal visual changes associated with aging include increased glare sensitivity, impaired night vision, reduced color discrimination, and reduced depth perception.
- Usually, hearing changes begin at the age of thirty.
- Aging-related changes include decreased hearing acuity and pitch discrimination.
- Low-pitched sounds are easier to hear, but it is difficult to hear conversations over background noise.
- There is a delay in reception and reaction to the speech.
- Gustatory and olfactory changes begin around age fifty and include a decrease in the number of taste buds and sensory cells in the nasal lining.
- Reduced sensitivity to odors and decreased taste discrimination are common during old age.
- After the age of sixty proprioceptive changes are common which include increased difficulty with balance and coordination.
- There are also tactile changes with aging, including decreased sensitivity to temperature, and pressure secondary to peripheral vascular diseases and neuropathies.

Presence of Meaningful Stimuli

- Meaningful stimuli reduce the incidence of sensory deprivation.
- Meaningful stimuli at home include pets, television, music, a clock, pictures of family members, etc.
- The same stimuli need to be present in the hospital.
- The presence of family members offers positive stimulation.
- The presence of meaningful stimuli influences alertness and the ability to participate in care.

Amount of Stimuli

- If the patient is in pain, has many tubes and dressings or restricted by cast or traction, overstimulation can be a problem.
- Patient's room near loud noises may contribute to sensory overload.
- Excessive stimuli in an environment causes sensory overload.
- The frequency of procedures performed in the health care setting is often stressful to patients.

Social Interaction

- The quality and amount of social contact with supportive family members and significant others influence sensory function.
- The absence of visitors during hospitalization influences the degree of isolation a patient feels.
- Visitors are often restricted in hospital intensive care units.
- The ability to discuss concerns with loved ones is an important coping mechanism for most patients.
- Therefore the absence of meaningful conversation results in a feeling of isolation, anxiety, and depression in patients.

Environmental Factors

- A person's occupation may influence visual, auditory, and peripheral nerve alterations.
- Persons with occupations involving exposure to high noise levels are at risk of noise induced hearing loss.
- Individuals who have an occupation involving the risk of exposure to chemicals are at risk for eye injuries and need to be screened for vision.
- Patients who are immobilized by bed rest or who have a chronic disability are unable to experience the normal sensations of free movement and unable to enjoy normal interactions with visitors.

Cultural Factors

- Certain sensory alterations occur more commonly in selected cultural groups.
- For example, non-Hispanic whites had a higher prevalence of age-related macular degeneration than non-Hispanic African-Americans but a lower prevalence of diabetic retinopathy and glaucoma.

Family interaction

- The amount and quality of contact with supportive family members and significant others can influence the degree of isolation that patient feels.
- The ability to discuss fears or concerns with loved ones is an important coping mechanism for most of the people.
- Absence of meaning full conversation cause sensory deprivation.

Disease Conditions

- Patient with hearing impairment tend to decrease time spent with social activities and with verbal communications.
- Children with hearing deficits will be inattentive, uncooperative and easily bored
- Patients with hearing impairment experience loneliness and low self-esteem.

Medications

Some medications like narcotics and sedatives have depressant effect on CNS thus the response to sensory stimuli is decreased.

ASSESSMENT OF SENSORY ALTERATIONS

Introduction

- In normal situations, individuals are adjusted to a certain level of sensory stimulation which varies both, in quantity and quality as compared to individuals who get admitted in hospital.

- Patients in hospitals are confronted with the different stimuli which directly or indirectly influence the sensory stimulation in several ways and can lead to sensory alterations.
- Carefully observing the factors which have impact on the hearing, visual and tactile stimulation of patients can help the patients in reducing the sensory disturbance.
- Assess the nature and characteristics of sensory alterations and include them in nursing history.
- When taking the history, consider the cultural background of the patient because certain alterations are higher in some cultural groups.
- During the history, it is useful to have a patient self-rate his or her sensory deficit by asking. "Rate your hearing as excellent, good, fair, poor, or bad."
- Then, based on the patient's self-rating, explore his/her perception of sensory loss. This provides an in-depth look at how sensory loss influences the patient's quality of life.
- In the case of hearing problems, a screening tool, such as the Hearing Handicap Inventory for the Elderly (HHIE-S) effectively identifies patients needing audiological intervention.
- A nursing history also reveals any recent changes in a patient's behavior.

Ask the family the following questions:
- Has your family member shown any recent mood swings (e.g., anger, nervousness, fear, or irritability?
- Have you noticed the family member avoiding social activities?

Assessment in General
- Assessment of mental status is valuable when you suspect sensory deprivation or overload.
- Observation of a patient during history taking, during the physical examination, and while providing nursing care offers valuable data about a patient's behaviors and mental status.
- Observe the patient's physical appearance and behavior, measure cognitive ability, and assess his or her emotional status.
- The Mini Mental State Examination (MMSE) is a tool you can use to measure disorientation, change in problem-solving abilities, and altered conceptualization and abstract thinking, e.g., a patient with severe sensory deprivation is not always able to carry on a conversation, attentive, or display recent or past memory.
- An important step toward preventing cognition-related disability is education by nurses about the disease process, available services, and assistive devices.
- To identify sensory deficits and their severity, use physical assessment techniques to assess vision; hearing; olfaction; taste; and the ability to discriminate light touch, temperature, pain, and position.
- In addition, rely on personal observation to detect sensory alterations.
- Patients with a hearing impairment may seem inattentive to others, respond with inappropriate anger when spoken to, believe people are talking about them, answer questions inappropriately, have trouble following clear directions, and have monotonous voice quality, and speak unusually loud or soft.
- An individual usually experiences discomfort and anxiety when subjected to a change in the type or amount of stimuli.
- A person can become confused as a result of either overstimulation or under stimulation.
- A person admitted to the healthcare agency experiences stimuli that are different from those usually encountered.
- As a result the hospital itself can become a stressor that negatively affects sensory, perceptual, cognitive functions
- These problems are manifested by four types of alterations:
  1. Sensory deficit
  2. Sensory deprivation
  3. Sensory overload
  4. Sensory poverty

Sensory Deficit
- A deficit in the normal function of sensory reception and perception is a sensory deficit.
- When a person loses hearing or visual acuity, he withdraws from others to cope with the sensory loss.
- It becomes difficult for the person to interact with the environment safely until he learns new skills.
- When a deficit develops gradually, a person learns to rely on unaffected senses.
- Some senses may even become more powerful to compensate for an alteration. For example, a blind person develops an acute sense of hearing to compensate for visual loss.
- Persons with sensory deficits may behave in adaptive or maladaptive ways. For example, a person with hearing impairment turns the unaffected ear towards others to hear better whereas the other person avoids people because he is embarrassed about not being able to understand while others communicating.
- A sensory deficit is a change in the perception of sensory stimuli.
- These deficits can affect all the senses.
- The patient's response to these losses usually depends on the time of onset and severity of condition.
- If the problem occurs suddenly and without warning the patient may have difficulty in adjusting to the loss of sensory and perceptual function.
- Inadequate functioning or impairment in any of the senses is known as sensory deficit-impairment of hearing and vision, taste alterations, and numbness.
- Such sensory deficits may be present at the time of birth or may develop suddenly due to any illness.
- These deficits may be permanent or temporary, reversible or irreversible.
- **Assessment of sensory deficit** is very important to understand the extent of deficit as it can help the health care worker to determine whether the person is able to cope the deficit.
- Normal adaptive or coping mechanism gets affected by any illness or unfavorable situation.

- During any stressful condition or hospitalization the normal coping mechanism gets threatened and it may require new self-care abilities and coping strategies.

Definition
Sensory deficit is defined as a deficit in the normal function of sensory reception and perception.

Causes of Sensory Deficit
The common causes of sensory deficit includes congenital (in most of cases the deficit is inborn), radical surgical procedures and disturbances or damages of CNS.

Sensory Deprivation
- Individuals can receive stimuli even while sleeping deeply because the reticular activating system in the brainstem mediates all sensory stimuli to the cerebral cortex.
- Sensory stimulation must be of sufficient quality and quantity to maintain a person's awareness.
- **There are three types of sensory deprivation:**
  1. Reduced sensory input due to visual or hearing loss.
  2. The elimination of patterns due to exposure to a strange environment.
  3. The restrictive environment is due to limited movement, e.g., bed rest.
- There are cognitive, affective, and perceptual effects of sensory deprivation.
- The person may experience disorientation, confusion, restlessness, increased anxiety, changes in visual and motor coordination.

Meaning of Sensory Deprivation
- Sensory deprivation is a state of reduced sensory input from the internal or external environment or isolation.
- A person experiencing sensory deprivation misinterprets the limited stimuli with a resultant impairment sensory deprivation.
- Decreased sensory input leads to insufficient quantity or quality of stimuli, which is known as sensory deprivation.
- The decreased sensory input disables reticular actively system (RAS) to an extent where RAS does not project a normal level of activation of the brain.
- Sensory deprivation can cause cognitive, emotional and perceptual damage to the person.
- Impairment of cognitive response involves the content of thought and the inability of the person to control the thought process.
- Patient may have some difficulty in memory, problem solving, and the performance of the person can deteriorate.
- The attention span and the concentration level of the person reduce with the impairment in cognition.
- Emotional responses are mainly as anxiety, fear, anger, depression, apathy and mood changes, which include ups and downs of mood and crying, irritability and annoying behavior.
- Disturbance of perceptual response will lead to inaccurate perception of the visual, hearing, kinesthetic and coordination tactile senses which will further create problems with the sight, sound, body position, balance or equilibrium and smell.
- The disturbance of the response varies from mild to severe level as from day dreaming to hallucinations and illusion.

Types of Deprivation
- Visual deprivation
- Auditory deprivation
- Tactile deprivation

Effects of Sensory Deprivation
Cognitive
- Reduced capacity to learn
- Inability to think or solve, poor task perform
- Disorientation
- Bizarre thinking
- Regression
- Increased need of socialization or altered mechanisms of attention.

Affective
- Boredom
- Restlessness
- Increased anxiety
- Emotional ability
- Panic
- Increased need for physical stimulation.

Perceptual
- Visual/motor coordination
- Color perception
- Apparent movement
- Tactile accuracy
- Ability to perceive size and shape
- Spatial and time judgment

Sensory Overload
Inability of a person to process or manage the intensity or quantity of incoming sensory stimuli, the person feel out of control and overwhelmed by the excessive input from environment and does not feel in control. —Lee, 1991

Meaning of Sensory Overload
- The sensory overload refers to the condition.
- When five senses the sight, hearing, smell, touch, and taste take in more information than your brain can process.
- When your brain is overwhelmed act by this input, it enters fight, flight, or freeze mode in response to what feels like a crisis, making you feel unsafe or even panicky.
- Common symptoms include—difficulty focusing, extreme irritability restlessness and discomfort, stress, fear, anxiety about surroundings.
- A person experiences sensory overload when he receives multiple sensory stimuli and cannot perceptually disregard or selectively ignore them.
- Excessive sensory stimulation prevents the brain from responding appropriately.
- Sensory overload prevents meaningful responses by the brain.

- The individual's attention scatters in many directions, anxiety and restlessness occur.
- A person's tolerance to sensory overload varies with the level of fatigue, attitude, and physical and emotional wellbeing.
- An acutely-ill patient in a critical care unit experiences sensory overload easily due to the performance of procedures sounds of machines, light, staff conversations, equipment alarms, etc.
- Sensory overload may cause confusion and disorientation.
- Hence constant reorientation and control of excessive stimuli become an important part of a patient's care.

Causes of Sensory Overload
Internal Factors
- It includes thinking about surgery or the meaning of a medical diagnosis, can contribute to anxiety and cognitive overload so that the person cannot process additional stimuli.
- Pain, medication, lack of sleep, worry, and brain injury also can contribute to a person's vulnerability to sensory overload.

Information
- It is imparting information to a patient may lead to sensory overload.
- Some examples include teaching a patient about a procedure, informing a patient about a diagnosis, making requests of a patient, or helping the patient solve a problem.
- Anxiety related to medical diagnosis, prognosis, and treatment can contribute to sensory overload.
- Lights and frequent activity may cause sensory overload in a premature newborn in the neonatal intensive care unit.

Environment
- The environment of the healthcare agency provides a higher than usual amount of sensory stimulation.
- A patient newly admitted to the hospital, for example, may have to cope with adjusting to a new roommate, having the television on more than usual, bright lights, paging systems, meeting many staff members, having the bed move up and down at someone else's bidding, waiting for someone to answer the call light, uncontrolled pain, and having strangers touch and not respect private body areas.
- Patients in intensive care units often exhibit symptoms of sensory overload because of the high degree of light, noise, and activity around the clock.

Signs
- Complaints of fatigue, sleeplessness
- Irritability
- Anxiety
- Restlessness
- Disorientation
- Reduced problem solving ability and task performance
- Increased muscle tension
- Scattered attention and racing thoughts.

Prevention of Sensory Overload
- Address the patient by name.
- Provide explanations of all procedures.
- Modify environment to reduce excessive multisensory stimulation; reduce distractions, loud noise, and excessive light.
- Use a calm, unhurried manner when communicating with the patient.
- Provide a private room.
- Plan the delivery of care to allow for rest periods with no stimulation.
- Use soft background music.
- Keep the environment free of strong odors.
- Limit the number and frequency of visitors.

Sensory Poverty
- Sensory poverty is learning about the world without experiencing it.
- The further we distance. ourselves from the spell of the present, explored by our senses, the harder it will be to understand and protect nature's balance.
- We are losing track of our senses, and spending less and less time experiencing the world firsthand.
- At some medical schools, it is even possible for future doctors to attend virtual anatomy classes, in which they can dissect a body by computer-minus that whole smelly, fleshy, disturbing human element.

MANAGEMENT
Promoting Meaningful Communication
- Patients with existing sensory deficits often develop alternative ways of communication.
- To interact with the patient nurse must understand patient's method of communication,

Patient with Aphasia
Aphasia is loss of the ability to understand or express spoken or written language. It commonly occurs after strokes or traumatic brain injuries. It can also occur in people with brain tumors or degenerative diseases that affect the language areas of the brain.
- Make sure you have the person's attention before you start
- Minimize or eliminate background noise (IV, radio, other people)
- Keep your own voice at a normal level, unless the person has indicated otherwise.
- Simplify your own sentence structure and reduce your rate of speech. Emphasize key words. Don't talk down" to the person with aphasia.
- Confirm that you are communicating successfully with "yes" and "no" questions.
- Listen to the patient and wait for the patient to communicate.
- Use simple short questions, and facial gestures to give additional clues
- If the patient has problem speaking, ask question that require simple yes or no answers or blinking of eyes.
- Communicate with drawings, gestures, writing and facial expressions in addition to speech.
- Give time to understand, be calm and patient.

- Engage in normal activities whenever possible. Do not shield people with aphasia from family or ignore them in a group conversation.
- Rather, try to involve them in family decision-making as much as possible.
- Keep them informed of events but avoid burdening them with day-to-day details.

Communication with Patient (with Artificial Airway)

- Patients are unable to vocalize during artificial airway such as patients with endotracheal intubation and tracheotomy tubes
- These patients suffer from a communication barrier which affects the communication.
- Patients may be sedated or have fluctuating consciousness; their ability to comprehend or attend to communications may also fluctuate.
- Writing may be impaired due to swollen hands/fingers, muscle weakness or lack of coordination

Following are some techniques for facilitating communication with patients with artificial airway:

- Patients with preserved cognition and fine motor abilities may be provided pen and paper to freely write.
- If fine motor abilities are preserved but the patient is unable to write, communication boards are available.
- These boards consist of icons and pictures representing basic needs.
- Speech-generating devices or voice-output communication aids are handheld devices that allow patients to touch a word or picture icon to generate pre-recorded messages.
- Use non-verbal method of communication.
- Use simple and short sentences while communicating with patient.

Visual Impairment

- Visual impairment is the functional limitation of eyes which leads to partial or complete reduction in vision.
- It is usually associated with age and ranges from mild to severe impairment.

Etiology

- Glaucoma, cataract, diabetes mellitus.
- **Possible causes:** Infections, injury or nutrition.
- **Other causes:**
  - Exposure of a pregnant woman to certain diseases can cause congenital eye problems.
  - Injuries to the eyes.
  - Disease in the brain or the optic nerves. Multiple sclerosis and similar nervous system diseases, brain tumors, diseases of the eye sockets and head injuries are rare causes of blindness.
- **Malnutrition:** Vitamin A deficiency.

Clinical Manifestations

- Lack of eye-to-eye contact
- Abnormal eye movement
- Failure to locate distant objects
- Squinting frequent blinking
- Frequent rubbing of eye
- Gray opacities in eyes
- Disorientation
- Anxiety
- Anger
- Visual distortions
- Incoordination of work
- History of falls, accidents

Related Factors

- Diabetes
- Glaucoma
- Cataract
- Ocular trauma
- Ocular infection
- Retinal detachment
- Advanced age

Communication with Patient having Visual Impairment

- Introduce self to patient and acknowledge visual impairment and ask for permission before touching the patient. This reduces patient's anxiety.
- Look directly at the patient while speaking.
- Stay in patient's field of vision if the patient has a partial vision loss.
- Orient patient to environment.
- Orientation reduces fear related to unfamiliar environment.
- Provide adequate lighting. The use of natural lighting is preferred to improve vision for patients with diminished vision.
- Keep furniture and other items in their usual place; orient the patient to the environment.
- Use normal tone, volume and rate of speaking
- Inform patient when you are entering or leaving the room.
- Place meal tray, tissues, water and call bell within patient's range of vision or reach. These ensure safety and sense of independence.
- Recommend use of visual aids when appropriate. Visual aids such as magnifying glass, large type printed books.
- Encourage use of sense of touch. Touch encourages patient to become familiar with unfamiliar objects.
- Encourage use of radios, tapes. Diversional activities should be encouraged. Radio and television increase awareness of day and time.
- Remove environmental barriers (furniture or waste baskets are moved) to ensure safety.
- Discourage doors from being left partially open. Fully open or closed doors reduce the risk for injury among the visually-impaired.
- Maintain bed in low position with side rails up, if appropriate rails help to remind patient not to get up without help when needed. Keep bed in locked position. This prevents falls.
- Guide patient when ambulating, if appropriate. Describe where you are walking identify obstacles.
- Instruct patient to hold both arms of chair before sitting and to feel for the seat on chairs or sofas without arms. These reduce the risk of falls.

- **Teach general eye care:**
  - Maintain sterility of all eye droppers, tubes of medications and other items. This reduces the risk of eye infection.
  - Care for contact lenses as recommended.
  - Do not rub eyes.
  - Demonstrate the proper administration of eye drops or ointments, allow for return demonstration by patient and/or caregiver.
  - Help family or caregiver to identify and make arrangements at home. This promotes patient's safety and sense of independence, as indicated.

Prevention of Blindness

In general, of blindness can be prevented as follows:
- Everyone should be aware of and follow personal and environmental hygiene.
- There should be health education program to prevent blindness.
- Teachers in schools should keep a watch on children.
- Those who have refractory error, refer them to hospital.
- All eye infections, errors should be treated without
- Avoid injury and burn of the eyes during festivals and parents should be vigilant when children play.
- Avoid using eye cosmetics. These can be dangerous.
- Do not make indiscriminate use of eye drops.
- Control program for cataract, glaucoma, trachoma, etc. should be carried out.

Hearing Impairment

- Hearing impairment is a hearing loss that prevents a person from totally receiving sounds through the ear.
- If the loss is mild in the person has difficulty in hearing or distant speech.
- If the hearing loss is severe the person may not be able to distinguish any sound

Types of Hearing Impairment

- **Conductive hearing loss:** It occurs due to an impairment of the external or middle ear or both. The sound vibrations do not go from the air around a person to the moving bones of the inner ear. It may be due to ear wax, fluid and impacted cerumen.
- **Sensorineural hearing loss (nerve deafness):** This hearing loss is due to disease of the inner ear or nerve pathways. Auditory nerve, which goes from the inner ear to the brain, fails to carry the sound or information to the brain.
- **Combined hearing loss:** Both conductive and neural hearing loss.
- **Psychogenic hearing loss:** Manifested as an emotional disturbance and unrelated to evident structural changes.

Characteristics of Hearing Impairment

- Inability to catch, recognize or understand words.
- Difficulty vocalizing words.
- Inability to recall familiar words, phrases or names of known persons, objects and places.
- Unable to speak dominant language.

Related Factors

- Brain injury that adversely affects the transmission, reception or interpretation of language or other forms of communication.
- Structural problem (e.g., cleft palate, laryngectomy, intubation or wired jaws).
- Cultural difference (e.g., speaks different language).
- Dyspnea.
- Fatigue.

Causes

Some of the causes include:
- Arteriosclerosis.
- Infectious disease, e.g., mumps, measles and meningitis
- Toxicity of drugs, e.g., quinine, neomycin, etc.
- Blows to the head or ear.

Clinical Manifestations

- Age-related hearing loss often starts at the high frequencies trouble in understanding women and children.
- Signs of deafness in young children include not responding to noises, responding slowly or not learning to speak by the expected age.
- A deaf child may also lag behind in developing motor skills and coordination or in learning how to balance, crawl or walk. Profoundly deaf children are usually diagnosed by the age of two.
- As the kid grows older, hearing loss impairs speech development.
- Presbycusis usually produces tinnitus and the inability to understand the spoken word.

Diagnostic Test

- History and complete audiologic examination.
- Weber's test
- Rinne tests

Management

- Hearing aids greatly improve the quality of life of hearing impaired persons.
- When speaking to a patient with hearing loss who can read lips, person can stand directly in front of him with the light on the face and speak slowly and distinctly
- Approach the patient within his visual range and get his attention by raising arm or waving
- Do not smile, chew gum or cover your mouth when talking. It makes lip reading more difficult
- Make other staff members and hospital personnel aware of the patient's handicap condition and his established method of communication.
- Carefully explain all diagnostic tests and hospital procedures in a way the patient understands
- Keep the patient with hearing loss in an area in which he can observe unit activities and can approach people.
- Speak slowly and distinctly in a low tone; avoid shouting
- Provide emotional support and encouragement to the patient who is learning to use a hearing aid.
- Educate him how the aid works and how to maintain it

- Patient may be referred to an audiologist or laryngologist for further evaluation.
- Help to prevent hearing loss, monitor for signs of hearing impairment in patients receiving, ototoxic drugs

Communication with Patients Having Hearing Impairment

- Anticipate patient's needs and pay attention to non verbal cues.
- Before initiating conversation, get the patient's attention. Do not approach a patient from behind.
- Maintain eye contact with patient when speaking; Stand close, within patient's line of vision (generally midline). Patients may have defect in field of vision or may need to see the nurse's face or lips to enhance understanding of what is being communicated.
- Face the patient and stand or sit on the same level.
- Decrease background noises.
- Talk at a moderate rate and at a normal tone of voice.
- The nurse should spare time to attend all of the details of patient care.
- Address the person directly; make sure that patient can see you and room should be well lighted.
- Avoid talking when you have something in mouth; avoid covering your mouth with hand.
- Keep your voice at the same volume through the sentence and do not drop it at the end of each sentence.
- Do not over articulate mouthing or overdoing articulation. Use shorter phrases and sentences.
- Place important objects within reach.
- Make efforts to enhance patient's sense of independence.
- Make efforts to enhance patient's sense of independence.
- Provide alternate means of communication for times when interpreters are not available (e.g., a phone contact who can interpret the patient's needs).
- Use written information to enhance the spoken word.
- Encourage patient's attempts to communicate, praise attempts and achievements.
- Listen attentively when patient attempts to communicate.
- Clarify understanding of the patient's communication with the patient or an interpreter.
- Keep distractions such as television and radio at a minimum when talking to patient. This will keep patient focused and enhance the nurse's ability listen.
- Change to a new subject at a slower rate, making sure the person follow the change in subject.
- Do not speak loudly unless patient's hearing is impaired. Loud talking does not improve the patient's ability to understand, if the barriers are primary language.
- If the patient's ability to speak is limited to yes and no answers, try to phrase questions accordingly so that the patient can use these responses
- Use short sentences and ask only one question at a time. This allows the patient to stay focused on one thought.
- Allow the patient to complete his/her sentence and thought, but if the patient appears to be having difficulty, ask the patient for permission to help them.
- Be calm and accepting during attempts.
- Provide patient with word and phrase cards, writing pad and pencil or picture board. This is especially helpful for intubated and tracheal patients or those whose jaws are wired.
- Consult a speech therapist for additional help. See that patient is well-rested before each session with the speech therapist. Fatigue may have an adverse effect on learning ability.
- Encourage family member/caregiver to talk to patient even though patient may not respond. This decreases patient's sense of isolation and may assist in recovery from aphasia.
- Encourage patient to socialize with family and friends.
- Communication should be encouraged despite impairment.
- Provide patient an appointment with a speech therapist.
- Deaf patients and their families should be referred to their local hearing society for community support, education and sign language training
- If the patient wear a hearing aid, make sure it is in place and in working order.
- Use visible expression, speak with your hands, your face, and your eyes.
- Talk toward the patient's best or normal ear
- **Do not restrict a deaf patient's hands:**
  - Get the patient's attention by touch and maintain eye contact.
  - Have glasses and hearing aids or amplifiers, large print, if needed.
  - Have notebook and marker available to write key words or phrases that emphasize or reinforce your message.
  - Use picture boards in addition to your words to explain medical procedures.
  - Use pointing and gestures as you speak
  - Speak slowly, enunciate, and in short sentences or phrases. Pause 10 seconds to wait for the patient's response before going on.
  - Consult with your hospital's speech language pathologists who are skilled at assessing communication impaired patients and can recommend low tech and electronic augmentative communication tools.

Aural Rehabilitation

- If hearing loss is permanent or cannot be treated by medical or surgical means or if the patient selects not to undergo surgery, aural rehabilitation may be beneficial.
- The purpose of aural rehabilitation is to maximize the hearing-impaired person's communication skills. Aural rehabilitation includes:
  - Auditory training to improve the listening skills.
  - Speech reading or lip reading to help in filling the gaps left by missed or misheard words
  - Speech training conserve, develop and prevent deterioration of current skills.
  - Use of hearing aids according to the degree of hearing impairment.

Prevention

- Many environmental factors have an adverse effect on the auditory system and with time it may result in permanent sensorineural hearing loss. The most common is noise.

- Try to prevent unnecessary noise.
- Do not put unnecessary things in ear as it is a delicate organ
- Clean the car carefully for impacted wax with soft ear buds
- Give health education to patients to seek proper medical advice when a child is complaining an earache.
- Hard articles such as glass medicine dropper, hairpin, toothpick or match stick should never be inserted into the car because it may perforate the eardrum.

People should be encouraged to seek medical advice, if they are experiencing the following:

- Increasing earache or headache even after application of heat
- Reddish fluid oozing from the ear (may indicate rupture of the eardrum).
- Temperature elevation greater than 30°C (120°F).
- Convulsive twitching of the facial muscles or dizziness.
- Children should be taught to avoid inserting hard articles into the ear canal.
- Avoid swimming in stagnant water or water identified as being polluted because this may lead to ear infection.
- Viral diseases, such as measles can cause hearing impairment in the fetus, immunization program and treatment of the pregnant woman who contracts the disease can prevent hearing loss in the infant.
- Good care is essential in preventing hearing loss in high-risk infants, e.g., prematured postnatally anoxic infants.
- Children under the age of 3 with upper respiratory infections should be seen by a physician. If they indicate any symptoms related to the ear.
- Prevent high intensity music
- Give health education to persons regarding exposure to industrial noise.
- Persons taking certain drugs that have ototoxic effects should give health education regarding the signs and symptoms to prevent hearing loss, e.g., dizziness, decreased hearing acuity or tinnitus.

Patient with Impaired Olfactory Senses

- Patient should be taught with the dangers of using chemicals like ammonia.
- Patient need to keep gas stove in good working condition, since leakage goes undetected.
- Food poisoning is a concern as patient would not be able to detect rotten food, instructs the patient to carefully inspect food for freshness.

UNCONSCIOUSNESS

- Unconsciousness occurs when an individual is unable to respond to other people and activities. According to doctors, it is also a comatose state.
- In other words, unconsciousness is a state of complete or partial unawareness or lack of response to sensory stimuli.

Definition of Unconsciousness

- Unconsciousness can be defined as, "A state in which the cerebral functions is decreased and the individual is unresponsive to sensory stimuli".
- "The part of mind not readily accessible to conscious awareness but whose existence may be manifested in symptom formation, in dream or under the influence of drugs".

Etiology

- **Structural:** Brain lesions that destroy tissue or occupy space that is normally occupied by the brain.
  - Epilepsy
  - Tumors
  - Trauma
- **Cardiovascular:** Temporary or permanent interruption in the blood supply to the brain.
  - Vasovagal response
  - Cerebrovascular Accident (CVA)
  - Hypertensive encephalopathy
  - Shock
  - Dysrhythmias
- **Metabolic:** Abnormally high or low levels of circulating metabolites.
  - Hypoxia
  - Hypoglycemia
  - Hyperglycemia
  - Renal failure (uremia)
  - Liver failure
  - Infection (sepsis)
- **Environmental:** External factors that cause deterioration of central nervous system function.
  - Overdose
  - Toxins
- **Behavioral:** Abnormal mental status that results from internal factors. Psychiatric disorders decreases the individual's to sensory stimuli.

Risk Factors

- Injury to head by fall or blow.
- Diabetes affects blood sugar.
- Substance abuse and alcohol abuse.
- Hepatic encephalopathy.
- Uremia
- Infection

Pathological Changes

See **Flowchart 10.1**.

Clinical Manifestations

Structural Changes

- Decreased wakefulness
- Decreased attention to surrounding environment
- Confusion
- Disorientation
- Agitation
- Poor memory
- Decreased ability to carry out activities of daily living
- Decreased mobility
- Incontinence
- Irritability
- Unwillingness to cooperate

Flowchart 10.1: Pathological changes in unconsciousness.

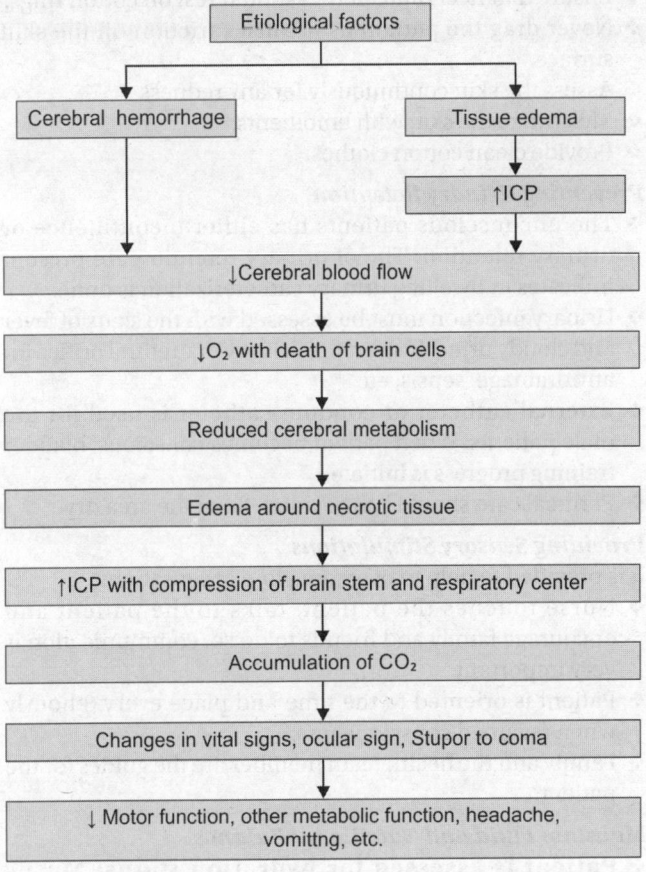

- Headache
- Disturbed vital functions

Sensory-perceptual Alterations
- Hallucination
- Delusions
- Illusion

Diagnostic Evaluation
- On physical examination including neurological assessment, physician will observe the patient's movement or reflexes, response to painful stimuli and the size of pupil.
- Observe the breathing pattern of patient which helps to diagnose the cause of coma.
- **Following laboratory tests are performed for the diagnosis of unconsciousness:**
  - Complete blood count (CBC), arterial blood gases (ABGs).
  - Carbon monoxide poisoning screen or alcohol overdose screening.
  - Electrolytes, glucose, thyroid, liver and kidney function tests.
  - Skull, chest and spinal X-ray studies.
  - ECG
  - CSF analysis
- **CT scan:** It is performed to rule out brain hemorrhage, tumors, strokes and other conditions.
- **MRI:** It is performed for the detection of brain tissue damaged by an ischemic stroke, brain hemorrhage or other conditions.
- **EEG:** It helps to measure the electrical activity inside the brain.

Management
Medical Management
First aid:
- The main aim of first aid is to ensure that patient's air passage remains open and clear.
- Note any alteration in the state of unconscious ness either improving or deteriorating
- If patient is unresponsive, there is no breathing only gasping. Then, activate emergency response and get defibrillator.
- Check pulse and initiate high quality CPR which improves patient's chance of survival.

CPR:
- **Compression:** Place hands on patient's chest. Push at least two inches deep on an adult breast bone and 100 times per minute to move oxygenated blood to the vital organs of patient.
- **Airway:** Open the airway and observe the breathing or blockage. Observe for chest rise and fall and listen the movement of air.
- **Breathing:** In this, tilt the chin of patient back for the unobstructed passing of air. Then, give two breaths and resume chest compressions.
- The primary focus of medical management is to maintain the oxygen supply and glucose to the brain.

Nursing Management
- A nurse should address the patient by his/her name.
- Note changes in response to stimuli.
- Note the return of protective reflexes, such as blinking the eyelids or swallowing saliva.
- Maintain a patent airway by proper positioning of the patient.
- Always observe the patient carefully when administering anything.
- Patient should be given a comfortable bath every other day. This prevents the drying of the skin.
- Change patient's position at least every two hours.
- Protect the patient from any injury.
- Provide passive exercises to the patient.
- Provide emotional and psychological support to the patient.

Complications
- Coma
- Brain damage
- Fractured ribs from the chest compression during CPR
- Choking

Nursing Care Plan
Nursing Assessment
- Monitor and record patient's vital signs.

- Assess respiratory rate pattern, papillary reaction, motor response and superficial reflexes.
- Assess patient's medical history.
- Assess level of consciousness using Glasgow Coma
- Scale (GCS)
- Assess self-care needs; self-care deficits of patient.

Nursing Diagnosis
- Ineffective airway clearance related to upper airway obstruction by tongue and soft tissues, inability to clear respiratory secretions.
- Risk for injury related to unconscious state.
- Risk for impaired skin integrity related to immobility.
- Impaired urinary elimination related to impairment in sensing and control.
- Disturbed sensory perception related to neurologic impairment.
- Interrupted family process related to health crisis.
- Risk for impaired nutritional status.

Planning
Nursing Goals
- To maintain airway clearance.
- To reduce risk for injury.
- To maintain skin integrity.
- To prevent urinary retention.
- To provide sensory stimulation.
- To maintain fluid balance and managing nutritional needs.

Nursing Interventions
Maintaining a Patent Airway
- Check the altered breathing pattern.
- Suctioning should be kept minimum
- Use an oral artificial airway to maintain patency.
- ABG results must be interpreted to determine the degree oxygenation by the ventilators or oxygen.
- Check vital signs and level of consciousness, pupils.
- Insert oral airway if patient's tongue is paralyzed or is obstructing the airway.
- Connect the patient to mechanical ventilator as needed.
- Auscultate patient's chest at least every 8 hours.
- Avoid restraints as far as possible.
- Provide oral hygiene 4 hourly.

Risk for Injury
- Side rails must be kept whenever the patient is not receiving direct care.
- Seizure precautions must be taken.
- Adequate support must be given to limbs and head.
- Assess the need for restrain.
- Over sedation should be avoided.

Maintaining Skin Integrity
- Provide back care and back massage observe.
- Pressure points for any pressure sores.
- Maintain proper body alignment.
- Use splints to prevent foot drops and contractors (deformities).
- Perform passive exercises of extremities.
- Ensure that heels and elbows should rest on cotton rings.
- Never drag the patient as it causes friction on the skin surface.
- Assess the skin continuously for any redness
- Moisturize the skin with emollients.
- Provide clean cotton clothes.

Preventing Urinary Retention
- The unconscious patients has either incontinence or urinary retention. The of urinary retention are present indicates in dwelling urinary catheterization is done.
- Urinary infection must be assessed with the signs of fever and cloudy urine. Inspect the urinary or urethral orifice for any drainage, sepsis, etc.
- External catheter or condom catheter is used for the male patients. When patient becomes conscious, bladder training progress is initiated
- Perineal care should be provided. Keep the area dry.

Providing Sensory Stimulations
It is provided to help to overcome loss of sensation.
- Nurse touches the patient, talks to the patient and encourage family and friends to do so, communication is very important.
- Patient is oriented to the time and place every 8 hourly when regained consciousness.
- Family and the health team member are the guides for the patient.

Maintain Fluid and Nutritional Balance
- **Patient is assessed for hydration status:** Mucus membrane, skin, skin turgor.
- I/V solutions and blood transfusions must be administered slowly as it could raise ICP.
- Nasogastric or gastrostomy feeding are given to meet nutritional needs.
- The fluid electrolyte balance is monitored by strict intake output recording.
- Patient education and health maintenance
- Instruct family members to protect the patient from falling off the bed.
- Regular change in position.
- Back massage.
- Avoid speaking negative about the patient.
- Keep bed and bedding free of moisture, dust and debris.
- Keep patient's nails short.

Evaluation: Expected Outcomes
- Airway clearance is maintained.
- Risk of injury is reduced.
- Skin integrity is maintained.
- Urinary retention is prevented.
- Sensory stimulation is provided.
- Fluid and nutritional balance is maintained.

Care of Terminally Ill, Death and Dying

CONCEPTS OF LOSS

A person experiences loss in the absence of an object, person's body part or function, or emotion that was formerly present.

Types/Categories of Loss

There are five categories of loss:

1. **Loss of external object:** It involves any possession that is worn-out, misplaced, stolen or ruined by disaster, e.g., jewelry, money, etc.
2. **Loss of a known environment:** It is a loss associated with separation from a known environment, includes familiar setting for a period or relocating permanently and transfers from place to place like hospitalization.
3. **Loss of significant others:**
   - It includes loss of parents, spouses, children, siblings, teachers, friends, neighbors and colleagues.
   - And also entertainment figures and well-known persons like cine actors, athletes, cricketers, popular figures of a particular field.
4. **Loss of an aspect of life:**
   - It includes loss of a body part, physiological function, or psychological function, e.g., loss of limb, eye, hair, teeth, breast, etc.
   - Loss of urinary or bowel control, loss of memory, humor of self-esteem, of self-confidence, of power of respect, of love, self-concept, self-Identity of job.
5. **Loss of life:**
   - Each person responds differently to death.
   - Some will welcome death as a relief; some will have fear of separation, abandonment, loneliness, or mutilation, etc.

Other Classifications of Loss

- **Actual loss:** It is easily identified and can be recognized by others as well as person sustaining the loss, loss of a limb, of a spouse, of an object and of a job.
- **Perceived loss:** It is felt by the person but is intangible or less intangible soothers. For example—Maceration loss, loss resulting from normal life transitions (loss of youth, of financial independence).
- **Situational loss:** Occurring suddenly in reference to a specific external event (sudden death of loved one)
- Other example of actual or perceived loss is physical loss, and psychological loss, e.g., losing limb from accident, limb leads to loss of self-image.
- **Anticipatory loss:** Anticipatory loss in which a person displays loss and grief behavior for a loss that has yet to take place, e.g., sickness or death.

GRIEF, BEREAVEMENT AND MOURNING

Grief

- Grief is the emotional response or reaction to a loss in a person's life.
- This loss can refer to a death but it can also refer to the loss of physical or cognitive abilities or the loss of something that was routine in his life such as a job
- It is manifested in a variety of ways that are unique to an individual and is based on personal experience, cultural expectations and spiritual beliefs.
- Bereavement includes grief and mourning the inner feelings and outwards reactions of the survivor.
- In addition to the emotional expression of grief, grief can be expressed in physical, behavioral, social, and cognitive ways.

Bereavement

- It is the inner feelings and outward reactions of the survivor.
- Bereavement refers to the time when a person experiences sadness after losing a loved one.
- It is the period after a loss during which grief and mourning occurs.
- The time spent in a period of bereavement depends on how attached the person was to the person who died, and how much time was spent anticipating the loss.
- Survivors go through a bereavement period that is not linear. It is the period during which the grief process unfolds.

Mourning

- Mourning is the process by which people adapt to a loss.
- Mourning can also defined as acts or outward expressions of grief.
- Mourning often goes along with grief

- Mourning involves religious beliefs or rituals, and may be affected by our ethnic background and cultural customs.
- Some common examples of mourning can include preparing for a funeral, wearing black or sharing memories or stories about a loved one.
- These parts of the mourning process can be impacted by cultural practices or rituals and can give structure to the grieving process.
- Losing someone can be considered a threat or risk of harm to the brain, so the process of mourning can help people to accept and emotionally process death or loss.
- The process of mourning allows people to form long-term memories of a loved one, and includes adapting and learning new ways to carry on without a person they cared deeply about.
- Mourning can be a lengthy and painful process, but it is a healthy part of bereavement.
- Mourning can help people preserve the memory of loved ones and feel hopeful about living a happy and fulfilling life without them.
- Although mourning can be painful, the mourning process allows people to re-engage with their daily life and to feel joy and happiness again.

TYPES OF GRIEF RESPONSES

Normal Grief

- Normal or uncomplicated grief consists of the normal feelings, behaviors, and reactions to losses.
- These might include resentment, sorrow, anger, crying, loneliness and temporarily withdrawal from activities.
- Often the normal grief response to a loss can prove positive, helping one to mature and develop as a person.
- As people mature they develop ways of dealing with losses and learn to maintain and enhance their feelings of safety and security.
- Many people define normal grief as the ability to move towards acceptance of the loss.
- With this comes a gradual decrease in the intensity of emotions.
- Those who experience normal grief are able to continue to function in their basic daily activities.

Anticipatory Grief

- The process of disengaging or "letting go" that occurs before an actual loss or death has occurred is called anticipatory grief.
- For example, once a person or family receives a terminal diagnosis, they begin the process of saying good bye and completing life affairs.
- The process becomes more stressful when the patient is unable to make decisions due to deterioration in health.
- Unless guided by a patient's explicit decision regarding end of life care, the family assumes the responsibility of deciding whether to continue life sustaining measures.
- For family caregivers, grieving can start long before the person you are caring for actually passes away.
- There are risks in anticipatory grieving.
- The family members may withdraw emotionally from the patient too soon, leaving the patient with no emotional support as death approaches.
- It can be difficult to speak with others about anticipatory grief because the person you care for is still alive and you may have feelings of guilt or confusion as to why you are feeling this kind of grief.

Disenfranchised Grief (Ambiguous)

- Disenfranchised grief can be felt when someone experiences a loss but others do not acknowledge the importance of the loss in the person's life.
- Others may not understand the importance of the loss or they may minimize the significance of the loss.
- Disenfranchised grief occur when someone experiences the loss of an ex-spouse, a pet, or a co worker.
- The other side of disenfranchised grief is when you experience a loss, such as when the person you are caring for has dementia or a decline in their physical abilities.
- The person is physically present but they are also absent in other significant ways.

Chronic Grief

- This type of grief can be experienced in many ways—through feelings of hopelessness, a sense of disbelief that the loss is real, avoidance of any situation that may remind someone of the loss, or loss of meaning and value in a belief system.
- At times, people with chronic grief can experience intrusive thoughts.
- If left untreated, chronic grief can develop into severe clinical depression, suicidal or self-harming thoughts, and even substance abuse.

Cumulative Grief

- This type of grief can occur when multiple losses are experienced, often within a short period of time.
- Cumulative grief can be stressful because you do not have time to properly grieve one loss before experiencing the next.

Complicated Grief (Traumatic or Prolonged)

- When a person has difficulty progressing through the normal phases or stages of grieving, bereavement becomes complicated.
- Complicated grief refers to normal grief that becomes severe in longevity and significantly impairs the ability to function.
- It can be difficult to judge when grief has lasted too long.
- Other contributing factors in diagnosing complicated or prolonged grief include looking at the nature of the loss or death (was it sudden? violent? multiple?).
- The relationship, personality, life experiences, and other social issues.
- Some warning signs that someone is experiencing traumatic grief include—self-destructive behavior, deep

and persistent feelings of guilt, low self-esteem, suicidal thoughts, violent outbursts, or radical lifestyle changes.
- In these cases, bereavement appears to go wrong and loss never resolves.

TYPES OF COMPLICATED GRIEF

Unresolved Grief
- It lasts much longer, at times for many years.
- It is much more severe and intense, not lessening with time but instead often worsening and interferes with a person's ability to function normally in daily life.
- Factors, it tends to be more common in people who have low self esteem, feel guilty about the loss, or struggle with their feelings about the deceased.
- It also tends to affect those experiencing an unexpected and perhaps violent death of a loved one or those suffering from a loss that others do not readily recognize, such as a miscarriage

Exaggerated Grief
- The persons become overwhelmed by grief, and they cannot function.
- This may be reflected in form of severe phobias or self destructive behavior, such as alcoholism, substance abuse, or suicide.

Inhibited Grief
- Appears when the griever avoids facing the realities of losing something or someone by turning their attention to other things.
- People may put all their time and energy into something that will keep them distracted and they hide their feelings in the hopes this will avoid pain.
- However, inhibited grief can lead to exhaustion and manifest itself in physical symptoms like migraines, digestive issues, nausea, etc.

Delayed Grief
- May result from pressing responsibilities (e.g., funeral arrangements) that the mourner needs to attend to, resulting in postponed grief that may last for years.
- An experience of grief may eventually be triggered by another loss or an event related to the original loss.
- Characterized by normal grief reactions that are suppressed or postponed and survivor consciously or unconsciously avoids the pain of the loss
- Active grieving is held back, only to resurface later, usually in response to a trivial loss or upset
- For example, a wife may only bereave a few weeks after the death of her spouse, only to become hysterical and sad a year
- Later when she attends a family gathering the extreme sadness is a delayed response to the death of her husband.

MANIFESTATIONS OF GRIEF

They can be classified in two ways:

I. First Classification
1. **Physical reactions:**
   - Loss of appetite
   - Weight loss
   - Insomnia
   - Fatigue
   - Decreased libido
   - Decreased immune function
   - Multiple somatic complaints
2. **Psychosocial reactions:**
   - Profound sadness
   - Helplessness
   - Hopelessness
   - Denial
   - Anger
   - Hostility
   - Guilt
   - Nightmares
   - Preoccupation with lost object
   - Loneliness
3. **Cognitive reactions:**
   - Inability to concentrate
   - Forgetfulness
   - Impaired judgment
   - Decreased problem solving ability
4. **Behavioral reactions:**
   - Impulsivity
   - Indecisive
   - Social withdrawal
   - Distancing

II. Second Classification

Worden (2005) identified four categories that demonstrate normal grief.

This includes ***feelings, cognitions, physical sensations and behaviors***.

It is also important to remember that these signs of grief will vary from individual to individual.

- **Feelings:**
  - Sadness is a common feeling experienced after the loss of a loved one.
  - This is often demonstrated by crying, a gesture that evokes a sympathetic and protective reaction from others.
  - Numbness or shock is often experienced immediately after a loss.
  - This serves as a defense to block pain and to protect the bereaved from being overwhelmed.
  - It allows opportunity to be gradually introduced to the reality of the loss.
  - Anger is frequently associated with loss.
  - It is not uncommon for the anger experienced to be directed at either the deceased of the bereaved, the bereaved themselves-or both.
  - The anger comes from a sense of frustration due to an inability to prevent the death and as a regressive experience that occurs after losing someone close.

- Guilt is also common in the process of grief
- The bereaved might feel guilty about being alive while he loved one is dead.
- Anxiety is a common feeling associated with loss and it comes primarily from; a fear that they will not be able to take care of themselves and a heightened sense of personal death awareness.
- The anxiety experienced may vary from mild anxiety to more extreme panic attacks. Other feelings associated with grief include loneliness, fatigue, helplessness.

❖ **Cognitions:**
- The most common cognitive response to death is a preoccupation with the deceased, which occurs as a form of obsessional thinking.
- This commonly occurs in the early stages of grief and disappears after a short while.
- Prolonged experience thoughts may trigger depression.
- Hallucination (visual and auditory) of the deceased loved one is also a frequent experience of the bereaved.
- Other cognitive responses may include confusion, disbelief, and passive suicidal thoughts.

❖ **Physical sensations:**
- In addition to feelings and cognitions associated with grief, there are also physical sensations that transpire during the grieving process.
- Although often overlooked, they may be key indicators of the individual's grief reaction.
- Examples of commonly reported physical sensations are listed below:
  - Physical sensations of grief:
    - Hollowness in the pit of the stomach
    - Tightness in the chest and throat
    - Oversensitivity to noise
    - Breathlessness
    - Lack of energy
    - Dry mouth
    - Muscular weakness

❖ **Behaviors:**
- There are a number of behaviors associated with a normal grief reaction too.
- These are often experienced immediately after a loss and correct themselves over time.
- Disturbances in sleep and eating patterns are very common during times of grief.
- Absent mindedness and social withdrawal are also common behaviors that are evident in the grieving process.
- Behaviors, such as dreams of the deceased and avoiding reminders of the deceased are also reported in the early stages following loss.

FACTORS INFLUENCING LOSS AND GRIEF RESPONSES

Human Development
❖ Persons of different ages and stages of development will show different and unique symptoms of grief.

❖ For example, toddlers are unable to understand loss or death, but they feel great anxiety over loss of an object and separation from parents.
❖ School-age children experience grief over the loss of a body part or function.
❖ They often associate misdeeds with causing death.
❖ Middle-age adults usually begin to re-examine life and sensitive to their own physical changes.
❖ Older adults often experience anticipatory grief because of aging and loss of self-care abilities.

Socioeconomic Status
❖ Socioeconomic status influence a person's ability to obtain options and use support mechanism when coping with loss.
❖ Generally an individual feels greater burden from a loss when there is lack of financial, educational or occupational resources.
❖ For example, a patient with limited finances may not be able to replace a home lost in a fire or may not be able to purchase necessary medications to manage a newly diagnosed disease.

Personal Relationship
❖ When loss involves a loved one, the quality and meaning of relationship are critical in understanding a person's grief experience.
❖ When a relationship between two individual is very close and well connected, it can be very difficult for the one left behind to cope.
❖ The support that the patient receives from the family and friends is based on part of their relationship with members of their social network and the manner and circumstances of their loss.

Nature of the Loss
❖ The ability to resolve grief depends on meaning of the loss and the situation surrounding the loss.
❖ The ability to accept help from others influences whether the bereaved will be able to cope effectively.
❖ The visibility of the loss influences the support a person receives.

Culture and Ethnicity
❖ Culture affects how patients and their support system or families respond to loss.
❖ For example, in western hemisphere, the grieving process is usually personal and private, with individual showing restrained emotions.
❖ However, ceremonies surrounding a person's death offer time for grief resolution and reminiscing
❖ In Eastern Nations, such as China, respect for dead is shown by wailing and physical demonstration of grief for a specified period of time.

Spiritual Beliefs
❖ Individual's spirituality significantly influences their ability to cope with loss.

- Patient who have a strong interconnections with a higher power or others are often very resilient and able to face death with relatively minimal discomfort.

THEORIES OF GRIEF AND LOSS—KUBLER ROSS

- **Dr Elisabeth Kubler Ross** has described the stages through which many terminally-ill patients progress.
- These are denial, anger, bargaining, depression and acceptance.
- These stages occur in progressive fashion or a person can move back and forth through the stages.

There is no specific time period for the completion of these stages:

The behavioral theory developed by psychiatrist Elisabeth Kubler Ross in 1969 suggests that people go through five distinct stages of grief after the loss of a loved one: *Denial, anger, bargaining, depression, and finally acceptance.*

The Five Stages of Grief is one of the best-known grief theories.

Kubler Ross's Five Stages of Dying

- Kubler Ross originally developed stages to describe the process patients with terminal illness go through as they come to terms with their own deaths; it was later applied to grieving friends and family as well, who seemed to undergo a similar process.
- People may not experience these stages in a particular order

The stages, popularly known by the acronym D-A-B-D-A, include:

Denial

- The first reaction is denial.
- It is a common defense mechanism used to protect oneself from the hardship of considering an upsetting reality.
- Kubler Ross noted that patients would often reject the reality of the new information after the initial shock of receiving a terminal diagnosis.
- Patients may directly deny the diagnosis, attribute it to faulty tests or an unqualified physician, or simply avoid the topic in conversation.
- A period of denial is quite normal in the context of terminal illness

Reactions: No-not ME

Nursing Implications

- Verbally support patient but do not reinforce denial.
- Try to avoid directly contradicting with patient.
- Find out what patient and family members were told.
- Examine your own behavior to ensure that you do not share in patient's denial.

Anger

- Anger is commonly experienced and expressed by patients as they concede the reality of a terminal illness.
- When the individual recognizes that denial cannot continue, they become frustrated, especially at proximate individuals.
- Certain psychological responses of a person undergoing this phase would be: "Why me? It's not fair!"; "How can this happen to me?"; "Who is to blame?"; "Why would this happen?"
- The anger may also be generalized and undirected, manifesting as a shorter temper or a loss of patience

Reactions: Why me

Nursing Implications

- Help patient to understand that anger is a normal response to feelings of loss and powerlessness
- Avoid withdrawal or retaliation; do not take anger personally.
- Deal with needs underlying any angry reaction.
- Provide structure and continuity to promote feelings of security

Bargaining

- The third stage involves the hope that the individual can avoid a cause of grief.
- Usually, the negotiation for an extended life is made in exchange for a reformed lifestyle.
- **People facing less:** Serious trauma can bargain or seek compromise.
- Examples include the terminally-ill person who "negotiates with God" to attend a daughter's wedding, an attempt to bargain for more time to live in exchange for a reformed lifestyle or a phrase, such as "If I could trade their life for mine".
- Many patients put their personals in order, make wills and fulfill lost wishes, such as trips, visiting relative, etc.
- It is important to meet these wishes if possible, because bargaining helps patients more into later stages of dying.

Reactions: Yes-but

Nursing Implications

- Listen attentively and encourage patient to talk to relieve guilt and irrational fear.
- If appropriate, offer spiritual support.

Depression

- Depression is perhaps the most immediately understandable of Kubler Ross's stages, and patients experience it with unsurprising symptoms, such as sadness, fatigue, and anhedonia (reduced ability to experience pleasure). "I'm so sad, why bother with anything?"; "I'm going to die soon, so what's the point?"; "I miss my loved one; why go on?"
- During the fourth stage, the individual despairs at the recognition of their death.
- In this state, the individual may become silent, refuse visitors and spend much of the time mournful and sullen.

Reactions: Yes, me

Nursing Implications

- Allow patient to express sadness.
- Communicate nonverbally by sitting quietly without expecting conversation.
- Convey caring by touch.

Acceptance

- Acceptance describes recognizing the reality of a difficult diagnosis while no longer protesting or struggling against it.
- Patients may choose to focus on enjoying the time they have left and reflecting on their memories.
- They may begin to prepare for death practically by planning their funeral or helping to provide financially or emotionally for their loved ones. "It's going to be okay."; "I can't fight it; I may as well prepare for it."

Reactions: I am ready

Nursing Implications

- Help family and friends to understand patient's decrease need to socialize.
- Encourage patient to participate as much as possible in treatment program.

THE R PROCESS MODEL (RANDO'S)

Rando's six "R" process of mourning

- Grief is not as simple as a list of steps or stages, and everyone grieves in their own unique way.
- Dr Therese Rando is the Clinical Director at the Institute for the Study and Treatment of Loss since 1970.
- It was her extensive research and experience in helping the bereaved that led her to develop her own grief model.

The Six R's of Mourning

- Dr Rando defines mourning as six distinct states (the six R's).
- She then groups each state into three emotional categories.

The Six R's are

- Recognize and accept the reality of loss
- React to the separation
- Recollect and re-experience
- Relinquish old attachments
- Readjust
- Reinvest

Rando contributed a stage model of the grief process that she observed people to experience while adjusting to significant loss.

She called her model the "Six R's":

- **Recognize the loss:** First, people must experience their loss and understand that it has happened.
- **React:** People react emotionally to their loss.
- **Recollect and Re-experience:** People may review memories of their lost relationship (events that occurred, places visited together or day to day moments that were experienced together).
- **Relinquish:** People begin to put their loss behind them, realizing and accepting that the world has truly changed and that there is no turning back.
- **Readjust:** People begin the processes of daily life and the loss starts to feel less acute and sharp.
- **Reinvest:** Ultimately, people re-enter the world, forming new relationships and commitments. They accept the changes that have occurred.

The three emotional categories are:
1. Avoidance Phase
2. Confrontation Phase
3. Accommodation Phase

Avoidance Phase

- Here the person tries to avoid the reality.
- The avoidance phase has one task-recognize the loss.
- This is the early part of mourning where we must accept the reality of a loss.
- Rando suggests that until we complete the first R where we recognize and acknowledge death has occurred, we'll remain in this phase of emotional avoidance.
- Once we are ready to accept the fact that our loved one has passed, we move into what Rando calls the confrontation phase.

Confrontation Phase

- The confrontation phase consists of dealing with our grief finding ways to in which we can express the complex set of emotions we feel. During this phase, there are three tasks.
- We must react to the separation.
- This process means w will react to our emotions, as well as the changes created by our loss.
- These changes are known as secondary losses. For example, a secondary loss includes the loss of a sense of security, identity, or traditions and routines.
- During the confrontation phase, we also recollect and re experience our relationship with the deceased.
- This process involves reviewing memories and experiences shared with the loved one.
- For example, it could be special places visited together, or even the small day-to-day moments shared together.
- As we go through this recollection phase, these memories become a critical part of how we continue our relationship with the loved one after they are gone.
- The last R in the confrontation phase involves relinquishing old attachments.
- This task is a long process.
- It involves accepting that our old life will never be the same after the loss, and we start processing the impact the loss has on us.

Accommodation Phase

- This phase features the final two R's of Rando's model.
- In this phase, we begin to find meaning-from both the loss and life again.
- It does not mean we would not experience some of the other R's again, such as the recollection or reactions to loss, but we do begin to move toward moments of happiness again.
- In this phase, we start to readjust to our new reality. We start to accept our new roles in life and our new responsibilities.
- For example, a widow or widower will start to take on their new roles as the sole caretaker of the household.
- Dr Rando describes this part as moving "adaptively into the new world without forgetting the old."
- We also reinvest our emotional energy. This means we begin to find a sense of happiness from life again.

- We might start a new hobby or project, or even find new sense of purpose.
- It is important to note that this does not mean closure or getting over a loss.
- Instead, Rando describes this stage as learning to live again.

DEATH

Definition

"Death is as the cessation of all vital functions of the body including the heartbeat, Brain activity (including the brain stem) and breathing." —**Medical dictionary**

"A permanent cessation of all vital functions: the end of life. The state of being no longer alive: the state of being dead" —**Merriam Webster's dictionary**

Meaning

Clinical death is the medical term for cessation of blood circulation and breathing, the two criteria necessary to sustain the lives of human beings and of many other organisms. It occurs when the heart stops beating in a regular rhythm, a condition called cardiac arrest.

Biological death: It occurs four-six minutes after clinical death. This is due to the fact that the heart is the main pumping machine of the body and without the blood coming from the heart, the brain gradually ceases to function until it achieves irreversible damage.

Uniform Determination of Death Act (UDDA)

"An individual who has sustained either:
1. Irreversible cessation of circulatory and respiratory functions,
2. Irreversible cessation of all functions of the entire brain, including the brain stem, is dead".

Death was defined in *1981 by the president commission for the study of ethical problems in medicine and biomedical and behavioral research as:* Death is present, if an individual has sustained:
1. Irreversible cessation of circulatory and respiratory functions
2. Irreversible cessation of all functions of entire brain, including the brainstem.

Death: Death is defined as a state when an individual has sustained either irreversible damage to circulatory and respiratory functions or irreversible malfunctioning of the entire brain, including the brain stems.

Types of Death

1. **Brain death:**
   - *Brain death* is sometimes used as a legal definition of death. The remains of a previously living organism normally begin to decompose shortly after death.
   - *Brain death:* It is the irreversible damage to cerebrum, cerebellum and midbrain. The damage is so severe that there is no hope for recovery and the patient life must be maintained with respiratory and vaso-active drugs.
   - *Brain death (also known as brain stem death):* Occurs when a person on an artificial life support machine no longer has any brain functions. This means he will not regain consciousness or be able to breathe without support. Brain death is the irreversible loss of function of the brain and brain stem. Brain death occurs when brain function ceases because the flow of blood to the brain is stopped permanently due to a severe injury to the brain.
   - The definition of **brain death** includes the absence of brainstem reflexes, the inability to breathe without a ventilator, and neurologic unresponsiveness. A person, whose brain is dead, is legally confirmed as dead such as before an organ donation.
   - *Clinical criteria for brain death:*
     - Unresponsive coma with absence of motor and reflex response.
     - No spontaneous respiration (apnea)
     - No occulocephalic or oculo motor response with dilated and fixed pupil. Isoelectric (flat) EEG.
     - Persistence of the above sign for 30 minutes to 1 hour and for 6 hours after the onset of coma and apnea.

2. **Circulatory/Cardiac death:**
   - **Circulatory death** is the irreversible loss of function of the heart and lungs.
   - **Cardiac death:** When person suffers a cardiac death, the heart stops pumping the blood. This will lead to lack of circulation of blood, to the vital organs. If CPR is performed with in 4–6 minutes of clinical death the patient can revive and the chances of brain death is minimal.

SIGNS OF IMPENDING DEATH

Although death is unique for each individual, common physical and psychological events occur when death approaches.

Physical Events

Death usually occurs gradually over hours or days. Cells deteriorate from underlying lack of sufficient oxygen; which leads to multisystem failure.

The following are signs of impending death that alert the nurse that patient will die shortly:

- **Facial appearance:**
  - Facial muscles relax
  - Checks flaccid
  - Facial structure changes
  - Facies hippocratica (prominent cheeks, chin pinched, sharp nose, pale skin, sunken eyes)
- **Change in sight:**
  - Gradually fails.
  - Pupils fail to react to light.
  - Sunken eyes or films appear
- **Change in speech:**
  - Speaking with difficulty
  - Confused
  - Unintelligent

- ❖ **Hearing:** Senses become impaired but hearing tends to remain intact.
- ❖ **Pulmonary function impairment:**
  - Failure of the heart pumping function causes fluid to collect in pulmonary circulation.
  - Shallow respiration, rate is irregular.
- ❖ **Peripheral circulation changes:**
  - Reduced cardiac output.
  - Compromised peripheral circulation.
  - Impaired cellular metabolism.
  - Skin becomes pale, cold.
  - Nail beds and lips appear blue.
- ❖ **Central nervous system alteration:**
  - Patient experiences period of apnea.
  - Pain perception is decreased.
  - Senses become impaired.
  - Restlessness.
- ❖ **Renal impairment:**
  - Low cardiac output.
  - Decreased urine volume.
  - Waste products accumulate in the body.
- ❖ **Gastrointestinal disturbance:**
  - Peristalsis decreases, causing intestinal content
  - Nausea/vomiting.
  - Abdominal distension.
  - Inability to swallow, gag reflex disappears.
- ❖ **Musculoskeletal changes:**
  - Reflexes become hypoactive.
  - Patient loses control over sphincters leading to incontinence.
  - Jaw and facial muscles relax.

Psychological Events

- ❖ Reaching the stage of acceptance, i.e., some terminally ill patients look forward to dying because it will end their suffering.
- ❖ Some are seen to forestall dying when they feel their loved ones are not prepared.
- ❖ This is waiting for permission phenomenon.

Signs of Clinical Death

- ❖ Cessation of breathing is generally considered ultimate sign of death.
- ❖ The signs of clinical death are absence of pulse, heartbeat, respiration, pupils are non-reactive to light and absence of all reflexes.

DYING PATIENT'S BILL OF RIGHTS

- ❖ The right to be treated as a living human being
- ❖ The right to maintain a sense of hopefulness, however changing its focus may be useful.
- ❖ The right to be cared for by those who can maintain a sense of hopefulness, however changing this may be.
- ❖ The right to express feelings and emotions about death in one's own way.
- ❖ The right to participate in all decisions concerning one's care.
- ❖ The right to be cared for by compassionate, sensitive, knowledgeable people who will attempt to understand one's needs.
- ❖ The right to expect continuing medical care, even though the goals may change from "cure" to "comfort goals.
- ❖ The right to have all questions answered honestly and fully.
- ❖ The right to seek spirituality
- ❖ The right to be free of physical pain.
- ❖ The right to express feelings and emotions about pain in one's own way.
- ❖ The right of children to participate in death.
- ❖ The right to understand the process of death.
- ❖ The right to die.
- ❖ The right to die in peace and dignity.
- ❖ The right not to die alone.
- ❖ The right to expect that the sanctity of the body will be respected after death.
- ❖ The right to be cared for by caring, sensitive, knowledge able people who will attempt to understand patient needs and will be able to gain some satisfaction in helping face death.

CARE OF DYING PATIENT

Immediate Signs of Death

- ❖ The respiration becomes labored, irregular, rapid or very slow, noisy breathing (death rattle) sound of secretions moving in the airway.
- ❖ There is a weak thready pulse and falling blood pressure
- ❖ The heart rate decreases. As the oxygen supply to the brain decreases, the patient may become restless.
- ❖ **Death rattle:** A rattling sound heard in throat caused by secretions as the patient cannot cough longer.
- ❖ The skin becomes pale and cool, there is peripheral cyanosis, and the skin loses its turgor and has mottled appearance. The extremities are cold to touch.
- ❖ The sight gradually fails, the pupils fail to react to light, and sunken eyes are present.
- ❖ Mental confusion arises.
- ❖ Urinary output may decrease in amount and frequency.
- ❖ There may be incontinence of urine and distension in bladder because of loss of sphincter control.
- ❖ Difficulty talking or swallowing.
- ❖ Dying may occur suddenly as a result of an accident, injury or pathologic crisis, such as heart attack; or it may occur as a prolonged experience of debilitating disease, such as cancer, AIDS or multiple sclerosis.
- ❖ Some choose to die at home surrounded by loved ones.
- ❖ Others die alone or in intensive care surrounded by health care professionals and technological equipment.

Physical Care

- ❖ As patients become weaker they find it increasingly difficult to take oral drugs.
- ❖ Non-essential drugs should be discontinued.
- ❖ Drugs that need to be continued, such as opioids, anxiolytics, and antiemetics, should be converted to the subcutaneous route or by continuous infusion, if appropriate.

- Inappropriate interventions, including blood tests should be discontinued.
- Few studies suggest that continuing artificial fluids in the dying patient is of limited benefit and should in most cases be discontinued.
- Patients who are in the dying phase should not be subjected to "cardiopulmonary resuscitation," as this constitutes a futile and inappropriate medical treatment.
- The patient may have an advance directive that can be used to facilitate discussion about care at this time
- Regular observations should be made and good symptom control maintained, including control of pain.
- Attention to mouth care is essential in the dying patient, and the family can be encouraged to give sips of water or moisten the patient's mouth with a sponge.
- If urinary incontinence or retention is a problem, catheterization may be needed.
- Good physical care is still mandatory for a dying patient.
- Simply because a patient is dying and may only have a few days left to live does not give medical staff a reason to stop performing the basic activities of daily living.
- Good physical hygiene and oral hygiene will provide a sense of comfort as the end draws near.
- A sponge bath may soothe aches and pains unlike any pain medicines are capable of doing.
- A hand massage with lotion is an amazing way to help someone to forget about his constant pain, at least temporarily but helps to connect with the patient while talking one on one.

Prevention of Pressure Ulcers

- Prevention requires relieving pressure by rotating the patient after every 2 hrs; a specialized mattress or continuously inflated air suspension bed may also help.
- Incontinent patients should be kept as dry as possible.

Safety

Our first priority is always to protect the patient, providing care and comfort in his or her final days, regardless of the type of person he or she may have been prior to arriving at death's doorway.

Psychological Support

- Most dying patients experience some depression
- Providing psychological support and allowing patients to express concerns and feelings are usually the best approaches.
- Meet their spiritual needs according to their religious customs.
- Patients' insight into their condition should be assessed.
- Issues relating to dying and death should be explored appropriately and sensitively.
- Spend time with them and answer to their questions honestly.

Environment

Establish and maintain a peaceful environment.

Nutrition

- Patients should be offered their favorite foods whenever possible.
- Conditions that may cause poor intake should be easily treated, for example. gastritis, constipation, toothache, oral candidiasis, pain and nausea should be treated.

Family Education

Notify and educate family about the possibility or probability of impending death.

Medications

- Review medications and other therapeutic interventions in light of the change in the patient's status.
- Are all the medicines being administered, still necessary?
- Generally speaking opioids and anticonvulsant medications should be continued, if possible.
- Adjust medication routes, as swallowing is likely to be lost.
- Consider adding a low opioid dose or increasing basal opioid by 259%, if dyspnea is present or probable.
- If the patient becomes anxious, give an anxiolytic.
- If respiratory secretions become troublesome, consider anticholinergic agents to dry them.
- Anticholinergic agents are likely to be more helpful if given early, as they prevent the production of secretions and do not remove existing secretions.
- If hydration via IV or nasogastric tube is being given, discuss discontinuation, because further hydration may contribute to respiratory secretions.

Oxygen

- Consider giving oxygen via nasal prongs or using a gentle fan.
- As a first intervention, O_2 helps to correct hypoxemia.
- Even when its oxygenating benefit is no longer certain, O_2 may continue to be psychologically comforting to patients and family members.

Care of Bowel

- Regular bowel movements are essential to the comfort of dying patients, at least until the last day or two of life.
- Laxatives help to prevent fecal impaction, especially in patients receiving opioids.
- Monitoring bowel function regularly is essential.
- Most patients do well on a twice/day regimen of stool softener.

Suctioning

- Occasionally, mouth suctioning of secretions can be helpful.
- Usually, deep suctioning is ineffective and unhelpful.

Counseling

- Counseling the family on the changes that are occurring.
- Coaching involves a process of sharing knowledge and working with families as they practice new skills in a supportive environment.

- Coaching of families should have parallel changes in the dying person.
- Changes are explained and suggestions are made for how the families can adjust to them.

Respect
- Finally, often a dying patient will not "leave" until everyone has come to say goodbye or until everyone has left the bedside.
- Provide psychological support to the dying patient in the absence of family members.
- Every patient deserves the utmost respect and the gentlest of care at the end of his or her life.

Social Care
- The family's insight into the patient's condition should be assessed.
- The family should be told that the clinical expectation is that the patient is dying and will die. Use of ambiguous language, such as "may not get better" can lead to misinterpretation and confusion.
- If relatives are told clearly that the patient is dying they have the opportunity to ask questions, stay with the patient, say their goodbyes, contact relevant people, and prepare themselves for the death.
- Relatives of patients dying in the community should be given contact telephone numbers so that they have access to help and advice on a 24 hour basis.

Spiritual Care
- Sensitivity to the patient's cultural and religious background is essential.
- Formal religious traditions may have to be observed in the dying phase and may also influence care of the body after death.
- After the patient's death, relatives should be dealt with in a compassionate manner.
- A leaflet explaining issues related to grieving can be helpful.

Assist with End of Life Decision Making
- Patients and family need proper explanations and time to take appropriate decisions.
- They face a range of difficult questions, such as: should the life extending treatments to be stopped? should artificial nutrition and hydration be provided when the patient is nearing death? etc.

Advance Directives
- The family members will face less stress, if the terminally ill person has placed an advance directive.
- Advance directives are legal documents that allow a person to spell out his decisions about end-of-life care ahead of time.
- It gives a way to tell the wishes to family, friends, and health care professionals to avoid confusion later on.
- A living will tells which treatments he wants if he is dying or becomes permanently unconscious.
- One can accept or refuse medical care.
- Will or testament is a legal declaration that permits a person (testator) to make decisions on how his property will be managed and distributed after his death.
- A will is effective only after the death of the testator. If a person does not leave a will, or the will is declared invalid, it results in the distribution of the property according to the laws of the state in which the person resided.

Dying Declaration
- Dying declaration is a statement by a person who is conscious and knows that death is imminent concerning what he/she believes to be the cause or circumstances of death.
- Dying declaration is a statement of a severely injured person who is aware that he/she is about to die, telling who caused the injury and possibly the circumstances.
- A dying declaration is considered credible and trustworthy based upon the general belief that most people who know that they are about to die do not lie.
- A person who makes a dying declaration must be competent at the time he makes a statement, otherwise, it is inadmissible.

PHYSIOLOGICAL CHANGES OCCURRING AFTER DEATH
- A body undergoes complex and intricate changes after death.
- These postmortem changes depend on a diverse range of variables.
- Factors, such as the temperature, season, sepsis/injuries, intoxication, presence of clothes/insulation over the body, etc. Determine the rate at which post-mortem changes occurs, physiological changes are immediate, early and late changes.

Immediate Changes
- Immediate changes include cessation of respiration, cessation of circulation, and cessation of nervous system functions.
- All of the muscles in the body relax, a state called primary flaccidity. Eyelids lose their tension and the pupils dilate.
- With the loss of tension in the muscles, the skin will sag, which can cause prominent joints and bones in the body, such as the jaw or hips, to become pronounced.
- As muscles relax, sphincters release and allow urine and feces to pass.

Early Changes
- Early postmortem changes are associated with cellular death.
- They include changes in the skin, eyes, postmortem cooling (algor mortis), postmortem rigidity (rigor mortis). and postmortem staining (livor mortis)
  - *Algor mortis:* Decrease in body temperature after death is termed as 'algor mortis, after death and cessation of circulation, no heat is being produced within the

body and it starts losing heat due to the temperature difference between the body and the surroundings. The body temperature falls at the rate of 1.5°F per hour and body becomes cool.
- *Rigor mortis:* In the third hour after death, chemical changes within the body's cells because all of the muscles to begin stiffening the first muscles affected will be the eyelids, jaw, and neck. Rigor mortis will spread into the face and down through the chest, abdomen, arms, and legs until it finally reaches the fingers and toes.
- *Livor mortis:* After the death, the circulation of blood stops, and the blood starts moving towards the dependant regions of the body due to gravity. This effect results in reddish-blue staining of those low-lying dependent regions of the body, known as the livor mortis or postmortem staining, during livor mortis the patches of discoloration start appearing in the dependent regions. These increase in size and spread all over the dependent regions in 4–6 hours and are fully developed within 6–8 hours. So, in case of the body of an individual lying on the floor of a room, the back of the individual will show postmortem staining.

Late Changes

- ❖ **Autolysis:** It is also termed as self-destruction is an intrinsic activity brought about by the breakdown of cells and tissues of the human body. After death, the cell membranes breakdown and release enzymes that start self-digestion. The first external sign of autolysis is the whitish appearance of the cornea.
- ❖ **Putrefaction (microbial action):** It is the decomposition of the body carried out by the microbial action. After cessation of homeostasis, the natural flora of the body migrates from the gut to the blood vessels and spreads all over the body.
- ❖ External microorganisms enter the body through the alimentary canal, respiratory tract, and open wounds. In the absence of body defenses/immune mechanisms, the microbes keep growing, as they feed upon the proteins and carbohydrates of the blood and body parts.

DYING DECLARATION

- ❖ Dying declaration is very important legal documentation.
- ❖ This is the recording of the dying patient to find out the cause behind the disease or injuries of the hospitalized patient.
- ❖ It is a verbal evidence of the patient even then it is given a lot of weightage in the courts.
- ❖ Recording of dying declaration is very important.
- ❖ If it is always recorded by a magistrate by keeping in mind the essential statements.
- ❖ Incomplete recording may save the offenders.
- ❖ Doctor or nurse should not involve themselves in dying declaration, in case where police records the dying declaration.
- ❖ Dying declaration is to be recorded by the magistrate.
- ❖ But, if condition of the patient becomes serious then medical officer can record it along with two nurses as witness.
- ❖ Dying declaration can be recorded by the nursing staff with two nurses as witness when medical officer is not present.
- ❖ Then the declaration to be sent immediately under sealed cover to the magistrate.
- ❖ Generally, a physician must make the determination that a person is dead.
- ❖ The physician makes a formal declaration of the death and a record of the time of death.
- ❖ In a hospital setting, the physician who declares the death may not be the one who signs the death certificate.
- ❖ A resident or the physician covering the emergency room may be asked to pronounce the death of a patient.
- ❖ The attending physician would be expected to determine the cause of death and file the death certificate. The physician who pronounces the death must simply determine that the patient is dead.
- ❖ If the determination of death is difficult, a physician should consult with others (i.e., a patient may be legally dead because of lack of brain function but still have a heartbeat when on a mechanical ventilator).
- ❖ Many accident victims are dead at the scene of the accident but are pronounced dead officially on arrival at a hospital because no physician was at the scene.
- ❖ When homicide is suspected or where the police handle large numbers of accidental deaths, a medical examiner may be on call to pronounce death at the scene and to determine the cause of death.

DEATH CERTIFICATE

- ❖ Law requires that a death certificate for each person who dies.
- ❖ The law specifies what information needs to be supplied.
- ❖ Death certificate is sent to local health departments, which compiles many statistics from the information.
- ❖ The mortician assumes the responsibility for handling and filling the death certificate with proper authorities.
- ❖ A physician's signature is required on the certificate, as well that of pathologist, the coroner and other in special cases.
- ❖ The nurse's responsibility is to ensure that a death certificate has been signed by the physician.

CARE OF DEAD BODY

Definition
Care of body in 30–45 minutes is following declaration of death by physician

Purposes
- ❖ To maintain normal body alignment before rigor mortis sets in
- ❖ To reduces mental distress of family
- ❖ To facilitate transportation to mortuary/residence.

Equipment
- ❖ Irony lined with towel
- ❖ Long artery clamp Bandage
- ❖ Absorbent and nonabsorbent cotton

- Hospital gown patient's clothes
- Mackintosh
- Mortuary cards in transplants plaster caver
- Valuable envelope
- Shroud/body-bag/gloves
- Clean disposable gloves
- Articles for leaving or booking the body.

Postmortem Care

When the patient has been pronounced dead by a physician or professional nurse, the nurse assumes the responsibility of caring for the body (postmortem care). During this phase of care, the nurse cleans, identifies and positions the body by following the formalities of procedure. At the time of death, the nurse must also make notation of any valuables, such as watch, rings, or money, and secure these articles so that they may be delivered to the family according to facility policy.

Postmortem Care of the Body

See **Table 11.1**.

TABLE 11.1: Postmortem care of the body.

Sl. No.	Preparations	Rationales
1.	Rearrange workload as needed	The nurse caring for the dead patient will have added time commitments with patient's family care of the body, and documentation in the chart, before transporting to the morgue. Other patients under this nurse's care may be neglected unless some of the work assignment is delegated to other capable people.
2.	Notify appropriate people: • In-charge nurse • Physician • Clergy • Morgue • Family	Notification of the nurse in charge of the medical area, the physician, and the morgue is important so hospital personnel can do their jobs effectively. The in-charge nurse can help with reassigning the nurse's workload and assuring hospital policy is followed. The physician will pronounce the patient dead and identify whether an autopsy is desired. Care and notification of the family may be shared by the nurse, and the physician.
3.	Review the institution's policy on postmortem care.	Each institution may have slightly different ways of caring for the body, there may be differences within the institution, depending on the age of the patient and cause of death.
4.	Talk with family about their wishes to spend time with the deceased or help in preparing the body. Find out if the family wants any religious activities before transporting the patient to the morgue.	Some family may want to see, touch and help in giving the final physical care. Offering the family some choices may help meet their needs. If the family feels the patient's religious needs were omitted, it can be further source for distress.
5.	Follow institutional policy for handling the patient's contamination if there was infection or isolation.	Possessions are very important to the family even when actual; value may be minimal. Giving the patient's belongings to identified relatives and having them sign for what they received will eliminate confusion and provide documentation for the institution.
6.	Consider any necessary precautions because of patient contamination if there was infection or isolation	If the patient was infected, the organisms are still present and could infect other people coming in contact with the body.
7.	Assemble equipment clean gown, envelope for valuable, container for personal possession, washbasin, towels body wrap, masking tape, identification tags, and dressings for draining wounds left when and if tubes are removed.	Organizing what will be needed ahead of time saves time and energy. Going in and out of the room can be distressing to family and other patients.
8.	If deceased patient had a room-mate, move that person to another room if possible.	The activities related to caring for the deceased patient may be very upsetting to another patient in the same room. It is also difficult to provide privacy for the family to be with the deceased.
9.	Provide privacy for the deceased	Care of the body to others is the last way the nurse can show respect. Other patients may also be upset by seeing a dead patient.
10.	Remove any valuables and place in envelope and seal. If the family wants the patient to keep a ring on, secure it with tape or according to institutional policy.	Valuables removed by the nurse should be identified on the envelope and sealed so there is no opportunity for theft or loss. Valuables should be locked in a safe place and this should be documented and signed in the patient's chart to protect the nurse.

Contd...

Contd...

Sl. No.	Preparations	Rationales
11.	Position the body in good alignment in the supine position with the head elevated slightly.	This will prevent possible problem with rigor mortis and liver mortis of the face and upper chest.
12.	Close eyelids if open by placing fingertips over each eyelid for a few seconds and gradually closing the eyes.	When rigor mortis sets in, the eyes will be held open, and this is usually undesirable for an open casket funeral.
13.	Place dentures in patient's mouth if possible. Send with body to mortician if unable to put in the patient's mouth.	Without the teeth in place the patient will have a sunken, altered appearance. The teeth are in place for an open-casket funeral. Rigor mortis may make it difficult to position dentures if not done shortly after death.
14.	Close patient's mouth if open by placing rolled towel under the chin.	The mouth is expected to be closed in death, and rigor mortis may make this difficult later.
15.	Remove all tubes and drains as identified in policies of institution.	This equipment is no longer needed and should be removed and disposed of appropriately.
16.	Soiled areas of the patient's body are washed, hairpins are removed, and the hair is combed. A clean gown is put on the patient if family is to view body. Some institutions do not use of gown under the morgue wrap.	Prevention of contamination and damage to the body by sharp objects. If family views body before it goes to the morgue, a clean gown and combed hair convey respect and optimum care.
17.	Place absorbent pad under buttocks	Relaxation of sphincters may cause release of stool or urine
18.	Attach identification tag to body. Leave hospital ID band in place.	Loss of outside tag could cause confusion on patient's identity if no identification is on the body.
19.	Wrap body as described for particular institution.	This serves to protect the body and provide privacy.
20.	Attach outside ID tag to wrapped body	This is for ease in identification by the morgue and mortuary. Make sure both tag are identical to name on hospital ID band.
21.	Pack all remaining personal belongings in a container for the relatives. Label accurately. Wash hands.	Patient's belongings can easily be forgotten if upset relatives collect them. Accurate labeling is helpful in getting the belongings to the right family members.
22.	Arrange for transportation of the body to morgue or mortuary.	
23.	Document care given in the patient's chart	This avoids confusion for the relatives and assures that no one arrives to claim the body before the nurse and family are ready for it to be moved
24.	After body is transported, the unit is stripped of linen and utensils. Wash hands. Notify housekeeping or appropriate personnel that the room is ready to be cleaned.	This is done to protect other patients and cleaning personnel from possible contamination.

Documentation

Documentation of the care given to the dying patient must be objective, complete, legible, and accurate. As death approaches, documentation should be frequent and include the signs of impending death as they occur. Recording by who was present at the time of the patient's death is important. The nurse should continue to chart until last entry states where and to whom the body was transferred.

■ AUTOPSY

Definition

"An autopsy, also known as a postmortem examination and necropsy is a medical procedure that consists of a thorough examination of a corpse to determine the cause and manner of death and to evaluate any disease or injury that may be present. It is usually performed by a specialized medical doctor called a pathologist"

Types According to Purpose

- ❖ Legal
- ❖ Medical—to find out a medical or clinical cause of death, academic purposes and research
- ❖ Forensic—when death is a criminal matter.

Types According to the Type of Examination

- ❖ External examination
- ❖ Internal examination

In this type of examination, the internal parts of the body are exposed and examination is done and the body is then sutured back. For this type of examination, a written consent from the relatives is required.

Meaning of Autopsy

The prefix 'auto-' means 'self', and so autopsy means 'to see for oneself'; it is used more broadly of personal examination of an object, as well as its specific usage for the postmortem examination of a human corpse.

History

The Egyptians were one of the first civilizations to practice the removal and examination of the internal organs of humans.

Value of Autopsy in Medicine

- Autopsies are important in clinical medicine as they can identify medical error and assist continuous improvement.
- The autopsies can detect medical diagnostic errors.
- Autopsies can help to detect whether the death certificates are incorrect and reveal the causes of death that were not suspected before the person died.
- The autopsies help to detect unexpected findings which could not be found out before the death of the client.

General Information

The term "autopsy" derives from the Greek for "to see oneself". "Necropsy" is from the Greek for "seeing a dead body"

Major Types of Autopsies

Forensic: This is done for medicolegal purposes, and is the one that is normally seen on television or in the news. This type depicts an extensive methodology and tends to be complete and comprehensive. No family permission is required to complete this type of autopsy.

Clinical/academic: This is usually performed in hospitals for research and study purposes. Prior to the start, of a clinical autopsy, a cause of death must have already have been established, and a death certificate completed. This usually is as comprehensive as it needs to be adequate. To complete this type of autopsy, permission from the deceased's legal next of kin is required.

Coroner's: In Great Britain, this type of autopsy encompasses cases where no medical cause of death is readily available. Cause, manner and mechanism of death are in question. Eventually, the prosecutors will identify whether the cases deserve comprehensive forensic autopsy or a routine postmortem. In the United States, each state has a set of guidelines defining a "coroner's case" for autopsy, for example, hospital deaths occurring within 24 hours of admission or within 24 hours of a major surgical procedure, with any history (current or remote) of illegal drug or alcohol abuse by the deceased, patients with certain communicable diseases (HIV, hepatitis C virus, etc.), patients with any previous history of violent injury (e.g., gunshot wound many years before death). These cases may/may not be also considered "forensic" in nature. They may be done by the hospital pathologist with the legal permission of the coroner or medical examiner for that county/parish and do not require permission from the deceased's legal next of kin.

Forensic Autopsy

A forensic autopsy is used to determine the cause of death. Forensic science involves the application of the sciences to answer questions of interest to the legal system. In United States law, deaths are placed in one of five manners:
1. Natural
2. Accident
3. Homicide
4. Suicide
5. Undetermined.

In some jurisdictions, the undetermined category may include deaths in absentia, such as deaths at sea and missing persons declared dead in a court of law; in others, such deaths are classified under "Other".

Following an in-depth examination of all the evidence, a medical examiner or coroner will assign a manner of death as one of the five listed above; and detail the evidence on the mechanism of the death.

Clinical Autopsy

Clinical autopsies serve two major purposes:
1. They are performed to gain more insight into pathological processes and determine what factors contributed to a patient's death. More importantly, autopsies are performed to ensure the standard of care at hospitals.
2. Autopsies can yield insight into how patient deaths can be prevented in the future.

Within the United Kingdom, clinical autopsies can only be carried out with the consent of the family of the deceased person as opposed to a medico legal autopsy instructed by a Coroner (England and Wales) or Procurator Fiscal (Scotland) to whom the family cannot object

The steps of procedure for conducting autopsy:
- The body is received at a medical examiner's office or hospital in a body bag or evidence sheet.
- A brand new body bag is used for each body to ensure that only evidence from that body is contained within the bag
- Evidence sheets are an alternate way to transport the body. An evidence sheet is a sterile sheet that the body is covered in when it is moved. If it is believed there may be any significant residue on the hands, for instance gunpowder, a separate paper sack is put around each hand and taped shut around the wrist.
- There are two parts to the physical examination of the body: the external and internal examination. Toxicology. Biochemical tests and/or genetic testing often supplement these and frequently assist the pathologist in assigning the cause or causes of death.

External Examination

- The person responsible for handling, cleaning and moving the body is often called a diener, the German word for servant.
- In the UK, this role is performed by an anatomical
- Pathology Technologist who will also assist the pathologist in eviscerating the deceased and reconstruction after the autopsy.

- After the body is received, it is first photographed.
- The examiner then notes the kind of clothes and their position on the body before they are removed.
- After this any evidence, such as residue, flakes of paint or other material is collected from the external surfaces of the body.
- Ultraviolet light may also be used to search body surfaces for any evidence not easily visible to the naked eye.
- Samples of hair, nails and the like are taken, and the body may also be radiographically imaged.
- Once the external evidence is collected, the body is removed from the bag, undressed and any wounds present are examined.
- The body is then cleaned, weighed and measured in preparation for the internal examination.
- The scale used to weigh the body is often designed to accommodate the cart that the body is transported on; its weight is then deducted from the total weight shown to give the weight of the body.
- If not already within an autopsy room, the body is transported to one and placed on a table.
- A general description of the body as regards ethnicity, sex, age, hair color and length, eye color and other distinguishing features (birthmarks, old scar tissue, moles, etc.) is then made.
- A handheld voice recorder or a standard examination form is normally used to record this information.

Internal Examination

- If not already in place, a plastic or rubber brick called a "body block" is placed under the back of the body, causing the arms and neck to fall backward whilst stretching and pushing the chest upward to make it easier to cut open.
- This gives the prosecutor, a pathologist or assistant, maximum exposure to the trunk.
- After this is done, the internal examination begins.
- The internal examination consists of inspecting the internal organs of the body for evidence of trauma or other indications of the cause of death.
- **For the internal examination there are a number of different approaches available:**
  - A large and deep Y-shaped incision can be made starting at the top of each shoulder and running down the front of the chest, meeting at the lower point of the breastbone. This is the approach most often used in forensic autopsies so as to allow maximum exposure of the neck structures for later detailed examination. This could prove essential in cases of suspected strangulation.
  - A T-shaped incision made from the tips of both shoulder, in a horizontal line across the region of the collar bones to meet at the sternum (breastbone) in the middle. This initial cut is used more often to produce a more esthetic finish to the body when it is reconstituted as stitching marks will not be as apparent as with a Y-shaped incision. A single vertical cut is made from the middle of the neck (in the region of the 'Adam's apple' on a male body).
- In all of the above cases the cut then extends all the way down to the pubic bone (making a deviation to the left side of the navel). Bleeding from the cuts is minimal, or nonexistent, due to the fact that the pull of gravity is producing the only blood pressure at this point, related directly to the complete lack of cardiac functionality. However, in certain cases there is anecdotal evidence to prove that bleeding can be quite profuse, especially in cases of drowning.
- An electric saw dubbed a "Stryker saw" after a common manufacturer of the tool, is most often used to open the chest cavity.
- However, in some cases, due to the large amount of dust created when the bone is cut by the saw, shears are used to open the chest cavity. It is also possible to utilize a simple scalpel blade.
- The prosecutor uses the tool to saw through the ribs on the lateral sides of the chest cavity to allow the sternum and attached ribs to be lifted as one chest plate; this is done so that the heart and lungs can be seen in situ and that the heart, in particular the pericardial sac is not damaged or disturbed from opening
- A scalpel is used to remove any soft tissue that is still attached to the posterior side of the chest plate. Now the lungs and the heart are exposed.
- The chest plate is set aside and will be eventually replaced at the end of the autopsy.
- At this stage, the organs are exposed. Usually, the organs are removed in a systematic fashion,
- Making a decision as to what order the organs are to be removed will depend highly on the case in question.
- **Organs can be removed in several ways:**
  - The first is the en masse technique of letulle whereby all the organs are removed as one large mass.
  - The second is the en bloc method of Ghon.

For Example

The pericardial sac is opened to view the heart. Blood for chemical analysis may be removed from the inferior vena cava or the pulmonary veins. Before removing the heart, the pulmonary artery is opened in order to search for a blood clot. The heart can then be removed by cutting the inferior vena cava, the pulmonary veins, the aorta and pulmonary artery and the superior vena cava. This method leaves the aortic arch intact, which will make things easier for the embalmer. The left lung is then easily accessible and can be removed by cutting the bronchus, artery, and vein at the helium. The right lung can then be similarly removed. The abdominal organs can be removed one by one after first examining their relationships and vessels.

Some pathologists, however, prefer to remove the organs all in one "block" Then a series of cuts, along the vertebral column, are made so that the organs can be detached and pulled out in one piece for further inspection and sampling. During autopsies of infants, this method is used almost all of the time. The various organs are examined, weighed and tissue samples in the form of slices are taken. Even major blood vessels are cut open and inspected at this stage.

Next the stomach and intestinal contents are examined and weighed. This could be useful to find the cause and time of death, due to the natural passage of food through the bowel during digestion. The more area empty, the longer the deceased had gone without a meal before death.

Reconstitution of the Body

An important component of the autopsy is the reconstitution of the body such that it can be viewed, if desired, by relatives of the deceased following the procedure. After the examination, the body has an open and empty chest cavity with chest flaps open on both sides, the top of the skull is missing, and the skull flaps are pulled over the face and neck. It is unusual to examine the face, arms, hands or legs internally. Normally, the internal body cavity is lined with cotton wool or an appropriate material; the organs are then placed into a plastic bag to prevent leakage and returned to the body cavity. The chest flaps are then closed and sewn back together and the skull cap is sewed back in place. Then the body may be wrapped in a shroud and it is common for relatives of the deceased to not be able to tell the procedure has been done when the deceased is viewed in a funeral parlor after embalming

Aim of Autopsy

- To determine the cause of death.
- To the state of health of the person before he/she died.
- To find out whether any medical diagnosis and treatment before death was appropriate.

When a person has given permission in advance of their death, autopsies may also be carried out for the purposes of teaching or medical research.

An autopsy is frequently performed in cases of sudden death, where a doctor is not able to write a death certificate, or when death is believed to be due to an unnatural cause. These examinations are performed under a legal authority (Medical Examiner or Coroner or Procurator Fiscal) and do not require the consent of relatives of the deceased. The most extreme example is the examination of murder victims, especially when medical examiners are looking for signs of death or the murder method, such as bullet wounds and exit points, signs of strangulation, or traces of poison.

■ EMBALMING

Introduction

Embalming is one of the earliest surgical procedures conducted to preserve the human bodies, since ancient times. The people of ancient times were very intelligent and emotional and believed in rebirth. So they invented the method of embalming for preserving the dead bodies of their near and dear ones. Embalming has a very long and cross cultural history, with many cultures giving the embalming processes a greater religious meaning.

Definition

"Embalming in most modern cultures is the art and science of temporarily preserving human remains to forestall decomposition and to make them suitable for display at a funeral."

Aims of Embalming

- Preservation of dead body
- Sanitization of dead body
- Presentation (or restoration) of a dead body.

History of Embalming

- In classical antiquity, perhaps the old world culture that had developed embalming to the greatest extent was that of ancient Egypt, who developed the process of mummification. They believed that preservation of the mummy empowered the soul after death, which would return to the preserved corpse.
- Other cultures that had developed embalming processes include the Incas and other cultures of Peru, whose climate also favored a form of mummification. The best preserved bodies in the world are from Han.
- Dynasty China, which preservation process is not still completely understood. It seems a special liquid, in which the bodies were embedded, was of major influence.
- Embalming in Europe had a much more sporadic existence. It was attempted from time to time, especially during the Crusades, when crusading noblemen wished to have their bodies preserved for burial closer to home. Embalming began to come back into practice in parallel with the anatomists of the Renaissance who needed to be able to preserve their specimens.
- Contemporary embalming methods advanced markedly during the American Civil War, which once again involved many servicemen dying far from home, and their family wishing them returned for local burial. Dr Thomas Holmes received a commission from the Army Medical Corps to embalm the corpses of dead Union officers to return to their families. Military authorities also permitted private embalmers to work in military-controlled areas. The passage of Abraham Lincoln's body home for burial was made possible by embalming and it brought the possibilities and potential of embalming to a wider public notice.
- In 1867, the German chemist August Wilhelm von Hofmann discovered formaldehyde, whose preservative properties were soon discovered and which became the foundation for modern methods of embalming.
- In the 19th and early 20th centuries, arsenic was frequently used as an embalming fluid but has since been supplanted by other mare effective and less toxic chemicals. There were questions about the possibility of arsenic from embalmed bodies later contaminating ground water supplies. There were also legal concerns as people suspected of murder by arsenic poisoning could claim that the levels of paisem in the deceased's body were a result of embalming postmortem rather than evidence of homicide.
- Embalming is distinct from taxidermy. Embalming preserves the human body intact, whereas taxidermy is the recreation of an animal's form using only the creature's skin.

Characteristics of an Embalmer

- The roles of a mortician and an embalmer are different.

- A mortician is a person who arranges for the final disposition of the deceased.
- An embalmer is someone who has been trained in the art and science of embalming.
- The embalmer needs a formal study in anatomy, thanatology, chemistry and specific embalming theory (to widely varying levels depending on the region of the world one lives in) combined with practical instruction in a mortuary with a resultant formal qualification granted after the passing of a final practical examination and acceptance into a recognized embalming body.
- Legal requirements about who can practice vary geographically.

Modern Trends in Embalming

Embalming as practiced in the funeral homes of the Western World (notably North America) uses several steps. Modern embalming techniques are not the result of a single practitioner, but rather the accumulation of many decades, even centuries, of research, trial and error, and invention. A standardized version follows below, but variation on techniques is very common.

Procedure for Embalming

- The first step in embalming is to check that the individual is in fact deceased, and then verify the identity of the body (normally via wrist or leg tags).
- At this point, embalmers commonly perform basic tests for signs of death, noting things, such as clouded-over corneas, lividity, and rigor mortis or by simply attempting to palpate a pulse in the carotid or radial artery.
- In modern times, people awakening on the preparation table is largely the province of horror fiction and urban myth. and
- Any clothing on the corpse is removed and set aside any personal effect, such as jewelry is inventoried.
- A molesty cloth is sometimes placed over the genitalia. The corpse is washed in disinfectant and germicidal solutions
- During this process, the embalmer bends, flexes and massages the arms and legs to relieve rigor mortis.
- The eyes are posed using an eye cap that keeps them shut and in the proper expression.
- The mouth may be closed via suturing with a needle and ligature, using an adhesive, or by setting a wire into the maxilla and mandible with a needle injector, a specialized device most commonly utilized in North America and unique to mortuary practice.
- Care is taken to make the expression look as relaxed and natural as possible and ideally a recent photograph of the deceased while still living is used as a template.
- The process of closing the mouth, eyes, shaving, etc., is collectively known as setting the features.

The actual embalming process usually involves four parts:
1. **Arterial embalming** involves the injection of embalming chemicals into the blood vessels, usually via the right common carotid artery. Blood is displaced from the right jugular vein. The embalming solution is injected with a centrifugal pump and the embalmer massages the corpse to break up circulatory clots as to ensure the proper distribution of the embalming fluid. In case of poor circulation, other injection points are used.
2. **Cavity embalming:** The suction of the internal fluids of the corpse and the injection of embalming chemicals into body cavities, using an aspirator and trocar. The embalmer makes a small incision just above the navel and pushes the trocar in the chest and stomach cavities to puncture the hallow organs and aspirate their contents. He then fills the cavities with concentrated chemicals that contain formaldehyde. The incision is either sutured closed or a "trocar button" is screwed into place.
3. **Hypodermic embalming:** The injection of embalming chemicals under the skin as needed.
4. **Surface embalming,** which supplements the other methods, especially for visible, injured body parts.

A typical embalming takes one to two hours. An embalming case that requires more attention could take longer. The repair of an autopsy case or the restorations of a long bone donor are two such examples.

Presentation of the Body after Embalming

- After the body is rewashed and dried, a moisturizing cream is applied to the face.
- The body will usually sit for as long as possible for observation by the embalmer. After being dressed for visitation/funeral services, cosmetics are applied to make it appear more lifelike and to create a "memory picture" for the deceased's friends and relatives.
- For babies who have died, the embalmer may apply a light cosmetic massage cream after embalming to provide a natural appearance; massage cream is also used on the lips to prevent them from dehydrating, and the infant's mouth is often left open a bit for a more natural expression
- If possible, the funeral director uses a light, translucent cosmetic, sometimes, heavier, opaque cosmetics are used to hide bruises, cuts, or discolored areas
- Make-up is applied to the lips to mimic their natural color
- Sometimes a very pale or light pink lipstick is applied on males, while brighter colored lipstick is applied to females.
- Hair gels or baby oil is applied to style the hair, especially for deceased who are male.
- Mortuary cosmetizing is not done for the same reason as make-up for living people; rather, it is designed to add depth and dimension to a person's features that the lack of blood circulation has removed.
- Warm areas where blood vessels in living people are superficial, such as the cheeks, chin, and knuckles have subtle reds added to recreate this effect, while browns are added to the palpabrae (eyelids) to add depth, especially important as viewing in a casket creates an unusual perspective rarely seen in everyday life.
- During the viewing, pink-colored lighting is sometimes used near the body to lend a warmer tone to the deceased's complexion.
- A photograph of the dead person in good health is often sought in order to guide the embalmer's hand in restoring the corpse to a more lifelike appearance.

- Blemishes and discolorations (such as bruises, in which the discoloration is not in the circulatory system and cannot be removed by arterial injection) occasioned by the last illness, the settling of blood, or the embalming process itself are also dealt with at this time (although some embalmers utilize hypodermic bleaching agents, such as phenol-based cauterants, during injection to lighten discoloration and allow for easier cosmetizing).
- Men are typically buried in semiformal clothing, such as a suit or coat and tie, and women in semiformal dresses or pant suits. In recent years, some individuals are now buried in less formal clothing that they would have worn on a daily basis.
- Clothing worn can also reflect the deceased person's profession or vocation. Priests and ministers are often dressed in their liturgical vestments and military personnel wear their uniform.
- The undergarments are also important. Funeral directors will suggest that when they bring the clothing to the funeral home, the family or other responsible parties should bring all undergarments as well. Underwear, t-shirts, bra, briefs and even hosiery are all used.
- The deceased are dressed just as they would be in life.
- The clothing is often cut down the back and placed on the deceased to ensure a proper fit
- In many areas of Asia and Europe, the custom of dressing the body in a especially designed shroud/funeral gown rather than in clothing used by the living, is preferred.
- After the deceased has been dressed, they are placed in the casket (the term casket is derived from older usage to refer to a "jewel box, it is called a coffin when the container is anthropoid (a stretched hexagon] in form) for the various funeral rites. It is common for photographs, notes, cards and favorite personal items to be placed in the casket with the deceased.
- Even bulky and expensive items, such as electric guitars, are occasionally interred with a body. In some ways this mirrors the ancient practice of placing grave goods with a person for the afterlife. In traditional Chinese culture, paper substitutes of the goods are cremated with the deceased instead, as well as Hell Bank Notes specifically purchased for the occasion.

Chemicals Used for Embalming

Embalming chemicals are a variety of preservatives, sanitizers, disinfectant agents and additives used in modern embalming to temporarily delay decomposition and restore a natural appearance for viewing a body after death

A mixture of these chemicals is known as embalming fluid and is used to preserve deceased individuals, sometimes only until the funeral, other times indefinitely.

Typical *embalming fluid* contains a mixture of formaldehyde, glutaraldehyde, methanol, ethanol, and other solvents. The formaldehyde content generally ranges from 5–35% and the ethanol content may range from 9–56%.

Advanced Method of Embalming

- Badly decomposing bodies, trauma cases, frozen and drowned bodies, and those to be transported for long distances also require special treatment beyond that for the "normal" case.
- The restoration of bodies and features damaged by accident or disease is commonly called restorative art or demisurgery and all qualified embalmers have some degree of training and practice in it.
- For such cases, the benefit of embalming is startlingly apparent. In contrast though, many people have unreal expectations of what a dead body should look like due to the unrealistic portrayal of "dead" bodies in movies and television shows.
- Viewers generally have an unreal expectation that a body going through decomposition should look as it did before death
- Ironically, the work of a skilled embalmer often results in the deceased appearing natural enough that the embalmer appears to have done nothing at all.
- Normally cosmeticians are very happy when someone can bring in a picture and the decedent's regular makeup. If worn, to help make their loved one to look as they did alive.
- Embalming autopsy cases differs from standard embalming because the nature of the postmortem examination irrevocably disrupts the circulatory system due to the removal of the organs and viscera
- In these cases, a six-point injection is made though the two iliac or femoral arteries, subclavian or axillary vessels, and common carotids, with the viscera treated separately with cavity fluid or a special embalming powder in a viscera bag.
- In many morgues in the United States (such as the Los Angeles County Coroners Office) and New Zealand, these necessary vessels are carefully preserved during the autopsy; in countries in which embalming has been less common, such as Australia and Japan, they are routinely excised.

Long-term Preservation

Long-term preservation requires different techniques, such as using stronger preservative chemicals and multiple injection sites to ensure thorough saturation of body tissues.

Embalming is meant to temporarily preserve the body of a deceased person. Regardless of whether embalming is performed the type of burial or entombment, and the materials used-such as wood or metal caskets and vaults the body of the deceased will eventually decompose.

Modern embalming is done to delay decomposition so that funeral services may take place or for the purpose of shipping the remains to a distant place for disposition.

Embalming for Anatomy Education

A rather different process is used for cadavers embalmed for dissection by medical and funeral service students. Here, the first priority is for long-term preservation, not presentation. As such, medical embalmers use embalming fluids that contain concentrated formaldehyde (37–40%, known as formalin) as well as phenol and are made without dyes or perfumes. Many embalming chemical companies make specialized anatomical embalming fluids. Anatomical embalming is performed into a closed circulatory system. The fluid is injected with an embalming machine into an artery under high pressure and flow and allowed to swell and saturate the tissues. After the deceased is left to sit for a number of hours, the venous system is opened and the fluid allowed draining out. This serves to replace any water in the tissues of the deceased with preservation. Excess water in the tissues can serve as a growth site for bacteria.

Anatomical embalmers may choose to use gravity feed embalming, where the container dispensing the embalming fluid is elevated above the body's level and fluid is slowly introduced over an extended time, sometimes as long as several days. Unlike standard arterial embalming, no drainage occurs and the body distends with fluid that eventually reduces, leaving a normal appearance. There is no separate cavity treatment of the internal organs anatomically embalmed cadavers have a typically uniform gray coloration due both to the high formaldehyde concentration and to the lack of red coloration (added normally to standard. nonmedical embalming fluids).

Religious Practices

There is much difference of opinion amongst different faiths as to the permissibility of embalming. A brief overview of some of the larger faiths positions are examined below:
- ❖ Some of the major branches of the Christian faith allow embalming, however, it is not a part of most mainstream European Christian traditions. Its popularity in North America owes more to marketing by the funeral industry than to any traditional or religious requirement (cf. Jessica Mitford, The American Way of Death). Some bodies within Eastern Orthodoxy maintain an absolute ban against embalming except when required by law or other necessity, while others discourage but do not prohibit it.
- ❖ The Book of Mormon and The Church of Jesus Christ of Latter-day Saints do not profess against embalming. Often, due to the custom of church members dressing the deceased, embalming is given preference.
- ❖ Many authorities hold Hinduism does not accept embalming. In practice, this is not an adamant prohibition and embalming for those of Hindu faith are known to happen, generally for repatriation to India or the South Pacific and for the purposes of viewing and funerary rites at the family home.
- ❖ Members of Bahá'í Faith are not embalmed. Instead the body is washed and then placed in a cotton, linen or silk shroud. The body is to be buried within one hour's journey from the place of death, if this will be feasible.
- ❖ Zoroastrians traditionally hold a type of sky burial within structures known as Towers of Silence in which the body is exposed to weathering and predation to dispose of the remains, and thus embalming the body is contrary to their funeral designs. This is due to the Zoroastrian belief that the dead body is unclean and the pure elements of earth and fire should not be allowed to come into contact with it. This practice is not universally performed any more, and many Iranian Zoroastrians perform traditional cremations and burials instead.
- ❖ Muslims are required to be buried within 24 hours of death if possible embalming is forbidden. The body is still washed and prepared specifically for interment. This procedure is to be done according to the last will of the deceased, usually by a close relative of the deceased who is of the same gender. He/she is then dressed in a plain white burial shroud (for women, the hair, ears and neck are covered as they were in life, preserving her dignity before men who are not closely related; men are buried in their ihram, or pilgrim garb, as worn during the Hajj in Mecca). Muslims believe that the spirit remains with the body from death until after burial, which is the reason for same day burial, as well as the aforementioned procedures; the body is treated with the same care and respect as in life so as to not cause undue stress to the deceased. For the same reason, cremation is also forbidden. Prayers and readings of the Qur'an are spoken aloud to give comfort to the deceased, and the body is not left alone even for a time following the burial, during which the deceased is buried (preferably without a casket) on his/her right side, facing Mecca.
- ❖ Traditional Jewish law forbids embalming, and burial is to be done as soon as possible-preferably within 24 hours. However, under certain circumstances, burial may be delayed if it is impossible to bury a person immediately, or to permit the deceased to be buried in Israel. Guidance of a Rabbi or the local chevra kadisha (Jewish Burial Society) should be sought regarding any questions, as particular circumstances may justify leniencies. Notably the Biblical Joseph was embalmed in the Egyptian fashion (Genesis 50:26).

Embalming in Popular Culture

Fictional works tend to portray the fantastic, extraordinary and often dysfunctional aspects of any profession or activity with which the public has little contact, and to ignore the mundane or routine. Embalming is no exception.

Examples of Embalming

- ❖ It was rumored that after her death Diana, Princess of Wales was hastily embalmed to cloud tests that she may have been pregnant. However, if this were the case an autopsy would still have easily been able to determine such an obvious condition and the rumor is just urban the dead body is unclean and the pure elements of earth and fire should not be allowed to come into contact with it. This practice is not universally performed any more, and many Iranian Zoroastrians perform traditional cremations and burials instead.

COUNSELING AND SUPPORTING GRIEVING RELATIVES

- ❖ Coping of the individuals and family with dying, death, grief, loss, and bereavement is as difficult experience.
- ❖ The response to the death of a family member, relative, or close friend places one in the category of "bereaved.
- ❖ "Those who are bereaved, experience grief (it is a person's response or reaction to loss).

- Counseling involves helping people facilitate normal or uncomplicated grief, to a healthy completion of the tasks of grieving within a reasonable time frame.
- How one copes with life events and adapts to one's present and future is also part of the grieving process.

Goals of Grief Counseling

The following are the goals of grief counseling:
- Accepting the loss and talking about it
- Identifying and expressing feelings related to the loss (anger, guilt, anxiety, helplessness, sadness).
- Living without the deceased and making decisions alone.
- Separating emotionally and forming new relationships.
- Identifying ways of coping that suit the bereaved.

Method of Grief Counseling

- Each counselor or therapist has his or her own techniques that he/she utilizes because they are effective, although counselors often refer different techniques that suit a particular person much better based on the individual's circumstances.
- Counseling and therapy techniques include art and music therapy, meditation, creation of personalized rituals, communication with the deceased (through writing, conversations, etc.), and role playing, bearing and participating in support groups.

PLACING BODY IN THE MORTUARY

- Mortuary is an important integral part of every hospital as it deals with the preservation of the dead body.
- Bodies may be kept until burial can be arranged.
- Mortuary complex consists of Autopsy room' postmortem room, and preservation room for dead body before disposal arrangement are made (Cold storage room) and ancillary areas.
- Make sure that the power supply is uninterrupted so that the body be kept undergoing any changes.
- Lots of sentiment values are attached to the dead body of the person with socio- and medicolegal importance attached to the mortuary of the hospital.
- Therefore, establishment and proper management of mortuary is of significance in every hospital.

Uses

- To preserve the dead body till the formalities of the handing over of deceased is completed.
- To keep the dead body unclaimed till the relative claim and take away for final disposal
- To receive and store dead body requiring postmortem examination To carry out medico legal postmortem work
- To impart teaching programs for undergraduates and post graduates.
- Transport of dead body from hospital to mortuary

Procedure

- After death, the body should be properly labeled mentioning the Name, Father's name, Admission number, ward, date & time of death etc by nursing staff on duty.
- In medicolegal cases, the letters 'MLC' should be put on the label prominently
- Nursing staff on duty in the ward should ensure that surgical operation drainage site if any is properly dressed before the body is wrapped in leak-proof sheets/plastic bag and handed over to next of kin or mortuary attendant
- The mortuary attendant on duty is informed that a pick up or removal is necessary from the wards
- The morgue attendant will receive the duly wrapped and labeled bodies in a courteous, sensitive and professional manner, along with the relevant records including death slip
- Record all identification of the body as far as possible.
- Noting down of identification features is carried out strictly in the register maintained for the said purpose.
- In case where death has occurred due to natural causes and there is no suspicion of any foul play, the dead bodies may be recorded with signatures of relatives or attendants

RELEASING BODY FROM THE MORTUARY

The steps that were taken to keep the body in mortuary have also to be followed to release the body from there:
- The person receiving the body should reveal his identity and relationship with the deceased.
- He/she should write full name with address and signature with date and Identification of dead body is very important.
- The identification marks of deceased should again be verified.
- The mortuary staff maintains a record of all events promptly.
- Follow hospital policy strictly for releasing the body.

Certificate of Death

- A death certificate is either a legal document issued by a medical practitioner who states when a person died, or a document issued by a Government Civil Registration Office, that declares the date, location and cause of a person's death, as entered in an official register of deaths.
- In India, a death certificate is a primary document on the basis of which inheritance of property, insurance settlement and a host of other legal claims are processed.
- A death certificate mentions the date and time of death and has the intrinsic capacity to relieve survivors of impending debts and obligations.
- The death in the house needs to be reported within 21 days of its occurrence by the head of the family.
- If the death happens in the hospital, it is the Medical in-charge/Chief Medical Officer who needs to report the same or the Jail in-charge, in case the deceased person breathes his/her last in a prison.

List of Documents Required to be Submitted

- Birth certificate, for proof of age
- Affidavit specifying the date and time of death
- Copy of Ration card
- Address proof (Electricity bills, etc.)
- The Registrar will enter the name of the deceased into records without any fee or reward.

ETHICAL AND LEGAL ISSUES IN DEATH AND DYING

As patient and family struggle with end of life treatment decision. They increasingly looking to nurses for information, advice and support. Patients have legally and morally protected right to consent and refuse any and all indicated medical therapies. A discussion of nurse's ethical and legal responsibilities in the end of life care follows

Advance Directives

- Decisions about health care are becoming increasingly complex. Some of most difficult cases involve patients who are no longer able to indicate their treatment preferences.
- Two kinds of advance treatment directives can minimize difficulties by allowing individual to state in advance of their choices.
- Living wills provide specific instructions about kind of health care they should be provided or foregone in a particular situation.
- A durable power of attorney for health care appoints an agent the person's trust to make decision in the event of the appointing person's subsequent incapacity.

Medicolegal Cases

- All cases where death has occurred due to accident, assault, burns, suicide, poison, rape or any other causes where it is suspected that death has not been due to natural causes, must be registered as medicolegal cases (MLC). The police authorities must be informed accordingly. In all the above cases, the out-patient paperwork and the death reports duly completed must be forwarded to the Medical Superintendent for onward transmission to the Medical Records Section and other concerned areas.
- Emphasis should be given to enter the name clearly and legibly, to enter the address, time of arrival of the patient and the cause and nature of injury. Signature should be in full with the name of CMO given in capital letters. At least two marks of identification should be carefully entered. A copy of the report should be handed over to the Police and the register should be kept under lock and key in the Casualty Department. No person, including the Police officer, should have access to the medicolegal record including medico-legal register without the written consent of Medical Superintendent or any other officer authorized by him.
- The following points may be considered while dealing with MLC cases:
  1. Each entry of identification data of patients in the MLC register should be made by the CMO and not by the Police Officer.
  2. The MLC reports should be prepared by the CMO's Residents and not by the Interns.
  3. Nature of injuries should be recorded in every MLC case.
  4. The CMO should write his/her full name in block letters along with the signature for adequate identification.

Do not Incubate/Do Not Resuscitate (DNI/DNR)

- A DNR order on a patient's file means that a doctor is not required to resuscitate a patient if his heart stops and is designed to prevent unnecessary suffering
- A do-not-resuscitate order (DNR) or allow natural death, is a legal order written or oral, depending on country, indicating that a person does not want to receive cardiopulmonary resuscitation (CPR) if that person's heart stops beating. Sometimes, it also prevents other medical interventions. The legal status and processes surrounding DNR orders vary from country to country.
- Most commonly, the order is placed by a physician based on a combination of medical judgments and patient wishes and values.
- The usual circumstances in which it is appropriate not to resuscitate are:
- if a patient's condition is such that resuscitation is unlikely to succeed when there is no benefit to the patient
- if successful resuscitation would not be in the patient's best interest because it would lead to a poor quality of life
- if a mentally competent patient has consistently stated or recorded the fact that he or she does not want to be resuscitated
- If there is advanced notice or a living will which says the patient does not want to be resuscitated Although DNRS can be regarded as a form of passive.
- Euthanasia, they are not controversial unless they are abused, since they are intended to prevent patients suffering pointlessly from the bad effects that resuscitation can cause: broken ribs, other fractures, ruptured spleen, brain damage.
- DNR orders should only be issued after discussion with patients or their family.

EUTHANASIA

- Euthanasia refers to the practice of intentionally ending a life in order to relieve pain and suffering.
- It is categorized as voluntary, non-voluntary and involuntary.
- Euthanasia can be further classified into active or passive ones.
- Active euthanasia is an intentional act to deliberately kill a terminally-ill patient using various means whereas passive euthanasia happens when medical treatment is removed purposefully resulting in a person's death to relieve him from unending pain.
- Until now euthanasia is not legalized in India.

Meaning

- The phrase "euthanasia" was coined by Sir Francis Bacon.
- It is also called as 'mercy killing'.
- The term "Euthanasia" has been derived from the two Greek words 'eu' and 'thanotos', which literally means 'good death'.
- Euthanasia is the practice of intentionally ending a life in order to relieve pain and suffering (provided motive should be good and death must be painless as much as possible) or

❖ "A deliberate intervention was undertaken with the express intention of ending a life, to relieve intractable suffering."
—*British House of Lords Select Committee on Medical Ethics*

Difference between Euthanasia and Physician-assisted Suicide

- ❖ Physician-assisted suicide is often misunderstood with euthanasia.
- ❖ The difference being in who administers the lethal drug.
- ❖ In euthanasia—a physician or third party administers it.
- ❖ In physician-assisted suicide, it is the patient himself administers it, though on the advice of the doctor.
- ❖ Assisted suicide and euthanasia are sometimes called under the umbrella term "assisted dying"

Classification

- ❖ **Voluntary euthanasia (with patients' consent):** Euthanasia is performed with the patients consent. It is legal in some countries like Belgium, Netherlands, etc.
- ❖ **Non-voluntary euthanasia (patient's consent unavailable):** Where a person is unable to give their consent (for example, the patient is in a state of coma or are severely brain-damaged) and another person takes the decision on their behalf, often because the ill person had expressed a wish previously to end their life in such circumstances.
- ❖ **Involuntary euthanasia (without asking consent or against the patient's will):** Euthanasia conducted against the will of the patient is termed involuntary euthanasia. It is also regarded as murder.
- ❖ **Active euthanasia:** Where a person intentionally intervenes to end someone's life with the use of lethal substances or forces. For example, administering a lethal injection to end life.
- ❖ **Passive euthanasia:** Where a person causes death by withholding or withdrawing treatment that is essential to maintain life. For example, stoppage of antibiotics treatment in certain cases where it is necessary for the continuance of life, removal of life support system, etc.

ORGAN DONATION

- ❖ A *'Green Corridor'* is a special route making the route of the hospital where an organ is harvested and the hospital where it is to be transplanted, traffic-free.
- ❖ It is a manually operated route.
- ❖ In India, the concept of Green Corridors has been since 2014.
- ❖ The functioning of this corridor is managed by transplant coordinators, local police, traffic police and airport staff that make this transfer of organs from the origin to destination quick and easy.

Green Corridor for Organ Donation

- ❖ A Green Corridor is a special route that is managed by different departments and authorities and ensures safe and quicker transfer of organs from one hospital to another by different modes of transport.
- ❖ It demarcates a special route for ambulances that can travel on traffic-free roads, which can reduce the total transfer time by 60–70%.
- ❖ The public's awareness of this Green Corridor is also of utmost importance.
- ❖ This will ensure that not just the concerned authorities but also the citizens of the country pave way for such a noble initiative of saving the lives of people.

Coordinating Authority

The National Organ and Tissue Transplant Organization (NOTTO) is the regulatory body for the Green Corridors.

Procedure of Organ Transfer through Green Corridor

- ❖ Once the doctor suggests an organ transplant and the patient's family also fills in their consent, the procedure for transplant begins.
- ❖ The authorities first check for organs within the hospital, and then as per the requirement look within the city, state, region and at the national level.

Need for Green Corridor

- ❖ As stated by experts, there is only time duration of four hours between which the harvesting and transplant of the organ must be done.
- ❖ In small cities and towns, this target can still be achieved, but in cities like Mumbai, Bengaluru, Delhi, etc., which are busy on roads, may not be able to fulfill this requirement.
- ❖ Thus, with a Green Corridor in every city, a lot of time can be saved in transferring the organ to the destination via traffic-free routes for the ambulance.

Significance of Green Corridor for Organ Transplant

- ❖ As per the latest government statistics, 17 people die each day waiting for an organ transplant.
- ❖ There are two main reasons for this:
  - The hesitation of people to donate their organs
  - Lack of provisions to deliver organs to the patient's destination
- ❖ With the help of Green Corridor, more lives can be saved by regulating the second cause of concern.
- ❖ If proper provisions are provided, the statistics of organ donation and the saving of people's lives can also be improved.
- ❖ In India, the National Organ and Tissue Transplant Program (NOTP) is being implemented by the Directorate General of Health Services under the Ministry of Health & Family Welfare.

- The program aims to improve access to life-transforming transplantation for needy citizens by promoting deceased organ donation.

Impact of Green Corridor for Organ Donation in India
- Cities across the country have started maintaining Green Corridors. Chennai was one of the first cities in India to have a Green Corridor.
- This system has also helped save lives in the cities of Mumbai, Gurugram, Hyderabad, Bengaluru, Kolkata, and Indore in the last two years.
- As of 2018, the city of Indore in Madhya Pradesh had 34 Green Corridors.
- In Chennai, the life of a 21-year-old was saved by transferring the organ in just 14 minutes, after travelling for 12 km.
- This initiative of Green Corridors has been taken under the terms and guidelines of the Transplantation of Human Organs Act, 1994.
- This Act provides regulation of removal, storage and transplantation of human organs for therapeutic purposes and for the prevention of commercial dealings in human organs and for matters connected therewith.

CHAPTER 12

Psychosocial Needs: Self-concept

INTRODUCTION

- Self-concept is one's mental image of oneself.
- A positive self-concept is essential to a person's mental and physical health Individuals with a positive self-concept are better able to develop and maintain interpersonal relationships.
- An individual possessing a strong self-concept should be better able to accept or adapt to changes that may occur over the lifespan. How one views oneself affects one's interaction with
- Self-concept involves all of the self perceptions, appearance, values and beliefs that influence behavior and referred to when using the word I for me.
- Self-concept is made up of one's self-schemas, and interacts with self-esteem, self-knowledge, and the social self to form the self as a whole.
- The perception people have about their past or future selves relates to their perception of their current selves.
- The temporal self-appraisal theory argues that people have a tendency to maintain a positive self-evaluation by distancing themselves from their negative self and paying more attention to their positive one.
- In addition, people have a tendency to perceive the past self less favorably (e.g., "I'm better than I used to be") and the future self more positively.
- Self-concept is the way people think about themselves.
- It is unique, dynamic and always evolving.
- This mental image of oneself influences a person's identity, self esteem, body image and role in society.
- As a global understanding of oneself, self-concept shapes and defines who we are, the decisions we make and the relationships we form.
- Self-concept is perhaps the basis for all motivated behavior.
- Self-concept is one's mental image of oneself.
- A positive self-concept is essential to a person's mental and physical health Individuals with a positive self-concept are better able to develop and maintain interpersonal relationships.
- An individual a strong self-concept should be better able to accept or adapt to changes that may occur over the lifespan.
- How one views oneself affects one's interaction with others

- Self-concept involves all of the self-perceptions, appearance, values and beliefs that influence behavior and referred to when using the word I for me,
- Self-concept is an individual's perception of self, including self-esteem, body image and ideal self.

Self-concept is Complex that Influences the Following

- How one thinks, talks and acts
- How one sees and treats another person
- Choices one makes
- Ability to give and receive love
- Ability to take action and to change things

Nurse and Self-concept

- A person's self-concept is often defined by self description such as "I am a mother, a nurse and a volunteer. Patient self descriptive statements, such as these help the nurse gain insight into the patient's perception of self.
- The nurse should be observant for self descriptive statements when assessing the patient's self-concept.
- A healthy self-concept is necessary for overall physical and mental wellness. Self-concept includes the ideal self, real self and public self.
- The ideal self is the person (the patient) would like to be, such as a good, moral and well respected person.
- Sometimes, this ideal view of how a patient would like to be conflicts with the real self (how the patient really thinks about oneself, such as "I try to be good and do what's right, but I'm not well respected").
- This conflict can motivate a patient to make changes toward becoming the ideal self. However, the view of the ideal self needs to be realistic and obtainable or the patient may experience anxiety or be at risk for alterations in self-concept.
- Public self is what the patient thinks of others, think of him and influences the ideal and real self.
- Positive self-concept and good mental health results when all three components are compatible.
- A positive self-concept is an important part of a patient's happiness and success.
- Individuals with a positive self-concept have self confidence and set goals they can achieve. Achieving their goals reinforces their positive self-concept.

- A patient with a positive self-concept is more likely to change unhealthy habits (such as sedentary lifestyle and smoking) to promote health than a patient with a negative self-concept.
- A person's self-concept is composed of evolving subjective conscious and unconscious self assessments. Physical attributes, occupation, knowledge and abilities of the person will change throughout the life span, contributing to changes in one's self-concept.

DIMENSIONS OF SELF-CONCEPT

There are four dimensions of self-concept:
1. **Self-knowledge:** Self-knowledge is the knowledge that one has about oneself, in including insights into one's abilities, nature and limitations.
2. **Self-expectation:** Self-expectation is what one expects of oneself, may be a realistic or unrealistic expectation.
3. **Social self:**
   - Social self is how a person is perceived by others and society.
   - *Social evaluation:* The appraisal of oneself in relationship to others, events or situations.
   - Many people are "me-centered", i.e., they value "how I perceive me."
   - They try hard to live up to their own expectations and compete only with themselves, not with the others.
   - On the other side, there are people who value "how other perceive me," they are other centered people who have a high need for approval from others, competing, and evaluating themselves in relation to others.
   - They are unable to assert themselves, and fear disapproval.
   - The positive self-concept, therefore, is me centered and is formed with minimal reference to others' opinions.
   - It is important for the nurse to promote a positive self-concept on the client.
   - A nurse's own self-concept is also important.
   - Nurses who understand the different dimensions of themselves are better able to understand the needs, desires, feelings, and conflicts of their clients.
   - Nurses who feel positive about themselves are more likely to help clients meet their needs.
4. **Self-awareness:**
   - *Self-awareness* refers to the relationship between one's perception of himself or herself and others perceptions of him or her. Becoming more self-aware has perceptions that are very congruent.
   - The nurse gains insight into the self through working with other nurses who serve as mentors and acting on the feedback obtained during regular performance reviews.
   - Once the nurse has developed a clear understanding and awareness of self, the nurse can respect and avoid projecting his or her own beliefs on others.

People are thought to base their self-concept on how they perceive and evaluate themselves in the following areas:
- Vocational performance
- Personal appearance and physical attractiveness
- Intellectual functioning
- Sexual attractiveness and performance
- Being liked by others
- Ability to cope with and resolve problems
- Independence
- Particular talents.

Self-concept and Health

- **Self-concept** in these areas also extends to the choices people make and perception they have about their health.
- Persons with strong positive self-concept about appearance are likely to value healthy behaviors and take action to maintain the health of their skin, hair, and body.
- Person with negative self-concept may be less proactive about health promotion and illness prevention activities.
- Maintaining and evaluating one's self-concept is an ongoing process.

COMPONENTS OF SELF-CONCEPT

- A positive and healthy self-concept generates stability and positive feeling towards self.
- There are four components of self-concept:
  1. Personal identity.
  2. Body image
  3. Role performance
  4. Self-esteem.

Personal Identity

- Personal identity is the unique numerical identity of a person over time.
- Personal identity is the concept one develops about self that evolves over the course of his life.
- This may include aspects of one's life that he has no control over, such as where he grew up or the color of the skin, as well as choices he makes in life, such as how he spends his time and what he believes.
- A person demonstrates portions of his personal identity outwardly through what he wears and how he interacts with other people.
- One may also keep some elements of his personal identity to himself even when these parts of self are very important.
- Personal identity is the conscious sense of individuality and uniqueness that is continually evolving throughout life.
- People often view their identity in terms of name, sex, age, race, ethnic origin or culture, occupation or roles, talents and other characteristics, such as marital status and education.
- Personal identity may also include beliefs, values, personality and character, e.g., the person is outgoing, friendly, reserved, generous, and selfish.
- Identity is what distinguishes self from others. The individual with a strong sense of identity sees himself or herself as a unique person.

Body Image

- The image of physical self is body image that bow a person perceives the size, appearance, and functioning of the body

and its parts. Body image has both cognitive and affective aspects
- The cognitive is the knowledge of the material body, the affective includes the sensations of the body, such as pain, pleasure, fatigue, and physical movement.
- Body image is the sum of these attitudes, conscious and unconscious, that a person has toward his/her body.
- Body image includes clothing, makeup, hairstyle, jewelry, and other things intimately connected to the person. It also includes body prosthesis, such as artificial limbs, dentures, as well as devices required for functioning such as wheelchairs, canes and eyeglasses.
- Body image is the perception that a person has of his physical self and the thoughts and feelings that result from that perception including physical appearance, structure or function.
- Body image is a person's thoughts, feelings and perception of the aesthetics or sexual attractiveness of his own body.
- The concept of body image is used in a number of disciplines, including psychology, medicine, psychiatry, psychoanalysis, philosophy, cultural and feminist studies.
- A healthy body image means that you see yourself as you really are and that you feel good in your own skin.
- Self image also involves how you feel about your strengths, weaknesses, and abilities. Because sex involves both the body and the mind, our self-image has a strong effect on our sexual health.
- Body image of a person develops partly from other's attitudes and responses to that person's body and partly from the individual's own exploration of the body.
- Body image develops in infancy as the parents or caregivers respond to the child with smiles, holding, and touching, and as the child explore its own body sensations during breastfeeding, thumb sucking, and the bath.
- Cultural and societal values also influence a person's body image
- Body image consists of the ways people view themselves; their memories, experiences, assumptions, and comparisons about their own appearances; and their overall attitudes towards their own respective heights, shapes, and weights.
- These feelings can be positive, negative or both. and are influenced by individual and environmental factors.
- **Body image is determined by four factors:**
    1. *SEE:* The way you SEE your body
    2. *FEEL:* The way you FEEL about your body. This relates to the amount of satisfaction or dissatisfaction you feel about your shape, weight, and individual body parts.
    3. *THINK:* The way you THINK about your body. This can lead to preoccupation with body shape and weight.
    4. *BEHAVIORS:* Behaviors in which you engage as a result of your body image encompass your behavioral body image. When a person is dissatisfied with the way he/she looks, he may isolate himself as he feels bad about his appearance.
- If a person's body image closely resembles with one's body ideal, the individual is more likely to think positively about self.
- A person with a healthy body image will normally show concern for both health and appearance.
- This person will seek for help if ill and will include health promoting practices in daily activities.
- A person who has an unhealthy body image is likely to be concerned about minor illness and neglect activities like sleep and a healthy diet that are important to health.
- The person who has a body image disturbance may hide or not look at or touch a body part that is significantly changed in structure by illness or trauma. Some individuals may also express feelings of helplessness, hopelessness, powerlessness, and vulnerability, and may exhibit self-destructive behavior, such as over- or under-eating, neglecting oneself or suicidal attempts.

Role Performance

- A role is a set of expectations about how the person occupies one position or behaves.
- Role performance relates what a person in a particular role does to the behaviors expected of that role.
- Each person usually has several roles, such as husband, parent, brother, son, employee, friend, and nurse.
- Some roles are assumed for only limited periods, such as client, student, and ill person.
- Role mastery means that the person's behaviors meet social expectations, expectations or standards of behavior of a role, are set by society.
- Role development involves socialization into a particular role.
- To act appropriately, people need to know who they are in relation to others and what society expects for the positions they hold.
- Role ambiguity occurs when expectations are unclear, and people do not know what to do or how to do it and are unable to predict the reactions of others to their behavior.
- Failure to master a role creates frustration and feelings of inadequacy, often with consequent lowered self-esteem
- Self-concept is also affected by role strain and role conflicts.
- People undergoing role strain are frustrated because they feel or are made to feel inadequate or unsuited to a role.
- It is often associated with sex role stereotypes, for example women in occupations traditionally held by men might be treated as having less knowledge and competence than man in the same roles.
- Role conflicts arise from opposing or incompatible expectations.
- In an interpersonal conflict, people have different expectations about a particular role. For example, a grandparent may have different expectations than the mother about how she should care for her children. Role conflicts can lead to tension, decrease in self-esteem and embarrassment if needs for achievement, independence and recognition are unmet.
- Role performance is the actual behavior and expression of an individual occupying a role.
- It is the way in which individual perceives his ability to carry out significant roles such as parent, student, teacher, friend, etc.

- Each individual has multiple roles and personal needs. Many times conflict occurs between these two.
- To function effectively the person must know the expected behavior and values and should be able to meet the role requirements.
- Fulfilling the expected role leads to an enhanced sense of self.

Self-esteem

- Self-esteem is one's judgment of one's own worth, that is, how that person's standards and performances compare to others and to one's ideal self.
- If a person's self-esteem does not match with the ideal self, then low self-concept results.
- There are two types of self-esteem: global and specific.
- Global self-esteem is how much one likes oneself as a whole.
- Specific self-esteem is how much one approves of a certain part of oneself.
- Global self-esteem is influenced by specific self-esteem.
- Self-esteem is derived from self and others.
- In infancy, self esteem is related to the caregiver's evaluations and acceptances.
- Later the child's self-esteem is affected by competition with others.
- As an adult, a person who has high self-esteem has feelings of significance, competence, the ability to cope with life, and control over one's destiny.
- The foundation for self-esteem is established during early life experiences, usually within the family structure.
- However, an adult's level of overall self-esteem may change markedly from day-to-day and moment to moment.
- Severe stress can substantially lower a person's self esteem, for example, stress related to prolonged illness or unemployment.
- It is important that both strengths and weakness be identified.
- Self-esteem (also known as self-worth) refers to the extent to which a person likes, accepts or approves him, or how much he values himself.
- Self-esteem refers to a person's feelings of self-worth or the value that he places on himself.
- Our self-esteem often depends on how we evaluate ourselves. In other words, we make personal comparisons and validate how others respond to us. For example, when our managers respond favorably to our achievements, we are encouraged by our performance and our self-esteem grows.
- Self-esteem always involves a degree of evaluation and the person may have either a positive or a negative view of self.

High self-esteem gives a positive view of self and confidence in our own abilities leads to:
- Self-acceptance
- Self-concept
- Not worrying about what others think
- Optimism

Low self-esteem means having a negative view of self. This leads to:
- Lack of confidence
- Want to be/look like someone else
- Always worrying what others might think
- Pessimism

Horse and Gergen (1970) showed that in uncertain or an anxiety arousing situations our self-esteem may change rapidly. For example, waiting for a job interview in a waiting room.

FACTORS THAT AFFECT SELF-CONCEPT

Stage of Development

- Growth and development begins at birth and continues into adulthood.
- Typically a person will achieve specific developmental tasks as one passes through each stage of life.
- The successful accomplishment of each task will influence and reinforce the development of a healthy self-concept.
- Individuals who experience developmental delays or situations in life that prevent or delay the accomplishment of developmental tasks can have an altered or negative self-concept.
- As an individual develops, the conditions that affect the self-concept change.
- For example, an infant enquires a supportive, caring environment, while a child requires freedom to explore and learn. Elder's self-concept is based on their experiences in progressing through life stages.

Family and Culture

- Individuals typically grow up learning and integrating their family's heredity and culture into their life.
- Beginning at birth, heredity and culture shape and influence a person's self-concept. Individuals who have integrated their heredity and culture into their life tend to have a healthier self identity and self-concept.
- A young child's values are largely influenced by the family and culture.
- Later on peers influence the child and thereby affect the sense of self.
- When the child is confronted by differing expectations from family, culture, and peers, the child's sense of self is often confused.
- For example, a child may realize that his parents expect he will not drink alcohol and attend religious services every Sunday.
- At the same time, his peers drink beer and encourage him to spend Sundays with them.

Resources

- An individual's resources are internal and external.
- Examples of internal resources include confidence and values, whereas external resources include support network, sufficient finances, and organizations.
- Generally, the greater the number of resources a person has and uses, the more positive the effect on the self-concept.

History of Success or Failure

- People with a history of success will have a more positive self-concept whereas people who have a history of failures see themselves as failures.
- People with positive self-concept tend to find contentment in their level of success while a negative self-concept can lead to viewing one's life situation as negative.

Illness

- Illness and trauma can also affect the self-concept. A woman who has mastectomy may see herself as less attractive, and the loss may affect how she acts and values herself.
- People respond to stressors such as illness and alterations in function related to aging in a variety of ways.
- Acceptance, denial, withdrawal, and depression are common reactions.
- Many researchers have shown that self-concept and health-related behavior are interwoven.
- People with positive elf-concept may enhance their health and are likely to follow health care plan.

Age

- Self-concept changes during the individual's life span, being its maximum peak of permeability from seven to twelve years old, and starts to decrease at adolescence.
- People tend to take their good health for granted.
- When they become ill, their altered health status can change their self identity and self-concept.
- Alterations in body image can result from such health issues as amputation, cancer, mastectomy, trauma or scarring.
- The nurse needs to monitor for changes in the patient's self-concept due to alterations in their health status.

Gender

- There are clear gender differences in self concept.
- The studies show that girls have a positive perception of themselves during primary education and around twelve it produces a decrease in self-confidence and acceptance of body image and tend to have worse self-concept than boys.
- Thus, according to research, age acts as a moderating variable of the differences between girls and boys (Orenstein, 1995).

Education

- Education is a vital feature for interpersonal development.
- Academic achievements in the school as well as parental guiding and social interaction, are factors conforming the individual's
- The role of education in the development of an individual's self-concept is that it not only intervenes the teacher-pupil relationship but also the rest of professionals within the educational system.
- Since education does not end in the school, family is key for a positive development of self-concept

Culture

Majority of the studies focus on the divergence between Western culture, characterized by a more dependent auto-conception of the self, and Asian culture, in which interdependence stands as the fundamental factor in the development of self-concept

Religion

Religion, its leaders and their teachings also influence the development of self-concept.

Media

- The media has played a fundamental role in how individuals perceive themselves.
- Marketing and advertising have contributed to a general attitude of compulsive consumption as well as to the creation of an ideal body image as a way to personal and professional success.
- Research shows that subjects with a positive self-concept are less vulnerable to the influence of the media than those with a lower self-esteem.

Stressors

- Stressors can strengthen self-concept as an individual copes successfully with his/her problems.
- On the other hand, over whelming stressors can cause maladaptive responses including substance abuse, withdrawal and anxiety.
- The ability of a person to handle stressors will largely depend on personal resources.
- Everyone experiences stress at some level each day. Common stressors include financial, work related, relationship and health issues.
- Individuals react and deal with stress in different ways depending on their past experiences and success and failure with dealing with stress.
- Individuals who learn and use effective coping strategies to deal with stress will most likely develop a positive self-concept.
- People who become overwhelmed with stress may feel hopeless and powerless, leading to a feeling of low self confidence and self-esteem.
- The nurse may need to teach the patient effective coping strategies and techniques for handling stress.
- **Different stressors includes:**
  - *Identity stressors:* Self-concept is affected by stressors that affect individual's identity throughout the life and it is seen more in adolescents. Adolescents try to adjust to physical, emotional and mental changes which may lead to insecurity and anxiety among them. As adults have more stable identity, they have firmly developed self-concept.
  - *Body Image stressors:* Any changes in the body structure, appearance or function lead to stress and needs adjustment, e.g., amputation of any body part, or disfigurement affect the body image.

- *Self-image stressors:* Loss of employment, breakups, and other life changes can cause fear or self-doubt. These feelings can affect one's self worth, confidence, and resilience. Once these factors are compromised, a person may be more prone to developing negative beliefs and self-talk patterns.
- *Role performance stressors:* Numerous role changes occur in a person throughout his life. A shift from one role to another creates stress especially situations like loss of breadwinner of the family. A person may have to assume two or more roles at a time.
- *Self-esteem stressors:* Individuals with positive self-esteem will be able to cope with the stressors of life as compared to the ones with low self esteem. Self-esteem stressors vary with developmental stages. Low self-esteem and stressful life events lead to suicidal tendency among adolescents. Some of the many causes of low self-esteem may include—unhappy childhood where parents (or other significant people, such as teachers) were extremely critical. Poor academic performance in school results in lack of confidence.

Life Experiences

- Life experiences, including success and failure, will develop and influence a person's self-concept.
- Experiences in which the individual has accomplished a goal and achieved success will positively reinforce the development of a healthy self-concept.
- Difficult experiences and/or failures can negatively impact a person's self-concept unless they have established coping strategies to deal effectively with these challenges to their self-concept.
- Coping strategies are learned as a person encounters and deals with various situations in life.

■ NURSING MANAGEMENT

The nursing process facilitates providing nursing care to patients at risk for alterations in self-concept, body image. Self-esteem and role performance.

Assessment

- A thorough assessment includes a psychosocial assessment of the client and the family support to provide clues to actual or potential problems.
- The nurse assessing self-concept focuses on the four components, personal identity, body image, role performance and self-esteem.
- Before conducting a psychosocial assessment, the nurse must establish trust and a working relationship with the client. Identify the stressor and coping style of the client
- Assessment data are the basis for prioritizing the patient's problems and the nursing diagnosis.
- Patients at risk for alterations in self-concept, identity, body image, and self-esteem and role performance require a health history and physical examination.
- Frequent reassessment may be necessary to facilitate appropriate changes in the plan of care and expected outcomes.

Health History

- The nurse begins gathering data for the health history by assessing the patient's perception of their identity, body image, and self-esteem and role performance.
- Patient verbalizations of feelings and perceptions that reflect an altered view of these areas of self-concept will need to be further evaluated.
- **The nursing history should elicit data in the following areas:**
  - Feelings or perceptions that reflect the patient's view of oneself.
  - Patient report of any changes in body image, self-esteem or role.
  - Feelings of powerlessness and/or hopelessness related to any of these changes.

Physical Examination

- A complete health assessment includes a physical examination to obtain objective data related to the patient's health status and presenting problems.
- When assessing the patient's self-concept, identity, body image, self-esteem and role performance, the nurse should focus the physical examination on:
  - Nonverbal actions and behaviors.
  - Withdrawal
  - Lack of appetite
  - Wanting to sleep all the time
  - Not participating in care
  - Intentional hiding not touching or not looking at the body part involved.
  - Isolation
  - Interaction with others.

Nursing Diagnosis

After data collection and analysis, identify a nursing diagnosis. The North American Nursing Diagnosis Association International (NANDA) identifies the nursing diagnosis related to self-concept.

Self-concept

Disturbed Body Image: Disturbed Body Image is defined by NANDA-1 (2018–2020) as:

"Confusion in mental picture of one's physical self".

Related factors to disturbances in body image are as follows:
- Injury
- Trauma
- Surgery
- Illness
- Illness treatment
- Perceptual
- Cognitive and spiritual
- Cultural
- Psychosocial
- Developmental changes
- Biophysical

Patients who are at risk for disturbances in body image may have other associated physiological and psychological concerns.

The common nursing diagnosis that often accompany *Disturbed Body Image* include:
- Readiness for enhanced self-concept
- Situational low self-esteem
- Chronic low self-esteem
- Ineffective role performance.
- Social isolation
- Powerlessness
- Hopelessness.
- Disturbed personal identity
- Risk for compromised human dignity.
- Risk for loneliness.
- Readiness for enhanced power.

The list identifies related diagnosis for alterations in self-esteem and role performance that must be considered when planning care for a patient at risk for alterations in self-concept.

Planning/Outcome

Identification
- Holistic nursing care requires collaborating with each patient to identify goals for each nursing diagnosis
- Planning and outcome identification for the patient focuses on promoting a healthy self-concept or facilitating change in an altered self-concept.
- These individualized goals should reflect the patient's abilities and limitations.
- Nursing interventions are selected and prioritized to support the patient's achievement of expected outcomes based on the goals.
- For example, if the patient states that she considers herself overweight, unattractive and undesirable to others, this leads to a nursing diagnosis of Disturbed Body Image and the goals might include expressing positive feelings about herself and integrating a realistic body image.

Implementation
Several interventions can promote a positive healthy self-concept in patients; they are as follows:
- Encourage patient to list past and current accomplishments.
- Ask patient to describe how they and others would describe them.
- Assess the patient's report of changes in their self-concept, body image, self-esteem or role performance.
- Encourage verbalization of the positive and negative feelings and perceptions of the changes that have occurred to their self-concept, body image, self-esteem or role.
- Acknowledge normalcy of changes in the emotional response and grieving stages to changes.
- Assist patient in incorporating the necessary changes into their daily life.
- Assist the patient in identifying methods of coping that have been useful in the past.
- Assist patient in contacting appropriate support groups and/or counseling as needed.

Evaluation
- Evaluation of the effectiveness of nursing care is based on the achievement of goals and expected outcomes.
- The plan of care must be updated on a regular basis with additional interventions used as needed.

Nurse's Responsibility
- Nurse's acceptance of a patient with altered self-concept helps to promote positive changes.
- Nurse should show a positive approach towards the patient especially on patients with disfigurement, so that patient gains confidence to accept his condition as it is.
- The nonverbal cues of the nurse matters a lot. Nurses need to be aware that majority of people whether men or women are dissatisfied about their appearance and over all self-concept.

Here are Some Ways to Develop a Healthy Self-concept

Look Within
- We can start by looking at our inner selves, our belief systems and daily thoughts.
- If we feel that our 'real' self (who we are) is vastly different from our 'ideal' self (who we want to be), we should invest time and to address the difference.
- We can make adjustments by setting realistic expectations.

Check Non-Verbal Cues
- Our bodies and minds are connected.
- Sometimes, what we feel may reflect in our body language.
- However, there are times when we can redirect our self-concept through our physical movements, e.g., some of us walk confidently to feel confident about ourselves.

Make Important Choices
- Lifestyles and habits impact our self-concept to a large extent.
- It is one of the factors that determine how we may reach our ideal selves, e.g., some of us make it a habit to sleep in time and wake up in time to remain productive throughout the day.

Following are seven ways to foster self-esteem and resilience in students:
1. Accept students as they are.
2. Help students develop a sense of responsibility.
3. Increase students' sense of ownership.
4. Help students establish self-discipline.
5. Promote self-advocacy skills.
6. Provide positive feedback and encouragement.
7. Teach students to cope with mistakes and failure.

Following are few ways to present a positive image:
- Stand straight and walk with confidence.
- Smile. You will appear more approachable and confident.
- Be the first to reach out.
- Look directly into someone's eyes.
- Do not chew gum.
- Speak clearly and pause.
- Be fully present.
- Ask questions about them instead of talking about yourself.

CHAPTER 13: Psychosocial Needs: Sexuality

INTRODUCTION

- Sexuality is part of a person's personality and is important for overall health.
- It is the process by which people experience and express themselves as sexual beings, which is determined by anatomy, physiology, relationships with others, the culture in which a person lives, and developmental experiences.
- Many values and issues surround sexuality. Religious teachings, cultural influences on gender roles, beliefs about sexual orientation and social and environmental climates influence the values systems for both patients and health care providers. Sexually healthy people have a positive and respectful approach to sexuality and sexual relationships.
- Sexuality is the crucial part of person's identity.
- Sex is central to who we are, to our emotional wellbeing and quality of our lives.
- Professional nurses, as healthcare providers focusing on the holistic nature of care, have a responsibility to provide effective sexual health care for their patients. In a holistic approach to the patient health care, all aspect of the being interacts

MEANING

- A word *Sexuality* is how one person understands our bodies and relationships.
- It includes all aspects like one's values, beliefs, bodies, desires, relationships, gender. Thoughts and feelings
- Sexuality contains different components, our concept of own sexuality is changing time and it is unique to each person.
- Sexuality is self-defined and every person has right to talk about and understand their own sexuality in their own way that makes sense to them. It is a key determinant of one's health and wellness.
- Sex is the term most commonly used to identify biologic male or female status. However most suitable term is gender. The term sex is also used to describe sexual behavior in general.
- **Sex roles/gender role behavior:** Culturally determined pattern associated with being male or female. It is the out ward expression of a person's sense of maleness or femaleness as well as the expression of what is perceived as gender appropriate behavior. Each society defines its roles for males and females. Boys are given reinforcement for behaving in "masculine" way and girls receive reinforcement for exhibiting "feminine" behaviors.

DEFINITION

- Sexuality is the quality or state of being sexual especially sexual orientation and behavior.
- Human sexuality refers to people's sexual interest and attraction to others, as well as their capacity to have erotic experiences and responses.
- It is the state or quality of being sexual. It includes how you feel about your body, interest in sexual activity, your need for touch, the ability to communicate your sexual needs to your partner.
- Human characteristics that refers not just to gender but to all the aspect of being male or female, including feelings, attitude, belief and behavior.

Nurses play an important role to help patients to achieve health by having sound scientific knowledge regarding sexuality.

A basic awareness regarding sexual development, sexual orientation, factors affecting sexuality, prevention of sexually transmitted infections is necessary to render quality client care.

SEXUAL HEALTH

- Sexuality differs from sexual health. According to the World Health Organization (WHO) sexual health is a state of physical, emotional, mental and social wellbeing in relation to sexuality; it is not merely the absence of disease, dysfunction or infirmity.
- It is essential to be well-informed about all aspects of sexual health. Similarly, it is important to be aware of factors that can complicate an individual's sexual health.
- Sexual health requires a positive and respectful approach to sexuality and sexual relationships, as well as the possibility of having pleasurable and safe sexual experiences, free of coercion, discrimination and violence.
- For sexual health to be attained and maintained, the sexual rights of all persons must be respected, protected and fulfilled.

Characteristics of Sexual Health

- One should have knowledge about sexuality and soul behavior.
- One should have ability to make autonomous decision about one's sexual life within a context of personal and social ethics.
- One should have experience of sexual pleasure as a source of physical, psychological, cognitive, and spiritual well-being.
- One should have capability to express sexuality through communication, touch, emotional expression, and love, etc.
- One should have right to make free and responsible reproductive choices.
- One should have ability to find sexual health care for the prevention and treatment of all sexual problems, and desire.

Rights of Sexual Health

- The highest attainable standard of health in relation to sexuality, including access to sexual and reproductive health care services.
- Seek, receive and impart information in relation to sexuality
- One should have right for sexual education.
- One should have right to respect for bodily integrity
- One should have right for choice of partner.
- One should have right to decide to be sexually active or not.
- One should have right to decide whether or not, and when to have children.
- One should have pursued a satisfying, safe and pleasurable sexual life.

Components of Sexual Health

Physical structure, variations in the internal sense of what is male and female, family values, and culture values all influence gender-role behavior.

Five critical components of sexual health are:
1. Sexual self-concept
2. Body image
3. Gender identity
4. Gender role behavior
5. Freedom and responsibilities

- **Sexual self-concept:** A positive sexual self-concept enable to people to form intimate relationships throughout life. A negative sexual self-concept may impede the formation of relationship.
- **Body image:** A central part of the sense of self, is constantly changing. Pregnancy, aging, trauma, disease, and therapies can alter an individual's appearance and function, which can affect body image. How a person feel about his body is related to one's sexuality. People who feel good about their bodies are likely to be comfortable with and enjoy sexual activity. People who are poor body image may respond negatively to sexual arousal.
- **Gender identity:** Gender identity is the result of a log series of developmental events that may not conform to one's apparent biologic sex. Once gender identity is established, it cannot be easily changed.
- **Gender role-behavior:** Gender role-behavior is the outward expression of a person's sense of maleness or femaleness as well as the expression of what is perceived as gender-appropriate behavior. Each society define its behaving in a "masculine" way, and girls receive reinforcement for exhibiting "feminine" behaviors.
- **Freedom and responsibilities:** Sexually healthy people engage in activities that are chosen, including both self-pleasuring and shared-pleasuring activities. Individuals also have freedom of their sexual thoughts feelings, and fantasies. Sexually healthy people are ethically motivated to exercise behavioral, emotional, economic, and social responsibility for themselves.

Sexual Development Throughout Life

Sexuality changes as a person grow and develop. Sexual functioning changes with each stage of development.

Infancy and Early Childhood

- While many people believe that sexual development does not become an important issue until puberty and adolescence, children begin showing sexual behavior and interest in their sexual functioning from infancy.
- Babies are continually exploring their bodies to learn about them.
- The first three years of life are very important in the development of gender identity.
- The child identifies with the parent of same sex and develops a relationship with the parent of the opposite sex.
- Children became aware of differences between the sexes and begin to perceive that they are either male or female.

Infancy (Birth to 12 Months)
Characteristics
- Given gender assignments of male and female.
- Differentiates self from others gradually.
- External genitals are sensitive to touch.

Nursing interventions
- Self-manipulation of the genitals is normal.
- Caregivers need to recognize these behaviors as common in children.

Toddler (1–3 years)
Characteristics
- Continues to develop gender identity.
- Able to identify own gender.

Nursing interventions
- Body exploration and genital fondling is normal.
- Use names for body parts.
- Children have contact with adults of both sexes

Preschooler (4–5 years)
Characteristics
- Becomes increasingly aware of itself.
- Explores own and playmates body parts
- Learns to control feelings and behaviors.
- Focuses love on parent of the other sex.

Nursing interventions
- Answer questions about "where babies come from honestly and simply.

- ❖ Parental overreaction should be avoided to exploration of genitals.
- ❖ Provide parents and children

School-age Years
- ❖ Sex education often begins as simple anatomy lessons during the toddler years.
- ❖ But during the school-age years, the child might start asking specific questions about the physical and emotional aspects of sex.
- ❖ They need accurate information from home and school about changes in their bodies and emotions during this period and what to expect as they move into puberty.
- ❖ Menstruation or nocturnal emission is sometimes frightening for children.
- ❖ Some children view them as dreadful diseases or disorders.

School age (6–12 years)
Characteristics
- ❖ Has strong identification with parent of same gender.
- ❖ Tends to have friends of same gender.
- ❖ Has increasing awareness of self.
- ❖ Increased modesty, desire for privacy
- ❖ Continues self-stimulating behavior.
- ❖ Learn the role and concepts of own gender as apart of the total self-concept.
- ❖ At About 8 or 9 years becomes concerned about specific sex behaviors and often approaches parents with explicit concerns about sexuality and reproduction.

Nursing interventions
- ❖ Provide parents and children with opportunities to express their concerns and ask questions.
- ❖ Answer all the questions with factual data.
- ❖ Provide parents and children with opportunities to express their concerns and ask questions.

Puberty/Adolescence
- ❖ Puberty is the process of physical changes through which a child's body matures into an adult body capable of sexual reproduction.
- ❖ It is initiated by hormonal signals from the brain to the gonads—the ovaries in a girl, the testes in a boy.
- ❖ During the teen years, the hormonal and physical changes of puberty usually mean persons start noticing an increase in sexual feelings.
- ❖ The adolescent functions within a powerful peer group.
- ❖ They have the anxiety of "Am I normal" "Will I be accepted".
- ❖ They need accurate information regarding body changes, sexual activity, emotional aspects, sexually transmitted infections (STIs), contraception and pregnancy.

Adolescence (12–18 years)
Characteristics
- ❖ Primary and secondary sex characteristics develop.
- ❖ Menarche usually takes place.
- ❖ Masturbation is common.
- ❖ May participate in sexual activity.

Nursing interventions
- ❖ Adolescents require information about body changes.
- ❖ Girls should be taught about subtle signs of impending menstruation.
- ❖ Educated regarding dysmenorrhea.
- ❖ Peer groups have great importance at this time and assist in forming gender roles.

Young Adulthood
- ❖ During the young adulthood period, youth engage in increased cross-sex interaction, experiment with adult sexualities, and begin to sort into different romantic and career trajectories.
- ❖ Although young adults have matured physically, they continue to explore and mature emotionally. Intimacy and sexuality are issues for all young adults.
- ❖ Sexual activity is often defined as a basic need and healthy sexual desire may be channelized into forms of intimacy throughout life.

Young Adulthood (18–40 years)
Characteristics
- ❖ Intimate relations develop.
- ❖ Sexual activity is common. Establish own lifestyles and values.
- ❖ Many couples financial obligations and household task.

Nursing interventions
- ❖ Couples need to communicate their needs to one another early in their courtship.
- ❖ Young adults often require information about measures to prevent unwanted pregnancies.
- ❖ Require information to prevent STDs.
- ❖ Regular communication is required to understand partner's sexual needs and to work through problems and stresses.

Middle Adulthood
- ❖ The period of middle adulthood cannot be defined under a specific time limit.
- ❖ Cognitive, physical and psychosocial changes take place all the time throughout one's lifespan, yet middle adulthood is a particularly sensitive time for both men and women as their bodies continue to change even more than usual.
- ❖ It is during this stage that they undergo the process of menopause in women and male menopause or andropause in men.
- ❖ Changes in physical appearance in middle adulthood may lead to concerns about sexual attractiveness.
- ❖ Decreasing levels of oestrogen in women lead to diminished vaginal lubrication and decreased vaginal elasticity.
- ❖ These often lead to dyspareunia.
- ❖ Decreased levels of oestrogen may result in decreased sexual desire.
- ❖ As men age, they are likely to experience an increase in the post-ejaculatory refractory period and delayed ejaculation.
- ❖ Some aging adults also need to adjust to the impact of chronic illness, medications, aches, pains and other health concerns about sexuality.
- ❖ Later in adulthood, some individuals have to adjust to the changes associated with children moving away from home.

- ❖ When children leave home, the intimate relationship of partners usually changes.

Middle Adulthood (40–65 years)
Characteristics
- ❖ Men and women experience decreased hormone production.
- ❖ The menopause occurs in women, usually anywhere between 40 and 55 years.
- ❖ Diminished vaginal lubrications and decreased vaginal elasticity, leads to dyspareunia.
- ❖ Individuals establish independent moral and ethical standards.

Nursing intervention
- ❖ Anticipatory guidance regarding these normal changes related to aging
- ❖ Women and men may need help in adjusting to new roles.
- ❖ Suggestions, such as using vaginal lubricants and HRT to eliminate symptoms of menopause.
- ❖ People may require counseling to help them reevaluate and direct their energies.
- ❖ Encourage couples to look at the positive aspect of this time of life.

Older Adulthood
- ❖ Many people want and need to be close to others as they grow older.
- ❖ For some, this includes the desire to continue an active, satisfying sex life.
- ❖ With aging, that may mean adapting the sexual activity to accommodate physical, health, and other changes.
- ❖ There are many different ways to have sex and be intimate alone or with a partner.
- ❖ Sexuality is an important aspect of health in older adults that is often overlooked by health care providers.
- ❖ Research studies showed a positive correlation between sexual activity and physical health among older adults.
- ❖ Older adult's sexual activity depends upon their health status, past and present life situations and status of marital relationships.
- ❖ For example, many older women are widowed or divorced and lack sexual partners which account for their decreased sexual activity.
- ❖ Older adults are usually reluctant to discuss their sexual problems with health care providers.
- ❖ Nurses working with older adults need to be aware of the sexuality of their patients.
- ❖ It is essential to have a nonjudgmental attitude towards the sexuality of older adults.

Late adulthood (65 years and over)
Characteristics
- ❖ Sexual activity is less frequent.
- ❖ Women's vaginal secretions diminished and breast atrophy.
- ❖ Men produce fewer sperm and need more time to achieve an erection and ejaculate.

Nursing intervention
- ❖ Couples may require counseling about adapting their affection and sexual needs to physical limitations.

SEXUAL ORIENTATION

Introduction
- ❖ One's attraction to people of the same sex, other sex, or both sexes is referred to as sexual orientation.
- ❖ Sexual orientation lies along a continuum with a wide range between the two extremes of exclusively heterosexual attraction and exclusively homosexual attraction.
- ❖ Individual who are attracted to of both genders are referred to as bisexuals.
- ❖ The origins of sexual orientation are still not well understood.
- ❖ Some biologic theories describe sexual orientation in term of the genetic composition of the individual.

Definition
- ❖ **The American Psychology Association:** Sexual orientation is an enduring pattern of emotional, romantic and/or sexual attractions to men, women or both sexes." This implies an interest in a person due to different factors—biological, psychological, economic, cultural, religious, and social.
- ❖ Sexual orientation is an enduring personal quality that inclines to feel romantic or sexual attraction to persons of the opposite sex or gender, the same sex or gender, or both sexes or more than one gender.
- ❖ Sexual orientation is a person's sexual identity or self-identification as bisexual, heterosexual, homosexual, pansexual, etc.
- ❖ People's sexual orientation is their emotional and sexual attraction to particular sexes or genders, which often shapes their sexuality.

Categories of Sexual Orientation
- ❖ **Heterosexual:** Person attracted to the opposite sex. This sexual preference means that an individual feels attraction on an emotional, romantic or sexual level to people of the opposite sex.
- ❖ **Bisexual:** Person attracted to either sex. Bisexual means when one feels emotional, romantic, sexual, or affective attraction towards both sexes.
- ❖ **Homosexual:** Person attracted to one's own sex. Homosexuality refers to those with a sexual preference for people of the same sex.
- ❖ **Pansexual:** Person attracted to any gender identity. Pansexual are not limited in the sexual choice concerning biological sex, gender, or gender identity. Pansexuality is sexual, romantic, or emotional attraction towards people regardless of their sex or gender identity. Pansexual people may refer to themselves as gender-blind, asserting that gender and sex are not determining factors in their romantic or sexual attraction to others.
- ❖ **Asexual:** Person who are not sexually attracted to other people.

Factors Affecting Sexuality
Various factors are affecting sexuality. They include sociocultural dimensions, decisional issues and alterations in sexual health.

Sociocultural Dimensions of Sexuality
- Cultural rules and regulations influence sexuality.
- Culture, gender, education, socioeconomic status and religion influence sexuality.
- Society plays an important role in shaping sexual values and attitudes.
- Cultural norms influence the selection of partners, how often they have sex and how they relate to one another.

Family
- Children view parents as their role models.
- If parents can share affection and with other family when children become adults, they can give and receive affection.
- The family is the earliest and most enduring social relationship.
- Families are the fabric of our day-to-day lives and shape the quality of our lives by influencing our outlooks on life, our motivations, our strategies for achievement, and our styles for coping with adversity.
- It is within our families that we develop our gender identity, body image, sexual self-concept, and capacity for intimacy.
- Through family interactions we learn about relationships and gender role and our expectations of others and ourselves.
- Children observe their parents and model themselves after these role models.
- If parents are able to share affection with one another and other family members, children will most likely become adult who are able to give and receive affection.

Culture
- Different cultures differ concerning which body part they find to be erotic or sexiest.
- In some cultures legs are erotic. Body weight may be a determinant of sexual attractiveness.
- Sexuality is regulated by the individual's culture.
- For example, culture, influences the sexual nature of dress, rules about marriage, expectations of role behavior and social responsibilities, and specific sex practices.
- Societal attitude vary widely.
- Premarital and extramarital sex and homosexuality may be unacceptable or tolerated.
- Polygamy or monogamy may be the norm.
- Gender behavior also varies from culture to culture.
- Culture is so much a part of everyday life that it is taken for granted.

Religion
- Religion provides guidelines for sexual behavior and influences sexual expression.
- Religion influences sexual expression.
- It provides guidelines for sexual behavior and acceptable circumstances for the behavior, as well as prohibited sexual behavior and consequences of breaking the sexual rules.
- The guidelines or rules may be detailed and rigid or broad and flexible, e.g., some religions view forms of sexual expression other than male-female intercourse as unnatural and hold virginity before marriage to be the rule.
- Many religious values conflict with the more flexible values of society that have developed during the last few decades, such as the acceptance of premarital sex unwed parenthood, homosexuality, and abortion.
- These conflicts create marked anxiety and potential sexual dysfunctional in some individuals.

Pregnancy and Menstruation
- Sexual interests of women and their partners vary during pregnancy and menstruation.
- Some cultures encourage sexual intercourse during pregnancy and menstruation, but other cultures strictly forbid it.
- In Hindu culture, women avoid cooking and worship during menstruation.
- Research findings revealed that there is no physiological contraindication for intercourse during menstruation and most pregnancies.
- Females have increased sexual interest during the second trimester and decreased interest during the first and third trimester.

Discussing Sexual Issues
- Sexuality is an important part of an individual's life but sexual assessment and interventions are not usually included in health care.
- The area of sexuality is emotionally charged for patients and health team members especially nurses.
- Nurses usually avoid discussing sexual issues with patients because they have different values than their patients.
- If nurses are uncomfortable in discussing a topic related to sexuality, the patient is unlikely to share their sexual issues.

Personal and Emotional Conflicts
- Sex is a natural and spontaneous act that passes easily through several physiological stages and ends in orgasms.
- Nurses meet patients who have problems with one or more of the stages of sexual activity.
- For example, some women and men who are on antidepressants usually report that their ability to reach orgasm is negatively affected.

Personal Expectations and Ethics
- Ethics is integral to religion, ethical thought and ethical approaches to sexuality can be viewed separately from religion.
- Cultures have developed written or unwritten codes of conduct based on ethical principles.
- Personal expectations concerning sexual behavior come from these cultural norms.
- Many people accept a variety of sexual expression if they are performed by consenting adults, are practiced in private, and are not harmful.
- Couples need to explore and communicate clearly about various type of acceptable sexual expression to prevent domination of sexual decision making by one member of the couple.

Decisional Issues
Individuals decide their sexuality. Nurses can help patients to make decisions regarding contraception and abortion.

Contraception
Choice for the methods of contraception varies concerning the age, income, marital status, education and previous pregnancies of the woman.

Abortion
Almost half of the unintended pregnancies end in abortion. Half of all pregnancies in the United States are unplanned. The majority of unplanned pregnancies occur in teenagers. Abortions are safer and less costly if it is performed in the early weeks of pregnancy. When a woman chooses abortion as a way of handling an unwanted pregnancy, she experiences a sense of loss, grief and guilt.

Alterations in Sexual Health

Infertility
- Infertility is the inability to conceive after one year of unprotected intercourse.
- Some experience a sense of failure and may feel their bodies are defective.
- With advances in reproductive technology, there are many choices for infertile couples like medical assistance with fertilization, adoption, etc.

Sexual Dysfunction
- Sexual dysfunction is defined as the inability to fully enjoy sexual intercourse.
- Sexual dysfunctions are disorders that interfere with a full sexual response cycle.
- These disorders make it difficult for a person to have sexual intercourse.
- Sexual dysfunction, also called psychosexual dysfunction, is the inability of a person to experience sexual arousal or to achieve sexual satisfaction under appropriate circumstances, as a result of either physical disorder or, more commonly, psychological problems.
- It may be an absence of complete sexual functioning.
- Sexual dysfunction is more prevalent in men and women with poor emotional and physical health.

Causes of Sexual Dysfunction
- **Biological contributions:**
  - Physical illness.
  - Prescription medications.
  - Use and abuse of alcohol and other drugs.
- **Psychological contributions:** The nature and components of performance anxiety.
- **Social and cultural contributions:**
  - Erotophobia—learned negative attitudes about sexuality.
  - Negative or traumatic sexual experiences.
  - Deterioration of interpersonal relationships
  - Lack of communication.

Sexual Dysfunction in Males
- **Primary erectile dysfunction:** Inability of the man to penetrate during sexual contact and to sustain an erection to point of penetration.
- **Secondary erectile dysfunction:** Inability of the man to maintain erection but with H/o penetration at least one time.
- **Premature ejaculation:** Consistent premature ejaculation. Premature ejaculation occurs when a man reaches orgasm and ejaculates too quickly and without control. In other words, ejaculation occurs before a man wants it to happen. It may occur before or after beginning foreplay or intercourse.

Sexual Dysfunction in Females
- **Preorgasmic (primary) dysfunction:** Impaired ability of women to have orgasm.
- **Secondary orgasmic dysfunction:** Impaired ability of women to have orgasm currently but with history of ability to have orgasm.
- **Dyspareunia:** Painful intercourse.

Prevention of Sexually Transmitted Disease
- **Avoid:** The most effective way to avoid sexually transmitted disease is to not have sex
- **Stay with one uninfected partner:** One should stay in a long-term relationship with one partner only
- **Wait and test:** One should wait for vaginal and anal intercourse with new person until tested for sexually transmitted disease.
- **Use of condoms:** To prevent from sexually transmitted disease one should use latex condoms to prevent skin to skin contact between genital mucosal membranes. Never use any lubricant with that.
- **Get vaccinated:** Before any sexual exposure one should get vaccinated to prevent human papillomavirus (HPV), A and hepatitis B.
- **Avoid drink alcohol excessively or drugs:** If person is under the influence of sexual drive, then avoid drink alcohol or taking drugs.
- **Communication:** If person wants to make serious sexual contact, then communicate with partner about practicing safer sex. Be sure that partner is specifically agree on what activities will and would not be OK.
- **Consider male circumcision:** Male circumcision may also help prevent transmission of genital HPV and genital herpes.

PREVENTION OF UNWANTED PREGNANCY
It has considered being the most effective strategy for decreasing the number of abortions.

Causes
- Wrong use of contraceptives
- Wrong calculation of safe days
- Irregular use of contraceptives
- Non-availability of emergency contraceptive pills
- Lack of knowledge
- Failure of contraceptive

Methods of Prevention of Unwanted Pregnancy

Reversible Methods of Birth Control

Copper T intrauterine device (IUD): The intrauterine device is a small device that is "T" shaped. It is placed inside the uterus to prevent pregnancy. It can remain in uterus for up to 10 years.

Hormonal Methods

- **Implant:** It is a single, thin rod that is inserted under the skin of a women's upper arm. It contains a hormone progestin that is released into the body over 3 years. It helps to prevent pregnancy.
- **Injection:** Women get injections of the hormone progestin after every three months to prevent pregnancy.
- **Combined oral contraceptives:** Combined oral contraceptives contain the hormones estrogen and progestin is taken at the same time each day.
- **Progestin only pill:** The progestin only pill contain only one hormone, progestin, is taken at the same time each day.
- **Patch:** The skin patch is worn on the upper body (but not on the breasts). Patch releases hormones progestin and estrogen into the bloodstream. This patch is pasted once a week for three weeks. During the fourth week, a patch is not wear, due to menstrual period.
- **Hormonal vaginal contraceptive ring:** This ring releases the hormones progestin and estrogen. It is placed inside your vagina. The ring is wear for three weeks and for the fourth week it will take out for menstruation period, and then after menstruation get over put in a new ring.

Barrier Methods

- **Diaphragm or cervical cap:** Diaphragm or cervical cap is barrier methods which are placed inside the vagina to cover the cervix to block sperm. The diaphragm is shaped like a shallow cup and the cervical cap is a thimble-shaped cup. It is inserted into vagina before sexual intercourse. Both are come in different sizes.
- **Sponge:** The contraceptive sponge contains spermicide and is placed in the vagina where it fits over the cervix, It works for up to 24 hours, and must be left in the vagina for at least 6 hours after the last act of intercourse, after that it is removed and discarded.
- **Male condom:** It is worn by the man, latex condoms, and the most common type; help prevent pregnancy, and HIV and other STDs.
- **Female condom:** It is worn by the woman and it prevents the sperms from getting into woman body. It is packaged with a lubricant and it can be inserted up to eight hours before sexual intercourse and also may help to prevent sexual transmitted disease.
- **Spermicides:** Spermicides helps to kill the sperms and it come in several forms like foam, gel, cream, film, suppository, or tablet, etc. They are placed in the vagina one hour before intercourse.

Fertility Awareness-based Methods

- Fertility awareness-based methods-woman should know their monthly fertility pattern it can help to avoid getting pregnant.
- If woman have a regular menstrual cycle then she will count their fertile days and do not have intercourse on the fertile days.

Emergency Contraceptives

Emergency contraceptives are not a routine method to prevent pregnancy. Emergency contraceptives can be used if no other contraceptives are used during intercourse, or if the other contraceptive methods get fails like if condom torn.

- **Copper IUD:** Woman can inserted copper T IUD into the cervix within five days of unprotected intercourse.
- **Emergency contraceptive tablets:** Women can take emergency contraceptive tablets within 24 hours after unprotected sex.

Permanent Methods of Birth Control

- **Female sterilization (Tubal ligation):** It is a small procedure in which a woman can have her fallopian tubes closed so that eggs and sperms cannot meet for fertilization.
- **Male sterilization (Vasectomy):** It is outpatient operation in which tubes are ligated so that in ejaculation never has any sperm in it that can fertilize an egg.

AVOIDING SEXUAL HARASSMENT AND ABUSE

Meaning of Sexual Harassment

- American Medical Association define sexual harassment as unwelcome attention or behavior that a person finds offensive and that makes feel unsafe and uncomfortable.
- Sexual harassment is unwelcome sexual behavior, i.e., offensive, humiliating or intimidating. It can be written, verbal or physical, and can happen in person or online. Both men and women can be victims of sexual harassment. it happens at work, school or college, it may consider as sex discrimination.
- Sexual harassment affects personnel and is defined as any unwelcome conduct of a sexual nature that causes offence or humiliation.
- Sexual harassment is any unwelcome conduct of a sexual nature that might reasonably be expected or be perceived to cause offense or humiliation, when such conduct interferes with work, is made a condition of employment or creates an intimidating, hostile or offensive work environment.
- Sexual harassment may occur in the workplace or in connection with work.
- While typically involving a pattern of conduct, sexual harassment may take the form of a single incident. In assessing the reasonableness of expectations or perceptions, the perspective of the person who is the target of the conduct shall be considered.

Sexual Exploitation

Any actual or attempted abuse of a position of vulnerability, differential power, or trust, for sexual purposes, including but not limited to, profiting monetarily, socially or politically from the sexual exploitation of another.

Sexual Abuse

- The actual or threatened physical intrusion of a sexual nature, whether by force or under unequal or coercive conditions.

- Sexual abuse means the actual or threatened physical intrusion of a sexual nature, whether by force or under unequal or coercive conditions. It includes sexual slavery, pornography, child abuse and sexual assault.
- Sexual abuse refers to sexual contact with any person incapable of giving consent. It may include unwanted touch, sexual assault or battery.
- Sexual abuse is a widespread health problem. Abuse occurs irrespective of age, sex, socioeconomic status and ethnic group. Sexual abuse has far-ranging effects on the physical and psychological functioning of individuals.
- Sexual abuse can include many different things, from sexually touching a victim, to forcing a victim to touch the perpetrator sexually, to making a victim look at sexual body parts or watch sexual activity.
- Child sexual abuse is a form of child abuse in which a child is abused for the sexual gratification of an adult or older adolescent. It includes direct sexual contact of theadult or older person engaging indecent exposure of the genitals to a child to gratify their sexual desires.
- Children who have been sexually molested need to understand that they are not at fault for the incident. The parents should realize that their response is very critical to determine how the child reacts and adapts. Sexual abuse of a child is a criminal act.

Rape

- Rape is a type of sexual assault usually involving sexual intercourse or other forms of sexual penetration carried out against a person without that person's consent.
- The act may be carried out by physical force, coercion, abuse of authority, or against a person who is incapable of giving valid consent, such as one who is unconscious, incapacitated, has an intellectual disability, or is below the legal age of consent.
- In 2012, the FBI (Federal Bureau of Investigation) issued a revised definition of rape as "penetration, no matter how slight, of the vagina or anus with any body part or object, or oral penetration by a sex organ of another person, without the consent of the victim." The revised law is gender-neutral, meaning that anyone can be a victim.

Sexual Assault

- Rape and sexual assault have been used interchangeably.
- Usually, a sexual assault occurs when someone touches any part of another person's body sexually, even through clothes, without that person's consent.
- Sexual assault takes many forms including attacks, such as rape or attempted rape, as well as any unwanted sexual contact or threats.
- Social and behavioral scientists often use the term "sexual violence."
- This term is far broader than sexual assault. It includes acts that are not codified in law as a criminal but are harmful and traumatic.
- Sexual violence includes using false promises, insistent pressure, abusive comments or reputational threats to coerce sex acts.

Prevention of Abuse

- If warning signs or risky behavior is suspected, raining concerns with other adults can be the first step for protection.
- Staying silent, because do not have proof, may leave an individual exposed to danger
- Finding allies like other trusted adults or professionals can help to figure out what is needed to address the situation and prevent harm.
- Speaking directly to the adult you are worried about can, in some cases, lead that person to seek specialized help.
- If abuse is suspected, reaching out to protective authorities could lead to the protection of individuals
- Filing a report can result in holding the person who is abusing and getting them treatment so that they will be able to stop abusive behaviors.

Dealing with Abuse

- Nurses offer an opportunity to talk about feelings and may also be able to suggest a referral to a counselor who is experienced in dealing with abuse victims.
- The nurse may also be the first person to recognize symptoms of depression or suicidal intent in an abuse victim.
- When a nurse recognizes abuse, mobilize support for the victim and the family.
- All family members require counseling
- To promote healthy interactions and relationships.
- The rape victim needs continuous support to overcome the crisis.
- Nurses are in an ideal position to assess occurrences of sexual abuse and violence, help patients confront the stressors and educate them regarding the available community services.
- Nurses must report suspected abuses to the proper higher authorities.

Dealing with Inappropriate Sexual Behavior

- Inappropriate sexual behavior is a disturbing thing that can happen when someone has Alzheimer's or dementia.
- It can be one of the most challenging to handle because it often makes caregivers feel uncomfortable, embarrassed, or frightened.
- Inappropriate sexual behavior could be caused by a need to feel intimacy again, needing comfort, or being bored.
- Sometimes, people with dementia may even take off their clothes or masturbate in public.
- This could be caused by disorientation-not knowing they are not in a private place.
- Or, it could be because they are uncomfortable or need to use the toilet.

To manage inappropriate behavior when it happens:
- Stay calm and be patient.
- Gently but firmly tell the person that the behavior is inappropriate.
- Match your body language to your words—frown and shake your head.

- People with dementia are better at reading nonverbal cues.
- Maintain consistent, firm boundaries.
- Do not accidentally encourage inappropriate behavior by sending mixed signals, like briefly allowing the behavior one time and then reacting negatively the next time.
- Be consistently firm every time, saying "No, stop. I do not like that." or "Stop, that's not right."
- Distract them and redirect them to a positive activity.
- To distract, ask a question, turn on the TV, or offer a snack.
- To redirect, turn on some music they like, go for a walk, bring out their favorite hobby.
- Move your older adult to another location.
- This takes them away from what is triggering their behavior.
- Guide them to a quiet area in a public place or to their bedroom.
- If nothing else works, shock them a bit by raising your voice and firmly saying "No!"
- Grab their hands and put them back in their lap.
- Look them in the eye, frown, and shake your head to let them know this behavior will not be tolerated.
- Inappropriate sexual behavior includes sexual conversation or content.
- Comments and jokes of a personal or sexual nature. Inappropriate touching or grabbing. Explicit sexual behavior.

NURSING MANAGEMENT

Assessment of Inappropriate Behavior

- **What form does behavior take?**
  - In what context?
  - How frequently?
  - What are contributing factors?
  - What are the risks involved? To whom?
- **Comprehensive exam including thorough history:**
  - Is this a new behavior?
  - Related to underlying cognitive changes or exacerbation of life-long characteristics related to underlying psychiatric disorder.

Management

- **Talk about behavior:**
  - Talk to the person about their behavior and what you or others expect.
  - Let them know if behavior is not appropriate, if they don't know, they can't change it.
  - Let them know how the behavior makes other feel.
- Provide feedback about behavior.
- Explain sexual behavior to other people. Let family, friends, and visitors know ahead of time that inappropriate behavior or sexual remarks
- Identify the triggers for the inappropriate behavior and try to prevent.
- Manage the environment (Some individuals have limited insight and awareness about sexually disinherited behavior, and/or very limited capacity to change behavior due to severe cognitive and behavioral impairments. If this is the case nurses need to use strategies to manage the environment.
- Provide supervision and structure. Provide one-to-one support and supervision in any "at risk" situations. Provide cues and prompts about appropriate or inappropriate behavior.
- Plan Ahead. If a person has a history of severe you disinherited sexual behavior, it is essential that plan ahead regarding personal safety.

Non-pharmacologic Interventions

- Distract/redirect modify environment.
- Reinforce positive behavior.
- Do not reinforce negative behavior.
- Treat co-morbid psychiatric disorders.
- Behavior management therapies includes; supportive. psychotherapy and behavior modification.

Pharmacological Management

Goal is to suppress sexual fantasies, sexual urges and behaviors, such as antidepressants, anticonvulsants, antipsychotics and hormonal agents.

Psychosocial Needs: Stress and Adaptation—Introductory Concepts

CHAPTER 14

INTRODUCTION

- Stress is a type of psychological pain.
- Small amounts of stress may be desired, beneficial, and even healthy.
- Stress is a universal phenomenon.
- Everybody experiences it
- Parents refer to the stress of raising children, working people talk about the stress of their jobs, and students talk about the stress they experience in schools and colleges.
- Stress can result in both positive and negative experiences.
- When the equilibrium of the body is disturbed, stress occurs.
- Positive stress plays a factor in motivation, adaptation, and reaction to the environment.
- Excessive amounts of stress may lead to bodily harm.
- Stress can increase the risk of strokes, heart attacks, ulcers, and mental illnesses, such as depression and also aggravate a pre-existing condition.
- Stress can be external and related to the environment, but may also be caused by internal perceptions that cause an individual to experience anxiety and discomfort.
- It is important to become familiar with stress to effectively assess and treat patients and families suffering from the impact of stress.
- **Hans Selye (1974)** proposed four variations of stress.
  - On one axis he locates good stress (eustress) and bad stress (distress).
  - On the other is over-stress (hyper stress) and under-stress (hypostress).
- **Selye** advocates balancing this ultimate goal would be to balance hyperstress and hypostress perfectly and have as much eustress as possible.
- The term "eustress" comes from the Greek root "eu" which means "good"
- Eustress results when a person perceives a stressor as positive.
- "Distress" stems from the Latin root dis- (as in "dissonance" or "disagreement").
- Medically defined distress is a threat to the quality of life.
- It occurs when a demand vastly exceeds a person's capabilities.
- Stress may cause a headache. Nurses need to recognizethe signs and symptoms of stress and understand stress management techniques to aid persons and families in coping with stress.

STRESS

Definition

"Stress is a state of psychological and physiological imbalance resulting from the disparity between situational demand and the individual's ability and motivation to meet those needs."

"Stress is a state of mental or emotional strain or tension resulting from adverse or demanding circumstances"

"Stress is an excessive burning of energy resources."
—**Selye**

"It is defined as an interference which disturbs the functioning of organism at any level and produces a situation natural for organism to avoid." —**Harry Gottesfeld**

"Stress is a state of strain, whether physical or psychological."
—**Atkinson, Berne and Woodworth**

"Stress is the arousal of mind and body in response to demands made upon them" —**Schafer**

"Stress is an internal state which can be caused by physical demands on the body or by environment and social condition which are evaluated as harmful and uncontrollable"
—**Lazarus and Folkman**

"One of the leading authorities on the concept of stress, described stress as "the rate of all wear and tear caused by life."
—**Dr Hans Selye**

Stress can be positive or negative:

- Stress is good when the situation offers an opportunity to a person to gain something. It acts as a motivator for peak performance.
- Stress is negative when a person faces social, physical, organizational, and emotional problems.

Types of Stress

- Stress is our built-in response to danger, a surge in hormones as we choose between fighting, fleeing, or freezing.

- ❖ The danger may be real or imagined, immediate or farther away; our bodies do not know the difference.

According to the American Psychological Association, the three types of stress, acute stress, episodic acute stress and chronic stress.

1. **Acute stress:**
   - Acute stress is the most common form of stress. It comes from demands and pressures of the recent past and anticipated demands and pressures of the near future.
   - Acute stress is thrilling and exciting in small doses, but too much is exhausting
   - The feeling of when you are behind on a seemingly all-important deadline.
   - Acute stress can crop up in anyone's life, and it is highly treatable and manageable.
   - Our heart might race and your blood pressure might rise.
   - Your sense of emergency might trigger a migraine or even chest pain.
   - Other possible symptoms include irritability, anxiety, sadness, headaches, back pain, and gut problems.
   - These may appear for a short time and subside when the stress cases.

2. **Episodic acute stress:**
   - Some people experience these mini-crises regularly and live in a state of tension.
   - They may be taking on too much or simply be overburdened by their lives.
   - If you tend to worry, your body will be tense or angry.
   - The symptoms are similar but occur more often and accumulate.
   - Over time, a pattern of episodic acute stress can wear away in your relationships and work.
   - That risk is greater if you turn to unhealthy coping strategies like binge drinking, overeating, or clinging to bad relationships.
   - Many people also slowly give up pursuing pleasurable activities or meaningful goals.
   - If poorly managed, episodic acute stress can contribute to serious illnesses like heart disease or clinical depression.

3. **Chronic stress:**
   - This is the grinding stress that wears us down over the years.
   - It arises from serious life problems that may be fundamentally beyond our control—poverty, war, etc.
   - The demands are unrelenting and you do not know when they will stop.
   - If you had a traumatic childhood, you may experience life as chronically stressful even when the surface appears okay.
   - You believe you are perpetually threatened by poverty or illness even when this is untrue.
   - Whether the cause lies in your mindset or difficult circumstances, many people stop fighting for change and begin to accommodate chronic stress.
   - Chronic stress comes when a person never sees a out of a miserable situation.
   - It is the stress of unrelenting demands and pressures for seemingly interminable periods.
   - With no hope, the individual gives up searching for solutions.
   - The worst aspect of chronic stress is that people get used to it.
   - They forget it is there.
   - People are immediately aware of acute stress because it is new; they ignore chronic stress because it is old, familiar, and sometimes, almost comfortable.
   - It is important to get all the help you can and not blame yourself. The blame will only grind you down further. Chronic stress feeds chronic and acute serious illness.

Another Classification
1. Acute
2. Chronic
3. Eustress
4. Distress
5. Developmental stress

Eustress
- ❖ A positive form of stress having a beneficial effect on health, motivation, performance, and emotional well-being
- ❖ Eustress, or positive stress, has the following characteristics:
- ❖ Motivates, focuses energy.
- ❖ Is short-term.
- ❖ Is perceived as within our coping abilities.
- ❖ Feels exciting
- ❖ Improves performance.

Distress
- ❖ Distress is an unpleasant emotion, feeling, thought, condition, or behavior, in which the person is unable to adapt the stressors and causes.
- ❖ Anxiety or concern.
- ❖ Feels unpleasant.
- ❖ Decreases performance.
- ❖ Distress can be short- or long-term, it is perceived as outside coping abilities and leads to mental and physical problems.

Developmental Stress
- ❖ This type of stress usually occurs with the normal growing process.
- ❖ This is based on the health needs (physical and emotional needs) of developmental stages of life.

■ STRESSOR

Definition
Stressors are situations that are experienced as a perceived threat to one's well-being or position in life, especially of the challenge of dealing with it exceeds a person's perceived and available resources. When an individual encounters stressors, the body's stress response is triggered, and a series of physiological changes take place to allow the person to fight or flight.

"A stressor is that which is perceived as challenging, threatening or demanding that triggers a stress reaction"

"A stressor is an event or stimulus that causes an individual to experience stress."

Stressors: "Stressors are agents that cause stress. It is an experience to which a person is exposed through a stimulus or stressor."

"Stressors are tension producing stimuli operating within or on any system or factors that are responsible for causing stress are called stressors."
—Newman and Fawcett, 2011

Type of Stressors

There are many kinds of stressors. A stressor is our experience of how much demand for adaptation that an event or situation puts upon us. Some stressors are different for different people.

1. **Ripple effect stressors:**
   - These are stressors that, like a stone thrown into the water, ripple off in response to a change or life event.
   - One occurrence can continue to cause other daily stressors e.g., divorce.
2. **Chronic stressors:** These are long-term stressful situations that have no resolution in sight. For example, constant deadlines, overcrowded working conditions, etc.
3. **Acute stressors:** These are short-term stressful situations that will soon be resolved. For example, short-term illness.
4. **Not knowing stressors:** These stressors are due to not knowing the who, what, where, or how of a situation. For example, traveling in an unfamiliar city, Being new on the job, etc.
5. **Personal or non-personal stressors:** These stressors are caused by things that cannot be controlled. For example, being stuck in a snowstorm.
6. **Trigger stressors:** These are reminders of past stress that produce a renewed stress response. For example, watching workmen on a tall building reminds you of your fear of heights.
7. **Daily hassles:** Those minor annoyances that happen daily can add up to become a big part of your stress load. For example, Concern about health, weight, or fitness; being lonely; performance anxiety, etc.

Examples of life stressors are:
- The death of a loved one.
- Divorce.
- Loss of a job.
- Increase in financial obligations.
- Getting married.
- Moving to a new home.
- Chronic illness or injury.
- Emotional problems (depression, anxiety, anger, grief, guilt, low self-esteem.)

Another Classification
Sources and Types of Stressor
- There are many sources of stress.
- They can be broadly classified as:
  - Internal or external stressors,
  - Developmental or situational stressors.
- **Internal stressors** originate within a person, for example, infection or feelings of depression.
- **External stressors** originate outside the individual, for example a move to another city, a death in the family, or pressure from peers.
- **Developmental stressors** occur at predictable times throughout an individual's life.
- **Situational stressors** are unpredictable and may occur at any time during life.
- **Situational stress may be positive or negative,** e.g., death of a family member, marriage or divorce, birth of a child, new job, illness, etc.

The degree to which any of these events has positive or negative effects can depend to some extent on an individual's developmental stage.

Stressor can also be classified as physiological or psychosocial:
- **Physiological stressors** are stressor that exerts strain on human body. They have both specific as well as generalized impact. The specific impact includes an alteration of normal body structure and function, whereas general impact includes response to the stress. Primary physiological stressors include physical agents (heat, cold, trauma and physical injury), chemical agents (drugs, toxins), infections agents (viruses, bacteria), genetic disorders, hypoxia, nutritional imbalance and immune disorders.
- **Psychosocial stressors** are events, situations, individuals, or anything a person explicate as negative, threatening or fearful. They involve both real and perceived threats. The person's responses are continuous and include individualized coping mechanisms. These coping mechanisms serve to maintain psychological homeostasis.

SOURCES/CAUSES OF STRESS

General Sources of Stress

Demographic Sources

Demographic differences, such as health, age, education and occupation are some of the common sources of stress.
- **Health:** Sound health enables a person to cope up the stress in better way. Physical conditions of the individuals like illness, disability leads to potential stress.
- **Age:** Age is positively related to stress. When a person grows old, his/her expectations and responsibilities also increases and same is with the level of stress.
- **Education:** Education provides an opportunity to understand things and decreases the stressful conditions
- **Occupation:** The nature of the occupation and stress are related to one another. For example, a factory worker is exposed to environmental stressors.
- **Lifestyle:** Lifestyle of individual can also leads to stress. Sedentary lifestyles or career changes leads to stress.
- **Physical environment:** Surrounding conditions like high temperature, improper sitting arrangement or noise.
- **Life events:** Major life events, such as divorce, changing job, shifted to new location, relationship problem can produce stress
- **Traumatic events:** Extreme events, such as fire, train accident or road accidents, robbery, or natural disasters
- **Type of personality:**
  - Stress can also be self-generated.
  - Each individual have their own personality traits.

- So individual basic dispositions can also be the source of stress, such as uncertainty, fear or worries, unrealistic expectations or belief, self-criticism, low self-esteem, excessive or unexpressed anger., lack of assertiveness.

The Major Sources/Causes of Stress at Work or in an Organization

- **Career concern:** If an employee feels that he/she is very much behind on the organizational ladder, then he/she may experience stress. If he/she seems that there are no opportunities for self-growth, he/she may experience stress. Hence, unfulfilled career expectations are a significant source of stress.
- **Role ambiguity:** It occurs when the person does not know what he/she is supposed to do, on the his/her tasks and responsibilities are not clear. The employee is not sure what he/she is expected to do. It creates confusion in the minds of the worker and results in stress.
- **Rotating work shifts:** Stress may occur in those individuals who work on different work shifts. Employees may be expected to work on the day shift for some days and then on the night shift. That may create problems in adjusting to the shift timings, and it can affect not only personal life but also family life.
- **Role conflict:** It takes place when people have different expectations from the person performing a particular role. It can also occur if the job is not as per expectation, or when a job demands a certain type of behavior that is against the person's moral values.
- **Occupational demands:** Some jobs are more demanding than others. Jobs that involve risk and danger are more stressful. Research findings indicate the job that causes stress needs constant monitoring of equipment and devices, unpleasant physical conditions, etc.
- **Lack of participation in decision-making:** Many experienced employees feel that management should consult them on matters affecting their jobs. In reality, the superiors hardly ask the concerned employees before taking a decision. That develops a feeling of being neglected, which may lead to stress.
- **Work overload:** Excessive workload leads to stress as it puts a person under tremendous pressure. Work overload may take two different forms:
  a. Qualitative work overload implies performing a job that is complicated or beyond the employee's capacity.
  b. Quantitative work overload is a result of many activities performed in a prescribed time.
- **Work under load:** In this, case, too little work or very easy work is expected on the part of the employee. Doing less work or jobs of a routine and simple nature would lead to monotony and boredom, which can lead to stress.
- **Poor working conditions:** Employees may be subject to poor working conditions. It would include bad lighting and ventilation, unhygienic sanitation facilities, excessive noise, and dust, the presence of toxic gasses and fumes, inadequate safety measures, etc. All these unpleasant conditions create a physiological and psychological imbalance in humans thereby causing stress.
- **Lack of group cohesiveness:** Every group is characterized by its cohesiveness, although they differ widely in their degree. Individuals experience stress when there is no unity among workgroup members. There is mistrust, jealousy, frequent quarrels, etc., in groups, and this leads to stress to employees.
- **Interpersonal and intergroup conflict:** These conflicts take place due to differences in perceptions, attitudes, values, and beliefs between two or more individuals and groups. Such conflicts can be a source of stress for group members.
- **Organizational changes:** When changes occur, people have to adapt to those changes, and this may cause stress. Stress is higher when changes are significant or unusual like the transfer or adoption of new technology.
- **Lack of social support:** When individuals believe that they have the friendship and support of others at work, their ability to cope with the effects of stress increases. If this kind of social support is not available, then an employee experiences more stress.

The Main Sources/Causes of Stress Outside Work or Organization

- **Civic amenities:** Poor civic amenities in the area in which one lives can be a cause of stress. Inadequate or lack of public facilities like improper water supply, excessive noise or air pollution, lack of proper transport facilities can be quite stressful.
- **Life changes:** Life changes can bring stress to a person. Life changes can be slow or sudden. Gradual life changes include getting older, and abrupt life changes include the death or accident of a loved one. Sudden life changes are highly stressful and very difficult to cope with.
- **Frustration:** Frustration is another cause of stress. It arises when goal-directed behavior gets blocked. Management should attempt to remove barriers and help the employees to reach their goals.
- **Racial, caste, and religious conflicts:** Employees living in areas, which are often prone to conflicts among people based on differences, were seen in their race, caste, and religion does suffer more from stress.
- **Personality:** We can classify people as 'Type A' and "Type B'.
  - *The Type A' people:*
    a. They feel guilty while relaxing.
    b. They get irritated by minor mistakes of themselves and others.
    c. They feel impatient and dislike waiting.
    d. They also multitask and prefer to do several things at one time.
  - *The 'Type B' people* are exactly opposite and hence are less affected by stress due to the above factors.
- **Technological changes:** When there are any changes in technical fields, employees are under the constant fear f losing jobs or need to adjust to new technologies. It can be a source of stress.
- **Career changes:** When a person suddenly switches to another job, he is under stress to shoulder new

responsibilities adequately under-promotion, over-promotion, demotion, and transfers can also cause stress.

EFFECTS OF STRESS

- ❖ People experience stress as a consequence of daily life events and experiences.
- ❖ How stress affects the body will differ from person to person. Some people may experience only psychological effects from feeling stressed, while others may also experience physical symptoms, such as headaches and heartburn.
- ❖ Some individuals may also be more sensitive to the effects of stress on the body and be more susceptible to complications.
- ❖ Learning to recognize symptoms and exploring stress reduction strategies can help a person manage stress and reduce its effects on the body.

Stress Effects on the Body

Stress can affect the major systems in the body. Stress affects the central nervous system, immune system, and digestive system.

- ❖ **Central nervous system:** The central nervous system comprises the brain and spinal cord. Stress effects on the central nervous system may be manifested as:
  - *Headaches:*
    - Stress can be a trigger for tension headaches and migraines in some people.
    - About 70% of people who experience migraine headaches report stress as the trigger.
  - *Depression:*
    - Many experts suggest that stress may cause depression.
    - Some researchers have proposed the term stress-induced depression to refer to depression that occurs when people have a history of stress before their diagnosis.
    - Continual work-related stress can contribute to depression.
  - *Insomnia:*
    - The hypothalamus is one of the key structures involved in the sleep-wake cycle.
    - During stressful experiences, the body activates the hypothalamic pituitary-adrenal axis and the sympathetic nervous system.
    - These systems release hormones that stimulate attention and arousal, causing issues with sleep.
    - People experiencing stress may develop insomnia or have worsening sleep issues.
- ❖ **Immune system:**
  - Stress may cause decreased immune function.
  - In moments of acute stress, the body prepares for the possibility of injury or infection by activating the immune system, which protects it from outside dangers.
  - If stress becomes persistent, the long-term release of immune factors, such as pro-inflammatory cytokines, can cause chronic inflammation.
  - Chronic inflammation is a risk factor for diseases, such as atherosclerosis.
- ❖ **Digestive system:**
  - Stress affects the interactions between the brain and the gut. Some of the changes may affect:
    - Deep gut sensations
    - Smooth muscle movements
    - Stomach acid secretion
    - Permeability (potentially leading to the leaky gut syndrome)
    - Cell reproduction and blood flow in the gut
  - These changes lead to or exacerbate several digestive problems, including irritable bowel syndrome, heartburn, ulcers, and inflammatory bowel disease. People can also experience changes in appetite when they feel stressed.
- ❖ **Reproductive system:**
  - Stress can affect both the male and female reproductive systems, potentially leading to issues with the libido, orgasms, and sustaining an erection.
  - Stress may also affect sperm production and the maturation of sperm.
  - In women, stress during or the postpartum period can have a significant impact on health?
  - People trying to conceive may have difficulty if one or both partners are experiencing a stressful life event.
  - Some people may experience changes in the menstrual cycle due to stress.
  - Periods may stop or become irregular, and premenstrual symptoms can become more severe.
- ❖ **Musculoskeletal system:**
  - Researchers have identified a link between work related stress and the development of chronic pain.
  - Monotonous work and lack of social support are possible risk factors for musculoskeletal issues, such as lower back pain.
- ❖ **Cardiovascular system:**
  - During acute stress, the cardiovascular system prepares the body for the fight or flight response.
  - **These preparations involve an increase in the following:**
    - Release of epinephrine, norepinephrine, and cortisol
    - Heart rate
    - Contraction strength of the heart
    - Blood flow to the major muscle groups
  - When a person experiences long-term stress, these responses persist and can also lead to inflammation.
  - Chronic stress can lead to high blood pressure, heart attack, and stroke.
  - Before reaching menopause, people have lower cardiovascular risks because estrogen helps with stress management.
  - After menopause, when estrogen levels drop, the cardiovascular risks relating to stress rise.
- ❖ **Endocrine system:**
  - Researchers have identified that stress can reduce insulin sensitivity.

- An increase in the hormones epinephrine and cortisol during stress affects the body's response to insulin.
- Cortisol can also lead to increased fat accumulation in the abdomen.
- The effects of stress might differ between people in good health and those with insulin resistance or obesity. People living with obesity may be more sensitive to the effects of stress on metabolism.

❖ **Respiratory system:**
- Some people may experience breathing difficulties during a stressful response.
- Breathing difficulties, such as shortness of breath and rapid breathing, can occur with stress and strong emotions.
- When a person is in good health, these effects are usually not dangerous, but they may significantly affect people with breathing problems, such as asthma, emphysema, and chronic bronchitis.
- Research findings indicate that children with asthma experiencing a stressful event may have a higher risk of asthma attacks.
- Stress does not directly cause asthma attacks, though experts suggest that stress increases the frequency, duration, and severity of symptoms by increasing the extent of the body's inflammatory response to irritants, allergens, and pathogens.

INDICATORS OF STRESS

Common physical, physiological, and psychological indicators of stress are:

A. Physical and physiological indicators/Problems:
- Muscle tension—neck, back, legs, etc.
- Shaking, trembling, spasms.
- Headache—tension/migraine
- Enuresis and encopresis
- Digestion—nausea, acid, ulcers, gas, gurgling, cramps, pains
- Eating—compulsive, tasteless, loss of appetite
- Elimination—diarrhea, constipation
- Sleep problems—insomnia, early awakening, nightmares, excessive sleep.
- Pain—backache, the pain of shoulders and arms
- Teeth grinding/jaw aching
- Excessive sweating—palms, body
- Heart problems—palpitations, rapid, variable heartbeat, chest pain
- Breathing—difficulty catching breath, deep sighs, chest pain
- High blood pressure
- Skin eruptions—rash, hives, itching, eczema patches
- Sexual difficulties-impotence, low libido (desire), non-orgasmic
- Absence of menstrual period

B. Psychological indicators/Problems:
- Depression, distress, and lack of caring.
- Irritability, hyperactivity, impatience, restlessness.
- Anger, table-pounding.
- Nervous mannerisms, tics, facial, finger tapping, drumming.
- Speech difficulties—stuttering, stammering, halting.
- Tiredness-boredom, low energy state, inefficiency, fatigue, lack of concentration, loss of memory, confusion, disorganization.
- Passivity, lack of assertiveness.
- Difficulty making decisions, immobility.
- Being late, being too early.
- Self-consciousness, constant awareness of others' responses or reactions.
- Rigidity, inability to change or be flexible.
- Feeling overwhelmed, not in control.
- Unproductiveness, impaired performance, reduced problem-solving ability.

ADAPTATION

Definition

"The action or process of adapting or the state of being adapted or adjusted."

"Adaptation is defined as the physical or behavioral characteristic of an organism that helps an organism to survive better in the surrounding environment."

Types of Adaptation

❖ **Behavioral adaptation:** Responses made by an organism that help it to survive/reproduce, e.g., migration.
❖ **Physiological adaptation:** A body process that helps an organism to survive/reproduce, e.g., sweating, tough skin, etc.
❖ **Structural adaptation:** A feature of an organism's body that helps it to survive/reproduce, e.g., body color, Giraffe's long neck.
❖ **Spiritual adaptation:** It involves belief about a supreme being and a positive sense of life's purpose and meaning
❖ **Physiological adaptation:** The way in which body responses to stressors affecting the functioning of body.
❖ **Social adaptation:** Social and personal relationships with family, friends and co-workers; who support in the time of stress
❖ **Cognitive adaptation:** Involves education, communication, problem solving ability and perception of people and world.
❖ **Psychological adaptation:** Involves the use of defense mechanisms and learning to mentally accept new situations.

STRESS ADAPTATION

Definition

❖ It refers to the ability of an individual to adapt to changing stress in the environment.
❖ The initial stress response involves activation of the sympathetic system, a pattern known as the fight or flight response.

- Three structures control the response of the body to a stressor:
  1. **Medulla oblongata** controls heart rate, blood pressure, and respiration. Impulses traveling to and fro from the medulla oblongata increase or decrease these vital functions, e.g., sympathetic or parasympathetic nervous system impulses traveling from the medulla oblongata to the heart control regulation of the heartbeat. The heartbeat increases in response to impulses from sympathetic fibers and decreases with impulses from parasympathetic fibers.
  2. **Reticular formation** is a small cluster of neurons in the brainstem and spinal cord that continuously monitors the physiological status of the body through connections with sensory and motor tracts, e.g., certain cells in the reticular formation cause a person to regain consciousness from the sleeping stage
  3. **The pituitary gland** produces hormones necessary for adaptation to stress such as adrenocorticotrophic hormone, which in turn produces cortisol. The pituitary gland also. regulates the secretion of thyroid, gonadal and parathyroid hormones. A feedback mechanism continuously monitors hormone levels in the blood and regulates hormone secretion. When hormone levels drop, the pituitary gland receives a message to increase hormone secretion, when they rise, the pituitary gland decreases the hormone secretion.

GENERAL ADAPTATION SYNDROME

Definition

- General adaptation syndrome (GAS), is a term used to describe the body's short-term and long-term reactions to stress.
- Originally described by Hans Selye (1907-1982), an Austrian-born physician who emigrated to Canada in 1939, the general adaptation syndrome represents a three-stage reaction to stress.
- **Selye explained his choice of terminology as follows:**
  - "I call this syndrome general because it is produced only by agents which have a general effect upon large portions of the body."
  - "I call it adaptive because it stimulates Defense...."
  - "I call it a syndrome because its manifestations are coordinated and even partly dependent upon each other."
- The general adaptation syndrome involved two major systems of the body, the nervous system, and the endocrine (or hormonal) system.
- The general adaptation syndrome is also influenced by such universal human variables as overall health and nutritional status, sex, age, ethnic or racial background, level of education, socioeconomic status (SES), genetic makeup, etc.
- Some of these variables are biologically based and difficult or impossible to change.
- For example, recent research indicates that men and women respond somewhat differently to stress, with women being more likely to use what is called the "tend and befriend" response rather than the classical "fight or flight" pattern.
- These researchers note that most of the early studies of the effects of stress on the body were conducted with only male subjects.
- Selye's observation that people vary in their perceptions of stressors was reflected in his belief that the stressors themselves are less dangerous to health than people's maladaptive responses to them.
- He categorized certain diseases, ranging from cardiovascular disorders to inflammatory diseases and mental as "diseases of adaptation," regarding them as "largely due to errors in our adaptive response to stress" rather than the direct result of such outside factors as germs, toxic substances,

Three Distinctive Stages in the Syndrome's Evolution

Hans Selye called these stages the:
1. Alarm reaction (AR),
2. The stage of resistance (SR),
3. The stage of exhaustion (SE).

Stage 1: Alarm reaction (AR)

- The first stage of the general adaptation stage, the alarm reaction, is the immediate reaction to a stressor.
- In the initial phase of stress, humans exhibit a "fight or flight" response, which prepares the body for physical activity.
- During the alarm stage, the central nervous system is aroused, and body defenses are mobilized, during this stage, rising hormone levels results in increased blood volume, blood glucose levels, epinephrine and norepinephrine amounts, heart rate, blood flow to muscles, oxygen intake, mental alertness, and pupils of the eye dilate to produce a greater visual field. If the stressor poses an extreme threat to life or remains for a long time, the person progresses to the second stage.

Stage 2: Stage of resistance (SR)

- Stage 2, the stage of resistance also named the stage of adaptation.
- During this phase, if the stress continues, the body adapts to the stressors it is exposed to.
- Changes at many levels take place to reduce the effect of the stressor, e.g., if the stressor is starvation, the person might experience a reduced desire for physical activity to conserve energy and to maximize the absorption of nutrients from food.

Stage 3: Stage of exhaustion (SE)

- At this stage, continuous stress causes a progressive breakdown of compensatory mechanisms.
- This occurs when the body is no longer able to resist the effects of the stressor and has depleted the energy necessary to maintain adaptation.
- Generally, this means the immune system, and the body's ability to resist disease may be almost eliminated.
- Patients who experience long-term stress may succumb to heart attacks or severe infections due to their reduced immunity. For example, a person with a stressful job may experience long-term stress that might lead to high blood pressure and an eventual heart attack.

Causes and Symptoms

- Stress is one cause of general adaptation syndrome.
- The results of unrelieved stress can manifest as fatigue, irritability, difficulty concentrating, and difficulty sleeping
- Persons may also experience other symptoms that are signs of stress.
- Persons experiencing unusual symptoms, such as hair loss, without another medical explanation might consider stress as the cause.

Diagnosis

- GAS by itself is not an official diagnostic category but rather a descriptive term.
- A person who consults a doctor for a stress-related physical illness may be scheduled for blood or urine tests to measure the level of cortisol or other stress-related hormones in their body, or imaging studies to evaluate possible abnormalities in their endocrine glands if the doctor thinks that these tests may help to establish or confirm a diagnosis.
- The American Psychiatric Association (APA) recognizes stress as a factor in anxiety disorders, particularly post traumatic stress disorder (PTSD) and acute stress disorder (ASD).
- These two disorders are defined as symptomatic reactions to extreme traumatic stressors (war, natural or transportation disasters, criminal assault, abuse, hostage situations, etc.) and differ chiefly in the time frame in which the symptoms develop.
- The APA also has a diagnostic category of adjustment disorders, which are characterized either by excessive reactions to stressors within the normal range of experience (e.g., academic examinations, relationship breakups, being fired from a job) or by significant impairment in the person's occupational or social functioning.

Treatment

- Treatment of stress-related illnesses typically involves one or more stress reduction strategies.
- Stress reduction strategies generally fall into one of three categories—avoiding stressors; changing one's reaction to the stressor(s), or relieving stress after the reaction to the stressor(s).
- Many mainstreams as well as complementary or alternative (CAM) strategies for stress reduction, such as exercising, listening to music, aromatherapy, and massage relieve stress after it occurs.

Following habits can remarkably help to relieve stress:
- Regular meditation.
- Physical exercise.
- Balanced diet.
- Focused thinking.
- Control of anger.
- Managing depression.
- Maintaining calmness in stressful situations.
- Having a positive attitude towards life.
- Harmony towards self and others, etc.

■ LOCAL ADAPTATION SYNDROME

- Local Adaptation Syndrome (LAS) is the response of body tissue, organ, or part to the stress of trauma, illness, or other physiological change.
- According to Selye's theory, a local adaptation syndrome occurs and includes the inflammatory response and repair processes that occur in the local site tissue injury.
- The syndrome occurs in small, topical injuries, such as contact dermatitis, if the local injury is severe enough, the general adaptation syndrome is activated as well.

Acute Local Adaptation

In the Alarm Phase, the body reacts to a local stressor, e.g., postural distortions, trauma, reflex activity, etc., with an increase in local muscular tone.

Local Adaptation Syndrome—Acute Phase

- When the local muscular tone is increased for any length of time, the affected tissues suffer from
- Local ischemia due to increased muscular tone and demand
- Restricted elimination leading to the retention of metabolic wastes
- This may be considered the beginning of the *Adaption/Resistance Phase*
- The combination of ischemia and retention of metabolites leads to fatigue then irritation and may cause inflammation.
- The pain and discomfort that are likely to arise can lead to further increases in tone and pain via the Pain-Spasm cycle.
- Palpation at this time would show tissues to be warmer than other tissues. The tissues could be edematous, and would usually be very sensitive.

Chronic Local Adaptation

- If the adaption phase lasts longer than a few weeks, the sustained stresses stimulate the production of collagen. The body uses this collagen to lay down bands of fibrous tissue in support of the hypertonic muscle. This point could be considered the transition from an acute condition to a chronic condition.

Local Adaptation Syndrome—Chronic Phase

- Ischemia, lack of oxygen, and the retention of metabolites continue to increase, and myofascial trigger points begin to develop.
- At this point, taut bands are palpable in the local muscle tissues, and satellite trigger points begin to develop.
- The effects of increased muscular tone also begin to be felt at the muscle's tendonous insertions. This increased tone may lead to
- LAS of the tendon ORLAS of the tendoperiosteal junction or Early-stage joint dysfunction
- When the body's adaptive capacities are exhausted (which may take many years), the exhaustion or collapse stage sets in.
- This may be characterized by arthritic joint changes or chronic muscular/soft-tissue dysfunction.

❖ The progression of tissue changes in an individual body through these three stages depends on age, exercise, and nutritional status among other things.

MANIFESTATIONS OF STRESS

❖ Stress can affect all aspects of your life, including your emotions, behaviors, thinking ability, and physical health.
❖ Symptoms of stress can vary.
❖ Symptoms can be vague and maybe the same as those caused by medical conditions.

Psychological/Emotional Symptoms of Stress

❖ Becoming easily agitated, frustrated, and moody.
❖ Feeling overwhelmed, like you are losing control or need to take.
❖ Having difficulty relaxing and quieting your mind.
❖ Low self-esteem, worthlessness, and depression.
❖ Avoiding others.

Physical Symptoms of Stress

❖ Low energy.
❖ Headaches.
❖ Upset stomach, including diarrhea, constipation, and nausea
❖ Aches, pains, and tense muscles pain and rapid heartbeat.
❖ Insomnia.
❖ Frequent colds and infections.
❖ Loss of sexual desire and/or ability.
❖ Nervousness and shaking, ringing in the car, cold or sweaty hands and feet
❖ Dry mouth and difficulty swallowing.
❖ Clenched jaw and grinding teeth.

Cognitive Symptoms of Stress

❖ Constant worrying.
❖ Forgetfulness and disorganization.
❖ Inability to focus.
❖ Poor judgment.
❖ Being pessimistic or seeing only the negative side.

Behavioral Symptoms of Stress

❖ Changes in appetite—either not eating or eating too much.
❖ Procrastinating and avoiding responsibilities.
❖ Increased use of alcohol, drugs, or cigarettes.
❖ Exhibiting more nervous behaviors, such as nail-biting, fidgeting, and pacing.

Consequences of Long-term Stress

Ongoing, chronic stress, can cause or exacerbate many serious health problems, including:

❖ Mental health problems, such as depression, anxiety. and personality disorders.
❖ Cardiovascular disease, including heart disease, high blood pressure, abnormal heart rhythms, heart attacks, and stroke.
❖ Obesity and other eating disorders.
❖ Menstrual problems.

❖ Sexual dysfunction, such as impotence and premature ejaculation in men and loss of sexual desire in both men and women.
❖ Skin and hair problems, such as acne, psoriasis, and eczema, and permanent hair loss.
❖ Gastrointestinal problems, such as GERD, gastritis, ulcerative colitis, and irritable colon.
❖ Stress is a normal part of life and something you cannot control, however, you can control your stress response.

Ways to Deal with Stress

1. **Keep a positive attitude:** Sometimes the way you think about things can make all of the difference. Your attitude can help offset difficult situations.
2. **Accept that there are events you cannot control:** When you know there are times when you have given all that you can to a situation, it allows you to expend energy where it can be more effective.
3. **Learn to relax:** Purposeful relaxation, such as deep breathing, muscle relaxation, and meditation is essential in training your body to relax. Relaxation should be a part of your daily regimen.
4. **Be active:** Regularly being active also helps your body more easily fight stress because it is fit.
5. **Eat well:** Balanced meals staying on track with healthy eating habits is a great way to manage stress.
6. **Rest and sleep:** Your body needs time to recover from stressful events, so sleep is an important part of caring for yourself.
7. **Find your and effective ways to cope with them:** Remember that you can learn to control stress because stress comes from how you respond to stressful events.

NURSING THEORY AND ROLE OF STRESS

Many nursing theories explain and describe stress.

1. **Betty Newman's system model:** It explains individual responses to stressors and families" and community responses. A systems approach explains that a stressor at one place in a system affects other parts of the system. A system is a person, family, or community. Every person develops a set of responses to stress that constitute the "normal line of Defense". This line of Defense maintains health and wellness.
2. **Pender's health promotion model:** Focuses on promoting health and managing stress.

FACTORS INFLUENCING STRESS AND COPING

❖ Potential stressors and coping mechanisms vary across the life span. For example, adolescence, adulthood and old age bring different stressors.
❖ Situational and social stressors place vulnerable people at higher risk for prolonged stress.

Situational Factors

❖ Situational stress arises from personal, job, or family changes.

- Work-related stressors include promotions, transfers, changes in supervisors, and responsibilities.
- Work stress manifests as burnout among healthcare workers. It is common in an emergency, oncology, and critical care setting but can occur in any setting.
- Another stressor in the healthcare workplace is changing work shifts.
- Chronic, such as cancer, cardiac disease, diabetics, and depression are examples of stress producing illnesses.
- Job-related proactive coping strategies, such as resilience training for nurses working with trauma and critically-ill patients.
- Prepare nurses to tackle critical situations, provide time to practice stress management techniques, and manage job-related stress.

Maturational Factors
- Stressors vary with the life stage.
- Children identify stressors related to physical appearance, families, friends, and school.
- Pre-adolescence experiences stress related to self-esteem issues, changing the family structure as a result of divorce or death of a parent, or hospitalization.
- Adolescence identifies with peer groups. They experience stress related to Job, sex, school, and carrier choices.
- Adults experience stress related to losing parents, seeing children leave home, and accepting physical aging.
- In old age, stressors include the loss of autonomy and mastery resulting from health problems that limit stamina, strength, and cognition.

Sociocultural Factors
- Environmental and social stressors often lead to developmental problems.
- Children become vulnerable when they lose parents and caregivers through divorce, imprisonment, or death or when parents have mental illness or substance abuse disorders.
- Homelessness, living under conditions of continuing violence affects people of any age, especially young people.

■ COPING
- Coping means investing one's conscious effort, to solve personal and interpersonal problems, in order to try to master, minimize or tolerate stress and conflict.
- The psychological coping mechanisms are commonly termed coping strategies or coping skills.
- A coping mechanism is a psychological strategy of adaptation that a person relies on to manage stress.
- Sometimes, coping mechanisms are intentional choices, while other times a person may be unaware that they're using them.

Mechanism of Coping
- **Psychologists Richard Lazarus and Susan Folkman** scientifically defined coping as the sum of cognitive and behavioral efforts, which are constantly changing, that aim to handle particular demands, whether internal or external, that are viewed as taxing or demanding.
- Simply put, coping is an activity we do to seek and apply solutions to stressful situations or problems that emerge because of our stressors.
- The term "coping" is more associated with "reactive coping", because in general, we see coping as a response to a stressor.
- On the other hand, there's also what we call "proactive coping", wherein the coping response is aimed at preventing a possible encounter with a future stressor.
- While coping mechanisms are brought about by a person's conscious mind, it does not mean that all of them bring about positive coping; there are some types of coping mechanisms which are maladaptive.
- Other psychologists say that maladaptive coping is also synonymous with "non coping", since a person who responds to a stressor using a coping mechanism but isn't able to positively ward off the stressor or solve the stressful situation has not coped with the stress at all.
- The availability of coping resources affects an individual's ability to cope with stressful situations.
- Coping resources are characteristics or actions to manage stress which include health status, problem-solving skills, social skills, belief systems, social support, and financial resources.

Coping with stress is achieved:
- By removing stressors changing the environment.
- By developing proficiency in dealing with conditions we do not want to avoid finding adequate specific response.
- Seeking relaxation or diversion from the demand.

Factors Affecting Coping
- Degree of danger (perceived by individual).
- Immediate needs of individuals.
- Amount of support from others.
- Individual's belief (in own ability).
- Individual's previous experience (previous success or failure to ups).
- Number of concurrent or cumulative stress.

Positive Coping Skills
- Ability to orient oneself rapidly.
- Planning of decisive action.
- Mobilization of emergency problem-solving mechanisms.
- Appropriate use of resources.
- Ability to deal simultaneously with the affective dimensions of the experience and the tasks.
- Appropriate expression of painful emotions.
- Acknowledgment of pain, without obsessing over troubled feelings.
- Development of strategies to convert uncertainty into manageable risk.
- Acknowledgment of increased dependency needs and seeking, receiving assistance.
- Tolerance of uncertainty without resorting to impulsive action.

- Reaction to environmental challenges and recognition of their positive value for growth.
- Use of non-destructive defenses and modes of tension relief to cope with anxiety.

Negative Coping Skills

- Excessive denial, withdrawal, and avoidance.
- Frequent use of fantasy, poor reality testing.
- Impulsive behavior.
- Venting rage on weaker individuals.
- Over-dependent, clinging behavior
- Inability to evoke caring feelings from others
- Emotional suppression, leading to "hopeless helpless-giving up" syndrome
- Fatigue.
- Addiction
- Inability to use support systems.

COPING STRATEGIES

Coping strategies are psychological patterns that individuals use to manage thoughts, feelings, and actions encountered during various stages of ill health and treatments.

Types of Coping Strategies

- Over the years, psychologists and researchers have identified 400–600 coping strategies, and yet there are so many other potential coping strategies that are still under research.
- Because of this, the classifications of coping strategies vary
- One of the recognized groupings of coping strategies is that which was written by **Wayne Weiten,** which includes the appraisal-focused or adaptive cognitive, the problem focused or behavioral, and the emotion focused
  1. *The appraisal-focused coping strategies:* Are those coping mechanisms that involve the change of mindset or a revision of thoughts Denial is the most common coping mechanism under this category.
  2. *The problem-focused coping strategies:* It attempts to find solutions to resolve the problems causing the stress. For example, setting priorities. The problem focused coping strategies are those that modify the behavior of the person. A good example of this is learning how to cook a family dinner upon knowing that your spouse's family would come over to your house this weekend.
  3. *The emotion-focused coping strategies:* It involves managing the emotions that an individual feels when a stressful event occurs, for example, discussing with a close friend. It includes the alteration of one's emotions to tolerate or eliminate the stress. Examples include distraction, meditation, and relaxation techniques.

When a situation is unchangeable or uncontrollable, emotion-focused coping may predominate. If a problem can be changed or controlled, problem-focused coping is the most helpful coping strategy. Many psychologists also contributed to the study of coping mechanisms by grouping mechanisms or strategies according to their manifestations and purposes.

Classifications of Coping Mechanisms

- **Defense** the unconscious ways of coping with stress, e.g., reaction formation, regression
- **Adaptive:** Tolerate the stress, e.g., altruism, symbolization.
- **Avoidance:** Keeps self away from stress, e.g., denial, dissociation, fantasy, passive aggression, reaction formation.
- **Attack:** Diverts one's consciousness to a person or group of individuals other than the stressor or the stressful situation, e.g., displacement, emotionality, projection.
- **Behavioral:** Modifies the way we act to minimize or eradicate stress, e.g., compensation, sublimation, undoing.
- **Cognitive:** Alters the way we think so that stress is reduced or removed, e.g., compartmentalization, intellectualization, rationalization, repression, suppression.
- **Self-harm:** Intends to harm self as a response to stress, e.g., introjection, self-harming
- **Conversion** changes one's thought, behavior, or emotion into another, e.g., somatization.

STRESS MANAGEMENT

Stress management is a wide spectrum of techniques and psychotherapies aimed at controlling a person's level of stress, especially chronic stress, usually for the motive of improving everyday functioning.

Stress management strategies requires the following steps:
1. Identification of the root cause or source of stress
2. Device ways to reduce stress
3. Create and implement techniques for managing stress

Stress Management Strategies/Techniques

- **Mindfulness-based stress reduction (MBSR):**
  - SBMR meditative practices are effective in reducing psychological and physical symptoms or perceptions.
  - One of the most widely used techniques across the world, 'meditation' offers relaxation to mind and body.
  - It is a powerful technique to overcome stress.
  - Based on deep breathing, meditation gives peace of mind and improved focus.
  - Through MBSR patients can control their stress response to illness and treatments, employees can manage job-related stress and students can learn to manage stress and anxiety.
- **Exercise/Yoga:**
  - Regular work-out/exercise is good for the body and keeps stress levels in control.
  - Physical activities like lifting weights, walking release stress-combating hormones and have contradictory effects of putting physical stress on the body and relieving mental stress.
  - Regular exercise helps to effectively manage stress and reduce feelings of anxiety.
  - Yoga too is one of the popular methods of stress management practiced across the globe by all age groups.

- Yoga helps to raise body and breath awareness and is a great stress buster.
- Many other physical activities, such as Pilates, Tai Chi, or sports help to effectively reduce stress.

❖ **Guided imagery and visualization:**
- Guided imagery is based on the belief that a person significantly reduces stress with imagination.
- This method uses soothing and pleasant images such as that of nature and by visualizing a calming image and controlling breaths, it offers deep relaxation.
- It is a convenient method and easy to implement.

❖ **Time-management:**
- The majority of stress results from poor time management and planning.
- So, it is essential to create a timetable or schedule of tasks and prioritize them to effectively balance time and work.
- In many cases, setting priorities helps individuals identify tasks that are not necessary or can be delegated to someone else.

❖ **Self-care:**
- The well-known saying, Health is Wealth, is so true as without taking good care of health, one cannot work properly.
- So, when it comes to managing stress, taking care of yourself is vital.
- One needs to maintain a healthy diet and take adequate sleep to function properly and to keep physical ailments at bay.
- Resorting to substance abuse, such as alcohol or drugs should be prohibited as it further worsens stress.
- Thus, the role of a healthy lifestyle and good habits cannot be excluded from curbing stress.

❖ **Maintain a stress diary:**
- It is important to emit out the negative emotions and one can write down all the negative feelings in a diary as a way to let them go.
- Also, listing down positive emotions would help to shift the attention and one can think of memories to be grateful for.
- In this way, negativity is ward off and replaced by optimistic thoughts.

❖ **Assertiveness training:**
- Assertiveness includes skills for helping individuals communicate effectively regarding their needs and desires.
- The ability to resolve conflict with others through assertiveness training is important for reducing stress.

❖ **Aromatherapy:**
- Aromatherapy uses essential oils/scents to treat one's mood.
- So, the use of essential oils or aroma candles helps in reducing stress.
- Many research studies have shown that aroma oils having a calming effect and help in lowering anxiety and improving sleep.

❖ **Tune into music:** Researchers identified that listening to calm and soothing music helps to lower down the heart rate and blood pressure, thus reducing 'cortisol, the stress hormone. Therefore, listening to good music is an easy escape from stress.

❖ **Reading books:**
- What better way to stay away from the stressors, than picking up a good book to read.
- Reading improves concentration and keeps the mind away from stressful thoughts.
- It diverts the mind and thus is an effective method to lessen stress.

❖ **Socializing with friends and family:**
- Being in the company of loved ones helps to relax and enables one to share their concerns or problems.
- This allows for freeing up the feelings and garnering emotional support.
- Studies reveal that socializing helps in the release of the hormone called "Oxytocin which is a stress reliever.

❖ **Get a hobby:** Getting your time into some good hobby like painting, dancing or fishing enables your mind to take a break from stressful thoughts and keeping it engaged. Thus, it not only acts as a de-stressor but also engages your mind to use the time productively

❖ **Befriend nature:** Exposure to nature helps reduce anger, anxiety, and stress. Being in the company of nature enhances pleasant and positive feelings, thus, reducing stress hormones.

❖ **Progressive muscle relaxation exercise:**
- Muscle tension is a universal reaction to stress. Therefore, muscle relaxation is a common method of eliciting the relaxation response.
- Progressive muscle relaxation (PMR) involves the tensing and relaxing of muscles. The PMR is based on the principle that when muscles are relaxed, the mind will relax.

❖ **Massage:**
- It involves the systematic manipulation of the soft tissues of the body to reduce tension and enhance health and healing.
- Massage can be implemented as backrubs for patients.

❖ **Consult a psychologist/counselor:**
- Nowadays, many people seek professional help to manage stress.
- Therefore, seeking treatment or getting counseling sessions can also prove beneficial to manage stress.

❖ **Keep a positive mindset:**
- Many times, 'stress' is a result of our thoughts and therefore, one has to train the mind to adopt a new perspective and develop a positive attitude.
- Self-affirmation takes away unnecessary stress.
- Although, stress and feelings of worry can arise in personal and professional life, tackling stress by implementing the above-listed tips can help to keep the stressors away.

ASSIST WITH COPING AND ADAPTATION FOR STRESS MANAGEMENT

In assisting people with coping and adaptation, the nurse is concerned with helping these individuals learn to develop increased self-awareness, learn to modify the number and intensity of existing stressors, and develop effective, healthy, and potential coping skills.

To accomplish this nurse uses the nursing process:
1. Assessment
2. Nursing diagnosis
3. Planning
4. Implementation
5. Evaluation

Assessment

The nurse should assess for:
- Intensity of stress
- Duration of exposure to stress
- Risk to the patients' wellbeing
- Recurring nature of stress
- Signs of adaptive and maladaptive coping

Nursing Diagnosis

The stress response is viewed as an individual response. The nursing diagnosis can be framed as:
- Ineffective coping
- Anxiety
- Denial
- Fear
- Powerlessness
- Stress overload
- Situational low self-esteem
- Risk for post-trauma syndrome

Planning

- Plan for identifying the individuals, families, or group's perceptions of the stressors.
- To develop expected outcomes.

Implementation

Nurse can facilitate:
- Health promotion measures- exercise, relaxation measures, etc.
- Utilization of support systems of family, friends, and colleagues.
- Explore community resources to reduce stress.
- Facilitate self-directed change in individuals, families, or groups to promote healthy living

Evaluation

The nurse evaluates the stress management technique to:
- Promote patient's attainment of the expected outcome.
- Inhibit the patient's attainment of the expected outcome.
- Patient's self-awareness level
- Patients' personal strength to cope with stress.
- The patients' satisfaction with his problem solved.
- Patients' change in lifestyle to cope and adapt.

CREATING A THERAPEUTIC ENVIRONMENT FOR STRESS MANAGEMENT

Definition

"A scientific structuring of the environment to bring behavioral changes and to improve psychological health and functioning of individual."
—BF Skinner (1979)

"A therapeutic environment can be defined as the total of all external conditions and influences affecting an individual in the illness situation."

Purposes

- A therapeutic environment is an environment provided to patients which aims at effective and fast recovery of patients.
- A patient may be anxious before or during an appointment in a clinical setting.
- A therapeutic environment has a calming effect, reduces stress, and makes the patient feel comfortable with the care.

For Patients to have a Positive Experience, Consider the Following

- A therapeutic environment promotes healing, supports the needs of the patient and staff, and provides a measurable impact on patient outcomes.
- Adequate space should be provided in public areas and waiting rooms to avoid crowding.
- Perceived waiting time can be mitigated by positive distractions.
- Visual and noise privacy.
- Odors that are objectionable can create stress.
- Some basic factors to consider when it comes to creating a therapeutic environment.

Choose the Right Colors

- Your room colors and furniture should promote peace and tranquillity.
- Various shades of blue can help you create a calming effect.
- White walls offer a neutral feel and leave room for some paintings or a bolder color statement with furniture.

Reduce Environmental Stressors

- Practitioner's waiting room should always be clean and uncluttered.
- Offer patients a variety of reading materials to make their wait more convenient but keep them organized and presentable.
- If you have a children's waiting area, make sure that the books and toys are routinely packed up and put away.
- Make sure that furniture is routinely dusted, and floors are routinely swept and vacuumed
- Other environmental stressors may include glare from the lights or poor air quality.
- When these are eliminated, the patient experience can improve.
- These may seem like smaller details, but they make a significant difference in inpatient care.

Noise Reduction
- Noise reduction plays a significant role in creating a therapeutic environment.
- If the sound is already a factor within your office, white noise machines may help.
- They create a stronger sense of calm amongst your patients, and they can show that you value patient privacy

Exposure to Nature
Whenever possible you can design your office with a view of nature. Interior or exterior gardens, aquariums, and artwork with a natural theme all offer a soothing feel.

Give a sense of control:
- The ability of patient to control the environment directly contributes to successful patient outcomes.
- Private patient rooms result in better outcomes as nursing care is individualized and leads to better patient health.
- Give the patient as much privacy and control over it as is consistent with the need for nursing supervision.

Enable social support: Social support is essential factor for maintaining therapeutic environment in hospital, for example, provide places where patient can engage socially with family and other caregivers. Ensure culturally appropriate environment.

RECREATIONAL AND DIVERSIONAL THERAPIES FOR STRESS MANAGEMENT

Recreational and Diversional Therapies play an important role in reducing stress, as they help in diverting the mind of the person to different situations from the existing one.

Following recreational and diversional therapies help in reducing stress:
- **Play activities:** Playing carom-board, chess, and badminton. Involve the client to play just for fun and enjoyment.
- **Play therapy:** Play therapy is a natural part for normal development. Patient will be able to learn, master experiences, express themselves, cope with anxiety, create, achieve, and develop skills through play and recreational activity. Play and recreation can be therapeutic by giving patient the opportunity to explore, express and process their healthcare experiences in a safe and non-threatening environment.
- **Music therapy:** Music can be given as therapy as per clients' likings, e.g., religious cassettes. It consists of using selected musical composition to produce distinct sensory stimuli for varied periods of time. The sensory stimuli from music may produce counter stimulation to the pain stimuli, resulting in decreased pain perception.
- **Reading:** Create interest in reading religious books and happy ending novels.
- **Involve in hobbies:** Encourage the client to do activities related to his or her hobby.
- **Painting:** This helps reduce stress. Provide colors, sketches, and other materials that are needed for the painting. The client may express the situations of stress/causes of stress by painting or drawing.
- **Yoga:** Yoga helps in keeping a person physically as well as mentally fit. Encourage the client for performing yoga asanas by stating their positive consequences. Yoga includes simple breathing, movement and stretching exercises that are available to anyone regardless of age, fitness or health. The objective of yoga is to integrate the physical, mental and spiritual energies that enhance health and well-being.
- **Exercise:** A healthy body keeps a healthy mind. Exercise is very beneficial in reducing stress. So, a client is encouraged for doing a morning walk, performing simple exercises. Exercise means exertion of muscles or limbs especially for the sake of healthy bodily, mental and spiritual training. Exercises increase the efficiency of functioning of all body processes. Relaxation produces physiological effects opposite to those of anxiety, i.e., slowed heart rate, and increased peripheral blood flow and muscular stability.
- **Group activities:** They provide emotional support that helps a person to identify and verbalize feelings associated with stress. Families and support groups provide an accepting environment, allowing the person to explore problem solving methods and try out new coping skills Group activities like making masks, candles, making toys with clay in a group. By participating in a group, the group members will share their feelings, and their home/family condition that will divert their minds from their stressful conditions and they feel happy.
- **Progressive muscle relaxation:** The technique involves learning to monitor tension in each specific muscle group in the body by deliberately inducing tension in each group. This tension is then released, with attention paid to the contrast between tension and relaxation. Each muscle group is tensed for 5–7 seconds and then relaxed for 20–30 seconds, during which time, the individual concentrates on the difference in sensations between the two conditions. Soft, slow background music may facilitate relaxation.
- **Mind body relaxation:** The goal of mind body relaxation is to relax both the body and mind. The basic idea is that it is easier to relax your mind, if you first relax your body. There are a variety of mind body relaxation techniques including yoga and meditation. Mind body meditation goes by many different names, including mindfulness-based stress reduction and mindful meditation. The term "mind body" is spelled either as "mind-body" or as "mind body", to emphasize the connection between the body and mind.
- **Deep breathing:** Diaphragmatic breathing, abdominal breathing, belly breathing or deep breathing is breathing that is done by contracting the diaphragm, a muscle located horizontally between the chest cavity and stomach cavity. Air enters the lungs and the belly expands during this type of breathing. This deep breathing is marked by expansion of the abdomen rather than the chest when breathing
- **Meditation:** Meditation is a practice in which an individual trains the mind or induces a mode of consciousness, either

to realize some benefit or as an end in itself. The term meditation refers to a broad variety of practices (much like the term sports) that include techniques designed to promote relaxation, build internal energy or life force and develop compassion, love, patience, generosity and forgiveness.

CONCLUSION

- Life is more hectic with the advancement in technology.
- Stress-related diseases are on the rise.
- Coping and adaptation are the abilities that help the person to adjust to the situation.
- If the client cannot adapt or cope with the situation, the disease results.
- Nurses play a vital role in preventing the occurrence of disease.

Psychosocial Needs: Concepts of Cultural Diversity and Spirituality

CHAPTER 15

■ CULTURAL DIVERSITY

Introduction
- It is nursing that seeks to provide care that acknowledges and is congruent with a patient's culture, values, beliefs and practices—the crux of which is good communication between the healthcare professional, the patient and their family.
- Indian Culture essentially preaches peaceful coexistence, potential divinity of an individual and freedom of thought, Indian Culture is like a huge tree with its branches representing various systems of religious thoughts.

Cultural Concepts
- Culture is an umbrella term which encompasses the social behavior and norms found in human societies, as well as the knowledge, beliefs, arts, laws, customs, capabilities, and habits of the individuals in these groups.
- A culture is described as the thoughts, communications, actions, customs, beliefs, values, and institutions of racial, ethnic, religious or social groups.

Subculture
- A subculture is a group of people within a culture that differentiates itself from the parent culture to which it belongs, often maintaining some of its founding principles.
- Subcultures develop their own norms and values regarding cultural, political, and sexual matters.

Multiculturalism
- The term multiculturalism has a range of meanings within the contexts of sociology, of political philosophy, and of colloquial use.
- Various ethnic groups collaborate and enter into a dialogue with one another without having to sacrifice their particular identities.
- It can describe a mixed ethnic community area where multiple cultural traditions exist or a single country within which they do.

Cultural Diversity
- Cultural diversity is the quality of diverse or different cultures, as opposed to monoculture, the global monoculture, or a homogenization of cultures, akin to cultural evolution.
- The term cultural diversity can also refer to having different cultures respect each other's differences.
- It is often used to mention the variety of human societies or cultures in a specific region, or in the world as a whole.

Diversity
- Diversity refers to the attributes that people use to confirm themselves with respect to others, "that person is different from me."
- These attributes include demographic factors (such as race, gender, and age) as well as values and cultural norms.
- The many separate societies that emerged around the globe differ markedly from each other, and many of these differences persist to this day.
- The more obvious cultural differences that exist between people are language, dress, and traditions.
- There are also significant variations in the way societies organize themselves, such as in their shared conception of morality, religious belief, and in the ways they interact with their environment.
- Cultural diversity is vital for the long-term survival of humanity; and that the conservation of indigenous cultures may be as important to humankind as the conservation of species and ecosystems is to life in general.
- With the onset of globalization, traditional nation-states have been placed under enormous pressure.
- Today, with the development of technology, information and capital are transcending geographical boundaries and reshaping the relationships between the marketplace, states, and citizens.
- In particular, the growth of the mass media industry has largely impacted individuals and societies across the globe.
- Although beneficial in some ways, this increased accessibility has the capacity to negatively affect a society's individuality.
- With information being so easily distributed throughout the world, cultural meanings, values, and tastes run the risk of becoming homogenized.
- As a result, the strength of the identity of individuals and societies may begin to weaken.

- With the advent of globalism, a decline in cultural diversity is inevitable because information sharing often promotes homogeneity and in a society where many people from different cultural backgrounds are living, mutual understanding is essential to promote a future with appreciative cultural diversity.
- The intangible cultural heritage, transmitted from generation to generation is constantly recreated by communities and groups in response to their environment, their interaction with nature and their history, and gives them a sense of identity and continuity, thus promoting respect for cultural diversity and human creativity.

Race

- A race is a grouping of humans based on shared physical or social qualities into categories generally viewed as distinct by society.
- Race is a human system that is socially constructed to distinguish between groups of people who share phonotypical characteristics.
- Race is the group of people who have differences and similarities in biological traits.
- The human species is divided into distinct groups on the basis of inherited physical and behavioral differences for example; the term race generally refers to a group of people who have in common some visible physical traits, such as skin color, hair texture, facial features, and eye formation.
- Such distinctive features are associated with large, geographically separated populations such as races, as the "African race," the "European race and the "Asian race".

Acculturation

- Acculturation is a process of social, psychological, and cultural change that stems from two cultures while adapting to the prevailing culture of the society.
- It is defined as the exchange of cultural features (traditions, values, or religious beliefs comprising the way of life) which results when groups of individuals from different cultures come into continuous direct contact, resulting in an alteration in the cultural patterns of one or both groups.
- While, theoretically, acculturation can work in both directions, the norm is that the minority population is assimilated into the population's dominant majority.
- It is the process of cultural and psychological changes that takes place as a result of contact between cultural groups and their individual members.
- Acculturation follows migration and continues in culturally plural societies among ethno cultural communities.
- Adaptation to living in culture contact settings takes place over time.
- It results in some form of mutual accommodation.

Cultural Assimilation

- Cultural assimilation is the process in which a minority group or culture comes to resemble a society's majority group or assume the values, behaviors, and beliefs of another group whether fully or partially.
- There are different forms of cultural assimilation.

Transcultural nursing

- Transcultural nursing is how professional nursing interacts with the concept of culture.
- It is supported by nursing theory, research, and practice.
- It is a body of knowledge that assists in providing culturally appropriate nursing care.

Cultural Competence

- Cultural competence, also known as intercultural competence, is a continuous and life long journey to increase people's skills in being proficient in intercultural and intracultural knowledge which can improve the ability to work with people with different culture.
- Cultural competence is the ability of a person to effectively interact, work, and develop meaningful relationships with people of various cultural backgrounds.
- Cultural background can include the beliefs, customs, and behaviors of people from various groups.
- It demonstrates knowledge and understanding of the client's culture; accepting and respecting cultural differences; adapting care to be congruent with the client's culture.
- In other words, cultural competence is learning how cultural differences may impact healthcare decisions and how to modify care to align with that patient's culture.

PROVIDING CULTURALLY RESPONSIVE CARE

There are many things nurses can do to provide culturally sensitive care to clients from different cultural background.

Awareness

- The nurse needs to have awareness about the need for culturally competent care.
- Encourage your co-workers to provide more culturally competent care.

Avoid Making Assumptions

- It is important that nurses avoid making assumptions about cultures that are not familiar with.
- This can lead to a breakdown of trust and rapport between the nurse and their patients and reduce treatment acceptance.
- If you are unsure about something, simply the client.
- Most people of different cultures will happily educate a healthcare provider who is willing to listen and understand their cultural differences.
- When asking questions, make sure your body language communicates openness and intent to truly hear the patient.

Learn About Other Cultures

- As a nurse, part of your responsibility to your patient is to learn about him. Often this aspect is neglected.
- In reality, healthcare only reaches its full potential when the whole patient is considered, including their family, their day to day life, and their culture.
- Make an effort to learn about other cultures by becoming immersed in them.

- Visit the area where that culture is dominant and read about the culture from reputable books and online sources,

Build Trust and Rapport
- It is essential for nurses to build trust with their patients, regardless of ethnic or racial backgrounds.
- Treating culturally diverse patients require a heightened level of trust to be established, which can become even more difficult when there is a language barrier.
- Ask for a translator, but do not be tempted to look at the translator when speaking.
- Look at the patient and speak to them as if no language barrier existed.
- The translator will relay the information to the patient and then their response back to you.
- Body language and eye contact become much more important, so be sure to display open and kind body language and look the patient in the eyes when speaking to him or his family members.

Overcome Language Barriers
- Language barriers exacerbate all other challenges nurses face when providing care for culturally diverse patients.
- To effectively communicate with a patient to ask them about their health history or to educate them about a procedure, the language barrier must be broken in some way.
- Ask your facility if a translator is available. Most hospitals do have translator staff.
- Explore translation technology while it may not be 100% accurate, it can help you better understand your patients and your patients better understand you. Use pictures or hand gestures to communicate when necessary, and remember to be patient.
- Language barriers are frustrating for both you and your patient, but your patient is at a distinct disadvantage.

Educate Patients about Medical Practices
- It is critical that every patient, regardless of their cultural or racial background, give informed consent for any medical procedures.
- If they are unfamiliar with a medical practice, nurses often have the job of explaining in detail why the procedure is needed and what to expect during and after the procedure.
- Additionally, patients from some cultural backgrounds need further education on how to manage at home on their own.
- They may need to blend new practices with cultural traditions to maintain their health, and education is a key component of that process
- When communicating with a patient, ask him to repeat back to you what you said, in his own words. If there is a language barrier, a translator can help.
- Essentially, this will help you determine how much of what you are saying has been understood and how you might be able to change the way you communicate to improve the patient's understanding.
- Continue until you are reasonably confident that the patient has enough clarity about the next step to willingly and knowingly consent to it.

Practice Active Listening
- Active listening in the healthcare community is imperative, especially when individuals of different racial or cultural backgrounds are involved.
- It is important that patients feel that they are heard and validated, particularly when they are in a vulnerable position.
- After asking a question to your patient, take the time to really listen.
- Sit down with him, make eye contact.
- Reassure him that you're there and ready to hear what he has to say.
- If you need clarity, ask.
- If your patient becomes frustrated by a language barrier, remain calm and let him know it is okay to take his time when communicating with you.
- Repeat back to him what he said in your own words, so he can also have confidence that you have understood him.

Spirituality
- Concepts—faith, hope, religion, spirituality, spiritual wellbeing
- Factors affecting spirituality
- Spiritual problems in acute, chronic, terminal illnesses and near-death experience
- Dealing with spiritual distress/problems

▌SPIRITUALITY

Introduction
- Spirituality is a broad concept with room for many perspectives.
- In general, it includes a sense of connection to something bigger than us, and it typically involves a search for meaning in life.
- As such, it is a universal human experience-something that touches us all.
- Emotional health is about cultivating a positive state of mind, which can broaden your outlook to recognize and incorporate a connection to something larger than yourself

▌CONCEPTS: FAITH, HOPE, RELIGION, SPIRITUALITY, SPIRITUAL WELLBEING

Faith
- Faith, derived from Latin 'fides' and Old French 'feid', is confidence or trust in a person, thing, or concept.
- In the context of religion, faith can be defined as "belief in a god or in the doctrines or teachings of religion".
- Religious people often think of faith as confidence based on a perceived degree of warrant, while others who are more skeptical of religion tend to think of faith as simply belief without evidence.

- It is a strong belief in the doctrines of a religion, based on spiritual conviction rather than proof.
- It is personal and means different to everyone.
- Faith includes a general religious attitude and personal acceptance of a specific set of beliefs.
- Both religion and spirituality require faith as a foundation.
- In other words, faith is the guiding principle by which individuals are either religious or spiritual.
- Faith serves as both the source and the target of their religion or spirituality.
- Devotion to religion or perception of growth in spirituality may be seen as a measure of understanding one's faith.

Hope

- Hope is an optimistic state of mind that is based on an expectation of positive outcomes with respect to events and circumstances in one's life or the world at large.
- It means "expect with confidence" and "to cherish a desire with anticipation" or to want something to happen.
- Spirituality and faith bring hope.
- Hope is anticipation of a continued good, an improvement or lessening of something unpleasant.
- It is multidimensional concept that is energizing and provides comfort while enduring life threats and personal challenges.
- Hope enhances coping skills and influences a person's survival.
- A person often reveals hope through an expression of expectations for life, the present and the future.
- Often in terminal illness, a patient focuses hope on milestones, significant events or for the relief of pain or other disabling symptoms.
- A person's spiritual distress is often based on his definition of hope. Person may view hope as encouragement to work toward recovery.
- Hope can be found in all aspects of life as a force that help person cope.
- It has a purpose and gives direction and gives reason for being.
- The existence and maintenance of hope depend on person having strong relationship and sense of emotional connectedness to others.
- Hopefulness offers an ability to see life as enduring and having sustained meaning or purpose.

Religion

- Religion refers to the system of organized beliefs and worship that a person practices to outwardly express spirituality.
- Religion is the belief in and worship of a superhuman controlling power, especially a personal God or Gods.
- Religion is a social-cultural system of designated behaviors and practices, morals, beliefs, worldviews, sanctified places, prophecies, ethics, or organizations that relates humanity to supernatural and spiritual elements.
- Different religions may/may not contain various elements ranging from the divine, sacred things, faith, a supernatural being or supernatural beings that will provide norms and power for the rest of life".
- Religious practices may include rituals, sermons, commemoration or veneration (of deities and/or saints), sacrifices, festivals, feasts, initiations, funerary services, matrimonial services, meditation, prayer, music, art, dance, public service, or other aspects of culture.
- Religions have sacred histories and narratives, which may be preserved in sacred scriptures, and symbols and holy places, that aim mostly to give a meaning to life.
- Religions may contain symbolic stories, which are sometimes said by followers to be true, that may also attempt to explain the origin of life, the universe, and other phenomena.
- Faith has been considered a source of religious beliefs.
- There are an estimated 10,000 distinct religions worldwide.
- About 84% of the world's population is affiliated with Christianity, Islam, Hinduism, Buddhism, or some form of folk religion.
- The religiously unaffiliated demographic includes those who do not identify with any particular religion, atheists, and agnostics. While the religiously unaffiliated have grown globally, many of the religiously unaffiliated still have various religious beliefs.

Spirituality

- Spirituality offers a sense of harmony and wholeness within self and with God, with ecosystem and with others.
- Spirituality is a worldview and a way of life based on the belief that there is more to life than what meets the senses, more to the universe than just purposeless mechanics, more to consciousness than electrical impulses in the brain, and more to our existence than the body and its needs.
- Spirituality usually involves the belief in a higher form of intelligence or consciousness running the universe, as well as life after death.
- Spirituality is about seeking a meaningful connection with something bigger than you, which can result in positive emotions, such as peace, awe, contentment, gratitude, and acceptance.

Spiritual Health and Wellbeing

- Health is defined as a state of wellbeing, resulting from harmonious interaction of body, mind, spirit and environment.
- Spiritual health refers to a state of wholeness of the spiritual dimensions which includes a sense of personal contentment, peace with the self and others, the ability to experience love, joy, place and contentment and live in wholeness consistent with the values of community and self.

Dimensions of Spiritual Health

- A sense of personal contentment.
- A sense of peace with the self and the world.
- A sense of fulfillment in life and interaction with self and others.
- The ability to discover and articulate a basic purpose in life.
- The ability to experience love, joy, place and contentment.

❖ The ability to live wholeness consistent with the values of community and self.

Factors Affecting Spiritual Well Being

Many factors affect our psychological and spiritual wellbeing. The spiritual needs of patient vary depending on his spiritual beliefs, faith, state of illness and adaptation to illness.

- **Cultural and religious background:** Culture means attitude, belief and values that arise from one's socio-cultural background that affects spiritual health. The culture and religion influence spiritual needs and preferences. All religious beliefs and practices are bound to the culture. The leadership pattern of the culture also affects client's spiritual needs. The leaders have great influence on the spiritual aspects.
- **Physiological factors:** Many illnesses affect the sense of wellbeing and may predispose to a spiritual conflict. When a life-threatening disease occurs one may even doubt the religion and its beliefs. He may even question the meaning purpose of disease. A patient with severe pain always not get involve in spiritual activities as usual.
- **Psychosocial factors:** Social support system and social roles can influence spiritual responses. The personality, outlook on life and coping styles also influence spirituality
- **Age:** Children do not have spiritual crisis as adults. Children usually follow the teachings of parents or teachers. But adolescents may question the religious beliefs and teachings, whereas religion and spirituality become more important as a person ages. Religion is the key to life satisfaction for many older adults.
- **Gender:** Each religion has its own expected behavior for male and female patients.
- **Crisis and change:** Usually people become more spiritual during crisis but in some cases like death of a dear one or life-threatening disease of a loved one make them distressed and may weaken the spiritual hope and faith (spiritual distress). Crisis most often strengthens an individual's spirituality, but in some cases it weakens one's spirituality.

Nurse's Responsibility

- The nurse has a responsibility to ensure that patient's spiritual needs are attended.
- Spiritual need represents a normal expression of a person inner being that seeks meaning in all experience and dynamic relationship with self, others, universe and to the Supreme Being.

Spiritual Need Includes the Following

- Need for love.
- Need for forgiveness, dignity and values.
- Need to be respected and valued.
- Need for creativity.
- Need to belong to a community and sense of purpose.
- Need for hope and trust.

In meeting spiritual needs nurses need to be sensitive to indications of the patient's spiritual needs and should respond appropriately

Specific interventions include facilitating expressions of feelings, prayer, meditation, reading and discussion with appropriate clergy or a spiritual advisor.

- Ask questions and show interest.
- Listen to patient with positive attitude.
- Respond naturally to spiritual concern.
- Help patient to face reality with hope.
- Encourage establishment of new relationship.
- Allow family to participate in care.
- Allow time to grieve.
- Avoid false assurance.
- Interpret normal behavior.
- Provide continuing support and be alert for signs of ineffective coping.

Spiritual Problems in Acute, Chronic and Terminal Illnesses

- Both chronic illness and life threatening diseases confront patients with the question of meaning and purpose in life
- In such times of need, several patients rely on external resources of help, i.e., medical doctors, alternative information and help, but also God's help.
- Studies have shown that spirituality/religiosity can be a source to rely on. An increasing number of published studies have examined the connection between spirituality/religiosity, health and quality of life, and its potential to prevent, heal or cope with disease. Most of these studies state that religious involvement is related to better mental and physical health, improved coping with illness, and improved medical outcomes.
- But a recent systematic review confirmed that spirituality/religiosity was associated with reduced mortality only in healthy population studies, but not in diseased population studies.
- Whatever the scientific evidence may prove, one cannot ignore that spirituality/religiosity is a relevant resource to cope for many patients.
- Particularly in cancer patients, spirituality/religiosity may be beneficial maintaining self esteem, providing a sense of meaning and purpose, giving emotional comfort and providing a sense of hope. In a recent study among advanced cancer patients, most (88%) considered religion to be important.
- This is of importance, particularly because spiritual support was associated with better quality of life
- A qualitative study by Grant et al. found that patient's spiritual needs addressed the loss of roles and self-identity and fear of dying; these needs were related to anxiety, sleeplessness, and despair. Many terminally-ill patients expressed needs for love, meaning, purpose and sometimes transcendence.
- *Hermann* measured the spiritual needs of patients near the end of life enrolling hospice patients and found that several patients reported a higher number of unmet spiritual needs. Enrolling cancer patients in hospice home care, it became evident that spiritual needs may exhibit a great variability; among these needs, family was the most frequently cited one (80%); attending religious services was the most frequently cited unmet need.

- Few studies identified 5 sub-constructs of spiritual needs is that love and connection, hope and peace, meaning and purpose, relationship with God, and acceptance of dying.

DEALING WITH SPIRITUAL DISTRESS (SPIRITUAL CARE INTERVENTIONS)

- Florence Nightingale wrote, "The needs of the spirit are as critical to health as those individual organs which make up the body".
- Ever since then, spiritual care has been part of nursing, **Oldnall (1996)** states that "each individual has spiritual needs regardless of whether the individual is religious or not.

Definition

- Spiritual Distress refers to a challenge to the spiritual wellbeing or to the belief system that provides strength, hope and meaning to life.
- Spiritual distress refers to challenge to the spiritual well being or to the belief system that provides strength, hope and meaning to life.
- Spiritual distress incorporates the five spiritual needs such as forgiveness, love, hope, trust and meaning of life. The patient may express the distress both verbally and behaviorally.

The Characteristics of Spiritual Distress Include

- Maladaptive behavior.
- Discomfort with self awareness.
- Ambivalent feeling about God.
- Valve conflict.
- Lacking commitment and vision of possible alternatives.
- Low self-esteem and lack of hope.
- Extreme anxiousness.

Role of Nurse in Maintaining Spiritual Health of a Patient

- **To identify spiritual needs:**
  - Be sensitive towards patient's spiritual needs
  - Show concern, empathy, a willingness to listen and no judgmental attitude.
  - Communication should be direct, specific and dear.
- **Establish a therapeutic environment:**
  - Establish a good interpersonal relationship with caring behavior.
  - Use observation and understanding as a therapeutic tool
  - Accept patients behavior and belief without judgment
- **Support religious practices of patient:**
  - Establish a trusting relationship with the patient.
  - Provide privacy and comfort measures prior to prayer on spiritual activities.
  - Do not discuss personal, spiritual belief with a patient unless the patient request
  - Respect and ensure safety of patient's religious articles.
  - Provide an opportunity to the patient to meet the religious leader when they want. Referrals can be made for hospitalized patients and their relatives through the hospital chaplain's office.
- **To ventilate patient's feeling:**
  - Encourage the patient to ventilate his/her feeling regarding illness, suffering of life.
  - Help the patient to examine his/her life experience to discover new meaning to reconnect the forgotten moments that represent significant morning, encourage the patient to review his/her life for better understanding his/her own life.

NURSING MANAGEMENT

Assessment

- Observation and discussion with the client; patient usually appears depressed.
- Collect history; medical conditions, stress producing situations at home or work place, separation from dear ones, etc.
- He may express hopelessness, sleeplessness and spiritual distress. It may be expressed both verbally and behaviorally.
- Assess for related factors, such as feeling of loneliness, fear of unknown, guilt, and anger towards God, etc.

Nursing Diagnoses

Various nursing diagnoses are:
- Spiritual distress
- Readiness for enhanced spiritual well being
- Ineffective coping
- Hopelessness

Planning

Establish expected outcome: The client will develop an inner spiritual peace and a sense of spiritual well-being.

Interventions

- Communicate about spiritual needs to patients
- Help the client to create, maintain and renew relationships.
- Create a sense of forgiveness and unconditional love towards others
- **Help the patient to maintain relationships:** Many disease conditions cause social isolation, e.g., AIDS, VDRL, Leprosy.
- Communicate with the family members and arrange for visits by them and by the religious leaders
- Create a trust relationship with the patient
- Create hope in him. Even a dying person can have hope for reunion with deceased loved ones, union with God.
- Arrange for nondenominational prayer services
- Provide a prayer corner in the family room, with increased availability of religious reading material
- A monthly calendar may be placed in each patient's room listing the holy days of many different religions
- Avail a spiritual well-being checklist with patient instructions on contacting a chaplain if they have checked any spiritual concerns.
- A book of prayers and meditations can be placed at the bedside in each room

Chapter 15: Psychosocial Needs: Concepts of Cultural Diversity and Spirituality 341

❖ Keep a monthly house-wide nursing newsletter that highlights spiritual-care nursing diagnoses and interventions.

Four Tools to Help Nurses Implement Spiritual Care

1. Listening in an authentic manner
2. Being present
3. Accepting what the patient says
4. Using of self-disclosure

■ THE FIVE R's OF SPIRITUAL CARE

❖ Reason and Reflection to find, meaning in life; the will to live; to meditate on one's existence (via art, music or literature)

❖ Religion to express spirituality through a framework of values and beliefs, often actively pursued in rituals and religious practices.
❖ Relationships to relate to one's self, others and a deity (via service, love, trust, hope and/or creativity
❖ Restoration—to positively influence the physical aspect of care (life events can result in spiritual distress).

■ CONCLUSION

❖ Spiritual aspect of human nature is an integral component of a person's sense of wellness.
❖ Facilitating spiritual wellbeing is an approach to attain and maintain holistic health.

Chapter 16: Nursing Theories: Introduction

INTRODUCTION

- ❖ The foundation of any profession is the development of a specialized body of knowledge.
- ❖ In the past, the nursing profession relied on theories from other disciplines, such as medicine, psychology, and sociology, as basis for practice.
- ❖ For nursing to define its activities and develop its research, it must have its own body of knowledge.
- ❖ This knowledge can be expressed as conceptual models and theories.
- ❖ **Nursing theories and models provide information about:**
  - Definitions of nursing and nursing practice.
  - Principles that form the basis for practice.
  - Goals and functions of nursing
  - Nursing theories and models are derived from concepts.
  - A concept is an idea of an object, property, or event and can be empirical or concrete (readily observable, such as a thermometer, bed, lesion, rash, or edema) inferential (indirectly observable, such as temperature or pain) or abstract (non-observable, such as health or stress).

Metaparadigm of Nursing

- ❖ Conceptual models and theories in nursing are based on the *nursing metaparadigm*.
- ❖ A *metaparadigm* is the most global conceptual or philosophical framework of a discipline or profession
- ❖ It defines and describes relationships among major ideas and values.
- ❖ It guides the organization of theories and models for a profession
- ❖ **The nursing metaparadigm comprises of four concepts:** person, environment, health, and nursing.
  - *Person* refers to the recipient of nursing care, including physical, spiritual, psychological and sociocultural components, and can include an individual, family, or community.
  - *Environment* refers to all the internal and external conditions, circumstances, and influences affecting he person.
  - *Health* refers to the degree of wellness of illness experienced by the person.
  - *Nursing* refers to the actions, characteristics, and attributes of the individual providing the nursing care.

Classification

Theories and models can be categorized according to how they describe, explain, and connect the four concepts of the nursing metaparadigm.

- ❖ **Developmental theories and models:**
  - It emphasizes growth, development, and maturation.
  - The primary focus is change in a particular direction.
  - This change is orderly and predictable, occurring in specific stages, levels, or phases.
  - The goal is to maximize growth.
- ❖ **Systems theories and models:**
  - It views persons as open systems.
  - Each open system can receive input from the environment, process it, provide output to the environment, and receive feedback while maintaining a dynamic tension of forces.
  - Each system strives for a steady state (balance between internal and external forces).
  - The goal is to view the whole rather than the sum of the parts
- ❖ **Interaction theories and models:**
  - These are based on the relationships among persons.
  - The primary focus is on the person as an active participant.
  - Emphasis is on the person's perceptions, self-concept and ability to communicate and perform roles.
  - The goal is achievement through reciprocal interaction.
- ❖ **The development of nursing theories and models:**
  - It is a relatively recent occurrence.
  - The nursing profession has not reached a consensus on the meaning and interpretation of concepts, theories, and models.
  - A lack of consensus also exists whether a single model or theory should be selected or whether multiple models and theories are more useful to nursing practice.
  - Areas of agreement among theorists include the importance of the four concepts of person, environment, health, and nursing, the goal of enhancing client comfort a holistic approach of nursing and a set of distinct values of nursing.
  - Like any discipline, nursing must have a theoretical base.

MODELS

General Information

- Describe a set of ideas that are connected to illustrate a larger, more general concept.
- Is a symbolic depiction of reality
- Provide a schematic representation of some relationships among phenomenon.
- Use symbols or diagrams to represent an idea.

Characteristics

- Attempt to describe, explain, and sometimes predict the relationships among phenomenon.
- They are composed of empirical, inferential, and abstract concepts.
- Provide an organized framework for nursing assessment, planning intervention and evaluation.
- Facilitate communication among nurses and encourage a unified approach to practice, teaching, administration, and research.

THEORIES

General Information

- They are a set of interrelated concepts that provide a systematic explanatory and predictive view of phenomenon.
- Can begin as an untested premise (hypothesis) that becomes a theory when tested and supported or can progress in a more inductive manner.
- Are tested and validated through researches and provide direction for this research.

Characteristics

- Must be logical, relatively simple, and generalizable.
- Are composed of concepts and propositions
- Interrelate concepts to create a specific way of looking at a particular phenomenon.
- Provide the bases for testable hypotheses.
- Must be consistent with other validated theories, laws, and principles but leave open unanswered questions for investigation.
- Can consist of separate theories about the same phenomenon that interrelate the same concepts but describe and explain them differently.
- Can describe a particular phenomenon (descriptive or factor-isolating theories), explain relationships among phenomenon (explanatory or factor-relating theories) predict the effects of one phenomenon on another (predictive or situation-relating theories) or be used to produce or control a desired phenomenon (prescriptive or situation-producing theories).
- Contribute to and assist in increasing the general body of knowledge within a profession through research implemented to validate them.
- Can be used by nurses to guide and improve their practice.
- Differ from conceptual models, both can describe, explain, or predict a phenomenon, but only theories provide specific direction to guide practice, conceptual models are more abstract and less specific than theories but can provide direction for practice.

Levels of Theory Development

- Meta-theories focus on broad issues, including analysis of the purpose and type of theory needed, proposal and critique of sources and methods for theory development, and proposal of criteria for theory evaluation (for example. J Dickoff's and P James's theory).
- Metaparadigm (sometimes referred to as grand theories) are abstract in content and broad in scope, they attempt to explain a global view useful in understanding key concepts and principles (for example. Orem's General Theory of Nursing or Roy's Adaptation Models).
- Middle-range theories specific phenomenon or concepts, such as pain and stress, they are limited in scope yet general enough to encourage research. Practice theories are narrowly defined, they address a desired goal and the specific actions needed to achieve it.

HISTORICAL PERSPECTIVE

1860–1959

- **In 1860** Florence Nightingale developed her Environmental Theory.
- **In 1952**, the Nursing Research Journal was established, encouraging nurses to become involved in scientific inquiry.
- In the same year, Hildegard Peplau published Interpersonal Relations in Nursing her ideas have influenced later nursing theorists.
- **In 1955**, Virginia Henderson published Definition of Nursing.
- **In the mid-1950s**, Teachers College, Columbia University, New York City, began offering master's and doctoral programs in nursing education and administration, resulting in student participation in theory development and testing.

1960–1969

- During the **1960s** Yale University School of Nursing, New Haven, Conn., defined nursing as a process, interaction, and relationship.
- Also during the **1960s**, the US Government began funding master's and doctoral education in nursing.
- **In 1960**, Faye Abdellah published Twenty-One Nursing Problems
- **In 1961**, Ida Orlando published her theory in The Dynamic Nurse-Patient Relationship: Function, Process, and Principles of Professional Nursing.
- **In 1962**, Lydia Hall published Core, Care, and Cure Model.
- **In 1964**, Ernestine Wiedenbach published her theory in Clinical Nursing A Helping Art.
- **In 1965**, the American Nurses Association Published a position paper stating that theory development was an important goal for nursing.

- **In 1966**, Myra Levine published Four Conservation Principles.
- **In 1969**, Dorothy Johnson published Behavioral Systems Model.

1970–1979

- **During the 1970s**, case Western Reserve University, Cleveland sponsored symposia to stimulate theory development.
- **During the mid-1970s**, the National League for Nursing established an accreditation requirement that nursing schools base their curricula on a nursing conceptual framework.
- **In 1970**, Martha Rogers published her model in An Introduction to the Theoretical Basis of Nursing
- **In 1971**, Dorothea Orem published Self-Care Deficit Theory of Nursing Imogene King published Theory of Goal Attainment, and Joyce Travelbee published Interpersonal Aspects of Nursing
- **In 1972**, Betty Neuman published Health Care Systems Models
- **In 1976**, Sister Callista Roy published Adaptation Model.
- **In 1976**, JG Paterson and LT Zderad published Humanistic Nursing
- **In 1978**, Madeleine Leininger published Cultural Care Theory.
- **In 1979**, Jean Watson published Nursing: Human Science and Human Care-A Theory of Nursing.

1980 to the Present

- **In 1980**, Evelyn Adam published to be a Nurse and Joan Richi-Sisca published Symbolic Interactionism.
- **In 1982,** Joyce Fitzpatrick published Life Perspective Model.
- **In 1983**, Kathryn Barnard published Parent-Child Interaction Model and Helen Erickson, Evelyn Tomlin, and Mary Ann Swain published Modeling and Role Modeling,
- **In 1984,** Patricia Benner published From Novice to Expert: Excellence and Power in Clinical Nursing Practice.
- **In 1985,** Ramona Mercer published Maternal Role Attainment.
- **In 1986,** Margaret Newman published Model of Health.

Predictions for Theory Development

- The number of theories and models will increase, especially in the middle-range level.
- The use of nursing theory will be challenged as a result of the nursing shortage and the decreased emphasis placed on nursing theory by the National League for Nursing.
- Clinical outcome research will become the leading stimulus to practice theory development.

Points to Remember

- Theories and models attempt to define and describe the discipline of nursing.
- Nursing theories and models provide information about the definition of nursing and nursing practice, principles that form the basis for practice, and the goals and function of nursing.
- The nursing metaparadigm consists of four concepts person, environment, health and nursing
- Both theories and models can describe, explain, or predict relationships among phenomena.
- Nursing practice must be theoretically based.
- The four levels of theory development are meta theory, metaparadigm (grand theory), middle-range theory, and practice theory.
- Florence Nightingale was the first nursing theorist.

THEORY

Definitions

"Theory is a set of concepts, definitions, relationships and assumptions or propositions that project a purposive, systematic view of a phenomenon, by designing specific interrelationship among concepts for the purpose of describing, explaining, predicting and/or prescribing."
—**Tomey and Alligood 1998**

"A nursing theory is a conceptualization of some aspects of nursing communicated for the purpose of describing, explaining, predicting and/or prescribing nursing care."
—**Barnum 1994, Meleis 1997**

Components of Nursing Theory

See **Flowchart 16.1**.

Concepts

The theory consists of interrelated concepts.
"Concepts are the mental formulations of an object or event that comes from individual perceptual experiences".
—**Torres 1986, Marriner Tomey and Alligood 1998**

Definitions

"The definitions included within the description of a theory convey the general meaning of concepts in a manner that they fit the theory".
—**Potter and Perry**

"Assumptions are the statements that describe the concepts or connect two concepts that are factual and are accepted as truth."
—**Potter and Perry**

Phenomenon: Nursing theories focus on the phenomenon are aspects of the reality that can be consciously sensual or experienced.
—**Melvis 1997**

Propositions: Are tentative statements about reality and its nature. They describe relationship, between events, situations or actions.
—**Melois 1991**

Model: Model is a representation of reality.
—**McFarlane 1986**

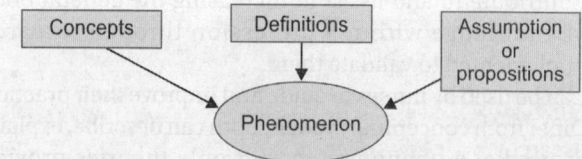

Flowchart 16.1: Components of nursing theory.

Model is a set of concepts and assumptions that integrate them into meaningful configuration. —Faweech 1992

Purposes of Theory
- To understand why and how the phenomenon of nursing are associated with one another.
- Predict the future relationships.

Classification of Theories
According to Level of Abstraction
- **Grand theories:** Broad in scope and complex and need further specification before they are tested and do not provide guidance for specific nursing intervention, but provide structural framework for broad, abstract ideas.
- **Middle range theories:** Limited in scope and less abstract they address specific nursing phenomenon or concepts and reflect nursing practice.

According to Goals of Theory
- **Descriptive:** 1st level of theory development. Describe why phenomenon have ability to explain and relate phenomenon.
- **Explanatory:** More complex, describe relationship among various phenomenons.
- **Predictive theory:** More powerful, predict, specific type of relationship between phenomenon.
- **Prescriptive theory:** Deals with nursing interventions and conditions which prescription is done and consequences of interventions.

Kinds of Theories
- **Stress theories:** Deal with how individual react psychologically and physiologically to stress.
- **Developmental theories:** Deal development of each family member and help to assess specific developmental levels and tasks for each member.
- **Family theories:** Deal with the family unit, interrelationship of a family group is reflected in theories. Interactive theories: Provide knowledge how to interact as nurse has to interact with patients, patient's relatives and other members of health team.
- **Adaptation theory:** Deal with how to adopt to various situations in life. Nurse has to teach patient about adapting themselves to various situations in life.
- **Other theories:** For example, role theories and change theories.

Nursing theories explain the phenomenon and guide nurses in giving care to the patients.

Basic Characteristics of Theory
- Theories can interrelate concepts in such a way as to create of different way of looking at particular phenomena.
- Theories must be logical in nature.
- Theories should be relatively simple yet generalizable.
- Theories can be basis for hypothesis that can be tested.
- Theories contribute to and assist in increasing the general body of knowledge within the discipline through the research implemented to validate them.
- Theories can be used by the practitioner to guide and improve their practice.
- Theories must be consistent with the other validated theories laws and principles but will leave open unanswered questions that need to be investigated.

Goals of Theoretical Models
- Identify the domain and goal of nursing.
- Provide knowledge to improve nursing administration, practice, education and research.
- Guide the research to establish empirical knowledge base for nursing.
- Identify areas to be studied.
- Identify research techniques and tools that will be validate nursing interventions used to
- Identify the nature of contribution to research will to advancement of knowledge. make
- Formulate legislation governing nursing practice, research and education.
- Formulate regulation interpreting nursing practice acts so that nurses and others better understand laws.
- Develop curriculum plans for nursing education.
- Establish criteria for measuring quality of nursing care, education and research.
- Guide development of nursing care delivery system.
- Provide systemic structure for and rationale for nursing activities.

NURSING THEORIES

Florence Nightingale 1860: Environmental Theory
Goal of nursing: To facilitate the body's reparative process by manipulating client's environment.

Framework for practice: Client's environment is manipulated to include appropriate noise, nutrition, hygiene, light, comfort, realization and hope.

Introduction
- Florence Nightingale was born on May 12, 1820, while her parents were on an extended European tour.
- Much attention has been to the "Calling" that Nightingale recorded in her diary in 1837, when she wrote that "God spoke to me and called me to his service".
- Florence Nightingale began her nursing training in 1851 in Germany.
- She pioneered the concept of formal education for nurses.
- She served the injured soldiers during the Crimean war which strongly influenced her philosophy of nursing.
- In 1859, she published her views on nursing care in notes on nursing.
- She is considered the first nursing theorist.
- She stated in her nursing notes that nursing "is an act of utilizing the environment of the patient to assist him in his recovery."
- Her contribution during Crimean war is well-known.
- She was a statistician, using bar and pie charts, highlighting key points.

- International Nurses Day, May 12 is observed in respect to her contribution to Nursing.
- Died—13 August 1910
- The foundation of Nightingale's theory is the environment-all the external conditions and forces that influence the life and development of an organism.
- According to her, external influences and conditions can prevent, suppress, or contribute to disease or death.
- Her goal was to help the patient retain his own vitality by meeting his basic needs through control of the environment.

Types of Environment
There are two types of environments:
1. **Physical environment:** Physical environment consists of physical elements where the patient is being treated. It affects all other aspects of the environment. Cleanliness of environment relates directly to disease prevention and patient mortality. Aspects of the physical environment influence the social and psychological environments of the person
2. **Psychological environment:** Psychological environment can be affected by a negative physical environment which then causes STRESS. It requires various activities to keep the mind active. It involves communication with the person, about the person, and about other people. It includes components of the physical environment—clean air, clean water, proper drainage. It consists of a person's home or hospital room, as well as the total community:
   - *Health of houses:* The importance of the health of houses as being closely related to the presence of pure air, pure water, efficient drainage, cleanliness and light. Cleanliness outside the house effected the inside.
   - *Ventilation and warming:* Nurses was "to keep the air he breathes as pure as the external air, without chilling". Nightingale was very concerned about "noxious air" or "effluvia" or foul odours that came from excrement. Nightingale stressed the importance of room temperature. The patient should not be too warm or too cold.
   - *Light:* She viewed that direct sunlight was what patients wanted. Although acknowledging a lack of scientific rationale for it, she noted that light has "quite real and tangible effects upon the human body".
   - *Noise:* She stated that patient should never be waked intentionally or accidentally during the first part of sleep. She asserted that whispered or long conversations about patients are thoughtless and cruel. Nurse's responsibility is to assess and stop different king of noise.
   - *Variety:* She believed that variety in the environment was a critical aspect of affecting the patients recovery. She discussed the need for changes in colour and form, including bringing the patient brightly colored flowers or plants.
   - *Bed and bedding:* She stated that dirty carpets and walls containing large quantities of organic matter and provided ready source of infection, just as dirty sheets and beds did.
   - *Personal cleanliness:* The need for cleanliness is extended to the patient, the nurse and the environment. Nightingale viewed the functions of the skin is important, believing that many disease "disorders" or caused breaks in the skin.
   - *Nutrition and taking food:* Nightingale addressed the variety of food presented to the patients and discussed the importance of variety in the food presented.
   - *Chattering hopes and advices:* False hope was depressing to patients, she felt and caused them to worry and become fatigued. She believed that sick persons should hear good news that would assist them in becoming healthier.
   - *Social considerations:* Nightingale supported the importance of looking beyond the persons to the social environments in which he or she lived. She observed that generations of families lived and died in poverty.

Four Major Concepts of Nightingale's Theory
1. **Nursing:** Nursing is different from medicine and the goal of nursing is to place the patient in the best possible condition for nature to act. Nursing is the "activities that promote health which occur in any care giving situation. They can be done by anyone."
2. **Person:** Nightingale referred person as a patient. Person is affected by environment. Person is multidimensional, composed of biological, psychological, social and spiritual components. He has a vital reparative power to deal with disease, recovery is within the person's power as long as a safe environment for recuperation exists.
3. **Health/disease:** Health is "not only to be well, but maintaining well-being by using a person's power to the fullest extent". Health is maintained by controlling the environmental factors to prevent disease. Disease is considered as disease or the absence of comfort. Health and disease are the focus of nurse, who helps a person through the healing process.
4. **Environment:** "Poor or difficult environments led to poor health and disease". "Environment could be altered to improve conditions so that the natural laws would allow healing to occur."

Relevance of Theory in Nursing Practice, Education and Research

Nursing Practice
- Disease control
- Sanitation and water treatment
- Utilized by modern architecture in the prevention of "sick building syndrome" applying the principles of ventilation and good lighting.
- Waste disposal
- Control of room temperature
- Noise management.

Education
- Principles of nursing training. Better practice result from better education.
- Skills measurement through licensing by the use of testing methods, the case studies.

Research
- Use of graphical representations like the bar, pie diagrams.
- Notes on nursing.

Application of Nightingale's Theory in Nursing Process

Assessment
The following information should be adequate:
- Adequacy of ventilation
- Cleanliness of environment
- Presence of draft
- Sudden noises
- Amount of sunlight and artificial light
- Variety of dietary offerings
- Odours present in throughout ward
- Methods of disposal of human waste and sputum
- Opportunity to communicate with others
- Insufficient warmth
- company from family and other patient
- Insufficient knowledge regarding disease

Nursing Diagnosis
Non-stimulating environment.

Implementation
- Provide adequate ventilation by opening doors and windows.
- Keep the surrounding environment clean (linen, bed, utensils)
- Keep the patient in warm and comfortable room, avoid unnecessary noise.
- Increase stimulus through a greater exposure to sunlight and fresh air.
- Provide nutritious diet and encourage for liquid diet frequently.
- Proper disposal of sputum, human excreta and other waste to remove odors.
- Proper dress-up, maintain room temperature and wear warm clothes.
- Isolate the patient from the children from the other patients but keep in touch and interaction with limited visitors.
- Keep in stimulating environment such as listening to radio, reading magazines and newspapers.
- Provide sufficient advice, information about disease, it is prognosis, course of treatment to the patient and family members.

Evaluation
It is based on observation on the effect of a changing environment on the health of a person specially focus on the vital signs and adequate knowledge about disease condition.

Dorothea Orem: Self-Care Deficit Theory

- Dorothea Orem is a nurse theorist who pioneered the Self-Care Deficit Nursing Theory.
- Get to know Orem's biography and works, including a discussion about the major concepts, sub concepts, nursing metaparadigm, and application of Self-Care Deficit Theory.
- Dorothea Elizabeth Orem (July 15, 1914 – June 22, 2007) was one of America's foremost nursing theorists who developed the Self-Care Deficit Nursing Theory, also known as the Orem Model of Nursing.
- Her theory defined Nursing as "The act of assisting others in the provision and management of self-care to maintain or improve human functioning at the home level of effectiveness."
- It focuses on each individual's ability to perform self-care, defined as "the practice of activities that individuals initiate and perform on their own behalf in maintaining life, health, and well-being."

Self-Care Theory
Dorothea Orem's Self-Care Deficit Theory focuses on each "individual's ability to perform self-care, defined as 'the practice of activities that individuals initiate and perform on their own behalf in maintaining life, health, and well-being."

The self-care or self-care deficit theory of nursing is composed of three interrelated theories:
- The theory of self-care
- The self-care deficit theory
- The theory of nursing systems, which is further classified into wholly compensatory, partially compensatory and supportive-educative.

Dorothea Orem's Self-Care Deficit Theory
- There are instances wherein patients are encouraged to bring out the best in them despite being ill for a period of time.
- This is very particular in rehabilitation settings, in which patients are entitled to be more independent after being cared for by physicians and nurses.
- Between 1959 and 2001, Dorothea Orem developed the Self-Care Nursing Theory or the Orem Model of Nursing.
- It is considered a grand nursing theory, which means the theory covers a broad scope with general concepts applicable to all instances of nursing.

Description
- Dorothea Orem's Self-Care Deficit Theory defined Nursing as "The act of assisting others in the provision and management of self-care to maintain or improve human functioning at the home level of effectiveness."
- It focuses on each individual's ability to perform self-care, defined as "the practice of activities that individuals initiate and perform on their own behalf in maintaining life, health, and well-being."
- "The condition that validates the existence of a requirement for nursing in an adult is the absence of the ability to maintain continuously that amount and quality of self-care which is therapeutic in sustaining life and health, in recovering from disease or injury, or in coping with their effects.
- With children, the condition is the parent's inability (or guardian) to maintain continuity for the child the amount and quality of care that is therapeutic." (Orem, 1991)

Assumptions of the Self-Care Deficit Theory
Dorothea Orem's self-care theory assumptions are:
1. To stay alive and remain functional, humans engage in constant communication and connect among themselves and their environment.

2. The power to act deliberately is exercised to identify needs and to make needed judgments.
3. Mature human beings experience privations in the form of action in care of self and others involving making life-sustaining and function-regulating actions.
4. Human agency is exercised in discovering, developing, and transmitting to others ways and means to identify needs for, and make inputs into, self and others.
5. Groups of human beings with structured relationships cluster tasks and allocate responsibilities for providing care to group members.

Major Concepts of the Self-Care Deficit Theory (Fig. 16.1)

Nursing
- Nursing is an art through which the practitioner of nursing gives specialized assistance to persons with disabilities, making more than ordinary assistance necessary to meet self-care needs.
- The nurse also intelligently participates in the medical care the individual receives from the physician.

Humans
Humans are defined as "men, women, and children cared for either singly or as social units" and are the "material object" of nurses and others who provide direct care.

Environment
- The environment has physical, chemical, and biological features.
- It includes the family, culture, and community.

Health
- Health is "being structurally and functionally whole or sound."
- Also, health is a state that encompasses both the health of individuals and groups, and human health is the ability to reflect on oneself, symbolize experience, and communicate with others.

Self-care
Self-care is the performance or practice of activities that individuals initiate and perform on their own behalf to maintain life, health, and well-being.

Self-care Agency
- **Orem's self-care theory:** Interrelationship among concepts. Click to enlarge.
- Self-care agency is the human's ability or power to engage in self-care and is affected by basic conditioning factors.

Basic Conditioning Factors
Basic conditioning factors are age, gender, developmental state, health state, sociocultural orientation, healthcare system factors, family system factors, patterns of living, environmental factors, and resource adequacy and availability.

Orem's Self-Care Theory—Conceptual Framework (Fig. 16.2)

Therapeutic Self-care Demand
Therapeutic Self-care Demand is the totality of "self-care actions to be performed for some duration to meet known self-care requisites by using valid methods and related sets of actions and operations."

Self-care Deficit
Self-care Deficit delineates when nursing is needed. Nursing is required when an adult (or in the case of a dependent, the parent or guardian) is incapable of or limited in providing continuous effective self-care.

Nursing Agency
Nursing agency is a complex property or attribute of people educated and trained as nurses that enables them to act, know, and help others meet their therapeutic self-care demands by exercising or developing their own self-care agency.

Nursing System
Nursing system is the product of a series of relations between the persons—legitimate nurse and legitimate client.

This system is activated when the client's therapeutic self-care demand exceeds the available self-care agency, leading to nursing.

Theories
The self-care or self-care deficit theory of nursing is composed of three interrelated theories:
1. The Theory of self-care
2. The self-care deficit theory

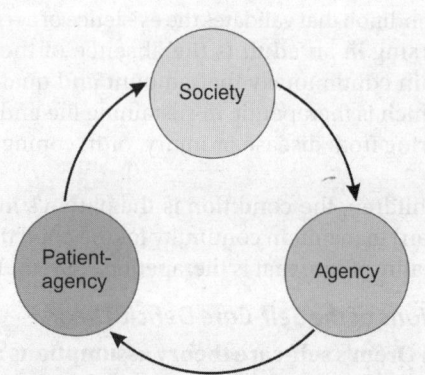

Fig. 16.1: Orem's self-care theory: Interrelationship among concepts.

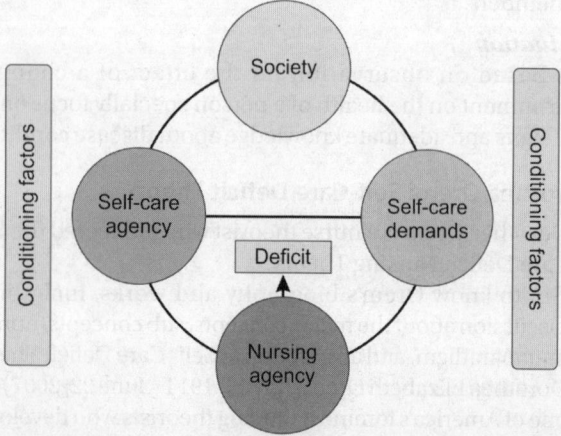

Fig. 16.2: Orem's self-care theory-conceptual framework.

3. The theory of nursing systems, which is further classified into wholly compensatory, partially compensatory and supportive-educative.

Theory of Self-care
This theory focuses on the performance or practice of activities that individuals initiate and perform on their own behalf to maintain life, health, and well-being.

Self-care Requisites
Self-care Requisites or requirements can be defined as actions directed toward the provision of self-care. It is presented in three categories:

1. **Universal self-care requisites:**
   - Universal self-care requisites are associated with life processes and the maintenance of the human structure and functioning integrity.
   - The maintenance of a sufficient intake of air
   - The maintenance of a sufficient intake of water
   - The maintenance of a sufficient intake of food
   - The provision of care associated with the elimination process and excrements
   - The maintenance of a balance between activity and rest
   - The maintenance of a balance between solitude and social interaction
   - The prevention of hazards to human life, human functioning, and human well-being
   - The promotion of human functioning and development within social groups in accord with human potential, known human limitations, and the human desire to be normal
   - Normalcy is used in the sense of that which is essentially human and that which is in accord with the genetic and constitutional characteristics and individuals' talents.

2. **Developmental self-care requisites:** Developmental self-care requisites are "either specialized expressions of universal self-care requisites that have been particularized for developmental processes or they are new requisites derived from a condition or associated with an event."

3. **Health deviation self-care requisites:**
   - Health deviation self-care requisites are required in conditions of illness, injury, or disease or may result from medical measures required to diagnose and correct the condition.
   - Seeking and securing appropriate medical assistance.
   - Being aware of and attending to the effects and results of pathologic conditions and states
   - Effectively carrying out medically prescribed diagnostic, therapeutic, and rehabilitative measures.
   - Being aware of and attending to or regulating the discomforting or deleterious effects of prescribed medical measures
   - Modifying the self-concept (and self-image) in accepting oneself as being in a particular state of health and in need of specific forms of health care
   - Learning to live with the effects of pathologic conditions and states and the effects of medical diagnostic and treatment measures in a lifestyle that promotes continued personal development

Theory of Self-Care Deficit
This theory delineates when nursing is needed. Nursing is required when an adult (or in the case of a dependent, the parent or guardian) is incapable of or limited in providing continuous effective self-care.

Orem identified 5 methods of helping:
1. Acting for and doing for others
2. Guiding others
3. Supporting another
4. Providing an environment promoting personal development about meet future demands
5. Teaching another

Theory of Nursing System
- This theory is the product of a series of relations between the persons—legitimate nurse and legitimate client.
- This system is activated when the client's therapeutic self-care demand exceeds the available self-care agency, leading to nursing.

Wholly Compensatory Nursing System
- This is represented by a situation in which the individual is unable "to engage in those self-care actions requiring self-directed and controlled ambulation and manipulative movement or the medical prescription to refrain from such activity. Persons with these limitations are socially dependent on others for their continued existence and well-being."
- **Example:** Care of a newborn, care of client recovering from surgery in a postanesthesia care unit

Partial Compensatory Nursing System
- This is represented by a situation in which "both nurse and perform care measures or other actions involving manipulative tasks or ambulation. Either the patient or the nurse may have a major role in the performance of care measures."
- **Example:** Nurse can assist the postoperative client in ambulating, Nurse can bring a meal tray for a client who can feed himself

Supportive-Educative System
- This is also known as a supportive-developmental system.
- The person "can perform or can and should learn to perform required measures of externally or internally oriented therapeutic self-care but cannot do so without assistance."
- **Example:** Nurse guides a mother on how to breastfeed her baby, counseling a psychiatric client on more adaptive coping strategies.

Dorothea Orem's Theory and the Nursing Process
The nursing process presents a method in determining self-care deficits and defining the roles of persons or nurses to meet the self-care demands.

Assessment
- Diagnosis and prescription; determine why nursing is needed.
- Analyze and interpret by making a judgment regarding care.

- Design of a nursing system and plan for delivery of care.
- Production and management of nursing systems.

Step 1—Collect data in six areas:
1. The person's health status
2. The physician's perspective of the person's health status
3. The person's perspective of his or health
4. The health goals within the context of life history, lifestyle, and health status.
5. The person's requirements for self-care
6. The person's capacity to perform self-care

Nursing Diagnosis and Care Plans

Step 2
- The nurse designs a system that is wholly or partly compensatory or supportive-educative.
- **The two actions are:**
  1. Bringing out a good organization of the components of patients' therapeutic self-care demands.
  2. Selection of a combination of helping methods will be effective and efficient in compensating for/overcoming the patient's self-care deficits.

Implementation and Evaluation

Step 3
- A nurse assists the patient or family in self-care matters to identify and describe health and health-related results. Collecting evidence in evaluating results achieved against results specified in the nursing system design.
- The etiology component of nursing diagnosis directs actions.

Analysis of the Self-care Deficit Theory
- There is a superb focus of Orem's work which is self-care.
- Even though there is a wide range of scope seen in the encompassing theory of nursing systems, Orem's goal of letting the readers view nursing care to assist people was apparent in every concept presented.
- From the definition of health which is sought to be rigid, it can now be refined by making it suitable to the general view of health as a dynamic and ever-changing state.
- The role of the environment in the nurse-patient relationship, although defined by Orem, was not discussed.
- Orem set nurses' role in maintaining health for the patient with great coherence following every individual's life-sustaining needs.
- Although Orem viewed the parent's or guardians' importance in providing for their dependents, the definition of self-care cannot be directly applied to those who need complete care or assistance with self-care activities such as the infants and the aged.

Strengths
- A major strength of Dorothea Orem's theory is that it is applicable for nursing by the beginning practitioner and the advanced clinicians.
- Orem's theory provides a comprehensive basis for nursing practice.
- It has utility for professional nursing in the areas of nursing practice, nursing education, and administration.
- The terms self-care, nursing systems, and self-care deficit are easily understood by the beginning student nurse and can be explored in greater depth as they gain more knowledge and experience.
- **She specifically defines when nursing is needed:** Nursing is needed when the individual cannot maintain continuously that amount and quality of self-care necessary to sustain life and health, recover from disease or injury, or cope with their effects.
- Her self-care approach is contemporary with the concepts of health promotion and health maintenance.
- Three identifiable nursing systems were clearly delineated and are easily understood.

Limitations
- Orem's theory, in general, is viewed as a single whole thing, while Orem defines a system as a single whole thing.
- Orem's theory is simple yet complex. The use of self-care in multitudes of terms, such as self-care agency, self-care demand, self-care deficit, self-care requisites, and universal self-care, can be very confusing to the reader.
- Orem's definition of health was confined to three static conditions, which she refers to as a "concrete nursing system," which connotes rigidity.
- Throughout her work, there is a limited acknowledgment of the individual's emotional needs.
- Health is often viewed as dynamic and ever-changing.

Conclusion
- Orem's theory is relatively simple but generalizable to apply to a wide variety of patients.
- It explains the terms self-care, nursing systems, and self-care deficit essential to students who plan to start their nursing careers.
- Moreover, this theory signifies that all patients want to care for themselves.
- They can recover more quickly and holistically by performing their own self-care as much as they're able.
- This theory is particularly used in rehabilitation and primary care or other settings where patients are encouraged to be independent.
- Though this theory greatly influences every patient's independence, the definition of self-care cannot be directly applied to those who need complete care or assistance with self-care activities such as infants and the aged.

Sister Callista Roy: Adaptation Model of Nursing
- Sister Callista L. Roy (born October 14, 1939) is a nursing theorist, professor, and author.
- She is known for her ground-breaking work in creating the Adaptation Model of Nursing.

Adaptation Model of Nursing
- Sr Callista Roy's Adaptation Model of Nursing was developed by Sister Callista Roy in 1976.
- The prominent nursing theory aims to explain or define the provision of nursing. In her theory, Roy's model sees the individual as a set of interrelated systems that maintain a balance between these various stimuli.

- The adaptation Model of Nursing is discussed further below.

Works

Callista Roy's Adaptation Model of Nursing
- The Adaptation Model of Nursing is a prominent nursing theory aiming to explain or define the provision of nursing science.
- In her theory, Sister Callista Roy's model sees the individual as a set of interrelated systems that maintain a balance between various stimuli.
- The Roy Adaptation Model was first presented in the literature in an article published in Nursing Outlook in 1970 entitled "Adaptation: A Conceptual Framework for Nursing."
- In the same year, Roy's Adaptation Model of Nursing was adapted in Mount St Mary's School in Los Angeles, California.
- Roy's model was conceived when nursing theorist Dorothy Johnson challenged her students to develop conceptual models of nursing during a seminar.
- Johnson's nursing model was the impetus for the development of Roy's Adaptation Model.
- Roy's model incorporated concepts from Adaptation-level Theory of Perception from renowned American physiological psychologist Harry Helson, Ludwig von Bertalanffy's System Model, and Anatol Rapoport's system definition.
- First, consider the concept of a system as applied to an individual. Roy conceptualizes the person in a holistic perspective.
- Individual aspects of parts act together to form a unified being.
- Additionally, as living systems, persons are in constant interaction with their environments.
- Between the system and the environment occurs an exchange of information, matter, and energy.
- Characteristics of a system include inputs, outputs, controls, and feedback.

Assumptions

Scientific Assumptions
- Systems of matter and energy progress to higher levels of complex self-organization.
- Consciousness and meaning are constructive of person and environment integration.
- Awareness of self and environment is rooted in thinking and feeling.
- Humans, by their decisions, are accountable for the integration of creative processes.
- Thinking and feeling mediate human action.
- System relationships include acceptance, protection, and fostering of interdependence.
- Persons and the earth have common patterns and integral relationships.
- Persons and environment transformations are created in human consciousness.
- Integration of human and environmental meanings results in adaptation.

Philosophical Assumptions
- Persons have mutual relationships with the world and God.
- Human meaning is rooted in the omega point convergence of the universe.
- God is intimately revealed in the diversity of creation and is the common destiny of creation.
- Persons use human creative abilities of awareness, enlightenment, and faith.
- Persons are accountable for the processes of deriving, sustaining, and transforming the universe.

Major Concepts of the Adaptation Model
The following are Callista Roy's Adaptation Model's major concepts, including the definition of the nursing metaparadigm as defined by the theory.

Person
- "Human systems have thinking and feeling capacities, rooted in consciousness and meaning, by which they adjust effectively to changes in the environment and, in turn, affect the environment."
- Based on Roy, humans are holistic beings that are in constant interaction with their environment.
- Humans use a system of adaptation, both innate and acquired, to respond to the environmental stimuli they experience.
- Human systems can be individuals or groups, such as families, organizations, and the whole global community.

Environment
- "The conditions, circumstances and influences surrounding and affecting the development and behaviour of persons or groups, with particular consideration of the mutuality of person and health resources that includes focal, contextual and residual stimuli."
- The environment is defined as conditions, circumstances, and influences that affect humans' development and behaviour as an adaptive system.
- The environment is a stimulus or input that requires a person to adapt.
- These stimuli can be positive or negative.
- Roy categorized these stimuli as focal, contextual, and residual. Focal stimuli are that confront the human system and require the most attention.
- Contextual stimuli are characterized as the rest of the stimuli present with the focal stimuli and contribute to its effect. Residual stimuli are the additional environmental factors present within the situation but whose effect is unclear.
- This can include previous experience with certain stimuli.

Health
- "Health is not freedom from the inevitability of death, disease, unhappiness, and stress, but the ability to cope with them in a competent way."
- Health is defined as the state where humans can continually adapt to stimuli.
- Because illness is a part of life, health results from a process where health and illness can coexist.

- If a human can continue to adapt holistically, they will maintain health to reach completeness and unity within themselves.
- If they cannot adapt accordingly, the integrity of the person can be affected negatively.

Nursing
- "The goal of nursing is the promotion of adaptation for individuals and groups in each of the four adaptive modes, thus contributing to health, quality of life, and dying with dignity."
- In Adaptation Model, nurses are facilitators of adaptation.
- They assess the patient's behaviors for adaptation, promote positive adaptation by enhancing environment interactions and helping patients react positively to stimuli.
- Nurses eliminate ineffective coping mechanisms and eventually lead to better outcomes.

Adaptation
Adaptation is the "process and outcome whereby thinking and feeling persons as individuals or in groups use conscious awareness and choice to create human and environmental integration."

Internal Processes
Regulator
- The regulator subsystem is a person's physiological coping mechanism.
- The body attempts to adapt via regulation of our bodily processes, including neurochemical and endocrine systems.

Cognator
The cognator subsystem is a person's mental coping mechanism. A person uses his brain to cope via self-concept, interdependence, and role function adaptive modes.

Four Adaptive Modes
Diagrammatic Representation of Roy's Human Adaptive Systems (Fig. 16.3)
The subsystem's four adaptive modes are how the regulator and cognator mechanisms are manifested; in other words, they are the external expressions of the above and internal processes.

Physiological-Physical Mode
- Physical and chemical processes are involved in the function and activities of living organisms.
- These are the actual processes put in motion by the regulator subsystem.
- This mode's basic need is composed of the needs associated with oxygenation, nutrition, elimination, activity and rest, and protection.
- This model's complex processes are associated with the senses, fluid and electrolytes, neurologic function, and endocrine function.

Self-Concept Group Identity Mode
- In this mode, the goal of coping is to have a sense of unity, meaning the purposefulness in the universe, and a sense of identity integrity.
- This includes body image and self-ideals.

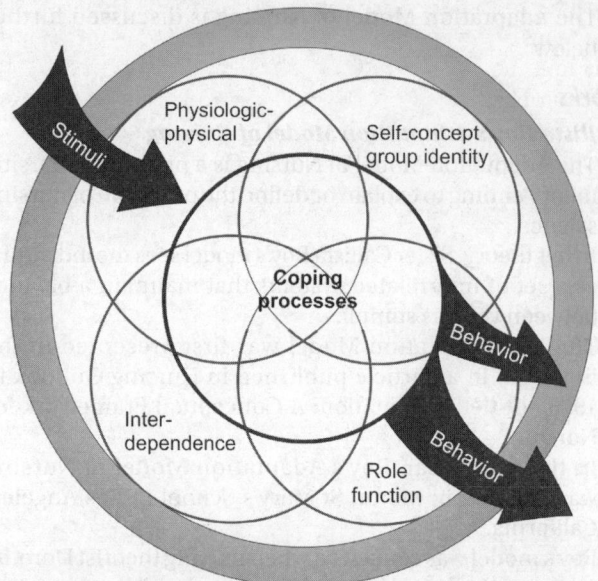

Fig. 16.3: Roy adaptation model.

Role Function Mode
This mode focuses on the primary, secondary, and tertiary roles that a person occupies in society and knowing where they stand as a member of society.

Interdependence Mode
- This mode focuses on attaining relational integrity through the giving and receiving of love, respect and value.
- This is achieved with effective communication and relations.

Levels of Adaptation
Integrated Process
The various modes and subsystems meet the needs of the environment. These are usually stable processes (e.g., breathing, spiritual realization, successful relationship).

Compensatory Process
The cognator and regulator are challenged by the environment's needs but are working to meet the needs (e.g., grief, starting with a new job, compensatory breathing).

Compromised Process
The modes and subsystems are not adequately meeting the environmental challenge (e.g., hypoxia, unresolved loss, abusive relationships).

Six-step Nursing Process
A nurse's role in the Adaptation Model is to manipulate stimuli by removing, decreasing, increasing, or altering stimuli so that the patient.
1. Assess the behaviors manifested from the four adaptive modes.
2. Assess the stimuli, categorize them as focal, contextual, or residual.
3. Make a statement or nursing diagnosis of the person's adaptive state.
4. Set a goal to promote adaptation.
5. Implement interventions aimed at managing the stimuli.
6. Evaluate whether the adaptive goal has been met.

Analysis
- As one of the weaknesses of the theory that applying it is time-consuming, applying the model to emergencies requiring quick action is difficult to complete, the individual might have completed the whole adaptation process without the benefit of having a complete assessment for thorough nursing interventions.
- Adaptive responses may vary in every individual and may take a longer time compared to others.
- Thus, the span of control of nurses may be impeded by the time of the patient's discharge.
- Unlike Levine, although the latter tackled adaptation, Roy focused on the whole adaptive system itself.
- Each concept was linked with the coping mechanisms of every individual in the process of adapting.
- When an individual presents an ineffective response during his or her adaptation process, the nurses' roles were not clearly discussed.
- The main point of the concept was to promote adaptation, but none were stated on preventing and resolving maladaptation.

Strengths of the Roy's Adaptation Model
- The Adaptation Model of Callista Roy suggests the influence of multiple causes in a situation, which is a strength when dealing with multi-faceted human beings.
- The sequence of concepts in Roy's model follows logically.
- In the presentation of each of the key concepts, there is the recurring idea of adaptation to maintain integrity. Every concept was operationally defined.
- The concepts of Roy's model are stated in relatively simple terms.
- A major strength of the model is that it guides nurses to use observation and interviewing skills in doing an individualized assessment of each person.
- The concepts of Roy's model are applicable within many practice settings of nursing.

Weaknesses
- Painstaking application of the model requires a significant input of time and effort.
- Roy's model has many elements, systems, structures, and multiple concepts.

Virginia Henderson's Nursing Theory

Introduction
- "The Nightingale of Modern Nursing"
- "Modern-Day Mother of Nursing."
- "The 20th century Florence Nightingale."
- Born in Kansas City, Missouri, in 1897.
- Diploma in Nursing from the Army School of Nursing at Walter Reed Hospital, Washington, DC in 1921.
- Worked at the Henry Street Visiting Nurse Service for 2 years after graduation.
- In 1923, started teaching nursing at the Norfolk Protestant Hospital in Virginia
- In 1929, entered Teachers College at Columbia University for Bachelor's Degree in 1932, Master's Degree in 1934.
- Joined Columbia as a member of the faculty, remained until 1948.
- Since 1953, a research associate at Yale University School of Nursing.
- Recipient of numerous recognitions.
- Honorary doctoral degrees from the Catholic University of America, Pace University, University of Rochester, University of Western Ontario, Yale University
- In 1985, honored at the Annual Meeting of the Nursing and Allied Health Section of the Medical Library Association.
- **Died:** March 19, 1996.
- In 1939, she revised: Harmer's classic textbook of nursing for its 4th edition, and later wrote the 5th; edition, incorporating her personal definition of nursing (Henderson,1991)

Theory Background
- She called her definition of nursing her "concept" (Henderson 1991)
- She emphasized the importance of increasing the patient's independence so that progress after hospitalization would not be delayed (Henderson,1991)
- "Assisting individuals to gain independence in relation to the performance of activities contributing to health or its recovery" (Henderson, 1966).
- She categorized nursing activities into 14 components, based on human needs.
- She described the nurse's role as substitutive (doing for the person), supplementary (helping the person), complementary (working with the person), with the goal of helping the person become as independent as possible.

Her definition of nursing was:
"The unique function of the nurse is to assist the individual, sick or well, in the performance of those activities contributing to health or its recovery (or to peaceful death) that he would perform unaided if he had the necessary strength, will or knowledge and to do this in such a way as to help him gain independence as rapidly as possible".
—Henderson, 1966

The 14 components:
1. Breathe normally. Eat and drink adequately.
2. Eliminate body wastes.
3. Move and maintain desirable postures.
4. Sleep and rest.
5. Select suitable clothes-dress and undress.
6. Maintain body temperature within normal range by adjusting clothing and modifying environment
7. Keep the body clean and well groomed and protect the integument
8. Avoid dangers in the environment and avoid injuring others.
9. Communicate with others in expressing emotions, needs, fears, or opinions.
10. Worship according to one's faith.
11. Work in such a way that there is a sense of accomplishment.
12. Play or participate in various forms of recreation.

13. Learn, discover, or satisfy the curiosity that leads to normal development and health and
14. Use the available health facilities.

Notes:
- The first 9 components are physiological.
- The tenth and fourteenth are psychological aspects of communicating and learning
- The eleventh component is spiritual and moral
- The twelfth and thirteenth components are sociologically oriented to occupation and recreation

Assumption
The major assumptions of the theory are:
- "Nurses care for patients until patient can care for themselves once again
- Patients desire to return to health, but this assumption is not explicitly stated.
- Nurses are willing to serve and that "nurses will devote themselves to the patient day and night"
- A final assumption is that nurses should be educated at the university level in both arts and sciences.

Henderson's Theory and the Four Major Concepts
1. **Individual:**
   - Have basic needs that are component of health.
   - Requiring assistance to achieve health and independence or a peaceful death.
   - Mind and body are inseparable and interrelated.
   - Considers the biological, psychological, sociological, and spiritual components.
   - The theory presents the patient as a sum of parts with biopsychosocial needs.
2. **Environment:**
   - Settings in which an individual learns unique pattern for living.
   - All external conditions and influences that affect life and development.
   - Individuals in relation to families
   - Minimally discusses the impact of the community on the individual and family.
   - Basic nursing care involves providing conditions under which the patient can perform the 14 activities unaided
3. **Health:**
   - Definition based on individual's ability to function independently as outlined in the 14 components.
   - Nurses need to stress promotion of health and prevention and cure of disease.
   - Good health is a challenge-affected by age, cultural background, physical, and intellectual capacities, and emotional balance.
   - Is the individual's ability to meet these needs independently.
4. **Nursing:**
   - Temporarily assisting an individual who lacks the necessary strength, will and knowledge to satisfy 1 or more of 14 basic needs.
   - Assists and supports the individual in life activities and the attainment of independence.
   - Nurse serves to make patient "complete" "whole", or "independent."

- The nurse is expected to carry out physician's therapeutic plan Individualized care is the result of the nurse's creativity in planning for care.
- "Nurse should have knowledge to practice individualized and human care and should be a scientific problem solver."
- In the Nature of Nursing Nurse role is," to get inside the patient's skin and supplement his strength will or knowledge according to his needs."

Comparison between Maslow's Hierarchy of Need and Henderson's Model (Table 16.1)

TABLE 16.1: Comparison between Maslow's Hierarchy of Need and Henderson's model.

Maslow's	Henderson
Physiological needs	- Breathe normally - Eat and drink adequately - Eliminate by all avenues of elimination - Move and maintain desirable posture Sleep and rest - Select suitable clothing - Maintain body temperature - Keep body clean and well groomed and protect the integument
Safety needs	Avoid environmental dangers and avoid injuring other
Belongingness and love needs	Communicate with others worship according to one's faith
Esteem needs	- Work at something providing a sense of accomplishment - Play or participate in various forms of recreation - Learn, discover, or satisfy curiosity

Henderson's 14 Components Model and Nursing Process (Table 16.2)

Characteristic of Henderson's Theory
- There is interrelation of concepts.
- Concepts of fundamental human needs, biophysiology, culture, and interaction, communication are borrowed from other discipline. For example, Maslow's theory.
- Her definition and components are logical and the 14 components are a guide for the individual and nurse in reaching the chosen goal.
- Relatively simple yet generalizable.
- Applicable to the health of individuals of all ages.
- Can be the bases for hypotheses that can be tested.
- Assist in increasing the general body of knowledge within the discipline.
- Her ideas of nursing practice are well accepted.
- Can be utilized by practitioners to guide and improve their practice.

Limitations
- Lack of conceptual linkage between physiological and other human characteristics.
- No concept of the holistic nature of human being.
- If the assumption is made that the 14 components prioritized, the relationship among the components is unclear.

Chapter 16: Nursing Theories: Introduction

TABLE 16.2: Comparison of Henderson's 14 components model and nursing process.

Nursing Process	Henderson's 14 components and definition of nursing
Nursing assessment	Henderson's 14 components
Nursing diagnosis	Analysis: Compare data to knowledge base of health and disease
Nursing plan	Identify individual's ability to meet own needs with/without assistance, taking into consideration strength, will or knowledge
Nursing implementation	Document how the nurse can assist the individual, sick or well
Nursing implementation	Assist the sick or well individual in to performance of activities in meeting human needs to maintain health, recover from illness, or to aid in peaceful death
Nursing process	Implementation based on the physiological principles, age, cultural background, emotional balance, and physical and intellectual capacities. Carry out treatment prescribed by the physician
Nursing evaluation	• Henderson's 14 components and definition of nursing • Use the acceptable definition of ;nursing and appropriate laws related to the practice of nursing • The quality of care is drastically affected by the preparation and native ability of the nursing personnel rather that the amount of hours of care • Successful outcomes of nursing care are based on the speed.with which or degree to which the patient performs independently the activities of daily living

- ❖ Lacks inter-relate of factors and the influence of nursing care.
- ❖ Assisting the individual in the dying process she contends that the nurse helps, but there is little explanation of what the nurse does.
- ❖ "Peaceful death" is curious and significant nursing role.

Conclusion
- ❖ Henderson provides the essence of what she believes is a definition of nursing.
- ❖ Her emphasis on basic human needs as the central focus of nursing practice has led to further theory development regarding the needs of the person and how nursing can assist in meeting those needs.
- ❖ Her definition of nursing and the 14 components of basic nursing care are uncomplicated and self-explanatory.

Hildegard Elizabeth Peplau: Interpersonal Relations Theory (Fig. 16.4)

Hildegard Elizabeth Peplau (September 1, 1909–March 17, 1999)
- ❖ She was an American nurse who is the only one to serve the American Nurses Association (ANA) as Executive Director and later as President.
- ❖ She became the first published nursing theorist since Florence Nightingale.
- ❖ Peplau was well-known for her Theory of Interpersonal Relations, which helped to revolutionize nurses' scholarly work.
- ❖ Her achievements are valued by nurses worldwide and became known to many as the "Mother of Psychiatric Nursing" and the "Nurse of the Century."

Interpersonal Relations Theory
- ❖ In 1952, Hildegard Peplau published her Theory of Interpersonal Relations influenced by Henry Stack Sullivan, Percival Symonds, Abraham Maslow, and Neal Elgar Miller. Her theory is discussed further below.
- ❖ Hildegard Peplau's Interpersonal Relations Theory emphasized the nurse-client relationship as the foundation of nursing practice.
- ❖ It emphasized the give-and-take of nurse-client relationships that was seen by many as revolutionary.
- ❖ Peplau went on to form an interpersonal model emphasizing the need for a partnership between nurse and client as opposed to the client passively receiving treatment and the nurse passively acting out doctor's orders.
- ❖ The four components of the theory are person, which is a developing organism that tries to reduce anxiety caused by needs; environment, which consists of existing forces outside of the person and put in the context of culture; health, which is a word symbol that implies a

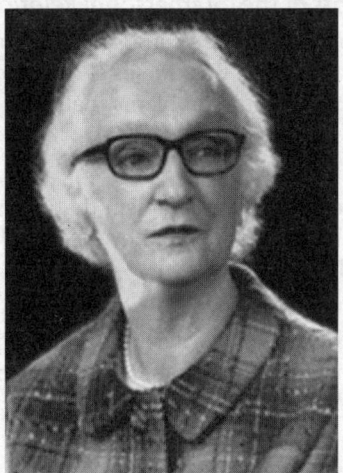

Fig. 16.4: Hildegard Elizabeth Peplau.

forward movement of personality and nursing, which is a significant therapeutic interpersonal process that functions cooperatively with another human process that makes health possible for individuals in communities.
- The nursing model identifies four sequential phases in the interpersonal relationship: orientation, identification, exploitation, and resolution.
- **It also includes seven nursing roles:** Stranger role, Resource role, Teaching role, Counseling role, Surrogate role, Active leadership, and Technical expert role.

Description
- Hildegard E Peplau's theory defined Nursing as "An interpersonal process of therapeutic interactions between an individual who is sick or in need of health services and a nurse especially educated to recognize, respond to the need for help."
- It is a "maturing force and an educative instrument" involving an interaction between two or more individuals with a common goal.
- In nursing, this common goal provides the incentive for the therapeutic process in which the nurse and patient respect each other as individuals, both of them learning and growing due to the interaction.
- An individual learns when she or he selects stimuli in the environment and then reacts to these stimuli.

Assumptions
1. Nurse and the patient can interact.
2. Peplau emphasized that both the patient and nurse mature as the result of the therapeutic interaction.
3. Communication and interviewing skills remain fundamental nursing tools. And lastly,
4. Peplau believed that nurses must clearly understand themselves to promote their client's growth and avoid limiting their choices to those that nurses value.

Major Concepts of the Interpersonal Relations Theory
The theory explains nursing's purpose is to help others identify their felt difficulties and that nurses should apply principles of human relations to the problems that arise at all levels of experience.

Man
Peplau defines man as an organism that "strives in its own way to reduce tension generated by needs." The client is an individual with a felt need.

Health
Health is defined as "a word symbol that implies forward movement of personality and other ongoing human processes in the direction of creative, constructive, productive, personal, and community living."

Society or Environment
Although Peplau does not directly address society/environment, she does encourage the nurse to consider the patient's culture and mores when the patient adjusts to the hospital routine.

Nursing
Hildegard Peplau considers nursing to be a "significant, therapeutic, interpersonal process." She defines it as a "human relationship between an individual who is sick, or in need of health services, and a nurse specially educated to recognize and to respond to the need for help."

Therapeutic nurse-client relationship:
- A professional and planned relationship between client and nurse focuses on the client's needs, feelings, problems, and ideas.
- It involves interaction between two or more individuals with a common goal.
- The attainment of this goal, or any goal, is achieved through a series of steps following a sequential pattern.

Four phases of the therapeutic nurse-patient relationship:
1. **Orientation phase:**
   - The nurse's orientation phase involves engaging the client in treatment, providing explanations and information, and answering questions.
   - Problem defining phase
   - It starts when the client meets the nurse as a stranger.
   - Defining the problem and deciding the type of service needed
   - Client seeks assistance, conveys needs, and asks questions, shares preconceptions and expectations of past experiences.
   - Nurse responds, explains roles to the client, identifies problems, and uses available resources and services.
   - The factors influencing the orientation phase are enlisted in **Fig. 16.5**.
2. **Identification phase:**
   - The identification phase begins when the client works interdependently with the nurse, expresses feelings, and begins to feel stronger.
   - Selection of appropriate professional assistance
   - Patient begins to have a feeling of belonging and a capability of dealing with the problem, which decreases the feeling of helplessness and hopelessness.
3. **Exploitation phase:**
   - In the exploitation phase, the client makes full use of the services offered.

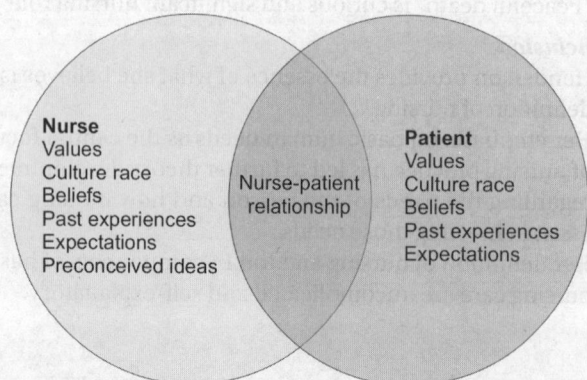

Fig. 16.5: Factors influencing orientation phase.

- In the exploitation phase, the client makes full use of the services offered.
- Use of professional assistance for problem-solving alternatives
- Advantages of services are used based on the needs and interests of the patients.
- The individual feels like an integral part of the helping environment.
- They may make minor requests or attention-getting techniques.
- The principles of interview techniques must be used to explore, understand and adequately deal with the underlying problem.
- Patient may fluctuate on independence.
- Nurse must be aware of the various phases of communication.
- Nurse aids the patient in exploiting all avenues of help, and progress is made towards the final step.

4. **Resolution phase:**
   - In the resolution phase, the client no longer needs professional services and gives up dependent behavior. The relationship ends.
   - In the resolution phase, the client no longer needs professional services and gives up dependent behavior. The relationship ends.
   - Termination of professional relationship
   - The patient's needs have already been met by the collaborative effect of patient and nurse.
   - Now they need to terminate their therapeutic relationship and dissolve the links between them.
   - Sometimes may be difficult for both as psychological dependence persists.
   - The patient drifts away and breaks the nurse's bond, and a healthier emotional balance is demonstrated, and both become mature individuals.
   - Sub concepts of the Interpersonal Relations Theory
   - Peplau's model has proved greatly used by later nurse theorists and clinicians in developing more sophisticated and therapeutic nursing interventions.

The following are the roles of the nurse in the therapeutic relationship identified by Peplau:

❖ **Stranger:** Offering the client the same acceptance and courtesy that the nurse would respond to any stranger
❖ **Resource person:** Providing specific answers to questions within a larger context
❖ **Teacher:** Helping the client to learn formally or informally
❖ **Leader:** Offering direction to the client or group
❖ **Surrogate:** Serving as a substitute for another such as a parent or a sibling
❖ **Counsellor:** Promoting experiences leading to health for the client, such as expression of feelings
❖ **Technical expert:** Providing physical care for the patient and operates equipment
   Peplau also believed that the nurse could take on many other roles, but these were not defined in detail. However, they were "left to the intelligence and imagination of the readers."
   —**Peplau, 1952**

Additional roles include:
❖ Technical expert
❖ Consultant
❖ Health teacher
❖ Tutor
❖ Socializing agent
❖ Safety agent
❖ Manager of environment
❖ Mediator
❖ Administrator
❖ Recorder observer
❖ Researcher

Anxiety
❖ Anxiety was defined as the initial response to a psychic threat.
❖ There are four levels of anxiety described below:

Four Levels of Anxiety
1. **Mild anxiety** is a positive state of heightened awareness and sharpened senses, allowing the person to learn new behaviors and solve problems. The person can take in all available stimuli (perceptual field).
2. **Moderate anxiety** involves a decreased perceptual field (focus on the immediate task only); the person can learn a new behavior or solve problems only with assistance. Another person can redirect the person to the task.
3. **Severe anxiety** involves feelings of dread and terror. The person cannot be redirected to a task; he/she focuses only on scattered details and has physiologic symptoms of tachycardia, diaphoresis, and chest pain.
4. **Panic anxiety** can involve loss of rational thought, delusions, hallucinations, and complete physical immobility and muteness. The person may bolt and run aimlessly, often exposing himself or herself to injury.

Interpersonal Theory and Nursing Process
❖ Peplau's Interpersonal Relations Theory and the Nursing Process are sequential and focus on the therapeutic relationship by using problem-solving techniques for the nurse and patient to collaborate on to meet the patient's needs.
❖ Both use observation communication and recording as basic tools utilized by nursing.
❖ Analysis
❖ Peplau conceptualized clear sets of nurse's roles that every nurse can use with their practice. It implies that a nurse's duty is not just to care, but the profession encompasses every activity that may affect the patient's care.
❖ The idea of a nurse-client interaction is limited to those individuals incapable of conversing, specifically those who are unconscious.
❖ The concepts are highly applicable to the care of psychiatric patients considering Peplau's background.
❖ But it is not limited to those sets of individuals. It can be applied to any person capable and has the will to communicate.

- The phases of the therapeutic nurse-client are highly comparable to the nursing process, making it vastly applicable.
- Assessment coincides with the orientation phase; nursing diagnosis and planning with the identification phase, implementation as to the exploitation phase, and evaluation with the resolution phase.

Strengths
- Peplau's theory helped later nursing theorists and clinicians develop more therapeutic interventions regarding the roles that show the dynamic character typical in clinical nursing.
- Its phases provide simplicity regarding the nurse-patient relationship's natural progression, which leads to adaptability in any nurse-patient interaction, thus providing generalizability.

Weaknesses
- Though Peplau stressed the nurse-client relationship as the foundation of nursing practice, health promotion and maintenance were less emphasized.
- Also, the theory cannot be used in a patient who doesn't have a felt need, such as with withdrawn patients.

Conclusion
- Peplau's theory has proved greatly used to later nurse theorists and clinicians in developing more sophisticated and therapeutic nursing interventions, including the seven nursing roles, which show the dynamic character roles typical in clinical nursing. It entails that a nurse's duty is not just to care, but the profession also incorporates every activity that may affect the client's health.
- The idea of nurse-client cooperation is found narrow with those individuals who are unfit and powerless in conversing, specifically those who are unconscious and paralyzed.
- Studying Peplau's Interpersonal Relations Theory of Nursing can be very substantial, especially to aspiring to be part of the profession.
- Knowing the seven nursing roles, future nurses can apply for different roles in different situations, which will guarantee their patients acquire the best care possible and ultimately speed along with treatment and recovery.

Linking Theories with Nursing Process
- Theory is the generation of nursing knowledge for use in practice.
- Process is the method for applying the theory for knowledge.
- The integration of the theory and process is the basis for professional nursing.
- The nursing process a tool for nursing practice, was introduced first by Orlando and is a framework for contemporary nursing practice.
- The nursing process is the procedure for organizing nursing care in which the first step, assessment initiates the act of nursing.
- The goals of the nursing process are noted in the theoretical work by Abdellah, Henderson, Orem, Orlando, Travelbee and (Meleis, 1997).
- Together they provide nursing with a perspective on assessment, diagnosis, planning implementation, and evaluation (Abdellah and other 1960; Henderson 1966); creates a process of defining and attaining goals (King 1981) and emphasize client's perceptions of their health.
- The nursing process offers a systematic approach for nursing practice an enhances research opportunities.
- The process is adaptable to different clients and different care settings.
- In addition, the nursing process is compatible with many other systems in the health care delivery system (e.g., computer-generated care plans, patient information systems, patient acuity systems) (Burnum,1994).
- The nursing process is central to the domain of nursing.
- The nursing process is central to the domain of nursing (Meleis 1997)
- However, the nursing process is not a theory. It provides the process for the delivery of nursing care, not the knowledge component of the discipline.
- There are however, attempts to build a comprehensive theory from the process.
- First there is an attempt to use the nursing process in conjunction with other theories that lack of process element.
- Second, there is an effort to organize nursing diagnoses and interventions as complementary places (Barnum, 1994).
- However, nurse theorists are divided as to whether the nursing process model is compatible with current and emerging theories (Meleis, 1997).

Index

Page numbers followed by *f* refer to figure, *fc* refer to flowchart, and *t* refer to table.

A

A1C level, diagnosis to 127*t*
A1C test 127
Abdomen 9, 10, 20
    general approach 20
    inspection 20
    trauma 108
Abdominal cramping 49
Ability, loss of 274
Abortion 316
Abstraction, level of 345
Abuse
    dealing with 318
    prevention of 318
    sexual 317, 318
Accidental disconnection 162
Acetone 68
    urine test for 136
Achilles reflex 26
Acid 173
    acetic 96
    acetoacetic 136
    amino 53
    buffered, strong 174
    gastric 120
    hydrochloric 120
    organic 189
Acid-base
    balance 171, 177
        regulating 118
        role of lungs in 174
    disturbance 173, 174
        primary 175*fc*
    status 174
Acidemia 173
Acid-fast bacillus 139
Acidic urine, causes of 137
Acidosis 173
Acoustic nerve, eighth 24
Acriflavin 96
Active transport 172, 176
Acute respiratory distress syndrome 164
Adaptation 320, 325, 352
    acute local 327
    behavioral 325
    chronic local 327
    cognitive 325
    levels of 352
    model, concepts of 351
    physiological 325
    psychological 325
    social 325
    spiritual 325
    structural 325
    theory 345
    types of 325
Addison's disease 188
Adhesive tape 89
Administer oral fluids 179
Adrenalectomy 188
Aerosol spray 261
Agranulocytes 116
Air
    embolism 197, 235
    lock method 231
Air-tight drainage system, maintenance of 159
Airway
    artificial 275
    collapse 143
    conditions affecting 144
    movement of 144
    obstruction
        causes of 150
        signs of 150
Alanine
    aminotransferase 122
    transaminase 122
Albumin 123
    indications 123
    urine test for 135
    water 42
Albuminuria 83
Aldosterone 173
Alkalemia 173
Alkaline
    fluids 77
    pH 136
    phosphatase 122, 123
    urine, causes of 136
Alkalosis 173
Allergy 144
    latex 87
Altered dietary intake 118
Aminophylline suppository 104
Ammonia buffer system 174
Ampoule 243, 246
    breaking 244*f*
    preparation 246
Analgesics 222
Anaphylaxis 207
Anatomy education, embalming for 298
Androgens 223
Anemia 150
Angioedema 207
Anorexia 44
    causes 44
Antacids 222
Antagonism 209
Anthropoid 298
Antiasthmatics 223
Antibiotics 222
Anticoagulants 222
Antidiarrheals 222
Anti-diuretic hormone 172
Antidote 222
Antiemetics 223
Anti-glare coatings 79
Antihistamine 45, 222
Anti-infection 223
Antipyretics 222
Antiseptic 75, 223
    lotion 73
Antitussives 223
Anuria 83
Anxiety 357
    levels of 357
    mild 357
    moderate 357
    panic 357
    severe 357
Aorta, contour of 21
Aortic valve, stenosis of 10
Aphasia 274
Aplastic anemia 208
Apnea 145
Appetite 328
Appraisal-focused coping strategies 330
Aromatherapy 331
Arousal mechanism 270
Arrhythmias 208
Arterial blood gas 189, 191, 192
    analysis 175*t*
Arterial embalming 297
Arterial puncture, sites for 268
Artery
    carotid 15
    ophthalmic 75
Ascending reticular activating system 270
Asepto syringe 91
Asparagus 82
Aspartate aminotransferase 122
Asthma 144
    bronchial 169
Astringent 75, 223
Atelectasis 145, 191
Atherosclerosis 126
Atrial natriuretic peptide 173
Attitude, positive 328
Auditory canal 76
Auditory deprivation 273
Aural rehabilitation 277
Auscultation 7, 10
Auscultatory gap 11
Automated cell counters 114
Autopsy 293
    aim of 296
    in medicine, value of 294
    room 300
    type of 294
        examination 293
Awareness 336
Axillary nodes 15

Index

B

Back
    care 58
    posterior 9
    rub 55
Bacteria 322
    fingernails transmitters of 68
Bandage, triangular 73
Bargaining 285
Barium chloride 132
Barley water 41
Bartter syndrome 190
Basic critical thinking 28
Basophils 116
Bath
    partial 55
    types of 55
Bathroom bath 55
Beating 59f
Bed and bedding 346
Bed bath 55
    scientific principles of 57
Bed shampoo, performing 71
Bedfast 64
Bedpan 77, 85, 86f
    types of 86
Bedsore 60
Belladonna, inhalation of 261
Benedict's test 133
Benzamide 46
Bereavement 281
Beta cholics 223
Betty Newman's system model 328
Bicarbonate 117, 121, 171
    ions 82
    level 121
Bile obstruction 132
Bilirubin fraction 123
Biochemical examination 39
Birth control
    permanent methods of 317
    reversible methods of 317
Bisacodyl 104
Bisexual 314
Bizarre thinking 273
Bladder
    irrigation 96, 259
    radiation injury to 95
Bleeding
    disorders 156
    external 202
    internal 202
Blindness, prevention of 276
Blood
    amino acid level 122
    ammonia 122
    buffers 174
    chemistry 10
    circulation 173
    collection of 126
    dyscrasias 208
    flow, insufficient 163
    increases, coagulability of 122
    urea 122
Blood glucose
    levels, long-term high 130
    technologies 126
    test 122
        lab-based 129
Blood pressure 11, 144
    high 325
Blood transfusion
    complications of 203
    indications of 202
    management during 204t
Blood vessels 13
    dilate 75
Blood volume
    decreased circulating 178
    maintaining 118
Bloodstream infection, catheter-related 198
Body
    after embalming 297
    block 295
    calcium 119
    fluid
        compartments and exchange 171
        homeostasis 173, 173fc
    image 34, 305, 306, 312
    inflammatory response 325
    pH balance of 117
    postmortem care of 292, 292t
    posture 144
    reconstitution of 296
    size 39
    stress effects on 324
    substances precautions, maintain 139
Boeck medium, modified 135
Bone soups 42
Boric acid 71, 75
    solution 96
Bowel elimination 96
    factors affecting 99
    physiology of 96
Bowel wash 106
    aftercare 107
    contraindications 106
    equipments 106
    procedures 106
Bowel, care of 289
Brachioradialis tendon 26
Braden scale 64, 64t
Brain death 287
Breast 16
    female 16
    male 16
    palpation 16
Breath
    focus technique 167
    humming bee 169
    lion's 168
    sitali 168
Breathing 165, 325
    coherent 168
    deep 169, 333
    diaphragmatic 167
    equal 168
    exercises 167
        deep 162
Breathlessness 150
Bristol stool chart 98f
Bronchospasm 170
Buccal cavity 70
Buccal mucosa 14
Burns, severe 53
Bypass gastrointestinal tract 52

C

Caffeine 132
Calcium 117
    absorption of 119
    gluconate 185
    in bone, deposition of 119
    values 119
Callista Roy's adaptation model 351
Campylobacter 132
Cancer 53, 95
Candida 110
Cannabinoids 45
Cannula
    gauge of 241
    selection 194
Capillary blood glucose
    monitoring 127
    test 127, 128
        advantages 127
        disadvantages 127
Carbohydrates 53, 195
Cardiac arrest 164
Cardiac atrial distension 173
Cardiac death 287
Cardiac manifestations 188
Cardiac output, decreased 178
Cardiac stimulant 223
Cardiac tonic 223
Cardiopulmonary resuscitation 301
Cardiovascular disease 328
    developing 124
Cardiovascular system 9, 142, 178, 192, 324
Care of dying 288
Care plans 350
Career changes 323
Caregiving roles 34
Carotid pulsation 19, 19t
Carpopedal spasmi 192
Cartilaginous ring 76
Cascade cough 166
Caste conflict 323
Catheter
    clamp 112
    color coding of 90t
    connect 92
    Coudé tip 90f
    embolism 198
    Foley's 90, 90f
    indwelling 83, 90f, 91
    method 103
    sterile suction 154
    straight 90f
    suprapubic 90
    triple lumen indwelling 90f
    tubing and funnel 96
    types of 90f
Catheterization 138
    types of 89
Cavity embalming 297
Cecum 97
Cell counter 114
Cellular metabolism, altered 118
Central nervous system 142, 192, 324
    alteration 288
Central parenteral nutrition 53
Cerebellar functions 25
Cerebral edema 175, 182
Cervical cap 317
Chemical agents 322
Chest
    catheter
        proper placement of 158
        removal 161
    drainage
        system 162
        types of 159
    percussion 156
    physiotherapy 156
    pressure in 162
    tube
        care of 162
        dressing 163

Cheyne-Stokes breathing 183
Chlorhexidine 68
Chloride 117, 171
    ions 82
Cholera 99
Cholesterol 124
    levels 125
Chronic obstructive pulmonary disease 145, 169, 191
Chvostek's sign 186, 192
Chyluria 83
Circulatory death 287
Circulatory fluid volume 83
Civic amenities 323
Clamp tubing 138
Clark's rule 217
Cleansing enema, rectal tube of 103
Client and unit, preparation of 56
Climate 39
Clinical autopsy 294
Clinical death, signs of 288
Clip fingernails straight 67
Clysis 97, 102
Coconut water 41
Coffee 41
Coffin 298
Cognition 33, 34
Cognitive 306
    function, function of 156
Colon
    cancer of 132
    descending 97
    sigmoid 97
    transverse 97
Colonic irrigation 98
Colostomy 107
    ascending 108
    descending 108
    permanent 108
    temporary 108
    types of 108
Colostomy bag 109*f*
    changing of 110, 111*f*
    regular emptying of 109
    with clamp 110*f*
Colostomy irrigation 109-111
    drain pouch 112
Combined oral contraceptives 317
Common cold 144
Communication 34, 275, 316
    non-verbal 2
Compensatory nursing system 349
Compensatory process 352
Complete blood count 114
    purposes of 115
Complex critical thinking 29
Compression 60
Computed tomography scan 140
Concentration techniques 133
Condom
    female 317
    latex-free 87
    male 317
    use of 316
Condom drainage 86
    catheter, insertion of 87*t*
    procedure of 87
Confusion 309
Congestive heart failure 164, 180
Conjunctiva
    bulbar 12
    palpebral 12
Conjunctivitis 12

Conn's syndrome 180
Connective tissue, band of 59
Conscious patient, oral hygiene for 68
Consciousness, level of 8
Constipation 97, 100
    assessment of 132
    untreated 100
Contact lenses and eyes, care for 79
Continent urinary reservoir 95
Continuous glucose monitoring 128
    advantages 128
    disadvantages 128
Contraception 316
Controlled coughing 166
    technique procedure 166
Coping mechanisms, classifications of 330
Coping responses 34
Coping skills
    negative 330
    positive 329
Coping strategy 330
    problem-focused 330
    types of 330
Copper T intrauterine device 317
Cornea 13
Coronary artery disease 124
Corticosteroid 223
    administration 180
    excess 187
    role of 173
Costal vertebral angle tenderness 21
Cough 144
    types of 144
Coughing techniques 166
Counseling 289, 299
Cranial nerve function 24
Creams 250
Critical thinking 27, 28
    attitudes for 27
    components of 27
    levels of 28
    meaning of 27
    standards for 28
Crohn's disease 53, 108
Crystals 133
Cultural assimilation 336
Cultural competence 336
Cultural diversity 335
    and spirituality, concepts of 335
Culture 308
    and ethnicity 284
Cupping 60*f*
Curd water 41
Cushing's syndrome 180, 187
Cyanosis 150, 162
Cystitis, chronic 95
Cystoscopy 83

D

Data
    collection, method of 2
    systematic collection of 29
Data base
    components of 29
    recording of 30
Dead body, care of 291
Death 287
    biological death 287
    care of 281
    certificate 291, 300
    clinical death 287
    ethical and legal issues in 301

    immediate signs of 288
    rattle 288
    signs of 296
    types of 287
Decongestant 223
Deep palpation 6, 6*f*
Defecation 97
    position during 99
Defensive coping 34
Dehydration 145, 179
    signs of 179
Demulcent 223
Denture
    care for removable 80
    good 80
Depression 324
    managing 327
Detergent 223
Developmental theory 345
    and models 342
Diabetes
    management 127
    role in 127
    type 2 127
    diagnose of 127
Diabetic acidosis 188
Diabetic ketoacidosis 129
Dialysis 176, 234
Diamond's medium 135
Diaphoretics 223
Diaphragm 317
    use 15
Diarrhea 49, 97, 99, 208
    assessment of 132
    severe 132
    symptoms of 100
Diet 99, 177, 212
    balanced 327
    clear fluid 40
    foodstuff liquid 40
    full 43
        fluid 40
    light 42
    liquid 40
    non-irritant 43
    soft 42, 43
Dietary management 180
Diffusion 143, 175
Digestion 325
Digestive system 324
Dilate vein 196
Discharge teaching 161
Disease 346
    alleviate 207
    conditions 271
    prevent 207
Dispensing oxygen, methods of 151
Disposable colostomy bag 109
Disposable drainage systems 160
Distress 320, 321
Diuretics 223
Divorce 322
Do-not-resuscitate order 301
Dopamine antagonists 45
Dorothea Orem's theory 349
    self-care deficit 347
    strength of 350
Dorsal gluteal site 230
Double boiled rice 42
Drainage
    apparatus, proper placement of 158
    lack of 161
    tubing, length of 158

Drip chamber 242
Droperidol 45
Drug 322
   action 211
   administration, routes of 225
   and fluids administered drugs, types of 230
   anesthetic 75
   dosage
      and applications 224t
      calculations 216
   idiosyncrasy 209
   incompatibility 209
   measurements, system of 214
   nomenclature 206
   on body, effects of 207
   preparation 209, 224, 224t
   recording of 217
   storage and maintenance of 220
   terminologies 222
Dry plastic bag 148
Dye excretion tests 121
Dying declaration 290, 291
Dying patient's bill of rights 288
Dyspareunia 316
Dysphagia 43
   nursing interventions for 44t
Dyspnea 144, 183
Dysuria 83

E

Ear 8, 256
   and hearing 13
   care of 76
      scientific principles of 76
   drops, instillation of 254
   drum 76
   irrigation 257
Edema 178, 181, 342
   generalized 182
   localized 181
   peripheral 180, 182
Edematous states 183
Education 322
   and health maintenance 46
Educational status 55
Effleurage 58, 59f
Effluent, type of 108
Effluvia 346
Egg flip 42
Ejaculation, premature 316
Electrolyte 171, 182
   and balance 177
   functions of 182
   imbalance 84, 182
      risk for 33
   regulation 182
   testing 191
Embalming 296
   advanced method of 298
   aims of 296
   characteristics of 296
   chemicals used for 298
   history of 296
   procedure for 297
Emergency contraceptive tablets 317
Emesis basin 68
Emetics 223
Emollient 69
Emotional status 8
Emotions 144
Empathy, validation and reassurance 2

Emptying colostomy bag, procedure for 110t
Enable social support 333
Encopresis 325
End of life, assist with 290
Endocrine
   disease 180
   disorder 132
   glands, secretion of 39
   system 324
Endolymph 77
Endoscopic procedures 141
   indications 141
Endotracheal tube occlusion 166
Enema 97, 102, 104
   administration of 103f
   anthelminthic 102
   astringent 102
   carminative 102
   classification of 102
   cold 102
   contraindications 102
   emollient 103
   evacuation 256
   glycerine 102
   medicated 102
   methods of 103
   nutrient 103
   oil 102
   phosphate 102
   purgative 102
   retention 102, 256
   sedative 102
   soap and water 102
   stimulant 103
Energy balance 33
Entamoeba histolytica, culture of 135
Enteral feeding 47
Enteric pathogens 131
Entero test 135
Enteroscopy 141
Enuresis 325
Environment 144, 346, 348, 351, 354, 356
   comfort 35
   hazards 35
   temperature 177
   theory 345
   types of 346
Eosinophils 116
Epidural route 264, 264f
Episiotomy patients 77
Epithelial cells 133
Epitrochlear nodes 15, 16
Equipment 13, 138, 239, 240
   cannula 240
Erb's point 10
Erectile dysfunction
   primary 316
   secondary 316
Erythrocytes 115
Esophagogastroduodenoscopy 45
Ethanol 132, 189
Ethnicity and culture 38
Ethyl acetate 68
Ethylene glycol 189
Eustachian tubes 76
Eustress 320, 321
Euthanasia 301
   active 302
   and physician-assisted suicide 302
   classification 302
   involuntary 302
   non-voluntary 302
   passive 302

   voluntary 302
Excess fluid retention 180
Exercise 33, 144, 330, 333
   regular 38
Exhaustion, stage of 326
Extracellular bicarbonate levels 121
Extracellular fluid 182
   compartment 171
   volume, loss of 178
Extracellular ions 171
Extremity 19
Eye 8, 256
   and vision 12
   care
      performing 74
      teach general 276
   cavities of 75
   contact 4
   drops, instillation of 254
   ears and nose 74
   irrigation 256
   pain in 80
   take care of 79
Eyeball, coats in 75
Eyelashes protect 75

F

Face mask 151
Facial expression 4
Facial nerve, seventh 24
Family and culture 307
Family education 289
Family interaction 271
Family relationships 34
Family theory 345f
Fat
   emulsification of 57
   emulsion 53
   metabolism 122t
Fatty acids, non-esterified 124, 125
Fecal consistency 132
Fecal impaction
   etiology of 107
   symptoms with 107
Fecal odor alterations 132
Feces 97
   abnormalities of 98
   blood in 98
   composition of 98, 130
   digital evacuation of 107
   mucus in 98
   parasites in 99
Feeding helpless patient
   articles 47
   procedure 47
   purposes 47
Feet and legs 10
Female catheterization, steps of procedure for 91t
Female genitalia 9, 21
   equipments 21
   procedure 21
Feminine 312
Ferricyanide 136
Fertility awareness-based methods 317
Filtration 172, 176, 234
Flash blood glucose monitoring 128
Flat vial insert 245f
Flatulence 98, 101
Flatus tube, passing 101
Floatation techniques 134
Flow rate calculation, formula for 195

Fluid 40, 171
   and electrolyte
      movements 172
         regulation of 172
   compartment 181
   constant bubbling of 162
   diets, types of 40
   homeostasis 171
   intake 83, 99
      enhancing 205
   management 178, 180
   mobilization of 181
   overload 49, 180
   pressures 172
   rate calculation 235
   restriction 204
   volume
      deficit 177-179
      disturbances in 178
      excess 177, 180
      overload, causes of 180
Food
   effect of 39
   intake assessment 40
Forceps, dissecting 69
Foreign body 77
Forensic autopsy 294
Formaldehyde 189
Formal-ether sedimentation techniques 134
Formalin 131
Forming clot 117
Fractured ribs 156
Fresh frozen plasma 200
Friction and shear 66
Fried's rule 217
Fruit 118
   juices 41
Funduscopic examination 13
Fungicides 223
Funnel and catheter method 103
Furosemide 184

G

Gag reflex 69
Galactose tolerance test 122
Gallipot 74
Gamma-glutamyl transferase 122, 123
   indications 123
Gargle 252
Gas exchange, impaired 178
Gastric emptying, delayed 49
Gastric mucosa, irritation of 208
Gastritis 132
Gastrointestinal diseases 130
Gastrointestinal disturbance 288
Gastrointestinal function 33
Gastrointestinal problems 328
Gastrointestinal system 141
Gastrointestinal tract 130
   role of 173
Gastrostomy 50, 51
   dressing 50
   tube feeding 51
   types 51
Gels 250
Gender identity 312
Gender role-behavior 312
General adaptation syndrome 326
General aesthetics, inhalation of 261
Genetic disorders 322
Genital care 87

female 88
male 88
Genitalia
   female 9, 21
   male 21
Germ cells 123
Germicides 223
Gingivitis 71
Girth measurements 182
Gitelman syndrome 190
Glacial acetic acid 135
Glass vials 244, 245f
Glomerular filtration 81
Glossopharyngeal nerve 25
Gloves
   clean 68
   remove 49
Glucophage 189
Glucose with insulin 185
Glycemic care 130
Glycerine 68, 71
   suppository 104
   syringe 103
Glycohemoglobin test 127
Glycosuria 83
Gonococcus 75
Gonorrheal ophthalmia, prevent 75
Gram's iodine 134
Granisetron 45
Granulating sugar 63
Granulocytes 116
Granulocytosis 208
Gravity, specific 133, 137
Green corridor organ transfer, procedure of 302
Grief 281
   and loss, theories of 285
   anticipatory 282
   chronic 282
   complicated 282
   counseling 300
      method of 300
   cumulative 282
   delayed 283
   disenfranchised 282
   exaggerated 283
   inhibited 283
   manifestations of 283
   normal 282
   responses, types of 282
   types of 283
Group activities 333
Group cohesiveness, lack of 323
Growth 35
   and development 82
   hormone, higher levels of 121
Guillain-Barre syndrome 191
Gums 14

H

Hacking 59, 59f
Hair 8
   care, scientific principles of 73
   problem 328
   wash 71
Halitosis, prevent 69
Haloperidol 45
Hands 9
HBA1C tests 129
Head 12
Headache 320, 324, 325
Head-to-toe physical assessment 5

Health 322, 342, 346, 348, 351, 354
   assessment 1, 4
      techniques, components of 1f
   awareness 32
   conditions 164
   deviation self-care requisites 349
   history 4
   level of 143, 177
   management 32
   promotion 32
   psychological 144
   status of 39
Hearing aid, care and maintenance of 80
Hearing impairment 276
   characteristics of 276
   communication with 277
   types of 276
Hearing loss
   combined 276
   conductive 276
   psychogenic 276
Heart 10, 18
   aortic area 10
   apical area 10
   attack 124, 326
   auscultation 19
   epigastric area 10
   failure 145
   inspections 18
   left ventricular 10
   palpations 18
   percussion 18
   problems 325
   pulmonary area 10
   right ventricular 10
   sounds–S1 and S2 9
Heat and moisture exchange humidifiers 166
Heated humidifiers 166
Hematinics 223
Hematocrit 114, 116
Hematoma formation 198, 234
Hematuria 83
Hemic hypoxia 145
Hemodynamic instability 164
Hemoglobin 114, 116, 127
   composition of 116
   functions of 116
   glycated 127
   normal values of 116
Hemolytic reaction 203
   delayed 204
Hemorrhage 162
Hemosiderosis 204
Hemostatic 223
   functions 121
Henderson's model 354, 354t
Henderson's theory 354
   characteristic of 354
Heparin 53
Hepatic dysfunction 84
Hernias, male 21
Heterosexual 314
Hirschsprung's disease 108
Histotoxic hypoxia 145
Holding sponge, steps of 69f
Holistic nursing care 310
Homeostasis 171
Homosexual 314
Hormonal methods 317
   implant 317
   injection 317
Hormonal vaginal contraceptive ring 317
Hormone secretion 326

Index

Huff cough 166
Huffing technique 167
Human development 284
Human immunodeficiency virus 116
Human papillomavirus, prevent 316
Humidification 165
    physiological concept 165
Humidifiers, types of 166
Hydration 165
    status 280
Hydrogen peroxide 63, 68, 77
Hydrostatic pressure 172, 176, 234
Hydroxyzine 45
Hygiene 55
Hygienic perineal care 87
Hygienic practice, factors influencing 55
Hyperaldosteronism 180, 187
Hypercalcemia 187
Hypercarbia 84
Hyperchloremic acidosis 188
Hyperemesis gravidarum, severe 53
Hyperglycemia 84, 129
Hyperkalemia 185
    spurious 185
    treatment 185
Hyperlipoproteinemia 126
Hypermagnesemia 188
Hypernatremia 183, 184
Hyperosmolar dehydration 49
Hyperosmolar diuresis 84
Hyperosmolar state 129
Hyperparathyroidism 187
Hyperphosphatemia 121
Hypersensitivity reaction 208
Hypertension 208
Hyperventilation 145
Hypervolemia 84, 183
Hypnotics 223
Hypocalcemia 186
Hypodermic embalming 297
Hypoglossal nerve 25
Hypoglycemia 84, 130
    causes of 130
    symptoms of 130
Hypoglycemics 223
Hypokalemia 184
Hypomagnesemia 187
Hyponatremia 182
Hypotension 208
    orthostatic 9
    postural 9
Hypothalamus 172
Hypoventilation 145
Hypovolemia 145, 178
Hypoxemia 192
Hypoxia 145, 322, 352
    circulatory 145
    demand 145
    types of 145
Hypoxic hypoxia 145

I

Ileal conduit 95
Illness 177, 308
Immune
    disorders 322
    system 324
Immunization shots 249
Impending death, signs of 287
Inappropriate behavior, assessment of 319
Incentive spirometer 169, 170f
Incontinence 66, 83, 98
Indwelling urinary catheter, removing 94t
Ineffective activity planning, risk for 34
Infancy 312
Infection
    droplet 57
    prevention of 241
    prominent sign of 62
    risk for 35
    signs of 62
    transmission of 249
    widespread 52
Infectious diseases 204
    toxins of 76
Infertility 316
Infiltration 234
Inflammation, chronic 324
Inflammatory bowel disease 132
Information 274
Infraclavicular nodes 15
Infusion
    disconnecting 54
    set 242
    stopping 54
Inguinal nodes 15, 16
Inhalation 145, 261
    carbon dioxide 261
    deep 166
    drugs used 261
    dry 146, 261
    moist 146, 261
    oxygen 261
Injection 229
    administration, route of 229f
    angle of 229f
    complications of 229
    selection of site for 230
    types of 229
    use correct technique of 230
Inorganic substances 130
Insomnia 324
Insulin 53, 63
Integrity 28
Integumentary function 33
Integumentary system 178
Intellectual standards 28
Interaction theories and models 342
Interpersonal conflict 323
Interpersonal relations theory 355
    concepts of 356
Interpersonal theory 357
Interview
    phases of 1f
    technique, strategies of 1
Intestinal placement 49
Intestinal protozoa, morphology of 135
Intestinal secretions 130
Intoxication 189
Intra-abdominal pressure 84
Intra-arterial cannulation steps 268
Intra-arterial route 267
Intracellular fluid 182
Intradermal injection 238
    administration, steps of procedure for 238t
Intramuscular injection 230
Intraosseous route 265
Intraperitoneal route 266, 266f
Intrapleural drain 162
    falls out 162
Intrapleural route 267, 267f
Intraprocedural steps 54, 153, 170
Intrathecal administration 264, 264f
Intravenous administration, types of 232
Intravenous cannula 240
    parts of 240f
Intravenous drip rates, calculation of 216
Intravenous fluid
    calculation for 194
    therapy, complications of 197
    types of 194
Intravenous infusion 193, 234
    flow rates for 196t
Intravenous injection 232
Intravenous set
    parts of 242, 242f
    principle of 242
Intravenous therapy 193
    solutions 195, 195t
Intravenous tubing calibration 243
Ions, types of 118
Iris 12
Iron
    hematoxylin 135
    overload 204
Irritability 274
Isoenzymes 123
Isosthenuric specific gravity, causes of 137
Isotonic fluid volume deficit 178
Itching, severe 72

J

Jaw produces facial twitching 186
Jejunostomy 51
    indications 51
    purpose 51
    tube feeding 51
        steps of procedure 51
Jelly 43
Jet medication nebulizer 147, 147f
Jewel box 298
Jugular pulsation, internal 19, 19t
Jugular vein 19
    dissipation 9
    distension 197
    pulsations 19

K

K-basin 69
Kelly's pad 72
Keratin 68
Keratolytics 223
Kerosene 74
Kidney 20
    problems 177
    proximal tubules of 123
    role of 173
    tray 69
Kneading (petrissage) 59, 59f
Known environment, loss of 281
Kubler Ross's five stages of dying 285
Kussmaul's respirations 189

L

Label specimen containers 139
Labia minora 88
Lacrimal tearing 207
Lactated ringer's solution 195
Lactic acidosis 188
Lactobacillus acidophilus 71
Language barriers 337
Laryngeal spasm 192

Latent tetany, provocative tests for 186
Laxatives 223
Left upper quadrant 20
Lens 13
Lesion 342
Leukocyte 115, 116
    depleted red cell 200
Leukocytosis 185
Leukopenia 116, 208
Lid
    lower 12
    margins 12
    upper 12
Liddle syndrome 190
Life
    changes 323
    events 322
    experiences 309
    loss of aspect of 281
    principles 34
Lifestyle 39, 177, 322
Life-threatening 124
    disorder, sign of 100
    scenario 129
Light
    interference of 164
    palpation 6, 6f
    sensitivity 80
Lip, inspect integrity of 69
Lipid 53, 124
    intolerance 84
    metabolism 121
    particulate aggregation 84
    profile
        normal 124
        tests for 126
    types of 124
Lipoprotein 125
    classes of 124
    high-density 124, 126
    intermediate density 124, 125
    low density 124, 125
    profile 124
    very low density 124, 125
Liquid
    direct application of 252
    form, milk products in 41
    paraffin 68
Listening
    practice active 337
    skill, components of active 2f
Listerine 68
Liver 20
    border, lower 20
    cirrhosis of 180
    damage 208
    enzymes estimation 122
    function tests 121, 122
        components of 122t
    functions of 122
Livor mortis 291
Lobe
    left upper 157, 157f
    lower 156f, 157, 157f
    right middle 157, 157f
    upper 157, 157f, 158, 158f
Local adaptation syndrome 327
Loop stoma 108
Loss
    actual 281
    anticipatory 281
    categories of 281
    classifications of 281
    concepts of 281
    nature of 284
    perceived 281
    situational 281
    types of 281
Lotions 250
Low flow systems 151
Low specific gravity urine, causes of 137
Lower extremity 9, 26
Lower urinary tract infection 84
Luer connector 243
Lugol's solution 133, 134
Lung 10, 16
    anterior 9, 17
    disease 192
    resonance, point of 20
    role of 173
    sounds 17t
Lymph nodes 15
Lymphedema 182
Lysozyme 75

M

Mackintosh 73
Macro drip 243
Macula 13
Magnesium 117
Male catheterization, steps of procedure for 92t
Malnutrition 53
Mammary glands, lactating 123
Mammography 140
Mandrel vial insert 246f
Mantoux test 238
Masculine 312
Maslow's hierarchy 354, 354t
Massage 331
    technique 59
Maturational factors 329
Meat and fish 118
Meatal care 77
Mechanical test 14
Meclizine 45
Media 308
Medical diagnosis 35, 36t
Medication 99, 271
    action dose 213
    administration 206, 224, 227
    carefully check 221
    dose 214
        calculation 216
    forms of 209
    interaction 208
    placement of 221
    storage system of 221
Medication error
    administration errors 220
    classification of 219
    dispensing error 220
    sources of 219
    transcribing error 219
Medication order
    and prescriptions 213
    components of 213
    types of 214
Medication storage
    conditions 221
    light 222
Medicolegal cases 301
Meditation 333
Medulla oblongata 326
Melena 98
Membranes, selective permeability of 176
Meniere's disease 45
Menstrual period, absence of 325
Menstrual problems 328
Mental condition 66
Mental health problems 328
Mental preparation 8
Mentally challenged 55
Merthiolate
    iodine formalin 135
    tincture of 135
Metabolic acidosis 188
Metabolic alkalosis 190
Metabolic syndrome, prevent 38
Meta-theory 343
Meteorism 98
Metered-dose nebulizer 146, 146f
    parts of 146f
Methanol 189
Microbial action 291
Microorganism, development of 76
Micturition 83
    reflex discharges urine 81
Mid-deltoid site 231, 231f
Mind body relaxation 333
Mini infusion pump 243
Mini mental state examination 272
Mobility 66
    completely immobile 66
    no limitations 66
    slightly limited 66
    very limited 66
Moisture 63, 64
    exchange humidifiers 166
Moisturize oral mucous membrane 69
Molecules, diffusion of 176
Moral distress 35
Mortuary
    placing body 300
    releasing body 300
Motor 24
Motor function 24
    findings 25
Mourning, six R's of 286
Mouth 8, 14
    breathers 68
    equipments 14
    gently swab roof of 70
    inspection 14
    mucous membrane of 69
    wash, scientific principles of 70
Movement, increased 164
Mucous membranes 14, 178
Multigrain roti 43
Multiple electrolyte solution 195
Murmurs 10
Muscle
    relaxants 223
    strength 24
    tension of 59, 325
    tone 83
Muscular strength 15
Musculoskeletal changes 288
Musculoskeletal structure 156
Musculoskeletal system 23, 178, 324
Music therapy 333
Mydriatics 223
Myocardial infarction 164

N

Nabilone 45

Nail 8
   and foot care, performing 67
   cutting, scientific principles of 67
   improper care of 67
   inspect 67
   polish 68, 164
Narcotics 223
Nasal cannula 151, 151f
Nasal drops, instillation of 255
Nasal irrigation 258
Nasal septum 14
Nasal spray 260
Nasogastric intubation 47
Nasogastric tube
   fasten end of 49
   measurement and insertion of 48f
Nature
   befriend 331
   exposure to 333
Nausea 44, 49, 207, 208
   causes 44
Nebulization therapy 146
Nebulized b-adrenergic agonists 185
Nebulizer
   kit 147
   solution, prescribed 147
Neck 8, 15
   equipment 15
   inspections 15
   palpations 15
Needle
   cutters 248
   parts of 240f
   size and specifications of 240t
Needlestick injury 248
   management 249
   prevention of 248
Needlestick Safety and Prevention Act 249
Nelson's inhaler 149f
   method 149
Neobladder 95
Nephron 81
   structure of 82f
Nerve
   cells 75
   damage 130
      severity of 109
   deafness 276
   impulses 142
Neurogenic bladder 95
Neurogenic hyperventilation 183
Neurologic examination, basic principles 23
Neurologic system 23
Neurological injury 144
Neuromuscular manifestations 188
Neuromuscular system 192
Neuropathy, peripheral 130
Neutrophils 116
Night blindness, prevents 75
Nightingale's theory
   application of 347
   concepts of 346
Nitrogenous substance, insoluble 68
Noise reduction 333
Non-hemolytic febrile reactions 203
Nonrebreather mask 151, 152f
Non-vegetarian soup 42
Non-verbal cues 310
Normal tears, pH of 75
Norton pressure sore 66
Nose 8
   and sinuses 14
   care of 77

Nostril breathing, alternate 168
Noxious air 346
Nuclear medicine 140
   indications 140
Numerous bacteria 130
Nurse's implement spiritual care 341
Nurse's responsibility 55, 73, 139, 339
Nursing 346, 354
   action 92
   adaptation model of 350
   agency 348
   care 50
      plan 33
   diagnosis 30, 35, 36t, 340, 332, 347
   evaluation 355
   goal of 345
   interventions classification 67
   interviews, phases of 1
   management 46, 340
   metaparadigm 342
   practice 346
   process 27, 29, 36, 355
      six-step 352
   system 348
      theory of 349
   theory 328, 342, 345
      components of 344, 344fc
      development of 342
Nutrition 33, 66, 289, 346
   imbalance 33, 46
Nutritional assessment, importance of 38
Nutritional imbalance 322
Nutritional needs 37
Nutritional status 38, 39
Nystagmus 12
   convergence 12

O

Observation
   levels of 3
   non-participant 2
   participant 2
   practice of nursing 3
   techniques 3
   types 2
Occult blood, stool test for 132
Occupation 322
   exposure asbestos 144
Ointments 250
Olfactory nerve 24
Olfactory senses, impaired 278
Oliguria 83
Oncotic pressure 172
Ondansetron 45
One-point cut ampoules 243
Ophthalmoscope, use of 13
Optic disc 13, 24
Optic nerve 75
Oral care
   artery forceps for 69f
   cleaning
      both sides in 70f
      roof of mouth, gums and cheeks in 70f
Oral cavity 70
Oral contraceptives 223
Oral glucose tolerance test 129
Oral infection, prevent and treat 69
Oral medication 226
Orbital cavity 75
Orem's self-care theory 348
   conceptual framework 348

Organ donation 302
   green corridor for 302, 303
Organ transplant, green corridor for 302
Orgasmic dysfunction, secondary 316
Orogastric feeding 49
Orthopnea 144, 183
Osmolarity 172
Osmosis 172, 175, 234
Osmotically active substance 132
Osteoporosis 156
Ostomy, care of 109
Oto-ophthalmoscope 11
Otoscope, examine with 13
Oxygen 289
   administration 150
      hazards of 153
   cylinder 147
   delivery systems 165
   mask, simple 151, 151f
Oxygenation
   alterations of 145
   needs 142
Oxytocin 223

P

Packed red cells 200
Pain 144, 325
   incision 162
Pancreatic deficiency 132
Pancreatitis, acute 53
Pansexual 314
Paralytic ileus 53
Parasites, recovering 135
Parasiticide, application of 73
Parathyroid
   gland loss, detect 119
   hormone 121
Parenteral medications 228
Parenteral nutrition
   indications for 52
   peripheral 53
   type of 54
Parenteral therapy
   routes of 228
   types of 228
Parotid glands 14
Paroxysmal coughing 170
Patch 317
Patent airway, maintenance of 150
Pathogenic organism 63
Patient and environment, preparations of 106
Pedal edema 182
Pediatric dosage, calculate 217
Pediculosis 72
Pediculus capitis 72
   treatment of 73
Pelvic examination, bimanual examination of 22
Pender's health promotion model 328
Penicillin 75
   test 238
Peplau's theory 358
Perception 33, 269
Percussion 6, 6f
Percutaneous endoscopic gastrotomy 141
Perfusion 143
Pericardial sac 295
Perilymph 77
Perineal care 77
Perineum
   for female, cleaning 89
   for male, cleaning 89

Peripheral venous access devices, types of 194
Peristomal skin 110
Personal and emotional conflicts 315
Personal habit 83, 99
Personal identity 305
Personal relationship 284
Personality 323
    disorders 328
    type of 322
Petrissage 59
pH 48, 81
    meter 136
Pharmacokinetics 210
Pharynx 8, 14
Phenol 71
Phosphate 117, 121
Phospholipid 124, 125
    estimation 125
Phosphorus 121
    excretion 121
    levels of 121
Physical activity
    degree of 64
    extent of 39
Physical care 288
Physical comfort 35
Physical condition 66
Physical environment 322, 346
Physical examination 5, 131, 309
Physical exercise 177, 327
Physical injury 35
Physical preparation 8
Physically challenged persons 55
Physics and chemistry 57
Physiological-physical mode 352
Piggyback infusion 243
Pinna 13
Pituitary gland 326
Planning 30
    steps of 31
Plantar reflex 26
Plasma
    drug concentration, graphical representation of 211f
    human 124
    osmolarity 184
    reduced blood 200
    volume expanders 195
Plastic vials 245, 245f
Platelet 117, 201
    distribution width 114
    functions of 117
    histogram 114
    plug, forming 117
    products 201t
Play
    activity 333
    therapy 333
Pneumococcus 76
Pneumothorax 170
Poached egg 42
Pocket vision screener 8
Polyuria 83, 180
Polyvinyl alcohol, mixture of 135
Porridge 42
Positron emission tomography 140
Postprocedural steps 153
Post-radiation enteritis 53
Post-trauma responses 34
Postural drainage 156
Potassium 117
    abnormal 118
    permanganate 68
    rich foods 118
Potential complication 178
Pounding 60f
Powders 250
Preanesthetic medication 266
Prediabetes, type 2 127
Pregnancy 99
    and menstruation 315
    test 45
Preorgasmic dysfunction 316
Preschooler 312
Pressure 63
Pressure sore 60
    mildest stage 61
    Norton rating for 66t
Pressure ulcer 61f
    prevention of 289
    recovery time 62
    stages of 61, 62f
Prochlorperazine 45
Professional standards 28
Progestin only pill 317
Progressive muscle relaxation 333
    exercise 331
Pro-inflammatory cytokines 324
Prokinetic agents 45
Promethazine 45
Prone position 61
Prophylaxis, post-exposure 249
Protein 82, 122
    metabolism 121
Proteinuria 83
Prothrombin time 124
    INR, normal range of 124t
Protozoa, cysts of 135
Pruritis 207
Pseudohyperkalemia 185
Psychological environment 346
Psychological factors 83, 99
Psychology 74
Psychosocial needs
    self-concept 304
    sexuality 311
Ptosis 12
Puberty 313
Pulmonary aspiration 49
Pulmonary circulation 142
Pulmonary edema 145, 182, 197
Pulmonary function
    impairment 288
    test 191, 193
Pulmonary responses 33
Pulse 11
    examination of 9
    oximeters, types of 164
    oximetry 163
    soup 42
Pump bottle, steps for using 260
Pupils 12
Pursed lip breathing 167
Pus cells 133
Putrefaction 291
Pyuria 83

Q

Quad cough 166
Quadriceps reflex 26
Quality management 115

R

Race 336
Radiographic testing 45
Radiological examination 40
Radiological procedures 140
Rando's process model 286
Range of motion 15
    test 8
Rape 318
Rapid shallow breathing, signs of 162
Rash 342
Reaction 270
    alarm 326
    allergic 198, 203, 235
    formation 330
    pyrogenic 198, 235
    septic 203
Reading 333
    books 331
Reagent strip 136, 137
Rebreather mask, partial 151, 152f
Reception 269
Record procedure 67
Rectal aerosols 256
Rectal catheter, size of 103
Rectal cream 256
Rectal drip method 103
Rectal instillation 256
    steps of procedure for 256t
Rectal irrigation 259
Rectal liquids 256
Rectal semisolids 256
Rectal suppository 252
    insertion of 253f, 253t
Rectum 22, 97
    equipment 22
    techniques of male 22
Red blood cell 115, 127, 133
Red cell
    concentrate 200
    parameters and histogram 114
    suspension 200
Red retinal reflex 13
Reflex 84
Refractometer 137
Relapsing fever 72
Religion 308, 338
Religious
    conflict 323
    factor 38
    practices 299, 338
Relinquish 286
Renal failure 180, 188
Renal impairment 288
Renal tubular acidosis 188
Rennin-angiotensin-aldosterone system 177
Reproductive system 324
Research 347
Resolution phase 357
Resources 307
Respiration 11
    component of 142
    internal process of 142
Respiratory acidosis 191
Respiratory alkalosis 192
Respiratory exercises 167
Respiratory function 33, 144, 169
    alterations in 144
Respiratory illnesses 164
Respiratory mucous membranes 165

Respiratory physiology 142
Respiratory quotient, increased 49
Respiratory system 142, 325
    organs of 141
Respiratory tract
    infections 150
        secretions 165
Rest 33
    and sleep 328
Retention 83
Reticular activating system 270
Retina 13
Rhinitis 207
Rice water 42
Right quadrant
    lower 20
    upper 20
Rigor mortis 291
Ringer's solution 195
Rinne test 14
Roller clamp 243
Romberg test 24
Rotating work shifts 323
Roy's adaptation model 343, 352f
    strengths of 353
Roy's human adaptive systems 352
Rupture disk 243, 244f

S

Safety 289
    needs 354
Salbutamol 185
Salicylates 189
Salivary glands 14, 70
Salmonella 132
Saprophytic fungi, varieties of 57
Saturated salt floatation technique 134
Scabicides 223
Scapula, massage over 59
Schaudinn's solution 135
Schistosoma mansoni 135
Schlesinger test 133
School-age years 313
Scientific assumptions 351
Scissors 89
Sclera 12
Sclerosis, multiple 83
Scotch tape method 135
Scrambled egg 42
Sebaceous glands 57
Sedative 223
Sedimentation 133
    techniques 134
Self-awareness 305
Self-care 33, 331, 348
    ability 55
    agency 348
    deficit 348
    requisites 349
    theory 347, 349
Self-care deficit theory 347, 349
    analysis of 350
    assumptions of 347
    concepts of 348
Self-concept 34, 304, 309
    and health 305
    changes 308
    complex 304
    components of 305
    develop healthy 310
    dimensions of 305
    factors affect 307
    group identity mode 352
Self-esteem 34, 307
Self-expectation 305
Self-knowledge 305
Self-perception 34
Sensation 33
Sense of control 333
Sensorineural hearing loss 276
Sensory 24
    alterations, assessment of 271
    deprivation 273
    experience, components of 269
    needs 269
    perception 64
    poverty 274
    stimulations 280
Sensory deficit 272
    causes of 273
    effects of 273
    types of 273
Sensory function 25
    factors affecting 270
Sensory overload 273
    causes of 274
    prevention of 274
Sepsis 52, 53, 84
Serotonin-receptor antagonists 45
Serum
    albumin 122
    bicarbonate
        functions 121
        regulation 121
    bilirubin 121
    calcium 118, 187
    electrolyte 10, 117, 189, 190
        imbalance 49
    globulin 122
    hepatitis 198, 235
    magnesium 119
    phosphate 120
    potassium 118
    sodium 117
Seven nursing roles 356
Sexual assault 318
Sexual behavior, inappropriate 318
Sexual development throughout life 312
Sexual difficulties 325
Sexual dysfunction 34, 109, 316, 328
    causes of 316
Sexual exploitation 317
Sexual function 34
Sexual harassment and abuse 317
Sexual health 311
    alterations in 316
    characteristics of 312
    components of 312
    rights of 312
Sexual identity 34
Sexual issues, discussing 315
Sexual orientation 314
    categories of 314
Sexual self-concept 312
Sexuality 34, 311
    changes 312
    factors affecting 314
    sociocultural dimensions of 315
Sexually transmitted disease, prevention of 316
Shigella 132
Sigmoid colostomy 108
Sigmoidoscopy 141
Silica 144
Silicone vials 245
Silver nitrate 96
Simple gravity sedimentation technique 134
Sitting position 61
Situation-producing theories 343
Sitz bath 105
Skin 8
    and mucous membrane 251
    care of 55
    eruptions 325
    examination of 11
    friction of 63
    functions 57
    lesions, prevention of 67
    problem 328
    protects 57
    rashes 207
Slapping 59, 59f
Sleep 33
    apnea 145
    problems 325
Slipper pan 86f
Small bowel ulceration 208
Smears, stained 135
Snellen test 8
Soap and water, mild 112
Social care 290
Social comfort 35
Social evaluation 305
Social expectations 83
Social factors 38
Social interaction 271
Social support, lack of 323
Sociocultural factors 83, 329
Socioeconomic conditions 55
Socioeconomic status 284, 326
Sodium 117, 171
    bicarbonate 185
    chloride 68, 75
        solution 195
    food rich in 180
    functions 118
    ions 82
    levels, restoration of 183
    nitrate 96
    nitroprusside 136
    polystyrene sulphonate 185
    retention of 177
Soft drinks 41
Solution filter 242
Sorbitol 132
Sordes 71
Speech patterns 8
Spermicides 317
Spinal accessory nerve 25
Spiritual beliefs 284
Spiritual care 290
    five R's of 341
    interventions 340
Spiritual distress
    characteristics of 340
    dealing with 340
Spiritual health
    and wellbeing 338
    dimensions of 338
Spiritual need 339, 340
Spiritual problems
    acute illnesses 339
    chronic illnesses 339
    terminal illnesses 339
Spiritual well-being 337
    factors affecting 339
    physiological factors 339
    psychosocial factors 339

Spirituality 337, 338
Spirochaeta pallida 76
Spirometry 170
Spleen 20
Sponge 317
Spring, conical vial inserts with 245*f*
Sputum
    culture 139
    observation and collection of 139
    specimen 139
        collection of 139
Staphylococcus 75
    albus 57
    viridans 57
Steam inhalation 148
    articles required for 263*t*
    steps of procedure for 263*t*
Steam tent method 149
Steatorrhea 99
Stercobilin, test for 133
Sterile
    catheterization pack 96
    eye dressing pack containing 74
    kidney tray 89
    normal saline 91
    special mouth care 68
    swabbing solution 74
    tray 154
        containing 89, 96
    water 96
Sterilization
    tubal ligation 317
    vasectomy 317
Steroid suppository 105
Stimuli
    amount of 271
    presence of 271
Stoma 112
    construction of 108, 108*f*
    double-barrel 108
    end 108
    location of 108, 108*t*
Stomach, cancer of 132
Stool
    analysis 130
    cultures 135
    examination 130
    mucus in 132, 133
    specimen
        collection and transport of 131
        examination 101
        routine examination 101
Stramonium, inhalation of 261
Streptococcus 76
Stress 84, 320, 324, 328
    acute 321
    adaptation 325
    and coping, factors influencing 328
    behavioral symptoms of 328
    causes of 322, 323
    chronic 321
    cognitive symptoms of 328
    coping with 329
    demographic sources 322
    developmental 321
    diary, maintain 331
    effects of 324
    emotional symptoms of 328
    episodic acute 321
    general sources of 322
    hyper 320
    indicators of 325
    long-term 328
    manifestations of 328
    neurobehavioral 34
    physical symptoms of 328
    psychological symptoms of 328
    reduction, strategies for 327
    role of 328
    sources of 322
    theory 345
    tolerance 34
    types of 320
Stress disorder
    acute 327
    post-traumatic 327
Stress management 330
    adaptation for 332
    coping for 332
    therapeutic environment for 332
Stressful situations 327
Stressors 308, 321
    acute 322
    body image 308
    chronic 322
    developmental 322
    different 308
    external 322
    identity 308
    internal 322
    knowing 322
    life 322
    non-personal 322
    personal 322
    physiological 322
    psychosocial 322
    reduce environmental 332
    ripple effect 322
    role performance 309
    self-esteem 309
    self-image 309
    situational 322
    sources of 322
    trigger 322
    type of 322
Stretched hexagon 298
Stroke 83, 124
Stryker saw 295
Subcutaneous emphysema 162
Subcutaneous injection 236, 236*f*
    administration 236*f*
    steps of procedure for 237*t*
Substance filtered 82*t*
Substance, test for reducing 133
Suctioning 153, 289
Supine position 60
Support religious practices 340
Suppository 98, 104
    types of 104
Supraclavicular nodes 15
Sweat
    acidity of 57
    excessive 325
    glands 57
Symbolic depiction 343
Syndrome's evolution, distinctive stages in 326
Synergism 208
Synthetic drinks 41
Syringe
    and needle, selection of 233, 238
    disposal of 248
    parts of 239*f*
Systemic lupus erythematosus 116

T

Tachypnea 144, 183
Tactile deprivation 273
Taenia
    saginata 135
    solium 135
Tandem 243
Tapotement 59
    five types of 59
Tea 41
    and coffee 41
Tears lubricate 75
Technical skill needed 230
Teeth 14, 70
    grinding 325
Temperature 99
Tendon reflexes, deep 23, 26
Tenesmus 98
Terminally ill, care of 281
Test tube 89
Theory 343, 344, 348
    background 353
    classification of 345
    development
        levels of 343
        predictions for 344
Therapeutic communication techniques 30
Therapeutic diet 40
    responsibilities of 40
Therapeutic environment 340
Therapeutic nurse-client relationship 356
Therapeutic relationship, roles of nurse in 357
Therapeutic self-care demand 348
Thermoregulation 35
Thorax 16
    and lungs, posterior 16, 17
    anterior 9, 17
    posterior 9
Throat
    irrigation 260
    spray 261
Thrombocytes 117
Thrombocytopenia 208
Thrombocytosis 185
Thrombophlebitis 234
Thrombotic thrombocytopenic purpura 200
Thumb forceps 89
Thymol 68, 71
Thyroid 15
    turbidity test 122
Time-management 331
Tinctures 250
Tissue
    hypoxia 192
    injury, deep 62
    integrity, impaired 178
Toddler 143, 312
Tongue 14, 70
    blade, use 14
    clean 70
    depressor 69
Tonics 223
Tonsils 14
Topical medications, types of 250
Total parenteral nutrition 52, 53
Touch 4
Toxic effects 209
Toxicity 208
Toxins 322
Trachea 15

Index

Tracheostomy 153f
    collar 153
    suctioning 155
    tube 153
Tranquilizers 223
Transcultural nursing 336
Transdermal patch 250, 250f
Transverse colostomy 108
Trauma 95, 150
Traumatic events 322
Trendelenburg position 197
Triceps tendon 26
Trichrome staining 135
Tricuspid area 10
Trigeminal nerve, fifth 24
Triglycerides 124, 125
Trimethobenzamide 46
Trousseau's sign 186, 192
Tube
    displacement 49
    occlusion 49
    verify placement of 48
Tuberculin
    syringe, parts of 240f
    test 238
Tubing 243
    maintaining patency of 159
    protector 91
Tubular reabsorption 81
Tympanic cavity 76
Tympanic membrane 13
Tympanites 98
Typhus fever 72

U

Ulcer
    decubitus 60, 61
    peptic 132
    treatment of 63
Ulcerative colitis, chronic 99
Ulcerative disease 108
Ultrasonic nebulizer 148, 148f
Unclamp irrigating tubing 112
Unconscious patient, oral care for 69
Unconsciousness 278
    complications 279
    etiology 278
    management 279
    pathological changes 278, 279fc
    risk factors 278
Uniform Determination of Death Act 287
Unwanted pregnancy, prevention of 316, 317
Upper endoscopy 141
Upper extremities 8
Urethral area 138
Urethral meatus, expose 88
Urethrovaginal fistula 95
Urge 84
Urinals 85f
Urinalysis 189
Urinary bladder 81
    sizes 90
Urinary catheter, indwelling 94
Urinary catheterization 84, 88
Urinary disorders, common 84
Urinary diversion 95
    surgical management for 95f
Urinary drainage, care of 93, 93t
Urinary elimination 81
Urinary function 33
Urinary incontinence 84
    types of 84
Urinary output 199
Urinary retention 84
    preventing 280
Urinary system 81f
    organs of 81
Urination 83
    uncontrolled 83
Urine
    ammonia 122
    causes of high specific gravity 137
    composition of 81, 82t
    culture 137
    excreted in 82t
    involuntary passage of 84
    test for sugar in 136
    withdrawing 139
Urine elimination
    complications of 84, 84t
    facilitating 85
    physiology of 81
Urine pH 136, 190
    methods 136
Urine specimen 138
    collection of 138, 139
    midstream 138
    types of 139
Urinometer 137
    accuracy of 137
    cylinder 137
Urostomy, conventional 95
Urticaria 207
Uvula 14

V

Vaginal and anal intercourse, wait for 316
Vaginal cream 254
    application, steps of procedure for 254t
Vaginal irrigation 258
Vaginal medication 253
Vaginal orifice 88
Vaginal suppository insertion, steps of procedure for 254t
Vagus nerve 25
Vascular bed 123
Vasodilators 223
Vastus lateralis site 230, 231f
Venepuncture, performing 196
Venipuncture site 194f, 234
    peripheral 193
Venous blood sample 128
Ventilate patient's feeling 340
Ventilation 142
    and warming 346
    deep 170
Ventrogluteal site 230, 231f
Venturi mask 152, 152f
    adapter valves, color coding of 152f
Venturi system 152
Vermifuge 222
Vesicant 223
Vesicovaginal fistula 95
Vial 244
    and ampoules, types of 243
    caps and septa 246, 246f
    containing powder 248
    inserts 245
    materials 244
Vibration 60
    humming like 15
Virginia Henderson's nursing theory 353
Virus 322
Vision
    blurry 80
    peripheral 12
Visual acuity 8, 12, 24
Visual deprivation 273
Visual fields 24
    gross 12
Visual impairment 275
    etiology 275
Visual yellow 75
Vital functions 142
Vital signs 11, 184
Vitamin
    A 71, 75
    B 75
    B_1 97
    B_{12} 97
        deficiencies 116
    C 71, 75
    D 71, 75, 187
        metabolite of 119
    K 97
    synthetic 71
Voice 4, 14
Voiding 83
Volatile drugs, inhalation of 261
Vomiting 44, 49, 207, 208

W

Walks frequently 66
Walks occasionally 66
Wall outlet oxygen 151
Warm water, use basin of 251
Warmth 234
Wash hands 56, 57, 76
Waste treatment 248
Water
    and electrolytes 130
    homeostasis 171
    seal
        chest drainage, care of 158
        system 159, 159f
Waterproofing ointments 63
Weaknesses 353, 358
Weber test 14
White blood
    cell 114, 115
    contains 199
Wound healing 130

X

X-ray 140

Y

Yersinia 132
Yoga 330, 333
Young's rule 217

Z

Zephiran cetavlon 77
Zinc oxide ointment 109
Zinc sulfate
    drops 75
    floatation technique 134
Z-track method 231, 231f